INCREASING HEALTHY LIFE SPAN
CONVENTIONAL MEASURES AND SLOWING THE INNATE AGING PROCESS

ANNALS OF THE NEW YORK ACADEMY OF SCIENCES
Volume 959

INCREASING HEALTHY LIFE SPAN
CONVENTIONAL MEASURES AND SLOWING THE INNATE AGING PROCESS

Edited by Denham Harman

The New York Academy of Sciences
New York, New York
2002

Copyright © 2002 by the New York Academy of Sciences. All rights reserved. Under the provisions of the United States Copyright Act of 1976, individual readers of the Annals are permitted to make fair use of the material in them for teaching or research. Permission is granted to quote from the Annals provided that the customary acknowledgment is made of the source. Material in the Annals may be republished only by permission of the Academy. Address inquiries to the Permissions Department (permissions@nyas.org) at the New York Academy of Sciences.

Copying fees: For each copy of an article made beyond the free copying permitted under Section 107 or 108 of the 1976 Copyright Act, a fee should be paid through the Copyright Clearance Center, Inc., 222 Rosewood Drive, Danvers, MA 01923 (www.copyright.com).

♾ The paper used in this publication meets the minimum requirements of the American National Standard for Information Sciences—Permanence of Paper for Printed Library Materials, ANSI Z39.48-1984.

Library of Congress Cataloging-in-Publication Data

International Association of Biomedical Gerontology. International Congress (9th : 2002 : Vancouver, B.C.)
  Increasing healthy life span: conventional measures and slowing the innate aging process / Ninth Congress of the International Association of Biomedical Gerontology ; edited by Denham Harman.
      p. ; cm. — (Annals of the New York Academy of Sciences, ISSN 0077-8923; v. 959)
  Includes bibliographical references and index.
    ISBN 1-57331-360-2 (cloth: alk. paper) — ISBN 1-57331-361-0 (paper: alk. paper)
    1. Aging—Molecular aspects—Congresses. 2. Aging—Physiological aspects—Congresses. 3. Longevity—Examinations, questions, etc. I. Harman, Denham. II. Title. III. Series.
    [DNLM: 1. Aging—physiology—Congresses. 2. Longevity—Congresses. W1 AN626YL v.959 2002/WT 104 I587i 2002]
    Q11 .N5 vol. 959
    [QP86]
    550 s—dc21
    [612.6'8]   2002002394

GYAT/PCP
Printed in the United States of America
ISBN 1-57331-360-2 (cloth)
ISBN 1-57331-361-0 (paper)
ISSN 0077-8923

ANNALS OF THE NEW YORK ACADEMY OF SCIENCES

Volume 959
April 2002

INCREASING HEALTHY LIFE SPAN
CONVENTIONAL MEASURES AND SLOWING THE INNATE AGING PROCESS

NINTH CONGRESS OF THE INTERNATIONAL ASSOCIATION OF BIOMEDICAL GERONTOLOGY

Editor
DENHAM HARMAN

Conference Organizers
DENHAM HARMAN (CHAIR), JOHN W. BAYNES, MICHAEL FOSSEL, SATARO GOTO, LI LI JI, VALERIAN E. KAGAN, AND SANG CHUL PARK

Advisory Board
AUBREY D.N.J. DE GREY, KENICHI KITANI, ANTHONY W. LINNANE, IMRE ZS.-NAGY, AND EDUARDO A. PORTA

This volume is the result of a conference entitled **Increasing Healthy Life Span: Conventional Measures and Slowing the Innate Aging Process,** sponsored by the International Association of Biomedical Gerontology and held on June 27–30, 2001 in Vancouver, B.C, Canada.

CONTENTS

Preface. *By* DENHAM HARMAN	xi
Genetic and Environmental Influences on Exceptional Longevity and the AGE Nomogram. *By* THOMAS PERLS	1

Part I. Molecular and Cellular Changes with Age

Cell Senescence in Human Aging and Disease. *By* MICHAEL FOSSEL	14

Replicative Aging, Telomeres, and Oxidative Stress. *By* GABRIELE SARETZKI AND THOMAS VON ZGLINICKI 24

Are Changes of the Cell Membrane Structure Causally Involved in the Aging Process? *By* GERHARD SPITELLER 30

Down-regulation of Receptor-mediated Endocytosis Is Responsible for Senescence-associated Hyporesponsiveness. *By* SANG CHUL PARK, JEONG-SOO PARK, WOONG-YANG PARK, KYOUNG-A CHO, JEONG SOO AHN, AND IK SOON JANG 45

Dietary Restriction Initiated in Late Adulthood Can Reverse Age-related Alterations of Protein and Protein Metabolism. *By* SATARO GOTO, RYOYA TAKAHASHI, SACHIKO ARAKI, AND HIDEKO NAKAMOTO 50

Pigments in Aging: An Overview. *By* EDUARDO A. PORTA 57

Aging and the Role of Reactive Nitrogen Species. *By* BARRY DREW AND CHRISTIAAN LEEUWENBURGH 66

Part II. Exercise and Aging

Exercise-induced Modulation of Antioxidant Defense. *By* LI LI JI 82

The Role of Apoptosis in the Normal Aging Brain, Skeletal Muscle, and Heart. *By* MICHAEL POLLACK, SHARON PHANEUF, AMIE DIRKS, AND CHRISTIAAN LEEUWENBURGH 93

Generation of Reactive Oxygen and Nitrogen Species in Contracting Skeletal Muscle: Potential Impact on Aging. *By* MICHAEL B. REID AND WILLIAM J. DURHAM 108

Can Exercise Training Improve Immune Function in the Aged? *By* JEFFREY A. WOODS, THOMAS W. LOWDER, AND K. TODD KEYLOCK 117

Part III. Nutritional Intervention

Fruit Polyphenolics and Brain Aging: Nutritional Interventions Targeting Age-related Neuronal and Behavioral Deficits. *By* RACHEL L. GALLI, BARBARA SHUKITT-HALE, KURESH A. YOUDIM, AND JAMES A. JOSEPH 128

Delaying Brain Mitochondrial Decay and Aging with Mitochondrial Antioxidants and Metabolites. *By* JIANKANG LIU, HANI ATAMNA, HIROHIKO KURATSUNE, AND BRUCE N. AMES 133

Enhancing Cognitive Function across the Life Span. *By* DONNA L. KOROL 167

Ascorbic Acid, Blood Pressure, and the American Diet. *By* GLADYS BLOCK ... 180

Part IV. Antioxidants and Aging

Toward Mechanism-based Antioxidant Interventions: Lessons from Natural Antioxidants. *By* VALERIAN E. KAGAN, ELENA R. KISIN, KAZUAKI KAWAI, BEHICE F. SERINKAN, ANATOLY N. OSIPOV, ELENA A. SERBINOVA, IRA WOLINSKY, AND ANNA A. SHVEDOVA 188

Role of Mitochondria in Oxidative Stress and Aging. *By* GIORGIO LENAZ, CARLA BOVINA, MARILENA D'AURELIO, ROMANA FATO, GABRIELLA FORMIGGINI, MARIA LUISA GENOVA, GIOVANNI GIULIANO, MILENA MERLO PICH, UGO PAOLUCCI, GIOVANNA PARENTI CASTELLI, AND BARBARA VENTURA 199

Programmed Death Phenomena: From Organelle to Organism. *By* VLADIMIR P. SKULACHEV 214

Melatonin Reduces Oxidant Damage and Promotes Mitochondrial Respiration: Implications for Aging. *By* RUSSEL J. REITER, DUN XIAN TAN, LUCIEN C. MANCHESTER, AND MAMDOUH R. EL-SAWI 238

Metabolic Alterations and Shifts in Energy Allocations Are Corequisites for the Expression of Extended Longevity Genes in *Drosophila*. *By* ROBERT ARKING, STEVEN BUCK, DAE-SUNG HWANGBO, AND MARK LANE 251

Prevention of Mitochondrial Oxidative Damage Using Targeted Antioxidants. *By* GEOFFREY F. KELSO, CAROLYN M. PORTEOUS, GILLIAN HUGHES, ELIZABETH C. LEDGERWOOD, ALISON M. GANE, ROBIN A. J. SMITH, AND MICHAEL P. MURPHY 263

Cognitive Impairment of Rats Caused by Oxidative Stress and Aging, and Its Prevention by Vitamin E. *By* KOJI FUKUI, NAO-OMI OMOI, TAKAHIRO HAYASAKA, TADASHI SHINNKAI, SHOZO SUZUKI, KOUICHI ABE, AND SHIRO URANO 275

Reaction of Carnosine with Aged Proteins: Another Protective Process? *By* ALAN R. HIPKISS, CAROL BROWNSON, MARIANA F. BERTANI, EMILIO RUIZ, AND ALBERT FERRO 285

Part V. Pharmacological Intervention in Aging

Pharmacological Interventions in Aging and Age-associated Disorders: Potentials of Propargylamines for Human Use. *By* KENICHI KITANI, CHIYOKO MINAMI, TAKAKO YAMAMOTO, SETSUKO KANAI, GWEN O. IVY, AND MARIA-CRISTINA CARRILLO 295

Pharmacological Interventions against Aging through the Cell Plasma Membrane: A Review of the Experimental Results Obtained in Animals and Humans. *By* IMRE ZS.-NAGY 308

Nitrones as Neuroprotectants and Antiaging Drugs. *By* ROBERT A. FLOYD, KENNETH HENSLEY, MICHAEL J. FORSTER, JUDITH A. KELLEHER-ANDERSON, AND PAUL L. WOOD 321

Therapeutics against Mitochondrial Oxidative Stress in Animal Models of Aging. *By* SIMON MELOV 330

Part VI. Free Radical Diseases

A Unified Mechanism in the Initiation of Cancer. *By* ERCOLE L. CAVALIERI AND ELEANOR G. ROGAN 341

Coenzyme Q_{10} Protects the Aging Heart against Stress: Studies in Rats, Human Tissues, and Patients. *By* FRANKLIN L. ROSENFELDT, SALVATORE PEPE, ANTHONY LINNANE, PHILIP NAGLEY, MICHAEL ROWLAND, RUCHONG OU, SILVANA MARASCO, WILLIAM LYON, AND DONALD ESMORE 355

The Maillard Hypothesis on Aging: Time to Focus on DNA. *By*
JOHN W. BAYNES 360

Oxidative Stress and Programmed Cell Death in Diabetic Neuropathy. *By*
ANDREA M. VINCENT, MICHAEL BROWNLEE, AND JAMES W. RUSSELL ... 368

Alzheimer's Disease: Role of Aging in Pathogenesis. *By* DENHAM HARMAN .. 384

Part VII. Mitochondrial Changes with Age: Effect on Function

Human Aging and Global Function of Coenzyme Q_{10}. *By* ANTHONY W.
LINNANE, CHUNFANG ZHANG, NATALIA YAROVAYA, GEORGE
KOPSIDAS, SERGEY KOVALENKO, PENNY PAPAKOSTOPOULOS,
HAYDEN EASTWOOD, STEPHEN GRAVES, AND MARTIN RICHARDSON 396

Mitochondrial DNA Deletion Mutations and Sarcopenia. *By* JUDD AIKEN,
ENTELA BUA, ZHENG JIN CAO, MARISOL LOPEZ, JON WANAGAT,
DEBBIE MCKENZIE, AND SUSAN MCKIERNAN 412

Involvement of Mitochondria and Other Free Radical Sources in Normal and
Abnormal Fetal Development. *By* ALAN G. FANTEL AND
RICHARD E. PERSON 424

Frequent Intracellular Clonal Expansions of Somatic mtDNA Mutations:
Significance and Mechanisms. *By* HILARY A. COLLER, NATALYA D.
BODYAK, AND KONSTANTIN KHRAPKO 434

Mitochondrial Damage in Aging and Apoptosis. *By* JUAN SASTRE,
CONSUELO BORRÁS, DAVID GARCÍA-SALA, ANA LLORET, FEDERICO V.
PALLARDÓ, AND JOSÉ VIÑA 448

Part VIII. Slowing the Inherent Aging Process

Time to Talk SENS: Critiquing the Immutability of Human Aging. *By*
AUBREY D.N.J. DE GREY, BRUCE N. AMES, JULIE K. ANDERSEN,
ANDRZEJ BARTKE, JUDITH CAMPISI, CHRISTOPHER B. HEWARD,
ROGER J.M. MCCARTER, AND GREGORY STOCK 452

Nature of the Aging Process: Open Discussion. *By*
AUBREY D.N.J. DE GREY, MODERATOR 463

Oxidative Stress and Life Span Determination in the Nematode *Caenorhabditis elegans*. *By* YOKO HONDA AND SHUJI HONDA 466

Membrane Fatty Acid Unsaturation, Protection against Oxidative Stress, and
Maximum Life Span: A Homeoviscous-longevity Adaptation? *By*
REINALD PAMPLONA, GUSTAVO BARJA, AND MANUEL PORTERO-OTÍN 475

Mitochondrial Decay in the Aging Rat Heart: Evidence for Improvement by
Dietary Supplementation with Acetyl-L-Carnitine and/or Lipoic Acid. *By*
TORY M. HAGEN, RÉGIS MOREAU, JUNG H. SUH, AND FRANCESCO VISIOLI .. 491

Can Antioxidant Diet Supplementation Protect against Age-related Mitochondrial Damage? *By* JAIME MIQUEL 508

The First Six Years at the National Institute for Longevity Sciences, Japan. *By*
KENICHI KITANI 517

Index of Contributors 527

Financial assistance was received from:

- NOW FOODS
- THE GLENN FOUNDATION FOR MEDICAL RESEARCH
- WILD BLUEBERRY ASSOCIATION OF NORTH AMERICA

The New York Academy of Sciences believes it has a responsibility to provide an open forum for discussion of scientific questions. The positions taken by the participants in the reported conferences are their own and not necessarily those of the Academy. The Academy has no intent to influence legislation by providing such forums.

Preface

The International Association of Biomedical Gerontology (IABG) was organized in 1985 with a purpose (1) of making the public more aware of the potential that biomedical aging research has to increase the span of healthy productive life and to decrease the social and economic problems of age; and (2) of promoting greater communication in the worldwide community among individuals engaged in biomedical aging research. Beginning in 1985 in New York City, a congress has been held by the IABG every two years. The proceedings have been published (see below), with the exception of those from the first and third congresses. When the meeting year of the IABG coincides with that of the International Association of Gerontology (IAG), the IABG meeting is held just prior to that of the IAG.

The Ninth Congress of the IABG, held on June 27–30, 2001 (just prior to that of the IAG) at the Hyatt Regency Hotel in Vancouver, British Columbia, Canada, was entitled Increasing Healthy Life Span: Conventional Measures and Slowing the Innate Aging Process. Sang Chul Park from South Korea, President of the IABG, opened the meeting. Thomas T. Perls presented the introductory lecture, entitled "Genetic and Environmental Influences on Exceptional Longevity and the AGE Nomogram." This was followed by eight symposia: (1) Molecular and Cellular Changes with Age, (2) Exercise and Aging, (3) Nutritional Intervention, (4) Antioxidants and Aging, (5) Pharmacological Intervention in Aging, (6) Free Radical Diseases, (7) Mitochondrial Changes with Age: Effect on Function, and (8) Slowing the Inherent Aging Process.

This volume contains chapters by all but one of the speakers. Information in the missing lecture by G. Attardi is included in the article "Role of mitochondrial DNA in human aging," (*Mitochondrion* 2002, in press) and in the Proceedings of Euromit 5 (European Meeting on Mitochondrial Pathology, Venice, Italy, September 19–23, 2001). This *Annals* also includes the remarks made by Kenichi Kitani, M.D., Ph.D, the biennial luncheon speaker, about the founding of the Japanese National Institute for Longevity Sciences and its activities during his tenure (1995–2001) as the first director general.

The title of this congress reflects a shift in the focus of biomedical aging research to increased emphasis on the inherent aging process. This basic biological process increases exponentially with age, largely determining the chances for death after about age 28 and limits ALE-B (a measure of the average span of healthy, productive life in a population) to around 85 years and the maximum life span to approximately 122 years. Efforts to further increase the ALE-Bs of the developed countries from 75–80 years by the conventional measures, that is, by better nutrition, housing, and medical care, employed in the past are now being progressively nullified by the exponential increases of the innate aging process with age as the ALE-Bs approach the potential maximum.

Knowledge of the biochemical changes associated with age is extensive and steadily growing, as discussed in this volume. Many would argue that the present increasing ineffectiveness of efforts to raise the ALE-Bs is a result of inadequate knowledge of aging. This may not be the case; it may be the result of insufficient application of current knowledge.

A growing number of biomedical gerontologists attribute the biochemical changes associated with age to free radical reactions largely initiated by superoxide radicals formed by the mitochondria in the course of normal metabolism. Applications of this possibility have been fruitful. For example, it is a useful guide to efforts to increase the ALE-B as well as the maximum life span, and it provides plausible explanations for aging phenomena (e.g., the association of diseases with age as well as insight into pathogenesis, the gender gap, the association between events in early life and diseases of later life, and the shortening of telomeres with cell division).

The above efforts should be augmented by future attempts to increase the life span, for example, studies with stem cells and telomerase, work directed toward decreasing the fraction of O_2 used by mitochondria to superoxide radicals (akin to the decrease in pigeons compared to rats, and of the white-footed mouse with that of the common mouse), measures to prevent accumulation of age-associated damage, and work with genetic mutations (e.g., in the human equivalent of the mouse $p66^{she}$ gene).

The members of the organizing committee are very grateful to Mr. Elwood Richard, President of NOW Foods, for the generous sponsorship that made this important congress possible and for the additional contributions from the Glenn Foundation for Medical Research and the Wild Blueberry Association of North America.

We are also indebted to the speakers and to the audience for ensuring the success of the Congress. Discussions were frequent and animated throughout the meeting. The organizing committee wishes to express their deep appreciation to the editorial staff of the *Annals* for publishing the proceedings of the Ninth Congress of the IABG.

—DENHAM HARMAN

Department of Medicine,
University of Nebraska College of Medicine,
Omaha, Nebraska 68198-4635, USA

Past Published Proceedings

2nd Congress: Steinhagen-Thiessen, E. & D.L. Knook, Eds. 1988. Trends in Biomedical Gerontology. TNO Institute for Experimental Gerontology. Rijswijk.

4th Congress: Fabris, N., D. Harman, D.L. Knook, E. Steinhagen-Thiessen & I. Zs.-Nagy, Eds. 1992. Physiopathological Processes of Aging: Towards a Multicausal Interpretation. Annals of the New York Academy of Sciences. Vol. 673.

5th Congress: Zs.-Nagy, I., D. Harman & K. Kitani, Eds. 1994. Pharmacology of Aging Processes: Methods of Assessment and Potential Interventions. Annals of the New York Academy of Sciences.Vol. 717.

6th Congress: Kitani, K., A. Aoba & S. Goto, Eds. 1996. Pharmacological Intervention in Aging and Age-Associated Disorders. Annals of the New York Academy of Sciences. Vol. 786.

7th Congress: Harman, D., R. Holliday & M. Meydani, Eds. 1998. Towards Prolongation of the Healthy Life Span: Practical Approaches to Intervention. Annals of the New York Academy of Sciences.Vol. 854.

8th Congress: Park, S.C., E.S. Hwang, H-S. Kim & W-Y. Park, Eds. 2001. Healthy Aging for Functional Longevity: Molecular and Cellular Interactions in Senescence. Annals of the New York Academy of Sciences. Vol. 928.

Genetic and Environmental Influences on Exceptional Longevity and the AGE Nomogram

THOMAS PERLS

Beth Israel Deaconess Medical Center,
330 Brookline Avenue, Boston, Massachusetts 02215, USA

ABSTRACT: To live beyond the octogenarian years, population and molecular genetic studies of centenarian sibships indicate that genetic factors play an increasingly important role as the limit of life span is approached. These factors are likely to influence basic mechanisms of aging that in turn broadly influence susceptibility to age-related illnesses. Lacking genetic variations that predispose to disease as well as having variations that confer disease resistance (longevity enabling genes) are probably both important to achieving exceptional old age. The AGE (aging, genetics, environment) nomogram is introduced as an illustrative construct for understanding the influence of environmental and genetic factors on survival to various ages, depending on variations in the hypothesized relative importance of genes and environment to longevity. The rapid rise in the incidence of centenarians could indicate that many more people than we originally thought have the optimal set of genetic factors necessary to get to 100 and beyond. Recent studies indicate the likelihood that such factors will be elucidated in the near future.

KEYWORDS: aging; centenarian; oldest old; longevity; demographic selection; nomogram; genetics

The relative contributions of environment and genes to human aging have been studied primarily through twin studies. As discussed below, however, the dynamics between these two forces are quite different in considering exceptional longevity. The forces of demographic selection become intense with old age, resulting in a cohort of select survivors who, in order to achieve exceptional old age, must markedly delay or escape age-associated lethal illnesses. Evidence from centenarian studies reveals that much of this survival advantage is genetically based, and, in addition to lacking genetic variations that predispose to disease, there are likely to be variations that confer disease resistance and predispose to good health. The evidence for the genetic role in achieving exceptional old age is discussed below. The AGE (aging, genes, environment) nomogram is introduced as a means of exploring the impact on survival of genes playing an important role in achieving exceptional old age.

Address for correspondence: Thomas Perls, M.D., M.P.H., New England Centenarian Study, 88 E. Newton St., F-4, Boston Medical Center, Boston, MA 02118. Voice: 617-638-6688; fax: 617-638-6671.

thomas.perls@bmc.org

TWIN STUDIES HAVE ADDRESSED THE GENETIC CONTRIBUTION TO AVERAGE LIFE EXPECTANCY BUT NOT EXCEPTIONAL LONGEVITY

A Scandinavian study of monozygotic and dizygotic twins calculated the heritability of life expectancy to be 20–30%.[1–3] One study of the twins also indicated that shared environmental factors also appeared to play a minor role.[4] Many have interpreted these results to indicate that 70–80% of how well a person ages or how old they live to be depends mostly on their individual health-related behaviors and the remainder is up to one's genes.[5] However, the mean age of the subjects in the twin study were in their early seventies, with an average life expectancy similar to the general population at the time. This optimistic and empowering message is probably valid and germane for the average person, but the twin studies of average life expectancy do not address the genetic and environmental influences on survival to extreme old age—that is, to live another 20 to 30 years to age 100 and beyond.

DEFINING EXCEPTIONAL LONGEVITY IN TERMS OF DEMOGRAPHIC SELECTION

In 1825, Benjamin Gompertz proposed that mortality rate increased exponentially with age.[6] Since then, most researchers accept that this rule indeed applies at younger adult ages for many species; however, at extreme old age an exception to the rule exists. At very old age, mortality begins to decelerate in species such as medflies,[7] the nematode worm *Caenorhabditis elegans*,[8,9] and humans. Survival calculations from a European database of 70 million people who reached at least age 80, and of 200,000 who lived to at least 100 years of age were performed by Thatcher and colleagues.[10] These researchers observed a deceleration in mortality rate as age 100 was approached that was maintained up through age 105 for males and 107 for females. Beyond those ages, mathematical modeling predicted a decline in mortality rate with age beyond 110. Why does mortality decelerate? Most likely it is because frailer individuals drop out of the population, leaving behind a more robust cohort that continues to survive. Because these frail individuals drop out of the population, the distribution of certain genotypes and other survival-related attributes in a cohort changes with older and older age.[11–13] This selecting-out process is termed demographic selection.[14]

The effect of demographic selection is exemplified by the dropout with extreme age of the apolipoprotein E ε-4 allele.[15] Rebeck and colleagues noted the frequency of the ε-4 allele to decrease markedly with advancing age.[16] One of its counterparts, the ε-2 allele, becomes more frequent with advanced age among Caucasians. Presumably the dropout at earlier age of the ε-4 allele is because of its association with "premature" mortality secondary to Alzheimer's disease and heart disease.[17]

A similar trend exists in the case of the apolipoprotein B locus, where investigators from the Italian Centenarian Study, comparing 143 centenarians with younger controls, demonstrated an association between specific variations of the locus and extreme longevity.[18] In another study, nonagenarian subjects had an extremely low frequency of HLA-DRw9 and an increased frequency of DR1. A high frequency of DRw9 and a low frequency of DR1 are associated with autoimmune or immunodeficiency diseases, which can cause premature mortality.[19]

THE CENTENARIAN PHENOTYPE

As a result of demographic selection, centenarians markedly delay or even escape age-associated diseases. In a retrospective study of the New England population-based sample, 88% of centenarian females and 100% of centenarian males were independently functioning at an average age of 92 years. At the average of 97 years, 45% of the women and 75% of the men were still independently functioning at an average age of 97 years.[20] These findings are consistent with James Fries' compression of morbidity hypothesis, proposing that as the limit of human life span is approached, the onset and duration of lethal diseases associated with aging must be compressed towards the end of life.[21,22]

Given these preliminary findings suggesting that morbidity is relatively compressed in the centenarian cohort, centenarians may be a human model of disease-free or, at the least, disease-delayed aging. A number of studies have been performed to better quantify the centenarian phenotype and to search for factors that could play a role in such a survival advantage. These include studies of body fat and metabolism,[23] pedigree studies,[24–28] and cardiovascular risk factors.[29,30] Nir Barzilai and colleagues, studying Ashkenazi Jewish centenarians, recently not only noted that the centenarians had lipid profiles conducive to lower cardiovascular disease risk, but that their children also had significantly favorable profiles compared to controls.[31] Specific investigations of thyroid function,[32] immune function,[33,34] blood clotting,[35,36] and cognitive function[35–40] have been performed.[41] Pathological series have been conducted to determine cause of death among this cohort. Thus far, no particular environmental trait, such as diet, economic status, or level of education has been significantly correlated with the ability to survive to extreme old age.[42–48]

THE OCCURRENCE OF CENTENARIANS

The ages of the oldest humans have probably not changed substantially at least since the times of ancient Greece. The artist Tiziano Vecellio, more commonly known as Titian (1488–1576), lived to almost age 90. Leonardo da Vinci, born in 1452, known for his scientific accuracy, drew several pictures of a 100-year-old man. Andrea della Robbia, a Florentine artist famous for his terra cottas, reportedly lived to age 90 (1435–1525), and around the same time, Michelangelo (1475–1564) lived to age 91. Hippocrates reportedly died in his mid-80s (460–377 B.C.), while Sophocles died in his mid-90s.

The question of whether centenarians or even nonagenarians are only recent phenomena is important. If so, it would imply that recent environmental factor(s), not long-standing genetic ones, are responsible for their existence. Centenarians, though much more rare in the past, are not a new phenomenon. Thus, from a historical point of view, a significant genetic contribution to extreme longevity cannot be ruled out.

For the past two decennial U.S. census reports, centenarians have been reported to be the fastest growing segment of the population. According to the census, in 1990, there were approximately 30,000 centenarians and in 2000, that number is approximately 60,000. Among industrialized countries, the number of centenarians is increasing at an exceptionally rapid rate of about 8% per year. In comparison, population growth of 1% per year is the norm.[49] In 1900 in the United States, approxi-

extremely small (less than one per all the families that exist in the world today) if one assumes that these family members were exposed to the same environment as those individuals who did not make it to extreme old age. Of course such an assumption is incorrect. Certainly the collective ability of siblings achieving at least old age would be enhanced if, for example, they were better off socioeconomically, or if they did not live in an area that experienced a lethal epidemic. Thus, environmental factors that the siblings and other relatives achieving exceptional old age have in common must play a role in this observed clustering. However, the question remains as to what factors would enable them to live twenty-five years beyond average life expectancy to 100. We believe that such clustering is indicative of a substantial genetic influence and are in the process of searching for families with enough alive effected individuals to warrant an association study.

In a more standard approach to determining familial risk, a number of groups have been studying pedigrees of long-lived individuals. The results have induced at least four groups to pursue yet another approach to discovering genetic modulators of exceptional longevity, genetic linkage studies among long-lived sibships.[26,67,68] Geneticists associated with the French Centenarian Study performed a linkage study of 558 individuals representing 188 nonagenarian sibships using seven polymorphic markers in the region of the ApoE gene.[75] They concluded from their negative nonparametric analysis and prior simulation studies that such analyses are unlikely to be successful if exceptional longevity is a chance event among individuals not carrying deleterious alleles that are quite common in the general population and rare among centenarians. On the other hand, the rarity of alleles that significantly enhance the ability to survive to such old age would be sufficiently enriched among a centenarian sample that a nonparametric analysis of a genome-wide scan for such excess allele sharing would be worthwhile performing.

We recently performed just such a study. A genome wide scan for such predisposing loci was conducted using 308 individuals belonging to 137 sibships demonstrating exceptional longevity. Using nonparametric analysis, significant evidence for linkage was noted for the chromosome 4 locus at D4S1564 with an MLS of 3.65 ($P = 0.044$). The analysis was corroborated by a parametric analysis ($P = 0.052$). These linkage results indicate the significant likelihood that there exists a gene or genes that exert a substantial positive influence on the ability to achieve exceptional old age.[76] The next step will be to replicate this result with an independent set of families and to proceed with a single nucleotide polymorphism analysis of the locus in the attempt to capture the gene playing a significant role in the marked survival advantage of these individuals.

Thus, there is substantial evidence indicating the likelihood that genetics does play a relatively important role in the ability to achieve exceptional old age. Given the rising relative risks associated with older and older age (TABLE 1, above), it appears that not only does a genetic advantage play an important role, but that the relative importance increases with the age achieved.

FIGURE 2 provides an illustrative construct in which we can think about the relative importance of genes and the environment in determining survival to exceptional old age. Conveniently called the AGE (aging, genes, and environment) nomogram, this nomogram illustrates the proposed increasingly essential role genes play in the ability to achieve exceptional longevity. There are three crucial determinants of life expectancy: environmental exposure, genes, and the relative importance of environ-

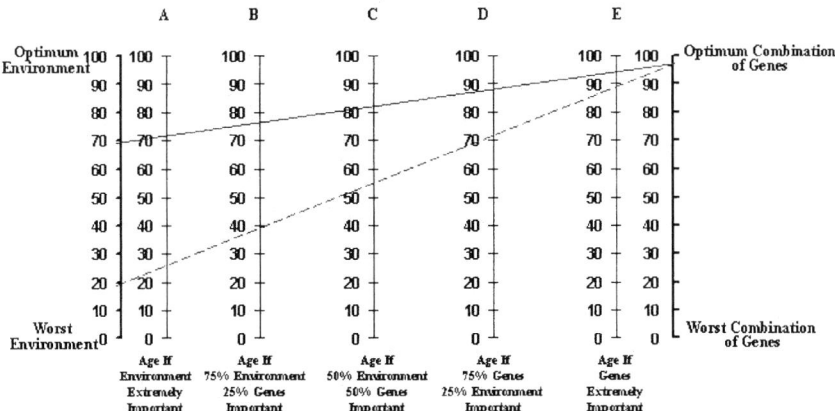

FIGURE 2. AGE (aging, genes, environment) nomogram. Three major factors contribute to survival: environment, genes, and the relative contribution of each and their interaction. The scale at the extreme left indicates the spectrum of environmental exposures related to longevity, from extremely poor at the bottom to optimal at the top. The scale at the extreme right indicates the spectrum of genetic variations that influence survival to very old age, ranging from a very poor, negative influence at the bottom, to optimal at the top. The vertical lines in between, lines A–E, vary according to the relative importance of environment and genes to achieving the age in question. Note that age 0 to 100 years, from bottom to top, appears on each of these lines. The nomogram can be used by selecting a level of environmental exposure (for example, poor, average, or optimal) on the extreme left and choosing a level of genetic exposure (for example, poor, average, or optimal) and connecting the two points with a line. Then, choose one of the lines, A–E, depending on the hypothesized relative contribution of genes and environment to survival to very old age. The hypothesized years of life can then be pinpointed where the line that you drew crosses the vertical line (A–E) you have chosen.

ment and genes in determining life expectancy. Vertical lines A through E illustrate a spectrum of this relative importance, line A indicating that environment is the predominant determinant and, at the other end of this continuum, line E indicating that genes are the predominant determinant.

If genes play the more important role (line E), a person endowed with an optimal set of genetic polymorphisms (who would be found high on the scale at the extreme right) would still be able to achieve relative old age, despite exposure to a very poor environment (low on the scale at the extreme left). This would explain the longevity of centenarians who were exposed to a terrible environment (e.g., smoking) and yet who still achieved extreme old age (represented by the dotted line). The solid line is an example of a person born with an optimal set of polymorphisms and exposed to an environment relatively conducive to survival.

As one can imagine there are a myriad of scenarios one can construct. Also imagine an individual with an optimal environment and a poor combination of polymorphisms. If environment is the predominant determinant of survival, then the individual will still be able to achieve very old age. If on the other hand genes are the critical player, then survival to even middle age is unlikely. Finally, if survival is

50% attributable to genes and 50% to environment, the person with an optimal environment and very poor genes will still find themselves living to age 50 or 60.

It is also interesting, using the nomogram, to consider potential interventions to improve survival. Such interventions as smoking cessation will move a person up the environment scale at the extreme left, or removing disease-enhancing genetic polymorphisms or adding longevity-enabling genetic polymorphisms will move a person up the scale at the extreme right. The effect on survival can be supposed based on the hypothesized relative roles of genes and environment.

As research progresses to further understand the factors that are important to achieving exceptional old age, their level of interaction and their mechanisms, it may be possible to construct a nomogram that is predictive rather than hypothetical. In the mean time, the study of potential factors among centenarians and their family members is increasingly contributing to the field. The discovery of key genetic factors is close at hand.

ACKNOWLEDGMENTS

This work was made possible by the generous support of the following: the Alzheimer's Association's Temple Early Discovery Award Award, the National Institute on Aging (1R01AG18721), the Institute for the Study of Aging, the Paul Beeson Faculty Scholar in Aging Research Award (administered by the American Federation of Aging Research and the Alliance for Aging Research), and the Retirement Research Foundation.

REFERENCES

1. MCGUE, M. *et al.* 1993. Longevity is moderately heritable in a sample of Danish twins born 1870–1880. J. Gerontol.: Biol. Sci. **48:** B237–B244.
2. HERSKIND, A.M. *et al.* 1996. Untangling genetic influences on smoking, body mass index and longevity: a multivariate study of 2464 Danish twins followed for 28 years. Hum. Genet. **98:** 467–475.
3. LJUNGQUIST, B. *et al.* 1998. The effect of genetic factors for longevity: a comparison of identical and fraternal twins in the Swedish Twin Registry. J. Gerontol. A. Biol. Sci. Med. Sci. **53:** M441–446.
4. HERSKIND, A.M. *et al.* 1996. The heritability of human longevity: a population-based study of 2872 Danish twin pairs born 1870–1900. Hum. Genet. **97:** 319–323.
5. FINCH, C.E. & R.E. TANZI. 1997. Genetics of aging. Science **278:** 407–411.
6. GOMPERTZ, B. 1825. On the nature of the function expressive of the law of human mortality, and on a new mode of determining the value of life contingencies. Philos. Trans. R. Soc. Lon. B. Biol. Sci. **115:** 513–585.
7. CAREY, J.R. *et al.* 1992. Slowing of mortality rates at older ages in large medfly cohorts. Science **258:** 457–461.
8. BROOKS, A. *et al.* 1994. Mortality rates in a genetically heterogeneous population of *Caenorhabditis elegans*. Science **263:** 668–671.
9. JOHNSON, T.E. 1990. Increased life-span of age-1 mutant in *Caenorhabditis elegans* and lower Gompertz rate of aging. Science **249:** 908–912.
10. THATCHER, A.R. *et al.* 1996. The force of mortality from age 80 to 120. University Press. Odense, Denmark.
11. VAUPEL, J.W. *et al.* 1979. The impact of heterogeneity in individual frailty on the dynamics of mortality. Demography **16:** 439–454.

12. VAUPEL, J.W. & A.I. Yashin. 1985. Heterogeneity's ruses: some surprising effects of selection on population dynamics. Am. Stat. **39:** 176–195.
13. VAUPEL, J.W. 1997. Kindred lifetimes: frailty models in population genetics. *In* Convergent Questions in Genetics and Demography. J. Adams, *et al.*, Eds.: 155–170. Oxford University Press. Oxford.
14. VAUPEL, J.W. *et al.* 1998. Biodemographic trajectories of longevity. Science **280:** 855–860.
15. SCHÄCHTER, F. *et al.* 1994. Genetic associations with human longevity at the APOE and ACE loci. Nat. Genet. **6:** 29–32.
16. REBECK, G.W. *et al.* 1994. Reduced apolipoprotein epsilon 4 allele frequency in the oldest old. Alzheimer's patients and cognitively normal individuals. Neurology **44:** 1513–1516.
17. GERDES, L.U. *et al.* 2000. Estimation of apolipoprotein E genotype–specific relative mortality risks from the distribution of genotypes in centenarians and middle-aged men: apolipoprotein E gene is a "frailty gene," not a "longevity gene." Genet. Epidemiol. **19:** 202–210.
18. DE BENEDICTIS, G. *et al.* 1997. DNA multiallelic systems reveal gene/longevity associations not detected by diallelic systems. The APOB locus. Hum. Genet. **99:** 312–318.
19. TAKATA, H. *et al.* 1997. Influence of major histocompatibility complex region genes on human longevity among Okinawan-Japanese centenarians and nonagenarians. Lancet **2:** 824–826.
20. HITT, R. *et al.* 1999. Centenarians: the older you get, the healthier you've been. Lancet **354:** 652.
21. VITA, A.J. *et al.* 1998. Aging, health risks, and cumulative disability. N. Engl. J. Med. **338:** 1035–1041.
22. PERLS, T.T. 1995. The oldest old. Sci. Am. **272:** 70–75.
23. PAOLISSO, G. *et al.* 1995. Body composition, body fat distribution and resting metabolic rate in healthy centenarians. Am. J. Clin. Nutr. **62:** 746–750.
24. BOCQUET-APPEL, J.P. *et al.* 1991. La transmission familiale de la longévité à Arthez d'Asson (1686–1899). Population **2:** 327–347.
25. PERLS, T. *et al.* 1997. Middle aged mothers live longer. Nature **389:** 133.
26. PERLS, T. *et al.* 1998. Siblings of centenarians live longer. Lancet **351:** 1560.
27. ALPERT, L. *et al.* 1998. Extreme longevity in two families. A report of multiple centenarians within single generations. *In* Age Validation of the Extreme Old. B. Jeune & J. Vaupel, Eds. Odense Monographs on Population Aging 4. Odense University Press. Odense.
28. PERLS, T. *et al.* 2000. Exceptional familial clustering for extreme longevity in humans. J. Am. Geriatr. Soc. **48:** 1483–1485.
29. BARBAGALLO, C.M. *et al.* 1995. Plasma lipid apolipoprotein and Lp(a) levels in elderly normolipidemic women: relationships with coronary heart disease and longevity. Gerontology **41:** 260–266.
30. BAGGIO, G. *et al.* 1998. Lipoprotein(a) and lipoprotein profile in healthy centenarians: a reappraisal of vascular risk factors. FASEB J. **12:** 433–437.
31. BARZILAI, N. *et al.* 2001. Offspring of centenarians have a favorable lipid profile. J. Am. Geriatr. Soc. **49:** 76–79.
32. MARIOTTI, S. *et al.* 1992. Thyroid and other organ-specific autoantibodies in healthy centenarians. Lancet **339:** 1506–1508.
33. EFFROS, R.B. *et al.* 1994. Decline in CD28(+) T cells in centenarians and in long term T cell cultures: A possible cause for both in vivo and in vitro immunosenescence. Exp. Gerontol. **29:** 601–609.
34. FRANCESCHI, C. *et al.* 1955. The immunology of exceptional individuals: the lesson of centenarians. Immunol. Today **16:** 12–16.
35. MARI, D. *et al.* 1995. Hypercoaguability in centenarians: the paradox of successful aging. Blood **85:** 3144–3149.
36. MANNUCCI, P.M. *et al.* 1997. Gene polymorphisms predicting high plasma levels of coagulation and fibrinolysis proteins: a study in centenarians. Arterioschler. Thromb. Vasc. Biol. **17:** 755–759.
37. SILVER, M. *et al.* 1998. Unraveling the mystery of cognitive changes in old age: correlation of neuropsychological evaluation with neuropathological findings in the extreme old. Int. Psychogeriatr. **10:** 25–41.

38. SILVER, M.H. *et al.* 2001. Cognitive functional status of age-confirmed centenarians in a population-based study. J. Gerontol. B. Psychol. Sci. Soc. Sci. **56:** P134–140.
39. HAGBERG, B. *et al.* 2001. Cognitive functioning in centenarians: a coordinated analysis of results from three countries. J. Gerontol. B. Psychol. Sci. Soc. Sci. **56:** P141–151.
40. ANDERSEN-RANBERG, K. *et al.* 2001. Dementia is not inevitable: a population-based study of Danish centenarians. J. Gerontol. B. Psychol. Sci. Soc. Sci. **56:** P152–159.
41. ISHII, T. *et al.* 1980. Cause of death in the extreme aged—a pathologic survey of 5106 elderly persons 80 years old and over. Age Ageing **9:** 81–89.
42. BEREGI, E. 1990. Centenarians in Hungary. A social and demographic study. Interdisciplinary topics in gerontology. Karger. Basel.
43. BEARD, B.B. 1991. Centenarians, the new generation. Greenwood Press. New York.
44. POON, L.W. 1992. The Georgian Centenarian Study. Baywood, Amytyville, New York.
45. KARASAWA, A. 1979. Mental aging and its medico–social background in the very old Japanese. J. Gerontol. **34:** 680–686.
46. ALLARD, M. 1991. A la recherche du secret des centeraires. Le Cherche-Midi, Paris.
47. LOUHIJA, J. 1994. Finnish Centenarians. Academic dissertation. University of Helsinki. Helsinki, Finland.
48. PERLS, T.T. *et al.* 1999. Validity of reported age and centenarian prevalence in New England. Age Ageing **28:** 193–197.
49. DEIANA, L. *et al.* 1999. AKEntAnnos. The Sardinia Study of Extreme Longevity. Aging (Milano) **11:** 142–149.
50. VAUPEL, J.W. *et al.* 1995. The emergence and proliferation of centenarians. *In* Exceptional Longevity: From Prehistory to the Present. B. Jeune & J.W. Vaupel, Eds.: 109–116. Springer. New York.
51. MANTON, K.G. & J.W. VAUPEL. 1995. Survival after the age of 80 in the United States, Sweden, France, England, and Japan. N. Engl. J. Med. **333:** 1232–1235.
52. CHRISTENSEN, K. & J.W. VAUPEL. 1996. Determinants of longevity: genetic, environmental and medical factors. J. Intern. Med. **240:** 333–341.
53. THATCHER, R. 1999. The demography of centenarians in England and Wales. Popul. Trends **96:** 5–12.
54. VAUPEL, J.W. 1997. The remarkable improvements in survival at older ages. Philos. Trans.: Biol. Sci. **352:** 1799–1804.
55. VAUPEL, J.W. *et al.* 1998. Biodemographic trajectories of longevity. Science **280:** 855–860.
56. PERLS, T. *et al.* 2001. Relative risk (λ_s) of achieving exceptional old age for siblings of centenarians. Submitted.
57. RYBICKI, B.A. & R.C. ELSTON. 2000. The relationship between the sibling recurrence-risk ratio and genotype relative risk. Am. J. Hum. Genet. **66:** 593–604.
58. PERLS, T.T. & R. FRETTS. 1998. Why women live longer than men. Sci. Amer. Presents **9:** 100–103.
59. KERBER, R.A. *et al.* 2001. Familial excess longevity in Utah genealogies. J. Gerontol. A Biol. Sci. Med. Sci. **56:** B130–139.
60. GUDMUNDSSON, H. *et al.* 2000. Inheritance of human longevity in Iceland. Eur. J. Hum. Genet. **8:** 743–749.
61. MARTIN, G.M. 1997. Genetics and the pathobiology of ageing. Philos. Trans. R. Soc. Lond. B.: Biol. Sci. **352:** 1773–1780.
62. MARTIN, G.M. 1979. Genetic and evolutionary aspects of aging. Fed. Proc. Fed. Am. Soc. Exp. Biol. **38:** 1962–1967.
63. SCHÄCHTER, F. 1998. Causes, effects, and constraints in the genetics of human longevity. Am. J. Hum. Genet. **62:** 1008–1014.
64. WACHTER, K.W. 1997. Between Zeus and the salmon: introduction. *In* Between Zeus and the Salmon. The Biodemography of Longevity, K.W. Wachter & C.E. Finch, Eds. National Academy Press. Washington, DC.
65. TOMITA-MITCHELL, A. *et al.* 1998. Single nucleotide polymorphism spectra in newborns and centenarians: identification of genes coding for rise of mortal disease. Gene **223:** 381–391.
66. FRISONI, G.B. *et al.* 2001. Longevity and the epsilon2 allele of apolipoprotein E: the Finnish Centenarians Study. J. Gerontol. A Biol. Sci. Med. Sci. **56:** M75–M78.

67. PERLS, T. 2001. Genetic and phenotypic markers among centenarians. J. Gerontol. A Biol. Sci. Med. Sci. **56:** M67–M70.
68. YASHIN, A.I. *et al.* 2000. Genes and longevity: lessons from studies of centenarians. J. Gerontol. A Biol. Sci. Med. Sci. **55A:** B319–B328.
69. MARTIN, G.M. *et al.* 1996. Genetic analysis of ageing: role of oxidative damage and environmental stresses. Nat. Genet. **13:** 25–34.
70. FINKEL, T. & N.J. HOLBROOK. 2000. Oxidants, oxidative stress and the biology of aging. Nature **408:** 239–106.
71. HAN, E. & S.G. HILSENBECK. 2001. Array-based gene expression profiling to study aging. Mech. Ageing Dev. **122:** 999–1018.
72. FOSSEL, M. 2000. Cell senescence in human aging: a review of the theory. In Vivo **14:** 29–34.
73. GUARENTE, L. & C. KENYON. 2000. Genetic pathways that regulate ageing in model organisms. Nature **408:** 255–262.
74. PAOLISSO, G. *et al.* 1998. Oxidative stress and advancing age: results in healthy centenarians. J. Am. Geriatr. Soc. **46:** 833–838.
75. NEMANI, M. *et al.* 2000. The efficiency of genetic analysis of DNA from aged siblings to detect chromosomal regions implicated in longevity. Mech. Ageing Dev. **119:** 25–39.
76. PUCA, A.A. *et al.* 2001. A genome-wide scan for linkage to human exceptional longevity identifies a locus on chromosome 4. Proc. Natl. Acad. Sci. USA **98**(18): 10505–10508.

Cell Senescence in Human Aging and Disease

MICHAEL FOSSEL

Michigan State University, Ada, Michigan 49301, USA

ABSTRACT: The most common causes of death and suffering, even in most underdeveloped nations, are age-related diseases. These diseases share fundamental and often unappreciated pathology at the cellular and genetic levels, through cell senescence. In cancer, enforcing cell senescence permits us to kill cancer cells without significantly harming normal cells. In other age-related diseases, cell senescence plays a direct role, and we may be able to prevent and reverse much of the pathology. While aging is attributed to "wear and tear," genetic studies show that these effects are avoidable (as is the case in germ cell lines) and occur only when cells down-regulate active (and sufficient) repair mechanisms, permitting degradation to occur. Aging occurs when cells permit accumulative damage by wear and tear, by altering their gene expression rather than vice versa. Using telomerase in laboratory settings, we can currently reset this pattern and its consequences both within cells and between cells. Doing so resets not only cell behavior but the pathological consequences within tissues comprising such cells. We can currently grow histologically young, reconstituted human skin using old human skin cells (keratinocytes and fibroblasts). Technically we could now test this approach in joints, vessels, the immune system, and other tissues. This model is consistent with all available laboratory data and known aging pathology. Within the next decade, we will be able to treat age-related diseases more effectively than ever before.

KEYWORDS: aging; telomeres; telomerase; cell senescence; gene expression

INTRODUCTION

Aging is frequently viewed, albeit with inadequate logical justification, as solely the result of "wear and tear," as though it were a set of generic processes, intrinsic to the passage of time. Bluntly, this point of view suggests that we get old because we "wear out." The stance is often assumed to be obvious, self-explanatory, and without any need for support, logical or factual. Accurate within a very narrow conceptual domain, the view is nonetheless parochial and fails when applied in a wider biological framework. It cannot explain aging—and the lack of aging—in any but the most common organisms. Even in such common organisms—for example, humans and mice—the view is neither robust nor consistent with known pathology and is incompatible with current data on germ cell survival, cancer, and telomere biology.

Address for correspondnece: Michael Fossel, M.D., PhD., Clinical Professor of Medicine, Michigan State University, Box 630, Ada, Michigan 49301. Voice: 616-676-8779; fax: 616-676-4099.

mfossel@earthlink.net

Ann. N.Y. Acad. Sci. 959: 14–23 (2002). © 2002 New York Academy of Sciences.

To achieve an accurate understanding of aging, wear and tear is almost certainly necessary but certainly not sufficient. Many cell lines and some multicellular organisms demonstrate indefinite maintenance in the face of such wear and tear, showing no accumulation of dysfunction. This is true of such cell lines as germ cell lineages, cancer cells, and telomerized human somatic cells. It is arguably true of some multicellular organisms such as the hydra. Despite the "slings and arrows" of a perennially hostile environment, there is a notable lack of aging in these cases. While it may be roughly accurate to say that homeostasis routinely wanes in *most* cell lines and in the *majority* of multicellular organisms (that is, most cell lines and most organisms age), a comprehensive understanding of aging requires that we explain the exceptions as well. We must account for *both* the maintenance of indefinite cellular and organismal homeostasis (that is, the lack of aging) and its far more common failure (that is, aging). Moreover, current laboratory evidence suggests that we might take lessons from the former and apply them to the latter with potentially unprecedented clinical benefits. Specifically, we may be able to take cells that would normally age and induce them to remain immortal by using the same mechanisms employed in, for example, germ cell lines and cancer cells. Maintaining indefinite cellular homeostasis is not so much a matter of redesigning cells as it is of adjusting their genetic expression. In the case of cells *in vitro* and *in vivo*, and in the case of reconstituted human tissue *ex vivo*, preventing aging is not a matter of replacing genes, but simply a matter of altering gene expression of those genes the cell normally possesses.

Indefinite maintenance of cellular function in the face of continual damage is a remarkably reliable biological phenomenon. It occurs in the germ cell lines of organisms whose somatic cells show aging changes, again suggesting that cellular aging may be not so much a matter of having the wrong genes as it is of expressing the ones you have poorly. Aging results from bad gene expression, not bad genes. The lessons of gene expression that we learn from understanding cellular senescence may be taken into clinical medicine,[1] allowing us to prevent and treat the diseases of aging and, perhaps, aging itself.

AGING: A DISEASE?

Although many would argue that aging is not a disease, it clearly results in disease and, from a purely sociological perspective, is generally treated as though it were one. Many biologists, for example, may be quick to disparage the notion of aging as being a disease, but may be the same individuals who dye their hair, use retinoids on their skin, and obtain face lifts. Whether or not we define aging as a disease, the association between aging and disease is chronological, behavioral, and pathologic. Denotational disputes notwithstanding, this last feature, the underlying pathology of age-related disease, is our major concern here.

Many diseases are not associated with aging per se, including strictly genetic disease (e.g., sickle cell), infectious disease (e.g., rabies), and trauma (e.g., motor vehicle accidents). However, the morbidity and mortality of these diseases may (and in many cases do) correlate with age. Other things being equal, older people are more likely to die of pneumococcal pneumonia or trauma than are younger people. This stems from age-related changes in the immune system in the former case and both an increased probability of falling and an increased frailty in the latter. Despite these rising correlative risks with age, these disease processes are not the result of aging itself. Their incidence may rise, their complications may become more likely, but the basic processes of infection and trauma are not the same as aging.

At the other extreme, could it be that perhaps there are diseases that are equivalent to aging itself? Here, we discover that that prim mythical biological etymologist is correct: aging is simply *not* any particular disease. There are no diseases that we define as being solely the result of aging, in the sense that the pathology lacks any other genetic or environmental component or interaction and is purely aging per se.

Although aging is not a disease, it contributes to many diseases. It often appears to drive the pathology, as though taking advantage of some genetic inadequacy, whether in atherosclerosis, Alzheimer's dementia, or osteoporosis. In each of these, and other aging-related diseases, there is strong evidence for genetic and often environmental components, but, at first sight, penetrance appears strongly influenced by chronological age as well. Those with a predilection for atherosclerosis express it more clearly as they grow older. The relationship is complex, however. Some of us age without any significant clinical evidence of atherosclerosis; there are centenarians without known atherosclerosis. At the other extreme, there are specific syndromes (e.g., Hutchinson-Gilford progeria) in which atherosclerosis occurs at such an early age[2] and in parallel with dermal changes[3] that we consider the syndrome as suggestive of early aging rather than simply a genetic syndrome with rampant atherosclerosis.[4] Aging (and in some altered form, perhaps early aging in progeria) appears to "unlock" or permit latent genetic risks—that is, genes that cause atherosclerosis—and thereby results in clinical disease. It is not aging that "causes" atherosclerosis, yet the clinical expression of such genes appears somehow dependent on not only chronological time, but aging itself. If aging is not a disease, then neither is it blameless. Perhaps aging is not a lone villain, but it is the primary contributor to a general "conspiracy of pathology." Whether in atherosclerosis, osteoarthritis, or Alzheimer's dementia, we do not see aging pure and simple, yet we see its mark in the rising incidence and in the functional decline of the organs involved.

Returning to the classic example of an age-related disease, that of atherosclerosis, we find pathology that is clearly the result of multiple genetic and environmental factors,[5] yet in which aging reliably and mysteriously insinuates itself.[6] In every aging organ, we find aging changes, sometimes blatantly—as in arteries[7]—and sometimes more subtly—as in the myocardium.[8] Basic gerontologic science has become a catalog of alterations that spans species, cell phenotypes, and the centuries. To an extent, we have learned a great deal about the specifics of aging, yet we find ourselves caught in our own assumptions and theories, unable to intervene effectively in the diseases of aging. Without exception, when we treat the diseases of aging, we are treating the outcomes not the causes. In atherosclerosis we lower serum cholesterol, arterial pressure, blood sugar, and tobacco intake, but we have been unable to lower the age of the tissues. It is aging that permits the genetic risks to express themselves in clinical risks. To date, we treat the outcomes of the slowly altered pattern of genetic expression that aging imposes on our cells, not the process of aging that drives that inexorable alteration. Yet there are hints that the process may not be inexorable at all, but that we might yet tease apart the process and intervene. In some cases, we find patients with none of the known risk factors, but with fulminant atherosclerosis;[9] in others, we find all the risk factors, but the absence of measurable disease. Our models, our understanding of both aging and the diseases that accompany it, are not so much wrong (for the bulk of the data says otherwise), as incomplete. We understand atherosclerosis, but only partially. We understand aging, but only partially. What have we left out?

AGING: IT'S THE GARDENER, NOT THE WEEDS

To most of us, aging is a gradual, erosive process that results in physiologic dysfunction.[8] Pressed, most of us would ascribe to the notion that aging results from the progressive accumulation of cell damage. More specifically, we might opine that mitochondrial dysfunction and free radical damage to proteins, DNA, lipid membranes, and larger cellular components is the essence of the aging process. Even in the absence of free radicals, a host of other processes (including simple biological error) might drive the leisurely cellular catastrophe that finally results in organismal aging. Undoubtedly this rough model parallels a great deal of biological reality, but—like our current model of atherosclerosis—it is not so much wrong as incomplete.[10] As in any scientific advance, the most useful considerations are in the exceptions to a model. We can only find enlightenment and progress by making the model robust enough to fit reality, not just a small, provincial part of reality.

Consider the problems with the simplistic notion that free radical damage simply "causes" aging. The major problem is that many cells do not age and that we would not be alive to consider this issue if they had. In short, you are here only because of cells that do not age, despite billions of years of free radicals. Despite equivalent genes in each of your cells, cell phenotypes vary markedly. A neuron differs from a fibroblast not in its genes, but in its gene expression. When a cell undergoes apoptosis, when it differentiates, when it senesces, it does not change its genes, but rather its pattern of gene expression. The difference between the embryonic stem cell from which you derive and the cells that populate your myocardium is not genetic, but a matter of how those genes are expressed. Similarly, cell senescence is not a matter of altered genes, but of altered expression.[11] In a broader evolutionary framework, consider a parallel case: the cell lines from which your embryo derives. You carry half of the genes from your mother and half from your father. Though reshuffled, those genes were not altered. The reason that you are not a precise replica of your great-great-grandparent is not due to altered, but to reshuffled, genes.

If we were to look at a gene that appears to play a prominent role in free radical metabolism, such as the SOD allele, that particular allele is not new with you, but inherited from one of your ancestors. In all likelihood, the SOD allele has been inherited unaltered with a provenance of several hundred million years. During that time, the cellular lineage from which you derive has been unbroken (though sexually reshuffled) until you branch off from it as an embryo and a collection of somatic cells. That cell line remained intact and maintained itself—essentially without accumulated damage (from free radicals or otherwise)—until your fertilization occurred. The same is true of every other gene and specific allele involved in free radical metabolism and cellular maintenance generally.

If we want to explain why free radicals cause accumulating damage in your somatic cells, we cannot place it at the doorstep of an inadequate SOD allele, which has functioned adequately for the millions of years or longer that the allele has been present in the human genome. Nor can we pretend that your genes are generally inadequate to maintain your cells indefinitely in the face of free radical attacks, which they have managed to deal with effectively for billions of years without accumulated damage. These genes are not only adequate to maintain cell homeostasis indefinitely, but they have already unarguably demonstrated their capability by still existing. Although some of us have inherited genetic defects and acquired genetic mutations, the survival of the germ cells from which we derive is an overwhelming argument that our genes are sufficient for indefinite cellular maintenance in the face of persistent free radical damage. We cannot blame aging on inadequate genes; we can ascribe it to an inadequate pattern of gene expression.

Indeed, gene expression does change as a cell senesces, and these changes result in inadequate responses to free radicals and free radical damage.[12] If we restrict our discussion only to free radicals, we would have to conclude that it is not so much that free radicals *cause* aging, as it is that a changing pattern of gene expression *permits* free radicals to cause aging. Our cellular mechanisms, and the genes that underlie them, can maintain our cells indefinitely, but not if gene expression changes prevent the cell from doing so adequately. If we want to prevent cell damage, we should not focus our clinical efforts on free radicals themselves or on replacing the genes we have, but on optimizing the expression of those genes to deal with free radicals and other biological insults.

Consider an analogy. A large flower garden, no matter how carefully planted, will have occasional weeds. While we cannot rely on a perfect weed-free garden to maintain itself without care, we can have maintenance mechanisms in place that are sufficient to deal with the weeds. If we have a gardener, they can maintain the apparent perfection of our garden indefinitely. Our garden is the cell, the weeds are free radical damage, and the gardener is the genes that sequester and trap free radicals and that repair free radical damage. As long as the genetic gardener is working, the cellular garden can be maintained indefinitely, as is the case in the germ cell lines. In somatic cells, however, we cut back on the gardener. In aging cells, this is precisely what happens. The weeds grow and cellular damage ensues not because the genetic gardener is inept or because the free radical weeds always destroy cellular gardens if a certain amount of time passes. The problem is that we fired the gardener.

Just as gardens can be maintained indefinitely *if cared for*, so too can cells be maintained indefinitely *if genetic expression is appropriate*. If we want to bring our weedy garden back to its previous state, the most effective intervention is not to study weeds or to find a more efficient gardener: we already know that our gardener is sufficient if we let him go back to the work he was previously doing. If we want to bring an aging cell back to its previous state, the most effective intervention is not to focus on the free radicals or to replace an SOD allele with a more active enzyme. Our derivation from an immortal germ cell line demonstrates that our SOD (and our other) alleles are sufficient for indefinite cell maintenance if expression is optimal. We need to understand how to reset gene expression to a pattern that effectively maintains our cells in the face of biological entropy.

This conclusion is not merely theoretical but well supported by data from several venues. For example, the approach suggested by this model works perfectly well in aging human somatic cells, which can be reset to function normally both *in vitro*[13–15] and *ex vivo*.[16] We can reset the pattern of gene expression from a senescent to a young cell pattern,[17] and when we do so, such cells are capable of indefinite maintenance and perfectly normal cell function. They function well as individual cells and are equally capable of reconstituting young human tissue.[16] The experimental support is unambiguous: resetting gene expression is necessary and sufficient to reset aging and to permit cell "immortality."

CELL IMMORTALITY

As they age, cells change their pattern of gene expression. Reasonably, however, and the above considerations notwithstanding, we might ask whether this is primary or secondary. Does the changing pattern of gene expression cause the cell to fail, or do the failing cells cause the gene expression to change? We know that the changing pattern of gene expression leaves the cell with failing defenses against "wear and tear," for example, free radicals, but might it not be that free radical damage prompts the changing pattern in the first place? This question is neither merely academic nor is it unanswerable. To answer this question, we need only try resetting gene expression and see what happens. If we can find a way to reset cell aging by resetting gene expression, the implication would be that we might be able to treat age-related diseases more effectively than ever before and perhaps even prevent aging itself. On the other hand, if the changes in gene expression were simply secondary to cell damage, then resetting gene expression would not affect the problem nor would it reverse aging in cells, tissues, or organisms. We would then have the vastly more difficult challenge of preventing cell damage in the first place. If true, this would suggest that to intervene in age-related disease and aging would be far more difficult as well.

The initial discussion—and the mere existence as the somatic cell derivative of an "immortal" germ cell line—argues strongly that cells accrue damage because they change their pattern of gene expression and not vice versa. The available data argues this conclusion even more forcefully. If we reset gene expression, we prevent the accrual of cell damage and cell aging.

From the standpoint of cell aging, gene expression appears to be under the direction of the telomere. Several misconceptions have arisen with regard to this point and require clarification. The first clarification is that telomeres do not directly control gene expression but do so through a barely understood series of mechanisms that may include a heterochromatin sheath and distant effects mediated by telomere binding proteins.[18] The second clarification is that telomere length per se is probably irrelevant to cell aging and cell function except at the extremes.[11] The alteration in gene expression that appears to define cell aging is likely the result of the relative change in telomere length that occurs postfertilization, rather than the result of absolute telomere length.[19] This not only explains the findings in murine telomere knockout studies[20,21] but is, in fact, predictable and consistent with what we know of embryology. Gene expression is essentially reset to a *tabula rasa* (or at least an undifferentiated cell phenotype) at the time of fertilization.[22] In the cases of both knockout mice and cloned animals, we would predict that absolute telomere length should be immaterial, as the linkage itself (between telomere and gene expression) must be entirely reset *regardless of actual telomere length*, or we would not have the proper resetting of gene expression and therefore would not have a viable fertilized cell. In summary, relative telomere length postfertilization rather than absolute telomere length must determine gene expression, or clones and telomere knockout mice would be totally infertile. The very existence of clones and multigenerational telomere knockout mice (far from arguing against the role of telomeres and cell senescence in aging) strongly supports this model.

The more interesting and suggestive data, however, come from telomerization studies in which we reset cell aging and gene expression by increasing telomere length. In general, this approach relies on the insertion of a normal human hTERT gene into human cells (typically fibroblasts), resulting in telomerase expression and activity, with consequent lengthening of telomeres and extension of the replicative limit.[13] Such studies show that cellular "life span" can be extended indefinitely and without loss of cell phenotype or malignant transformation.[23] The cells remain normal in all regards, except that they do not age. Moreover, telomerization does not cause cancer in these cells and may even make them more resistant to DNA damage and secondary malignant transformation.[24–26]

In the most important studies, however, human dermal cells (fibroblasts and keratinocytes) were telomerized. These cells showed renormalization of their patterns of gene expression[17] as well as indefinite cell life span and retention of normal cell phenotype. A portion of this study showed that senescent cells can be used to reconstitute normal young human tissue when the cell aging is reset with telomerization. The cells, grown on an immunocompromised mouse, formed simple human dermal tissue, complete with normal layering patterns and normal dermal-epidermal interdigitation.[16]

When the study was done with young human fibroblasts and keratinocytes, the result was what appeared to be young human dermal tissue. The skin layers were thick and the interdigitations complex and tight. When done with senescent cells, the result was what appeared to be old human dermal tissue. The skin layers were thin and the interdigitations simplified, loose, and characterized by easy sloughing and microbullae. When senescent cells were telomerized, however, and placed back on the immunocompromised mouse, the result was what appeared to be young human dermal tissue. Once again, the layers were thick and the interdigitations complex and tight, just as in young skin.

This study has remarkable implications both for our understanding of aging and, far more importantly, for potential interventions in human disease.[27] It suggests that by resetting cell senescence (by whatever means, telomerization, use of an hTERT promoter, or other approach), we may be able to prevent or treat human age-related disease in a more effective and fundamental fashion than we have ever done in the past. The limits depend on the accuracy of this model, our ability to find techniques that effectively reset cell senescence, and the degree to which cell senescence is the cause of age-related human clinical disease. To what extent does cell senescence contribute to age-related disease?

CELL SENESCENCE: DO OLD CELLS CAUSE OLD AGE?

The answer to the title question for this section is simple: we do not know. Appropriate criticism reflects this ignorance, rather than the more common ignorance of clinical pathology. In any case, we expect to test the model in human *in vivo* studies within the next few years.

Frequently and ironically, the criticisms leveled at this model tell us more about the ignorance of the critic than about the ignorance of our data. For example, the notion that cell senescence cannot cause heart disease because myocardial cells do not senesce, is fatuous. It is equivalent to saying that cholesterol accumulation cannot cause heart disease because myocardial cells do not accumulate cholesterol. Cholesterol accumulation *does* contribute strongly to heart disease, but does so by accumulating in the subendothelial layers of the coronary arteries. The fact that cholesterol does not accumulate in myocardial cells is a non sequitur. The fact that cell senescence does not occur in nondividing myocardial cells is likewise irrelevant and suggests that the critic has a closely circumscribed knowledge of human pathology.

In the case of atherosclerosis, the relevant pathology occurs in the coronary arteries. The endothelial cells, which line these arteries, play a clear role in the etiology of the cascade of pathology,[28] and these cells show profound senescent changes in patients with atherosclerosis.[29] The model that atherosclerosis is attributable to cell senescence is not only consistent with everything we know of the pathology involved, but it also has two added recommendations. First, it explains exceptions to the classic model of atherosclerosis, such as why progeric children, without any of the classic risk factors, die overwhelmingly of atherosclerosis. Second, and more importantly, it suggests a powerful point of clinical intervention: if we reset cell aging in endothelial cells, we might prevent or cure atherosclerosis and thereby heart disease, strokes, and aneurysms.[30]

In the case of Alzheimer's disease, although equally vacuous criticisms have been raised, the relevant pathology appears to involve microglial activation.[31] It might well be true that microglial or astrocytic cell senescence is the primary culprit in this complex pathology, the nondividing (and nonsenescing) status of adult neurons notwithstanding and being irrelevant to the model. This model of Alzheimer's dementia again is more comprehensive and consistent with the clinical data than are other current models. Likewise, if accurate, we might attempt to intervene in the disease by resetting cell senescence in the affected glial cells.

In each age-related disease—for example, immunosenescence, osteoarthritis, osteoporosis, endocrine aging, and dermal aging—the role of cell senescence as the trigger and driving force behind the pathology is entirely consistent with the clinical pathology.[32] The conceptual framework is conceptually elegant, consistent with the known pathology, and biologically sophisticated. More importantly, it offers testable points of intervention. In each case, cell senescence is a tempting target for therapeutic intervention, whether via direct transfection, viral or other carriers, or hTERT promoters. There remain significant technical, regulatory, and clinical hurdles to be overcome. Nonetheless, a growing number of clinical studies are focusing on the role of cell senescence in human aging and age-related disease, including cancer,[33,34] hepatitis,[35] dermal aging,[36,37] immunosenescence,[38,39] and ocular aging.[40] New financial resources are gradually coming into play, as are new organizations dedicated to supporting this work. Comprehensive reviews of the field are already in preparation.[41]

SUMMARY

Aging reflects the failure of otherwise previously balanced homeostatic biological mechanisms at the cellular level. This failure has profound intracellular and intercellular consequences for the organism. Age-related diseases represent the failure of these intercellular mechanisms at the tissue level, such as occurs in atherosclerosis where myocardial cells depend on aging vascular endothelial cells. These cellular mechanisms are rarely attributable to the failure of specific genes but generally reflect an altered and ineffective pattern of gene expression in aging cells. This pattern can be, and has been, reset in human somatic cells both *in vitro* and *ex vivo*. Results imply that we will potentially be able to intervene in age-related diseases at the level of gene expression and thereby prevent and/or cure such diseases. Using this approach, we will not only examine our ability to reset aging within human cells and tissues, but within organisms as a whole.

REFERENCES

1. FOSSEL, M. 1998. Implications of recent work in telomeres and cell senescence. J. Anti-Aging Med. **1:** 39–43.
2. BAKER, P.B., N. BABA & C.P. BOESEL. 1981. Cardiovascular abnormalities in progeria: case report and review of the literature. Arch. Pathol. Lab. Med. **105:** 384–386.
3. BROWN, W.T. 1992. Progeria: a human-disease model of accelerated aging. Am. J. Clin. Nutr. **55:** 1222S–1224S.
4. FOSSEL, M. 2000. Human aging and progeria. J. Ped. Endo. & Metab. **13:** 1477–1481.
5. HOEG, J.M. 1996. Can genes prevent atherosclerosis? JAMA **276:** 989–992.
6. BIERMAN, E.L. 1994. Aging and atherosclerosis. *In* Principles of Geriatric Medicine and Gerontology. W.R. Hazzard, E.L. Bierman, J.P. Blass, W.H. Ettinger Jr. & J.B. Halter, Eds.: 509–516. McGraw Hill. NewYork.
7. LAKATTA, E.G. 1994. Alterations in circulatory function. *In* Principles of Geriatric Medicine and Gerontology. W.R. Hazzard, E.L. Bierman, J.P. Blass, W.H. Ettinger Jr. & J.B. Halter, Eds.: 493–508. McGraw Hill. NewYork.
8. ARKING, R. 1998. Biology of aging. 2nd ed. Sinauer Associates. Sunderland, Massachusetts.
9. FOSSEL, M. 2000. Human aging and progeria. J. Ped. Endo. & Metab. **13:** 1477–1481.
10. FOSSEL, M. 2000. Emails to the editor. The function of mitochondrial dysfunction in aging. J. Anti-Aging Med. **3:** 103–104.
11. FOSSEL, M. 2001. The role of telomerase in age-related degenerative disease and cancer. *In* Interorganellar Signaling in Age-Related Disease. M.P. Mattson, Ed.: Chapter 6. Elsevier Science. Amsterdam.
12. FOSSEL, M. 1996. Reversing Human Aging. William Morrow and Company. New York.
13. BODNAR, A.G., C. CHIU, M. FROLKIS, *et al.* 1998. Extension of life-span by introduction of telomerase into normal human cells. Science **279:** 349–352.
14. VAZIRI, H. 1998. Extension of life span in normal human cells by telomerase activation: a revolution in cultural senescence. J. Anti-Aging Med. **1:** 125–130.
15. VAZIRI, H. & S. BENCHIMOL. 1998. Reconstruction of telomerase activity in normal cells leads to elongation of telomeres and extended replicative life span. Curr. Biol. **8:** 279–282.
16. FUNK, W.D., C.K. WANG, D.N. SHELTON, *et al.* 2000. Telomerase expression restores dermal integrity to in vitro-aged fibroblasts in a reconstituted skin model. Exp. Cell Res. **258:** 270–278.
17. SHELTON, D.N., E. CHANG, P.S. WHITTIER, *et al.* 1999. Microarray analysis of replicative senescence. Curr. Biol. **9:** 939-945.
18. FOSSEL, M. 2000. Cell senescence and human aging: a review of the theory. In Vivo **14:** 29–34.
19. FOSSEL, M. 2000. The Role of Cell Senescence in Human Aging. *In* Endocrinology of Aging. B. Bercu & R. Walker, Eds. Springer-Verlag. New York.
20. BLASCO, M.A., R.A. DEPINHO, C.W. GREIDER, *et al.* 1997. Telomere shortening and tumor formation by mouse cells lacking telomerase RNA. Cell **91:** 25–34.

21. HERRERA, E., E. SAMPER, J. MARTIN-CABALLERO, et al. 1999. Disease states associated with telomerase deficiency appear earlier in mice with short telomeres. EMBO J. **18:** 2950-2960.
22. HUMPHREYS, D., K. EGGAN, H. AKUTSU, et al. 2001. Epigenetic instability in ES cells and cloned mice. Science **293:** 95–97.
23. JIANG, X.R., G. JIMENEZ, E. CHANG, et al. 1999. Telomerase expression in human somatic cells does not induce changes associated with a transformed phenotype. Natl. Genet. **21:** 111–114.
24. COUNTER, C.M., A.A. AVILION, C.E. LEFEUVRE, et al. 1992. Telomere shortening associated with chromosome instability is arrested in immortal cells which express telomerase activity. EMBO J. **11:** 1921–1919.
25. OHYASHIKI, J.H., H. IWAMA, N. YAHATA, et al. 1999. Telomere stability is frequently impaired in high-risk groups of patients with myelodysplastic syndromes. Clin. Cancer Res. **5:** 1155–1160.
26. AMIT, M., M.K. CARPENTER, M.S. INOKUMA, et al. 2000. Clonally derived human embryonic stem cell lines maintain pluripotency and proliferative potential for prolonged periods of culture. Dev. Biol. **227:** 271–278.
27. FOSSEL, M. 1998b. Telomerase and the aging cell; implications for human health. JAMA **279:** 1732–1735.
28. COOPER, L.T., J.P. COOKE & V.J. DZAU. 1994. The vasculopathy of aging. J. Gerontol. **49:** 191–196.
29. CHANG, E. & C.B. HARLEY. 1995. Telomere length and replicative aging in human vascular tissues. Proc. Natl. Acad. Sci. USA **92:** 1190–1194.
30. BANKS, D.A. & M. FOSSEL. 1997. Telomeres, cancer, and aging; altering the human lifespan. JAMA **278:** 1345–1348.
31. MCGEER, E.G., P.L. MCGEER. 1999. Brain inflammation in Alzheimer disease and the therapeutic implications. Curr. Pharm. Des. **5:** 821–836.
32. FOSSEL, M. 2000. The role of cell senescence in human aging. J. Anti-Aging Med. **3:** 91–98.
33. SHAY, J.W. 1995. Aging and cancer: are telomeres and telomerase the connection? Mol. Med. Today **1:** 378–384.
34. CAMPISI, J. 1997. Aging and cancer: the double-edged sword of replicative senescence. J. Am. Geriatr. Soc. **45:** 482–488.
35. RUDOLPH, K.L., S. CHANG, M. MILLARD, et al. 2000. Inhibition of experimental liver cirrhosis in mice by telomerase gene delivery. Science **287:** 1253–1258.
36. CAMPISI, J. 1998. The role of cellular senescence in skin aging. J. Investig. Dermatol. Symp. Proc. **3:** 1–5.
37. MATSUI, M., J. MIYASAKA, K. HAMADA, et al. 2000. Influence of aging and cell senescence on telomerase activity in keratinocytes. J. Dermatol. Sci. **22:** 80–87.
38. EFFROS, R.B. & G. PAWELEC. 1997. Replicative senescence of T lymphocytes: Does the Hayflick limit lead to immune exhaustion? Immunol. Today **18:** 450–454.
39. PAWELEC, G. 1999. Importance of T-cell replicative senescence for the adoptive immunotherapy of cancer in humans? J. Anti-Aging Med. **2:** 115–120.
40. FARAGHER, R.G., B. MULHOLLAND, S.J. TUFT, et al. 1997. Aging and the cornea. Br. J. Ophthalmol. **81:** 814–817.
41. FOSSEL, M. Cell senescence in human aging and disease. Oxford University Press. New York. In preparation.

Replicative Aging, Telomeres, and Oxidative Stress

GABRIELE SARETZKI AND THOMAS VON ZGLINICKI

Department of Gerontology, University of Newcastle,
Newcastle upon Tyne NE6 4BE, United KIngdom

ABSTRACT: Aging is a very complex phenomenon, both *in vivo* and *in vitro*. Free radicals and oxidative stress have been suggested for a long time to be involved in or even to be causal for the aging process. Telomeres are special structures at the end of chromosomes. They shorten during each round of replication and this has been characterized as a mitotic counting mechanism. Our experiments show that the rate of telomere shortening *in vitro* is modulated by oxidative stress as well as by differences in antioxidative defence capacity between cell strains. *In vivo* we found a strong correlation between short telomeres in blood lymphocytes and the incidence of vascular dementia. These data suggest that parameters that characterise replicative senescence *in vitro* offer potential for understanding of, and intervention into, the aging process *in vivo*.

Keywords: senescence; telomeres; oxidative stress; dementia

TELOMERES AND REPLICATIVE SENESCENCE

In vitro aging of human fibroblasts is an established model for cellular aging, first described by Leonard Hayflick.[1] Explanted mammalian cells perform *in vitro* a limited number of cell divisions and arrest then (at the Hayflick limit) in a state known as replicative senescence. Such cells are irreversibly blocked, mostly in the G1 phase of cell cycle, and are no longer sensitive to growth factor stimulation. Thus, replicative senescence was defined as a permanent and irreversible loss of replicative potential of cells. The Hayflick limit is usually a constant number under standardized culture conditions. However, the external change of oxidative stress levels can modulate the replicative life span of a given cell culture.[2,3]

Telomeres are repetitive structures of the sequence $(TTAGGG)_n$ at the ends of mammalian chromosomes. It has been shown that the average length of telomere repeats in human somatic cells decreases by 20–200 base pairs with each cell division.[4,5] One reason for this shortening is the so-called "end replication problem": during the replication of the lagging strand, the RNA primer for the most distal Okazaki fragment cannot be replaced by DNA. Accordingly, the newly synthesized lagging strand is shorter by at least the length of the primer (less than 12 nt), resulting

---

Address for correspondence: Dr. Gabriele Saretzki, University of Newcastle, Department of Gerontology, Wolfson Research Centre, Newcastle General Hospital, Westgate Road, Newcastle upon Tyne NE6 4BE, UK.Voice: +44-0191 256 3384; fax: +44-0191 2195074.
gabriele.saretzki@ncl.ac.uk

in an overhang of the parental G-rich strand at one end of the chromosome. Experimentally, G-rich overhangs 100–500 nt long have been found. However, whether these overhangs exist on one (as predicted by the end replication problem), or on both chromosome ends, is not clear,[6,7] and neither is the contribution of a hypothetical 5′ exonuclease to telomere shortening.

On the basis of regular shortening, telomeres have been connected with replicative aging *in vitro* and *in vivo* and were characterized as a "mitotic clock."[8,9] Direct evidence linking telomere shortening causally to replicative senescence was given by overexpression of the telomere-elongating enzyme, telomerase, in mortal cells. In this case, telomeres are elongated and the transfected cells are immortalized without any evident karyotypic changes or perturbations of cell cycle checkpoints.[10,11]

DO EXTERNAL FACTORS CHANGE THE REPLICATIVE LIFE SPAN?

The answer is yes: this is accomplished by changing the rate of telomere shortening. The end replication problem suggests a constant shortening of telomeres. However, we could show for the first time that telomere shortening is stress dependent.[2] There is a minimal shortening of less than 20 bp per cell division[12] in cells with high antioxidative capacity, and telomere shortening rates are higher in cells with lower antioxidative defence.[5] Cultivating cells under enhanced oxidative stress like mild hyperoxia (40% normobaric oxygen) shortens the telomeres prematurely and shortens the replicative life span accordingly.[2] Most parameters of those prematurely aged fibroblasts are identical to normal fibroblast aging (e.g., morphology, lipofuscin accumulation, and specific changes in gene expression).[2,13] Radical scavengers like phenyl-butyl-nitrone are able to lower the telomere shortening rate.[14]

We uncovered the mechanism of the enhanced telomere shortening rate as damage of free oxygen radicals to the telomeric DNA. More specifically, an accumulation of single-stranded regions takes place in the telomeres, which is caused by lower repair of those lesions in the telomeric compartment in comparison to other repetitive nontranscribed regions in the genome, like minisatellite structures, and to the bulk of the genome.[15] The single-strand breaks in the telomeric regions result in telomere shortening after DNA replication.[16] The mechanism is probably the transient stalling of the replication fork.[17]

Telomeres are not simple linear stretches of DNA but are highly organized structures. The G-rich telomeric strand forms an overhang, which is more than 100 nt long. There is still controversy as to whether the length of these overhangs relates to telomere shortening rates in different cell lines.[14,18] When we treated fibroblasts with different concentrations of hydrogen peroxide and other agents that damage telomeric DNA preferentially, we could not find a difference in the overhang length.[14]

CAN THE G-RICH OVERHANG BE CONNECTED WITH SIGNALING PATHWAYS INITIATING SENESCENCE?

Not only the overhang, but also different telomere binding proteins, like TRF1 and TRF2, are responsible for a characteristic loop structure of telomeres[19] and are involved in telomere length control.[20] In this way the single strand sequence of the overhang is protected and probably not accessible to signal-transducing proteins and enzymes. Recently the existence of the overhang binding protein pot1 has been described,[21] but its function is not yet known.

There are at least three events that unfold the telomeric loop structure. The first one is the normal DNA replication. A second process takes place in cells with active telomerase during elongation of the G-rich overhang of a telomere. These two events are both regulated and coordinated. By contrast, unfolding of the loop structure due to critical telomere shortening or telomere-specific DNA damage is unscheduled and might activate a cell cycle checkpoint signal. We modeled this unscheduled exposure of the single-stranded overhang by treating cells with short oligonucleotides of telomeric G- and C-rich sequences and compared them with unrelated sequences like scrambled or minisatellite sequences. Those oligonucleotides (12mers) are fast internalized into the cell nucleus. Only the G-rich oligonucleotides cause a proliferation arrest, which is p53 dependent.[22] This arrest is long lasting in human fibroblasts but is of shorter duration in the telomerase-positive human glioblastoma cell line U87. U87 cells that overcome the arrest have activated telomerase above normal levels and elongated telomeres. The same effect was detected after arrests by hydrogen peroxide treatment or chronic hyperoxia. p53 seemed necessary for both the transient proliferation arrest and the telomere elongation by telomerase in cells overcoming the arrest, because both effects were abrogated in cells expressing a dominant negative p53 mutation.[22] The simplest interpretation of these findings is that treatment with G-rich oligonucletides mimics the unscheduled unfolding of the telomeric loop and that single-stranded G-rich overhangs activate p53 either directly or indirectly.

The telomeric loop structure might also be the cause for the decreased repair of telomeres, because it might make telomeres less accessible for repair enzymes than other parts of the genome. In this way the unrepaired single-strand breaks accumulated in the telomeres contribute to a telomere shortening, which is additional to the one caused by the end replication problem. Therefore, oxidative damage and free radicals can modulate the telomere length plus their structural and functional integrity. Additional evidence for the importance of a stabilized telomeric structure comes from telomerase inhibition experiments. Telomerase not only elongates telomeres but stabilizes the ends of chromosomes via a "capping" function as well.[23] Inhibition of capping, for instance, by prevention of the synthesis of the catalytic subunit of telomerase by a ribozyme approach[24] appears to destabilize the telomere structure in tumor cells. The surprising result of telomerase inhibition via viral transduction of an anti-hTERT ribozyme was the fast induction of apoptosis in the treated tumor cells, irrespective of their telomere length or p53 status.[25] We hypothesize that the withdrawal of telomerase in this model activates p53-independent apoptotic pathways.

TELOMERE SHORTENING AND ANTIOXIDATIVE DEFENCE

An age-dependent telomere shortening has been demonstrated in different self-renewing human tissues like peripheral blood monocytes, fibroblasts, endothelial cells, and others.[9,26] The variation of telomere length between different individuals seems to be mainly genetically determined.[27]

We measured telomere shortening rates over at least 20 population doublings in different fibroblast strains. From all examined strains, BJ foreskin fibroblasts had the longest replicative life span (80–100 PD) and maintained their telomeres best both under normoxic and hyperoxic conditions. By contrast, MRC-5 and WI38 displayed a high telomere shortening rate and shorter replicative life span under both conditions.[12] Measuring both telomere-shortening rate and antioxidative capacity (using DCF fluorescence as an indicator of intracellular peroxide levels), we found a significant inverse correlation between telomere-shortening rate and antioxidative capacity in more than 20 human fibroblast strains.[2] Fibroblasts with low antioxidative defence capacity shorten their telomeres faster and vice versa. These data are in good concordance with those showing an important role of the antioxidative enzymes gluthathione peroxidase and Cu/Zn-superoxide dismutase for the telomere shortening rate in human fibroblasts.[28] These data confirm that telomere length is mainly determined by the relation between oxidative stress and antioxidative defence capacity. Thus, the age-corrected telomere length is a cumulative measure of the history of oxidative damage a cell line has experienced over its life span. While this has been shown for *in vitro* experiments so far, it might hold true for the *in vivo* situation as well. A correlation between oxidative stress and enhanced telomere shortening rate has been shown earlier for inherited respiratory chain disorders[29] and for patients with Down syndrome.[30]

If antioxidative defence determines telomere length *in vivo* as well, one would expect a good correlation between telomere lengths in different tissues from the same donor, and such correlation should not deteriorate with age. In fact, telomere lengths in blood lymphocytes and fibroblasts from the same donor were significantly correlated irrespective of different replicative histories and the presence of telomerase in lymphocytes. Similar correlations were found between telomere lengths in four different tissues in cattle (Serra *et al.*, in prep.). There was no evidence for a deterioration of the correlations with age. Recently, these results were independently confirmed.[31] Taken together, our results suggest that telomere length in one (proliferating) tissue should be a cumulative indicator of the relative amount of oxidative stress even in other tissues, and of the ability of the individual to cope with such stress. In other words, the relative telomere length might indicate the probability of a successful defence against an oxidative insult.

TELOMERE LENGTH AND DEMENTIA

The involvement of telomeres has been implicated in several conditions: progeria, Werner syndrome,[32] and hyper- and hypoproliferative diseases.[33,34,26] We sought to examine whether degenerative neurological conditions might be related to telomeres and oxidative stress. To test the idea that telomere length is not only important for the replicative life span of a cell population *in vitro* but might represent a valuable diagnostic or even prognostic factor for an *in vivo* situation, we analyzed telomeres of lymphocytes from 186 individuals between 18–98 years of age. Among them were 16 patients with Alzheimer's dementia; 97 patients displayed severe vascular symptoms like stroke, myocardial infarction, severe peripheral arterial occlusions, coronary heart diseases, and other vascular risk factors. Out of these 97 patients, 56 were cognitively unimpaired, while a possible or probable vascular dementia was diagnosed in 41 cases. The estimation of telomere length revealed that none of the patients with vascular dementia had telomeres longer than the age-dependent average of the healthy study participants. The average telomere length in the vascular dementia group was about 400 bp shorter than in the control group.[2] This difference was highly significant ($P<0.001$), while telomere lengths in stroke or infarct patients without cognitive decline and in Alzheimer's patients were not significantly different from controls.

In our patients, there was no correlation between dementia and presence of the ApoEe4 allele or gluthation-S-transferase polymorphisms. So the conclusion is that the correlation between short telomeres in blood lymphocytes and vascular dementia is much more robust than that of established genetic risk markers for dementia. Telomere length might actually be a prognostic factor for vascular dementia. Oxidative stress and insufficient antioxidative defence is most probably an important pathogenetic factor for vascular as well as so-called mixed dementias.[35] The interesting question now is whether our *in vitro* data, which define telomere length as a marker for antioxidative defence capacity, can be confirmed *in vivo*. Experiments are in progress to test this suggestion.

REFERENCES

1. HAYFLICK, L. 1965. The limited in vitro lifetime of human diploid cell strains. Exp. Cell Res. **37:** 614–636.
2. VON ZGLINICKI, T., *et al.* 1995. Mild hyperoxia shortens telomeres and inhibits proliferation of fibroblasts: a model for senescence? Exp. Cell Res. **220:** 186–193.
3. TOUSSAINT, O., *et al.* 2000. Cellular and molecular mechanisms of stress-induced premature senescence (SIPS) of human diploid fibroblasts and melanocytes. Exp. Gerontol. **35:**927–945.
4. HARLEY, C.B., *et al.* 1990. Telomeres shorten during ageing of human fibroblasts. Nature **345:** 458–460.
5. VON ZGLINICKI, T., *et al.* 2000. Short telomeres in patients with vascular dementia: an indicator of low antioxidative capacity and a possible risk factor? Lab. Invest. **80:** 1739–1747.
6. MAKAROV, V.L., *et al.* 1997. Long G tails at both ends of human chromosomes suggest a C strand degradation mechanism for telomere shortening. Cell **88:** 657–666.
7. WRIGTH, W.E., *et al.* 1997. Normal human chromosomes have long G-rich telomeric overhangs at one end. Genes & Dev. **11:** 2801–2809.
8. HARLEY, C.B. 1991. Telomere loss: mitotic clock or time bomb? Mutat. Res. **256:** 271–282.
9. ALLSOPP, R.C., *et al.* 1995. Evidence for a critical telomere length in senescent human fibroblasts. Exp. Cell Res. **219:** 130–136.
10. BODNAR, A.G., *et al.* 1998. Extension of life-span by introduction of telomerase into normal human cells. Science **279:** 349–352.
11. JIANG, X.-R. 1999. Telomerase expression in human somatic cells does not induce changes associated with a transformed phenotype. Nat. Genet. **21:** 111–114.
12. LORENZ, M., *et al.* 2001. BJ fibroblasts display slow telomere shortening independent of hTERT transfection due to high antioxidant capacity. Free Radic. Biol. Med. **31:** 824–831.
13. SARETZKI, G., *et al.* 1998. Similar gene expression pattern in senescent and hyperoxic treated fibroblasts. J. Gerontol. A Biol. Sci. Med. Sci. **53A/6:** B438–B442.
14. VON ZGLINICKI, T., *et al.* 2000. Accumulation of single-strand breaks is the major cause of telomere shortening in human fibroblasts. Free Radic. Biol. Med. **28:** 64–74.
15. PETERSEN, S., *et al.* 1998. Preferential accumulation of single-stranded regions in telomeres of human fibroblasts. Exp. Cell Res. **239:** 152–160.

16. SITTE, N., et al. 1998. Accelerated telomere shortening in fibroblasts after extended periods of confluency. Free Radic. Biol. Med. **24:** 885–893.
17. VON ZGLINICKI, T. 2000. Role of oxidative stress in telomere length regulation and replicative senescence. Ann. N.Y. Acad. Sci. **908:** 99–110.
18. HUFFMANN, K.E. 2000. Telomere shortening is proportional to the size of the G-rich telomeric 3′-overhang. J. Biol. Chem. **275:** 19719–19722.
19. GRIFFITH, J.D., et al. 1999. Mammalian telomeres end in a large duplex loop. Cell **97:** 503–514.
20. SMOGORZEWA, A., et al. 2000. Control of human telomere length by TRF1 and TRF2. Mol. Cell. Biol. **20:** 1659–1668.
21. BAUMANN, P., et al. 2001. Po1, the putative telomere end-binding protein in fission yeast and humans. Science **292:** 1171–1175.
22. SARETZKI, G., et al. 1999. Telomere shortening triggers a p53-dependent cell cycle arrest via accumulation of G-rich single stranded DNA fragments. Oncogene **18:** 5148–5158.
23. BLACKBURN, E.H. 2000. Telomere states and cell fates. Nature **408:** 53–56.
24. LUDWIG, A., et al. 2001. Ribozyme cleavage of telomerase mRNA sensitizes breast tumor cells to inhibitors of topoisomerase. Cancer Res. **61:** 3053–3061.
25. SARETZKI, G., et al. 2001. Ribozyme-mediated telomerase inhibition induces immediate cell loss but not telomere shortening in ovarian cancer cells. Cancer Gene Ther. **8:** 827–834.
26. RUFER, N., et al. 1999. Telomere fluorescence measurements in granulocytes and T lymphocyte subsets point to a high turnover of hematopoetic stem cells and memory T cells in early childhood. J. Exp. Med. **190:** 157–167.
27. SLAGBOOM, P., et al. 1994. Genetic determination of telomere size in humans: a twin study of three age groups. Am. J. Hum. Genet. **55:** 876–882.
28. SERRA, V., et al. 2000. Telomere length as a marker of oxidative stress in primary human fibroblast cultures. Ann. N.Y. Acad. Sci. **908:** 327–330.
29. OEXLE, K., et al. 1997. Advanced telomere shortening in respiratory chain disorders. Hum. Mol. Genet. **6:** 905–908.
30. VAZIRI, H., et al. 1993. Loss of telomeric DNA during ageing of normal and trisomie 21 human lymphocytes. Am. J. Hum. Genet. **52:** 876–882.
31. FRIEDRICH, U., et al. 2000. Telomere length in different tissues of elderly patients. Mech. Ageing Dev. **119:** 89–99.
32. WYLLIE, F.S., et al. 2000. Telomerase prevents the accelerated cell ageing of Werner syndrome fibroblasts. Nat. Genet. **24:** 16–17.
33. CHANG, E., et al. 1995. Telomere length and replicative aging in human vascular tissues. Proc. Natl. Acad. Sci. USA **92:** 11190–11194.
34. PRESCOTT, J.C., et al. 1999. Telomerase: Dr. Jekyll and Mr. Hyde? Curr. Opin. Genet. Dev. **9:** 368–373.
35. FOY, C.J., et al. 1999. Plasma chain-breaking antioxidants in Alzheimer's disease, vascular dementia and Parkinson's disease. Q.J.M. **92:** 39–45.

Are Changes of the Cell Membrane Structure Causally Involved in the Aging Process?

GERHARD SPITELLER

Organische Chemie, Universität Bayreuth,
Universitätsstraße 30, 95440 Bayreuth, Germany

ABSTRACT: Lipid peroxidation is recognized by proliferation, wounding, and aging. The connecting link between these different events is a change in cell wall structure, which activates membrane bound phospholipases. These cleave phospholipids. Thus liberated polyunsaturated fatty acids (PUFAs) are substrates for lipoxygenases, which accept equally well linoleic acid and arachidonic acid and generate lipid hydroperoxides (LOOHs). If the amount of free PUFAs exceeds a certain amount, lipoxygenases commit suicide. The consequence is liberation of free iron ions that react with LOOHs by formation of radicals. These start a chain reaction. LOO• radicals produced in the course of this process attack proteins, nucleic acids, and also double bonds of all unsaturated compounds by epoxidation. Morever LOOHs are decomposed to toxic epoxy acids and $\alpha,\beta,\gamma,\delta$-unsaturated aldehydes. Both species react with glutathione. The resulting products seem to induce apoptosis. Since the products generated by wounding or aging are formed by decomposition of LOOHs the investigation of the aging processes can be simplified by studying the physiological action of artificially generated lipid peroxidation products derived from pure PUFAs. Degradation products of LOOHs are generated by thermal decompositon of fat-containing PUFAs. These products are induced into the body by adsorption in the intestine. They are at least partly incorporated in low density lipoproteins (LDLs). Primarily investigations seem to indicate that an overload of a diet rich in PUFAs induces only after two days an increase in oxidized LDL/PUFAs for a factor up to two in young people and for a factor of more than two in old individuals.

KEYWORDS: aging; lipid peroxidation; linoleic acid; atherosclerosis

INTRODUCTION

Aging is not only controlled by genetic disposition[1] but also by nutritive habits: in many experiments it was recognized that caloric reduction of about 40% increases the mean life span of animals by 25–30%. Furthermore many investigations suggest that aging is associated with an increase of oxidation products derived from nucleic acids,[2] proteins,[3] and fatty acids.[4]

Address for correspondence: Gerhard Spiteller, Organische Chemie, Universität Bayreuth, Universitätsstraße 30, 95440 Bayreuth, Germany. Voice: +49-921-552675; fax: +49-921-552671.
Gerhard.Spiteller@uni-bayreuth.de

SUPEROXIDE—THE SINGLE SOURCE OF OXIDATION?

These oxidation processes are seen as the consequence of "mitochondrial leakage":[5] mitochondria transform oxygen to water in a four-step electron transfer reaction. It was postulated that after the first electron transfer reaction the generated superoxide anion $O_2^{\bullet-}$ is able to escape from the complex prior to further electron uptake. $O_2^{\bullet-}$ reacts with water to become an $OH_2^{\bullet}$ radical, which is disproportionate to H_2O_2 and oxygen. H_2O_2 reacts in a Fenton reaction (SCHEME 1) to $OH^{\bullet}$ radicals. These are able to abstract hydrogen atoms from all types of molecules, for example, polyunsaturated fatty acids, proteins, and nucleic bases, and activate them to react with oxygen.

$$O_2 \xrightarrow{+e} O_2^{\bullet \ominus}$$

$$O_2^{\bullet \ominus} + H_2O \longrightarrow HO_2^{\bullet} + OH^{\ominus}$$

$$HO_2^{\bullet} + HO_2^{\bullet} \xrightarrow{SOD} H_2O_2 + O_2$$

$$HO-OH + Fe^{2+} \longrightarrow OH^{\ominus} + OH^{\bullet} + Fe^{3+}$$

SCHEME 1. Generation of $OH^{\bullet}$ radicals.

Superoxide anions are not chiral, nor are the other derived reactive oxygen species (ROS). Nonchiral products cannot produce chiral derivatives. Nevertheless chiral products are obtained from polyunsaturated fatty acids (PUFAs): PUFAs are oxidized first to lipid hydroperoxides (LOOHs); these are reduced by peroxidases to corresponding hydroxy acids (LOH) (SCHEME 2).

During the reduction the bond between carbon and oxygen is not involved; therefore no change at the chiral center is possible. Investigation of isolated hydroxy acids, derived from PUFAs were carried out by two independent groups in the United States[6] and in Germany.[7] They recognized a preponderance of the S isomers in atherosclerotic tissue samples. Thus at least a part of the LOOHs cannot be generated by superoxide anions and by leakage of mitochodria but by action of enzymes. As a consequence the first step in radical generation needs a reinterpretation.

INVOLVEMENT OF LIPOXYGENASES IN THE GENERATION OF LIPID HYDROPEROXIDES

Chiral LOOHs are generated in the body by the activation of lipoxygenases (LOX). With the exception of the 15-LOX all LOX require free PUFAs as substrates.[8] Free fatty acids are usually not present in healthy cells, but large amounts of fatty acids are in the cell wall in phospholipid form. When the cell wall is stimulated,[9] A2 phopholipases are activated. These phospholipases cleave the phospholipids exclusively in position 2 of the glycerol backbone where mainly PUFAs are

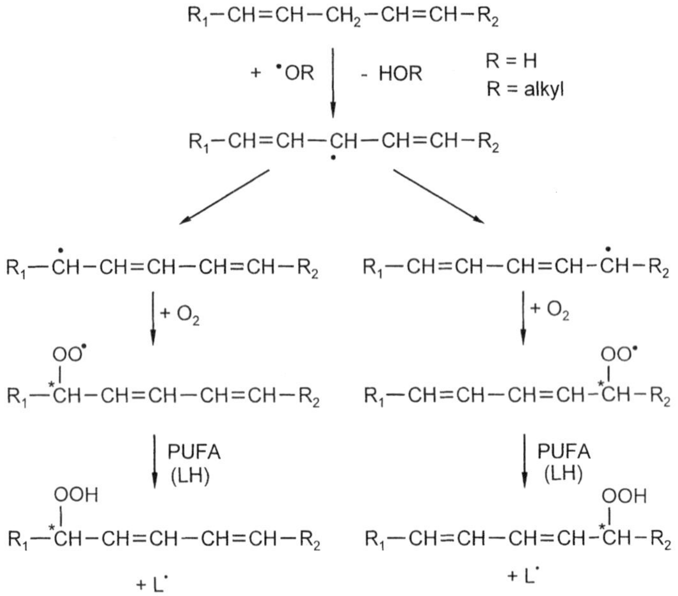

$$R_1-CH=CH-CH_2-CH=CH-R_2$$

$$+ \cdot OR \quad | \quad - HOR \qquad \begin{array}{l} R = H \\ R = alkyl \end{array}$$

$$R_1-CH=CH-\overset{\cdot}{C}H-CH=CH-R_2$$

$$R_1-\overset{\cdot}{C}H-CH=CH-CH=CH-R_2 \qquad R_1-CH=CH-CH=CH-\overset{\cdot}{C}H-R_2$$

$$\downarrow + O_2 \qquad\qquad\qquad \downarrow + O_2$$

$$\begin{array}{c} OO^{\cdot} \\ | \\ R_1-\overset{*}{C}H-CH=CH-CH=CH-R_2 \end{array} \qquad \begin{array}{c} OO^{\cdot} \\ | \\ R_1-CH=CH-CH=CH-\overset{*}{C}H-R_2 \end{array}$$

$$\downarrow \begin{array}{c} PUFA \\ (LH) \end{array} \qquad\qquad \downarrow \begin{array}{c} PUFA \\ (LH) \end{array}$$

$$\begin{array}{c} OOH \\ | \\ R_1-\overset{*}{C}H-CH=CH-CH=CH-R_2 \end{array} \qquad \begin{array}{c} OOH \\ | \\ R_1-CH=CH-CH=CH-\overset{*}{C}H-R_2 \end{array}$$

$$+ L^{\cdot} \qquad\qquad\qquad + L^{\cdot}$$

SCHEME 2. Generation of lipid hydroperoxides by radicals, for example, of OH• by hydrogen abstraction from a PUFA.

located.[10] These reactions are well known and well investigated initiating steps in the generation of leukotrienes, which are obtained by lipid peroxidation (LPO) of arachidonic acid.

STIMULATION OF MAMMALIAN AND PLANT CELLS CAUSE A SIMILAR RESPONSE: LIPID PEROXIDATION

Similar processes are reported from plants: stimulation of plant cells, for instance, by an attacking microorganism or an insect causes generation of jasmonic acid,[11] formed by cleavage of phospholipids followed by LPO of linolenic acid: plants contain linolenic acid instead of arachidonic acid. The similarity in the response of plant and mammalian cells to stimulation from outside has been recognized for about 10 years by plant chemists.[12,13] The similarities in the responses of plant and human cells to stimulation is further corroborated by the observation that both cell types respond equally to wounding: when plant or mammalian cells are homogenized—a severe type of wounding—large amounts of lipid peroxidation products are generated.[14-16]

Linolenic acid is exclusively generated in plant cells, whereas arachidonic acid is exclusively generated in mammalian cells. The precursor molecule of both acids is linoleic acid; enzymes in plants dehydrate linoleic acid in the direction to the alkyl residue, while in mammals, enzymes enlarge the fatty acid first for a two carbon unit and dehydrate it later in the reverse direction. Linoleic acid is the most abundant

PUFA in mammals and also in many plants. It is equally well susceptible to LPO by LOX as linolenic acid and arachidonic acid. Therefore any cell stimulation or any cell wounding, for instance, by homogenation of tissue in aqueous solution, generates LOOHs of all PUFAs, not only of arachidonic acid, as previously tacitly assumed.

Activation of lipases and LOX is not restricted to wounding or aging of cells: increased amounts of LPO products have been described also after induction of proliferation processes, for instance, in germinating cereals.[17]

IS A CHANGE IN CELL MEMBRANE STRUCTURE THE CAUSE OF LIPID PEROXIDATION?

Thus increased amounts of LPO products are formed in three different processes: by cell proliferation, cell injury, and aging. These three different processes seem to have a common link, the change in cell membrane structure.[18] The cell membrane is certainly involved by wounding, but also by shrinking in aging processes, and it is enlarged by proliferation. The membrane consists of a fatty phospholipid layer. The surface of a fat is influenced by contact with surfactants, and therefore compounds that act as surfactants, for instance proteins, change the cell wall structure. Phospholipases, incorporated in the cell wall, react in response to this change apparently by liberation of fatty acids. Thus the cell becomes acidic, and probably this causes the influx of Ca^{2+} ions. Ca^{2+} ions, together with adenosine cyclase, also activated by changes in the cell membrane structure, activate then cytosolic enzymes, for instance LOX. So far the processes are still physiological; enzymatic degradation of LOOHs probably generates signaling compounds that induce reinforcement of cell walls.

THE CHANGE FROM ENZYMATIC TO NONENZYMATIC LIPID PEROXIDATION

When the supply of substrate surmounts a certain level, for instance, caused by severe impact from outside, for example, by wounding or if the oxygen supply is too low[20] (infarction), LOX commit suicide. LOX have an iron ion in their active center. This iron ion is liberated by suicide. Iron ions react with LOOH—originally produced by LOX—and start a nonenzymatic LPO. The latter reaction differs from the enzymatic one in several crucial respects (SCHEME 3).

In an enzymatic LPO reaction, first iron ions that occur in the nonactivated enzyme in Fe^{2+} form are transformed to Fe^{3+}. In this form the enzyme reacts with a PUFA by removal of a hydrogen atom from a double allylically activated CH_2 group, transforming it by uptake of its electron to a proton. Thus Fe^{2+} ions are regenerated. In a following step the formed lipid radical (L•) reacts with oxygen to a peroxylradical (LOO•) in a regio- and stereospecific reaction. The generated LOO• radical is finally transformed within the enzyme by transfer of an electron from Fe^{2+} to a LOO⁻ anion, which combines with a proton.[19] The thus formed Fe^{3+} is then ready to undergo the next cycle if the substrate is still available.

By contrast, in a nonenzymatic reaction, Fe^{2+} ions generated by suicide of lipoxygenases[7,20] cleave formed LOOHs in a similar manner to H_2O_2 in a Fenton

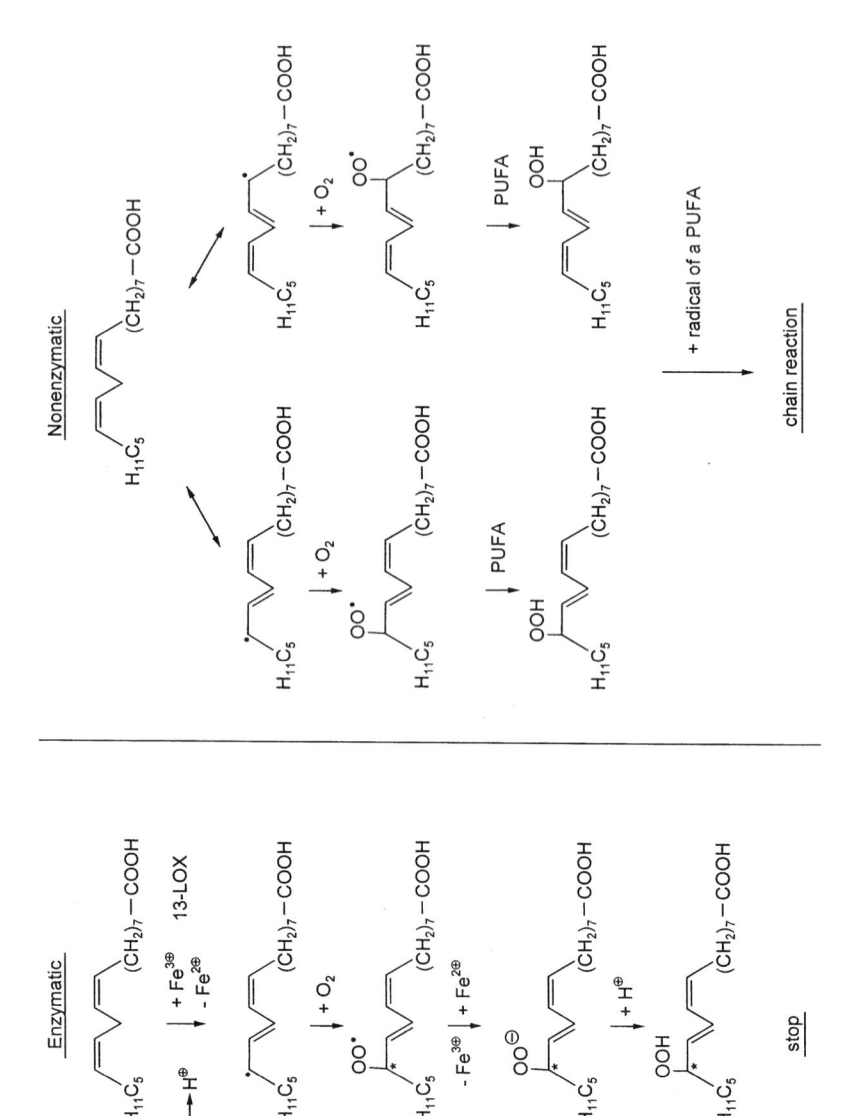

SCHEME 3. Comparison of the events occurring in enzymatic and nonenzymatic LPO processes.

reaction to alkoxylradicals (LO•). These LO• are only slightly less reactive than hydroxyl radicals. Therefore they react similarily to OH• by hydrogen abstraction from a double allylically activated CH_2 group. In contrast to enzymes, radicals recognize only the structural element $-CH=CH-CH_2-CH=CH-$. Thus they attack not only free PUFAs but also the $-CH=CH-CH_2-CH=CH-$ groups in phospholipids or PUFAs bound in the form of cholesterol esters. In contrast to enzymes, they do not produce a single stereospecific hydroperoxide. Each double allylically activated CH_2 group causes generation of two regioisomeric LOOHs, and these are split off in two enantiomeric products. The consequence is a mixture of isomeric products. Their number increases considerably with an increasing number of double allylically activated CH_2 groups. Therefore the number of isomeric LOOHs that are generated by nonenzymatic LPO of arachidonic acid is much larger than the number of isomers obtained from linoleic acid, which has only one double allylically activated CH_2 group.

The generated L• react with oxygen to LOO• like the radicals formed in LOX, but this LOO• lacks the possibility for transformation to an anion LOO⁻. Therefore LOO• have to abstract hydrogen from somewhere, usually from another PUFA, thus starting a chain reaction. This is the most serious difference between an enzymatic and a nonenzymatic induced LPO process.

Mitochondria must be stimulated to generate superoxide. The stimulating reagent, for instance, an antibiotic, behaves like a surfactant. Since the cell walls of mitochondria consist of layers of phospholipids, the membrane structure is changed, and this might induce an LPO reaction. Thus it is assumed that superoxide generation might be the consequence of a preceding LPO.

DECOMPOSITION OF LIPID HYDROPEROXIDES

LOOHs are rather unstable. They are reduced quickly in biological surroundings by peroxidases to corresponding LOHs.[21] Nevertheless in the presence of bivalent metal ions obtained by suicide of LOX, the generated LO• radicals may be sometimes too far away to generate LOOH by hydrogen abstraction from another PUFA. Thus they stabilize in a different way.

The most common stabilization reaction is the production of an epoxide with an adjacent double bond; the formed radical may take up another oxygen to form a LOO• radical, which then removes a hydrogen atom from another PUFA. The resulting new hydroperoxide is then transformed by reduction to an epoxyhydroxy acid (SCHEME 4). Alternatively the primarily generated alkoxyradicals may decompose by cleavage of the adjacent bond to generate $\alpha,\beta,\gamma,\delta$-unsaturated aldehydes (SCHEME 5). These decompose further in retroaldol reactions to smaller aldehydic compounds.

ARTIFICIAL GENERATION OF LIPID HYDROPEROXIDES

The number of LPO products formed by LPO processes is rather low compared to other compounds in tissue. The low number of LPO products formed in physiological processes (aging) is enhanced considerably by homogenation of tissue. This procedure can be even much more facilitated if the action of iron ions on pure hy-

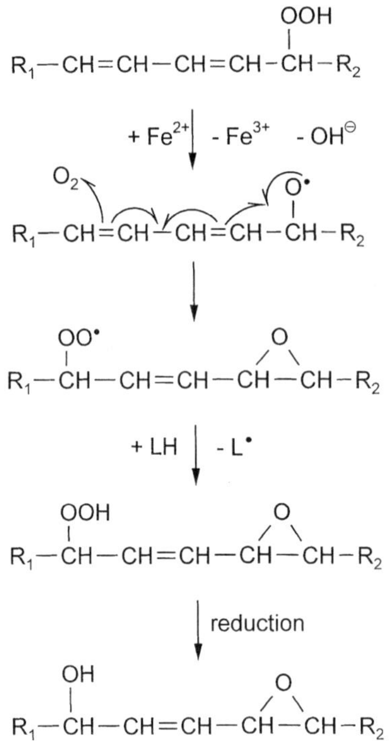

SCHEME 4. Generation of epoxyhydroxy acids from alkoxy radicals.

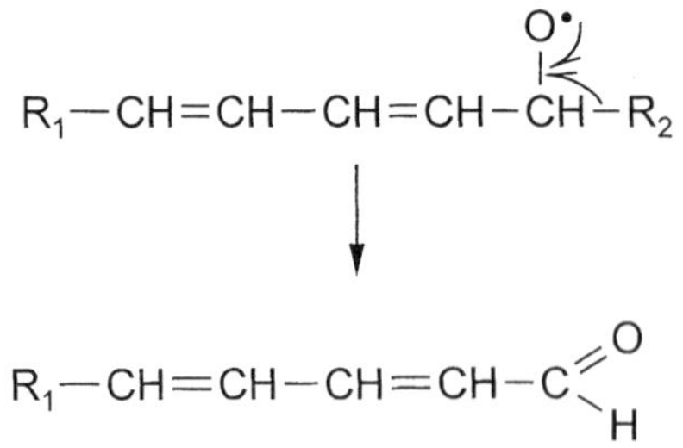

SCHEME 5. Generation of α,β,γ,δ-unsaturated aldehydes from alkoxy radicals.

droperoxides (derived by LPO of PUFAs) is studied (FIG. 1). The product spectrum (FIG. 1) allows identification of the main products that are necessary to elucidate the main degradation processes.[22] These reactions were investigated a long time ago by food chemists[23,24] who were interested in the process of rancidity, a natural or artificial induced LPO reaction.

The best method for identification of compounds was found to be a gas chromatographic separation of samples after appropriate derivatization—methylation of acids, followed by trimethylsilylation of hydroxy groups. Compound identification is then achieved by mass spectrometry.

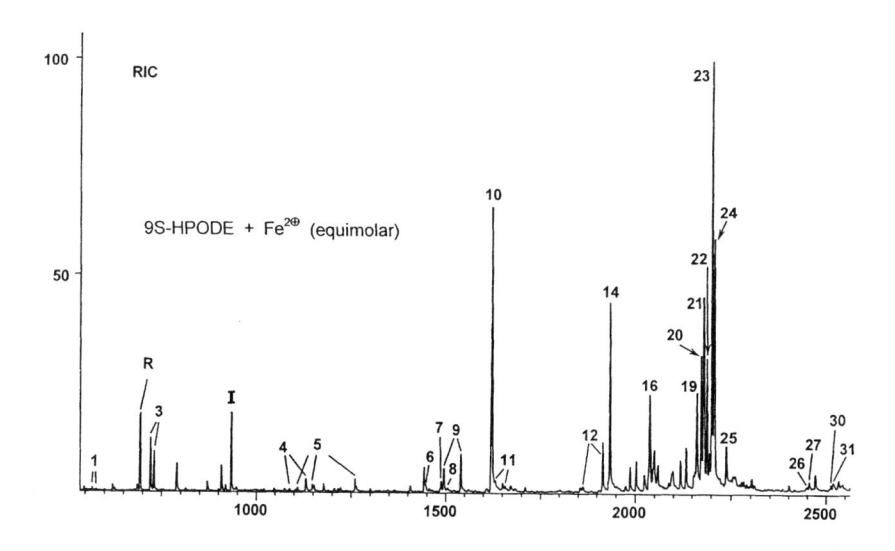

#		#	
1	H$_3$C-(CH$_2$)$_3$-CHO	16	H$_{11}$C$_5$—CH=CH—CH(OH)—CH—CH—(CH$_2$)$_7$—COOH (with epoxide O)
2	H$_{11}$C$_5$-CH(OH)-CH=CH-COOH	17	OHC-CH(OH)-CH=CH-(CH$_2$)$_7$-COOH
3	C$_5$H$_{11}$-CHO	18	H$_{11}$C$_5$-CO-CH=CH-CHO
4	H$_{11}$C$_5$-CH(OH)-CHO	19	H$_9$C$_4$-CH(OH)-(CH=CH)$_2$-CH(OH)-(CH$_2$)$_7$-COOH
5	H$_{11}$C$_5$-CH=CH-CHO	*	
6	OHC-CHO	20	H$_{11}$C$_5$-CH(OH)-CH=CH-[CH(OH)]$_2$-(CH$_2$)$_7$-COOH
7	HOOC-(CH$_2$)$_6$-CHO	21	H$_{11}$C$_5$-[CH(OH)]$_2$-CH=CH-CH(OH)-(CH$_2$)$_7$-COOH
8	H$_{11}$C$_5$-(CH=CH)$_2$-CHO	22	H$_{11}$C$_5$-[CH(OH)]$_2$-CH=CH-CH(OH)-(CH$_2$)$_7$-COOH
9	H$_{11}$C$_5$-CH(OH)-CH=CH-CHO	23	H$_{11}$C$_5$-CH(OH)-CH=CH-[CH(OH)]$_2$-(CH$_2$)$_7$-COOH
10	HOOC-(CH$_2$)$_7$-CHO	24	H$_{11}$C$_5$-CH(OH)-CH=CH-[CH(OH)]$_2$-(CH$_2$)$_7$-COOH
11	H$_{11}$C$_5$—CH—CH—CH=CH—CHO (with epoxide O)	25	OHC-CH=CH-CH(OH)-(CH$_2$)$_7$-COOH
12	OHC-CH(OH)-(CH$_2$)$_7$-COOH	26	H$_{11}$C$_5$-(CH=CH)$_2$-CO-(CH$_2$)$_7$-COOH
13	H$_{11}$C$_5$-CH(OH)-(CH=CH)$_2$-(CH$_2$)$_7$-COOH	27	H$_{11}$C$_5$-(CH=CH)$_2$-CO-(CH$_2$)$_7$-COOH
		28	H$_{11}$C$_5$-CO-(CH=CH)$_2$-(CH$_2$)$_7$-COOH
14	H$_{11}$C$_5$-(CH=CH)$_2$-CH(OH)-(CH$_2$)$_7$-COOH	29	H$_{11}$C$_5$-CO-(CH=CH)$_2$-(CH$_2$)$_7$-COOH
15	H$_{11}$C$_5$—CH—CH—CH(OH)—CH=CH—(CH$_2$)$_7$—COOH (with epoxide O)	30	H$_{11}$C$_5$-CH(OH)-CH=CH-CH$_2$-CO-(CH$_2$)$_7$-COOH
		31	H$_{11}$C$_5$-CH(OH)-CH=CH-CH$_2$-CO-(CH$_2$)$_7$-COOH
		I	Impurity

FIGURE 1. GC of appropriately derivatized LPO products obtained by artificial oxidation of linoleic acid, according to Spiteller.[22]

PRODUCTS DERIVED BY DECOMPOSITION OF LIPID HYDROPEROXIDES INDUCE APOPTOSIS

Comparison of product chromatograms of artificial oxidized pure linoleic acid and those obtained from biological material reveals that the main oxidation products are identical, with one exception: in biological samples unsaturated epoxyhydroxy acids and unsaturated aldehydes are much less abundant. It turned out that these compounds react easily with nucleophilic reagents, especially thiols. Such compounds are abundant in biological material in glutathione form. Therefore we suspect that the deficiency in epoxyhydroxy acids and unsaturated aldehydes in

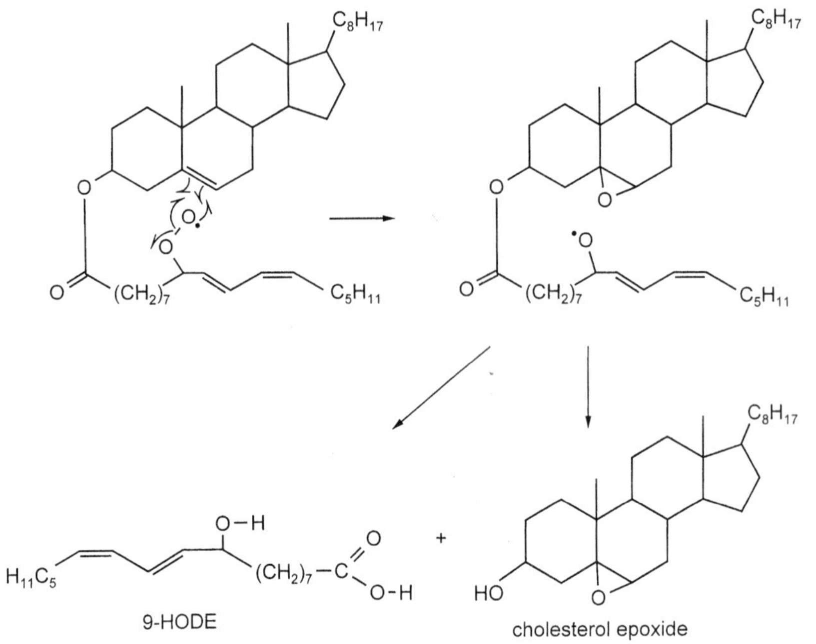

SCHEME 6. Generation of cholesterol epoxide from peroxidized cholesterol linoleate.

biological material is caused by further reactions. These compounds may develop physiological activity, given that leukotriene is the slow reacting factor of anaphylaxis and that α,β-unsaturated aldehydes were found to be highly toxic.[25] In this connection it might be of interest to mention the recent detection that 2,4-decadienal causes apoptosis.[26] The reduction products of the hydroperoxides derived from linoleic acid, 9-hydroxy-10,12-octadecadienoic acid (9-HODE) and 13-hydroxy-9,11-octadecadienoic acid (13-HODE), are also physiologically active: they induce cell differentiation,[27] for instance, the conversion of neutrophiles to macrophages, and induce the generation of cytokines, for instance, 1β-interleukin.[28]

PEROXYL RADICALS INDUCE EPOXIDATION AND OXIDATION OF PROTEINS AND NUCLEIC ACIDS

The action of LOO• radicals is not restricted to hydrogen abstraction from other molecules: LOO• radicals are well-known reagents in organic chemistry for epoxidation of double bonds. Such reactions are probably responsible for the the epoxidation of cholesterol: if in a nonenzymatic reaction cholesterol linoleate, the main compound in the low density lipoprotein, reacts with a radical, peroxyl radicals are generated that attack in an intramolecular reaction, the cholesterol moiety forming an epoxide[29] (SCHEME 6). Likewise other unsaturated acids, including PUFAs, are epoxidized (SCHEME 7).

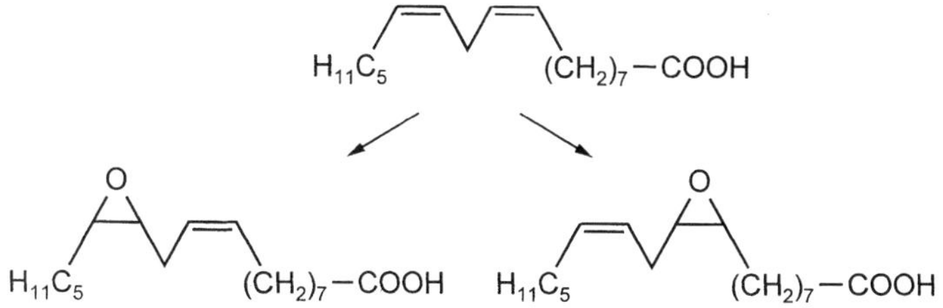

SCHEME 7. Generation of leukotoxines.

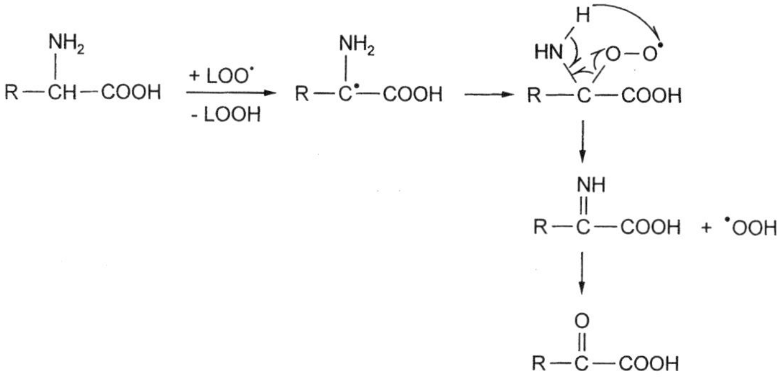

SCHEME 8. Generation of 2-oxo acids from α-amino acids.

These compounds have been detected in tissue after a myocardial infarction,[30] and after burn injury[31] they were found to be highly toxic, probably due to their ability to react with nucleophiles, for example, glutathione. Moreover LOO• radicals are able to remove hydrogens not only from PUFAs but also from secondary alcohols or amines (SCHEME 8) or nucleic acids with an imidazole residue. When these compounds react with LOO• radicals they are transformed to carbonyl groups, explaining the enrichment of oxidized proteins and nucleic acids in aged tissue.

In a similar way peroxyl radicals are able to oxidize amino acids and amino groups of lysyl residues. It seems that formation of LOX and LOO• radicals is not a late step but is in fact the initiating event for oxidation of all other compounds. Certainly proteins and nucleic acids are as sensitive or even more sensitive than PUFAs to oxidation by a reagent added from outside, but these oxidizing agents are not present in healthy tissue. By contrast, lipid LOO• radicals are generated in the moment when LOX commit suicide, and this does not require the presence of an oxidizing agent except oxygen.

TRAPPING OF LIPID HYDROPEROXYL RADICALS BY PHENOLIC COMPOUNDS

LOO• radicals react with all phenolic compounds (SCHEME 9) by preferential hydrogen removal. Long-living phenolic radicals tend to dimerize; the result is a con-

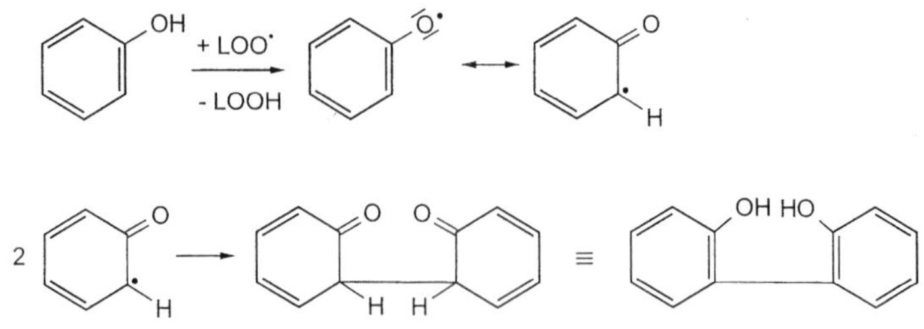

SCHEME 9. Phenolic radicals are removed by dimerization.

sumption of the radicals. Phenolic compounds are flavanoids, vitamin E, introduced with the nutrition, but also gluthathione and estrogens, synthetized in the body. These compounds react with radicals, but they are inactive against the enzymes that are liberated by cell injury, phospholipases, and lipoxygenases. Therefore the influence of drugs that prevent liberation of phospholipases and lipoxygenases, might help to retard the aging process.

MARKERS FOR LIPID PEROXIDATION PROCESSES

Many compounds are used as markers for LPO. The best markers seem to be those that are the most abundant ones. The quantity of a marker compound depends not only on how fast it is generated, but also how fast it suffers metabolism. In this respect LOOHs are not good markers because they are transformed very quickly to other compounds. Similarily, 4-hydroxynonenal is not well suited as a marker: it is generated only very late in the degradation cascade and suffers easily from further degradation. Isoprostanes are produced only from arachidonic acid in low yield; thus they are poor marker compounds, too. LOH and epoxyhydroxy acids are the most abundant degradation products of hydroperoxides. Epoxyhydroxy acids are degraded rapidly either by hydrolysis to trihydroxy compounds or attacked by nucleophiles (see above). Therefore the most useful markers seems to be the LOH. Nevertheless they suffer slow degradation. They are mainly degraded primarily by hydrogenation and not by oxidation, as might be assumed.[32] The ability to remove LOH by reduction decreases with increasing age. This might be an indication that with increasing age the amount of NADPH decreases. Thus the genetic equipment of NADPH producing enzymes and their impairment by influences of diet may be factors that are involved in the aging process.

LIPID HYDROPEROXIDES AND ATHEROSCLEROSIS

As already mentioned reduction of caloric intake influences considerably the average life span of animals. Considering that degradation products of hydroperoxides, especially polyunsaturated aldehydes and probably also epoxyhydroxy acids, apparently exert deleterious effects on cells, and that these products are generated by heating of fat containing PUFAs, we propose that the consumption of heated fat might induce cell destruction in the body. Fat is packed in the intestine in chylomicrones. These transport the fat into the bloodstream. In the bloodstream chylomicrones loose glycerolesters. The thus generated remnants are transformed in the liver to very low density lipoprotein (VLDL) and by further loss of gycerol esters to LDLs. LDLs consist of a core of cholesterol esters. The cholesterol is mainly bound to linoleic acid. The core is surrounded by a bilayer of phopholipids and a protein chain. The endothelial cells possess receptors that recognize the protein. The LDL molecule is then transferred together with its receptor by a process called endocytosis into the cell. There the receptor is separated and the LDL molecule is digested by hydrolysis of the protein to amino acids and the cholesterol esters to cholesterol and free fatty acids. This process is highly regulated.[33] By contrast, in atherosclerosis LDL molecules are partly "oxidized." Oxidized LDLs can be generated artificially by treatment with bivalent metal ions, for instance, copper ions.[34] This LDL is not longer recognized by the LDL receptor but by receptors of macrophages. The uptake of oxidized LDL is not longer regulated. The macrophages are filled with cholesterol esters and then are deposited in the form of plaque at the endothelial cell wall, and thus cause the phenomenon of atherosclerosis.

ARE THERE CONNECTIONS BETWEEN FAT CONSUMPTION AND ATHEROSCLEROSIS?

If oxidized fat is consumed it is incorporated as shown by Staprāns[35] and independently by Naruszewicz[36] in chylomicrons. Staprāns[37] detected that the oxidized fat is further transformed to VLDL. Oxidized fat appears in the VLDL only 8–12 hours after consumption. With this knowledge I and some friends consumed large amounts either of olive oil, known to be rich in oleic acid, and of sunflower oil, known to be rich in PUFAs. Blood withdrawn after 4-h time intervals was analyzed for hydroxyoctadecadienoic acids (HODEs) in the LDL fraction after appropriate derivatization. The investigation revealed that after two days the cholesterol level remained constant. The level of HODE increased dramatically in old individuals after consumption of sunflower oil and much less after consumption of olive oil. In young individuals only a moderate increase in HODE values was observed two days after consumption of food rich in olive oil. The increase after intake of sunflower oil was much higher, but only one half compared to old persons.

It must be emphasized that it is not easy to carry out such experiments: first, it is difficult to find students willing to fill up with fat-containing food; it is even more difficult to convince aged people to undergo such a treatment. Second the individual responses are different, dependent apparently on previous nutritional habits of the individual. Young people reach the climax of HODE values in LDL much faster than old people (about 12 to 16 hours after intake) and come back to normal levels after ending the experiment about 30 hours later. Old individuals reach much higher climaxes, and it lasts then a few days before the normal HODE level is reached again. This remaining level is in old individuals about 5 to 20 times higher than in young ones.

These observations were made with a small number of persons and deserve confirmation. Nevertheless the results seem reasonable: certainly LDL cholesterol is not involved *a priori* in oxidation.

LDL IS NOT OXIDIZED AT THE ENDOTHELIAL CELL WALL

In order to confirm that PUFAs can oxidize preferentially in LDL, we oxidized LDL artificially and investigated the obtained oxidized LDL for LPO products by comparing a sample before and after oxidation.[38] The oxidized sample showed all the oxidation products typical for oxidation of linoleic acid. Arachidonic acid oxidation products were detected, but in much reduced amounts compared to linoleic acid oxidation products, in agreement with the fact that the relationship of arachidonic acid to linoleic acid in LDL is 1:7. Thus this experiment revealed that in oxidized LDL linoleic acid oxidation products dominate, and not those of arachidonic acid. The same investigation was repeated with so called minimally oxidized LDL,[39] LDL that was just stored for some weeks. This LDL is known to be still accepted by the endothelial receptors. This minimally oxidized LDL showed an identical pattern of oxidation products,[38] compared to an artificially prepared oxidation sample. Therefore we must conclude that all the different linoleic acid oxidation products are transferred into the cell. This means that toxic products are able to pass the cell wall, and therefore they must be able to destruct the cell from inside.

Previously it was assumed that LDL is oxidized at the cell wall. This assumption was based on the observation that LDL is not oxidized if macrophages are added to LDL, but LDL suffers oxidation if macrophages together with endothelial cells are added. It was apparently overlooked in these experiments that the media in which the endothelial cells were grown usually contained traces of copper ions,[34] which induce LPO. Thus it seems that the age-dependent disease atherosclerosis is the result of the decreasing ability with age to remove oxidized PUFAs and their degradation products, but this ability seems to be also influenced by our nutritional habits: high fat consumption, which is increased by frying and other processes combined with heating.

CONCLUSION

Aging processes are connected to oxidation. They seem to be induced by changes in the structure of the cell membrane, which, in turn, induces enzymatic lipid peroxidation processes. When these switch to nonenzymatic LPO, LOO• radicals are generated. These attack proteins, sugars, and nucleic acid. Thus LPO is apparently located in the sequence of events before any other reaction, in contrast to previous assumptions.

ACKNOWLEDGMENTS

The experimental facts reported above were obtained by my collaborators: Dr. Andreas Batna, Dr. Angela Dudda, Dr. C. Fuchs, Dr. Wolfgang Jira, Dr. Michael Herold, Dr. Claus Hölzel, Dr. Uwe Kießling, Werner Kern, Dr. Christine Kraus, Dr. Rupert Kraus, Dr. Jochen Schmidt, Dr. Angelika Loidl-Stahlhofen, Dieter Spiteller (Dipl.-Chem.), and Dr. Peter Spiteller. I am very obliged to these collaborators for their help. I also appreciate the cooperation of Dr. K. Schubert (University Jena/Germany), Dr. J. Zapf (University Bayreuth/Germany), Dr. U. Pachmann (Blutspendedienst, Transfusionsmedizin Bayreuth/Germany), Dr. W. Carson, and Dr. A. Richter (Klinikum Bayreuth/Germany). I am obliged for financial support to Deutsche Forschungsgemeinschaft, Fonds der Chemischen Industrie, Schering AG (Berlin), and Fischer Stiftung (Kulmbach).

REFERENCES

1. VON ZGLINICKI, T. 1998. Telomeres: influencing the rate of aging. Ann. N.Y. Acad. Sci. **854:** 318–327.
2. YU, B.P. 1996. Aging and oxidative stress: modulation by dietary restriction. Free Radic. Biol. Med. **21:** 651–668.
3. HIRANO, T., Y. HOMMA & H. KASAI. 1995. Formation of 8-hydroxyguanine in DNA by aging and oxidative stress. Oxid. Stress Aging 69–76.
4. STADTMAN, E.R. & R.L. LEVINE. 2000. Protein oxidation. Ann. N.Y. Acad. Sci. **899:** 191–208.
5. SOHAL, R.S., H.-H. KU, S. AGARWAL, et al. 1994. Oxidative damage, mitochondrial oxidant generation and antioxidant defenses during aging and in response to food restriction in the mouse. Mech. Ageing Dev. **74:** 121–133.
6. FOLCIK, V.A., R.A. NIVAR-ARISTY, L.P. KRAJEWSKI & M.K. CATHCART. 1995. Lipoxygenase contributes to the oxidation of lipids in human atherosclerotic plaques. J. Clin. Invest. **96:** 504-510.
7. KÜHN, H., J. BELKNER, R. WIESNER, et al. 1992. Structure elucidation of oxygenated lipids in human atherosclerotic lesions. Eicosanoids **5:** 17-22.
8. YAMAMOTO, S. 1992. Mammalian lipoxygenases: molecular structures and functions. Biochim. Biophys. Acta **1128:** 117–131.
9. AARSMAN, A.J., H.B.M. LENTING, F.W. NEYS, et al. 1986. Some properties of membrane-bound phospholipases A2. NATO ASI Ser., Ser. A **116:** 139–143.
10. VONKEMAN, H. & D.A. VAN DORP. 1968. The action of prostaglandin synthetase on 2-arachidonyl lecithin. Biochim. Biophys. Acta **164:** 430–432.
11. SEMBDNER, G. & B. PARTHIER. 1993. The biochemistry and the physiological and molecular actions of jasmonates. Annu. Rev. Plant Physiol. Plant Mol. Biol. **44:** 569–589.
12. FARMER, E.E. & C.A. RYAN. 1992. Octadecanoid-derived signals in plants. Trends Cell Biol. **2:** 236–241.
13. MÜLLER, M.J., W. BRODSCHELM, E. SPANNAGL & M.H. ZENK. 1993. Signaling in the elicitation process is mediated through the octadecanoid pathway leading to jasmonic acid. Proc. Natl. Acad. Sci. USA **90:** 7490–7494.
14. WILLS, E.D. 1966. Mechanisms of lipid peroxide formation in animal tissues. Biochem. J. **99:** 667–676.
15. GALLIARD, T. 1975. Degradation of plant lipids by hydrolytic and oxidative enzymes. Annu. Proc. Phytochem. Soc. (Recent Adv. Chem. Biochem. Plant Lipids, Proc. Symp.) **12:** 319-357.
16. KIESSLING, U. & G. SPITELLER. 1998. The course of enzymatically induced lipid peroxidation in homogenized porcine kidney tissue. Z. Natforsch. Sect. C Biosci. **53:** 431–437.
17. FEUSSNER, I., T.J. BALKENHOHL, A. PORZEL, et al. 1997. Structural elucidation of oxygenated storage lipids in cucumber cotyledons. Implication of lipid body lipoxygenase in lipid mobilization during germination. J. Biol. Chem. **272:** 21635–21641.
18. SPITELLER, G. 2001. Peroxidation of linoleic acid and its relation to aging and age dependent diseases. Mech. Ageing Dev. **122:** 617–657.
19. DE GROOT, J.J.M.C., G.A. VELDINK, J.F.G. VLIEGENTHART, et al. 1975. Demonstration by EPR spectroscopy of the functional role of iron in soybean lipoxygenase-1. Biochim. Biophys. Acta **377:** 71–79.
20. FUCHS, C. & G. SPITELLER. 2000. Iron release from the active site of lipoxygenase. Z. Natforsch. Sect. C Biosci. **55:** 643–648.
21. WANG, T. & W.S. POWELL. 1991. Increased levels of monohydroxy metabolites of arachidonic acid and linoleic acid in LDL and aorta from atherosclerotic rabbits. Biochim. Biophys. Acta **1084:** 129–138.

22. SPITELLER, P., W. KERN, J. REINER & G. SPITELLER. 2001. Aldehydic lipid peroxidation products derived from linoleic acid. Biochim. Biophys. Acta **1531**: 188–208.
23. GARDNER, H.W. 1997. *In* Advances in Lipid Methodology Four. W.W. Christie, Ed.: 24-25. The Oil Press. Dundee.
24. FRANKEL, E.N. 1998. *In* Lipid Peroxidation. 187–248. The Oily Press. Dundee.
25. KANEKO, T., S. HONDA, S.I. NAKANO & M. MATSUO. 1987. Lethal effects of a linoleic acid hydroperoxide and its autoxidation products, unsaturated aliphatic aldehydes, on human diploid fibroblasts. Chem.-Biol. Interactions **63**: 127–137.
26. MIRALTO, A., G. BARONE, G. ROMANO, *et al.* 1999. The insidious effect of diatoms on copepod reproduction. Nature (Lond.) **402**: 173–176.
27. NAGY, L., P. TONTONOZ, J.G.A. ALVAREZ, *et al.* 1998. Oxidized LDL regulates macrophage gene expression through ligand activation of PPAR-γ. Cell **93**: 229–240.
28. THOMAS, C.E., R.L. JACKSON, D.F. OHLWEILER & G. KU. 1994. Multiple lipid oxidation products in low density lipoproteins induce interleukin-1 beta release from human blood mononuclear cells. J. Lipid Res. **35**: 417–427.
29. SPITELLER, G. 1998. Linoleic acid peroxidation—the dominant lipid peroxidation process in low density lipoprotein—and its relationship to chronic diseases. Chem. Phys. Lipids **95**: 105-162.
30. DUDDA, A., G. SPITELLER & F. KOBELT. 1996. Lipid oxidation products in ischemic porcine heart tissue. Chem. Phys. Lipids **82**: 39–51.
31. OZAWA, T., S. SUGIYAMA, M. HAYAKAWA & F. TAKI. 1988. Neutrophil microsomes biosynthesize linoleate epoxide (9,10-epoxy-12-octadecenoate), a biological active substance. Biochem. Biophys. Res. Commun. **152**: 1310–1318.
32. HECHT, S. & G. SPITELLER. 1998. Linoleic acid peroxidation products are metabolized by hydrogenation in porcine liver tissue. Eur. Mass Spectrom. **4**: 393–399.
33. GOLDSTEIN, J.L. & M. BROWN. 1977. The low density lipoprotein pathway and its relation to atherosclerosis. Annu. Rev. Biochem. **46**: 897–930.
34. STEINBRECHER, U.P., S. PARTHASARATHY, D.S. LEAKE, *et al.* 1984. Modification of low-density lipoprotein by endothelial cells involves lipid peroxidation and degradation of low-density lipoprotein phospholipids. Proc. Natl. Acad. Sci. USA **81**: 3883–3887.
35. STAPRĀNS, I., J.H. RAPP, X.-M. PAN, *et al.* 1994. Oxidized lipids in the diet are a source of oxidized lipid in chylomicrons of human serum. Arterioscler. Thromb. **14**: 1900–1905.
36. NARUSZEWICZ, M., E. WOZNY, E. MIRKIEWICZ, *et al.* 1987. The effect of thermally oxidized soybean oil on metabolism of chylomicrons. Increased uptake and degradation of oxidized chylomicrons in cultured mouse macrophages. Atherosclerosis **66**: 45–53.
37. STAPRĀNS, I., J.H. RAPP, X.-M. PAN, *et al.* 1996. Oxidized lipids in the diet are incorporated by the liver into very low density lipoprotein in rats. J. Lipid Res. **37**: 420-430.
38. SPITELLER, D. & G. SPITELLER. 2000. Oxidation of linoleic acid in low-density lipoprotein: an important event in atherogenesis. Angew. Chem., Int. Ed. **39**: 585–589.
39. BERLINER, J.A., M.C. TERRITO, A. SEVANIAN, *et al.* 1990. Minimally modified low density lipoprotein stimulates monocyte endothelial interactions. J. Clin. Invest. **85**: 1260–1266.

Down-regulation of Receptor-mediated Endocytosis Is Reponsible for Senescence-associated Hyporesponsiveness

SANG CHUL PARK, JEONG-SOO PARK, WOONG-YANG PARK, KYOUNG-A CHO, JEONG SOO AHN, AND IK SOON JANG

Department of Biochemistry and Molecular Biology,
Seoul National University College of Medicine, Seoul, South Korea

ABSTRACT: Human diploid fibroblasts (HDF) do not divide indefinitely and eventually lead to an arrest of cell division by a process termed cellular or replicative senescence. Irreversible growth arrest of senescent cells is strongly related to the attenuated response to growth factors. Recently, we reported that up-regulation of caveolin in the senescent cells is responsible for the attenuated response to growth factors. Senescent cells did not phosphorylate Erk-1/2 after EGF stimulation, whereas young cells did. In those senescent cells, we found an increased level of caveolin proteins and strong interactions between caveolin-1 and EGFR. When we overexpressed caveolin-1 in young HDF, the activation of Erk-1/2 on EGF stimulation was significantly suppressed. These results suggest that the hyporesponsiveness of senescent fibroblasts to EGF stimulation might be due to the overexpression of caveolin. In addition, the clathrin-dependent endocytosis system plays the more active and dominant role over the caveolae system. Therefore, we monitored the efficiency of clathrin-dependent receptor-mediated endocytosis in the senescent cells in order to elucidate the exact mode of the attenuated response to growth factors in the senescent cells. Using a transferrin-uptake assay and Western blot analysis of endocytosis-related proteins, we found a significant decrease of amphiphysin-1 in human diploid fibroblasts of multipassages. By adjusting the level of amphiphysin, we could modulate the efficiency of receptor-mediated endocytosis either in young or old cells toward growth factors: that is, a dominant negative mutant of amphiphysin-1 blocked the endocytosis in the young cells, while microinjection of the gene resumed its activity in the old cells. Taken together, we conclude that the loss of endocytotic activity of senescent cells is directly related to the down-regulation of amphiphysin-1 and/or up-regulation of caveolins. This opens a new field of functional recovery of the senescent cells simply through adjusting the receptor-mediated endocytosis capacity.

KEYWORDS: hyporesponsiveness; endocytosis; amphiphysin-1; caveolin

Address for correspondence: S.C. Park, Department of Biochemistry and Molecular Biology, Seoul National University College of Medicine, 28 Yongondong, Chongnogu, Seoul, 110-799, South Korea. Voice: +82-2-740-8244; fax: +82-2-744-4534.
scpark@snu.ac.kr

```
┌─────────────────────┐  ┌─────────────────────┐
│  Overexpression of  │  │   Down-regulation   │
│     Caveolins       │  │    of amphiphysin   │
└─────────────────────┘  └─────────────────────┘
              ↘              ↙
        ┌──────────────────────────────┐
        │   Loss of endocytotic activity│
        │  and reduced signal transduction│
        │      in the senescent cells   │
        └──────────────────────────────┘
                      ⇓
┌─────────────────────┐  ┌─────────────────────┐
│   Down-regulation   │  │  Induced expression │
│    of caveolins     │  │    of amphiphysin   │
└─────────────────────┘  └─────────────────────┘
              ↘              ↙
        ┌──────────────────────────────┐
        │ Functional recovery in endocytosis│
        │     and signal transduction   │
        │      in the senescent cells   │
        └──────────────────────────────┘
```

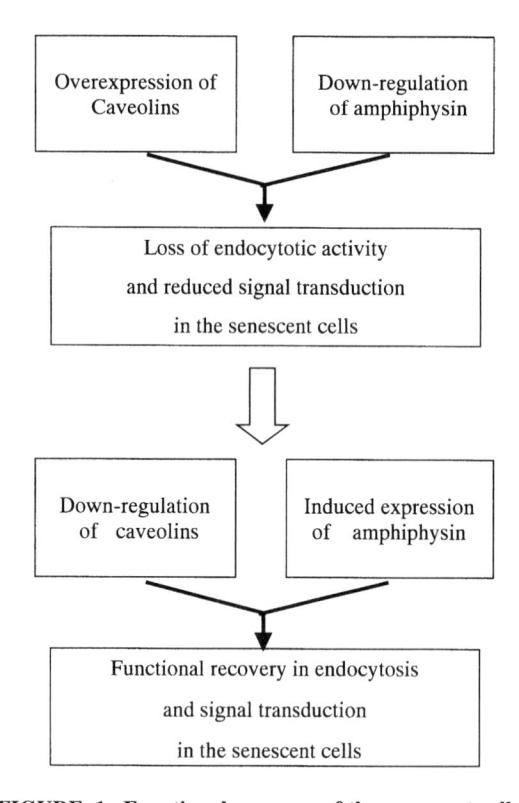

FIGURE 1. Functional recovery of the senescent cells.

The aging process accompanied by multiple functional deteriorations results in various age-related diseases. To overcome such diseases, it is primarily important to elucidate the basic mechanisms underlying functional deteriorations. Using a replicative senescence model of HDF that has long been used as an *in vitro* model for aging research,[1,2] we tried to identify the mechanism of senescence-related hyporesponsiveness toward growth factors. After a finite number of divisions, senescent cells do not grow or respond to growth factors or even to apoptotic stimuli such as UV or TNFα.[3,4]

UP-REGULATION OF CAVEOLIN AND HYPORESPONSIVENESS OF SENESCENT CELLS

Recently, we reported that up-regulation of caveolin in senescent cells is responsible for the attenuated response to growth factors through suppression of the downstream signal pathway.[5,24] Caveolae are vesicular invaginations of the plasma membrane with a diameter of 50–100 nm,[6,7] and they regulate signal transduction, potocytosis, and transcytosis.[8,9] Caveolin, a 21–24 kDa integral membrane protein, is a principal structural component of caveolae structures.[10] Caveolin functions as a scaffolding protein within the caveolae membrane and interacts with a variety of signaling proteins, namely EGFR (epidermal growth factor receptor), G proteins, Src-like kinases, H-Ras, PKC, eNOS, and integrin, which results in inactivation of downstream signaling.[11–16] We found that the old cells as well as the old tissues were enriched with caveolins.[5,24] Therefore, we tried to analyze the relationship of enriched caveolins with signaling systems in the old cells, especially for its hyporesponsiveness to growth factors. As an example, we examined the mode of Erk activation after EGF stimulation in the old cells. Interestingly, the attenuated responses in signaling behaviors were consistent with the expression of caveolins in senescent cells. To know the direct effect of caveolin in HDF, we overexpressed caveolin-1 in young HDF. The phosphorylation of Erk-1/2 upon HGF stimulation was significantly blocked by caveolin-1 expression in young HDF. Our results suggest strongly that the expression of caveolin and the consequent formation of caveolae might be responsible for the attenuation of EGF signaling in the aged cells.

ALTERATION OF CLATHRIN-DEPENDENT RECEPTOR-MEDIATED ENDOCYTOSIS IN SENESCENT CELLS

For the receptor-mediated endocytosis, the clathrin-dependent endocytosis system plays the more active and dominant role over the caveolae system. Therefore, it is necessary to monitor the efficiency of clathrin-dependent receptor-mediated endocytosis in the senescent cells. By use of the transferrin uptake model, illustrating functional efficacy of receptor-mediated endocytosis via clathrin-coated vesicle,[17] it was shown that the senescent HDF would not uptake transferrin readily in contrast to their presenescent counterparts. It suggests that efficacy of clathrin-dependent receptor-mediated endocytosis in the senescent cells was significantly deteriorated.

DOWN-REGULATION OF AMPHIPHYSIN-1 PROTEIN IN SENESCENT CELLS

The process of clathrin-dependent receptor-mediated endocytosis is composed of several steps, which include recruitment of the clathrin coats and fission of the coated buds.[18] After the receptor conjugation by ligand, such as EGF, receptor tyrosine kinase phosphorylates clathrin, which can provide a binding site for the Src-homology-3 (SH3) domain of amphiphysin.[19,20] Amphiphysin-1 is suggested to be involved in the recruitment and oligomerization at the neck of endocytotic buds. Amphiphysin-1 bridges the AP-2/clathrin coat and dynamin-1 to make an endosomal vesicle. The carboxy-terminal domain of amphiphysin recruits GTPase dynamin to pinch off the coated buds.[21,22] Disruption of the interaction of amphiphysin with either dynamin, clathrin, or AP-2 inhibits clathrin-mediated endocytosis. These findings indicate that amphiphysin may act as a regulation linker protein that couples clathrin-mediated budding of endocytotic vesicles to dynamin-mediated vesicle fission.

To identify the molecular mechanism for the reduced clathrin-dependent receptor-mediated endocytotic function of senescent cells, the expression level of several proteins associated with receptor-mediated endocytosis were compared among early-, middle-, and late-passaged fibroblasts. Interestingly, only amphiphysin-1, but none of the other endocytotic proteins tested, was significantly reduced during the cellular senescence. These results suggest that amphiphysin-1 may play a critical role in the alteration of receptor-mediated endocytosis of the senescent fibroblasts.

FUNCTIONAL RECOVERY OF RECEPTOR-MEDIATED ENDOCYTOSIS IN SENESCENT CELLS

To clarify the functional significance of the amphiphysin in receptor-mediated endocytosis, we checked the effect of the inhibition of amphiphysin-1 protein in presenescent cells. In order to inhibit the function of amphiphysin-1 protein, a dominant negative mutant of amphiphysin-1 that encoded the middle portion (amino acids 250–588) containing the AP-2 and clathrin binding sites was transfected into presenescent fibroblasts. Following transfection, cellular capacity to internalize the transferrin was monitored with rhodamine-conjugated transterrin. Those cells that overexpressed the dominant negative mutant of amphiphysin-1 protein could not uptake transferrin, in contrast to neighboring nontransfected cells. However, mock transfected cells revealed no functional alteration in uptake of transferrin. In this experiment, we clearly demonstrated that the functional incompetence of amphiphysin-1 could inhibit receptor-mediated endocytosis in human diploid fibroblasts. Moreover, we were interested in whether the microinjection of the amphiphysin-1 gene with cytomegalovirus (CMV) promoter could resume the endocytotic capacity in the senescent cells. The expression of amphiphysin-1 was detected in the injected cells by immunofluorescent staining against amphiphysin-1 as well as by coinjected markers, such as rabbit IgG. Those wild type amphiphysin-1 reconstituted-senescent cells were challenged with fluorescence-conjugated transferrin to check the clathrin-dependent receptor-mediated endocytosis activity. The endocytotic activity of senescent cells was sharply increased by introduction of amphiphysin-1 cDNA. These results suggest that supplementation of amphiphysin-1 is sufficient for the restoration of functional endocytosis of the senescent fibroblasts. The functional recovery of the transtferrin uptake in the senescent cells by simple microinjection of the amphiphysin-1 gene suggests the possibility of resuming receptor-mediated endocytotic activity in the senescent cells. The other aspects of the biological effects of amphiphysin-1 gene transfection on senescent cells should be studied in detail, such as, for example, the responsiveness to growth factors, cellular replicability, and extension of the *in vitro* life span of the senescent cells; these aspects are under study in our laboratory. Nonetheless, with the present data, the role of amphiphysin-1 in receptor-mediated endocytosis of the senescent cells has been clearly analyzed, and the possibility of the application of amphiphysin-1 for the functional recovery of the senescent cells, especially in relation to receptor-mediated endocytosis, has been suggested.

Taken together, we conclude that the loss of endocytotic activity of senescent cells is directly related to the down-regulation of amphiphysin-1 and up-regulation of caveolins, which suggests the strong possibility of opening a new field for functional recovery of the senescent cells, simply by adjusting the cellular level of those elements.

ACKNOWLEDGMENTS

This work was supported by the BK21 program of the Ministry of Education (to Dr. J.-S. Park and Ms. K.-A. Cho), the Ministry of Health and Welfare (to Dr. W.-Y. Park), and by KOSEF (to Dr. S.C. Park).

REFERENCES

1. HAYFLICK, L. & P. MOORHEAD. 1961. Exp. Cell Res. **25:** 585–621.
2. HAYFLICK, L. 1965. Exp. Cell Res. **37:** 614–636.
3. SESHADRI, T. & J. CAMPISI. 1990. Science **247:** 205–209.
4. RIABOWOL, K., J. SCHIFF & M.Z. GILMAN. 1992. Proc. Natl. Acad. Sci. USA **89:** 157–161.
5. PARK, W.Y., J.S. PARK, K.A. CHO, et al. 2000. J. Biol. Chem. **275:** 20847–20852.
6. SEVERS, N.J. 1988. J. Cell Sci. **90:** 341–348.
7. ANDERSON, R.G. 1993. Proc. Natl. Acad. Sci. USA **90:** 10909–10913.
8. ENGELMAN, J.A., C. CHU, A. LIN, et al. 1998. FEBS Lett. **428:** 205–211.
9. LISANTI, M.P., P.E. SCHERER, J. VIDUGIRIENE, et al. 1994. J. Cell Biol. **126:** 111–126.
10. LIPARDI, C., R. MORA, V. COLOMER, et al. 1998. J. Cell Biol. **140:** 617–626.
11. LI, S., J. COUET & M.P. LISANTI. 1996. J. Biol. Chem. **271:** 29182–29190.
12. KO, Y.-G., J.-S. LEE, Y.-S. KANG, et al. 1999. J. Immunol. **162:** 7217–7223.
13. KO, Y.-G., P. LIU, R.K. PATHAK, et al. 1998. J. Cell. Biochem. **71:** 524–535.
14. GARCIA-CARDENA, G., P. MARTASEK, B.S. MASTERS, et al. 1997. J. Biol. Chem. **272:** 25437–25440.
15. COUET, J., M. SARGIACOMO & M.P. LISANTI. 1997. J. Biol. Chem. **272:** 30429–30438.
16. OKAMOTO, T., A. SCHLEGEL, P.E. SCHERER & M.P. LISANTI. 1998. J. Biol. Chem. **273:** 5419–5422.
17. ROTHENBERGER, S., B.J. IACOPETTA & L.C. KUHN. 1987. Cell **49:** 423–431.
18. SCHMID, S.L. 1997. Annu. Rev. Biochem. **66:** 511–548.
19. WANG, L.H., T.C. SUDHOF & R.G. ANDERSON. 1995. J. Biol. Chem. **270:** 10079–10083.
20. SLEPNEV, V.I., G.C. OCHOA, M.H. BUTLER, et al. 1998. Science **281:** 821–824.
21. DAVID, C., P.S. MCPHERSON, O. MUNDIGL & P. DE CAMILI. 1996. Proc. Natl. Acad. Sci. USA **93:** 331–335.
22. URRUTIA, R., J.R. HENLEY, T. COOK & M.A. MCNIVEN. 1997. Proc. Natl. Acad. Sci. USA **94:** 377–384.
23. PAK, J.S., W.Y. PARK, B.H. JEON, et al. 2001. FASEB J. **15:** 1625–1627.
24. PARK, W.Y., K.A. CHO, J.S. PARK, et al. 2001. Ann. N. Y. Acad. Sci. **928:** 79–84.

Dietary Restriction Initiated in Late Adulthood Can Reverse Age-related Alterations of Protein and Protein Metabolism

SATARO GOTO, RYOYA TAKAHASHI, SACHIKO ARAKI, AND HIDEKO NAKAMOTO

Department of Biochemistry, School of Pharmaceutical Sciences, Toho University, Funabashi, Chiba, 274-8510 Japan

ABSTRACT: Many reports have been published on the effects of lifelong dietary restriction (DR) on a variety of parameters such as life span, carcinogenesis, immunosenescence, memory function, and oxidative stress. There is, however, limited available information on the effect of late onset DR that might have potential application to intervene in human aging. We have investigated the effect of DR initiated late in life on protein and protein degradation. Two months of DR in 23.5-month-old mice significantly reduced heat-labile altered proteins in the liver, kidney, and brain. DR reversed the age-associated increase in the half-life of proteins, suggesting that the dwelling time of the proteins is reduced in DR animals. In accordance with this observation, the activity of proteasome, which is suggested to be responsible for degradation of altered proteins, was found increased in the liver of rats 30 months of age subjected to 3.5 months of DR. Thus, DR can increase turnover of proteins, thereby possibly attenuating potentially harmful consequences by altered proteins. Likewise, DR in old rats reduced carbonylated proteins in liver mitochondria, although the effect was not observed in cytosolic proteins. Fasting induced apoA-IV synthesis in the liver of young mice for efficient mobilization of stored tissue fats, while it occurred only marginally in the old. DR for 2 months from 23 months of age partially restored inducibility of this protein, suggesting the beneficial effect of DR. Taking all these findings together, it is conceivable that DR conducted in old age can be beneficial not only to retard age-related functional decline but also to restore functional activity in young rodents. Interestingly, recent evidence that involves DNA array gene expression analysis supports the findings on the age-related decrease in protein turnover and its reversion by late-onset DR.

KEYWORDS: aging; dietary restriction; late onset; altered protein; protein turnover; proteasome; fasting; apoprotein

INTRODUCTION

Lifelong dietary restriction (DR) or caloric restriction is a well established and perhaps the only reliable means to delay the functional decline of cells and tissues

Address for correspondence: S. Goto, Department of Biochemistry, School of Pharmaceutical Sciences, Toho University, Miyama 2-2-1, Funabashi, Chiba, 274-8510 Japan. Voice & fax: +81-474-72-1531. goto@phar.toho-u.ac.jp

Ann. N.Y. Acad. Sci. 959: 50–56 (2002). © 2002 New York Academy of Sciences.

with age and the onset of age-associated diseases, and to extend the life span of a variety of animals.[1,2] In the majority of reported cases, DR is initiated early in life, that is, soon after weaning or at early growth stages. Some of the antiaging effects of DR can be observed even in animals like nematodes, fruit flies, spiders, and water fleas.[3] In rodents, DR initiated much later in life was also demonstrated to have a beneficial effect: reduction of tumor incidence, resulting in the extension of life, albeit less remarkable compared with earlier onset.[4] In view of the wide range of beneficial effects, long-term DR is likely to influence "public" mechanism(s) of aging, such as increased resistance against oxidative stress.[5] We are particularly interested in the mechanism of antiaging effects, if there are any, of adult-onset short-term rather than lifelong DR in animals because it could be extended to humans in a practical manner.

Many theories have been proposed to explain the mechanism of the antiaging effect of DR, including attenuation of oxidative stress,[6] lowering of energy metabolism,[7] hormesis effect due to mild stress as reflected in elevated plasma glucocorticoid concentration,[8] and reduced glycation due to low plasma glucose level[9], which are not necessarily independent. Regardless of the primary mechanism(s) of the antiaging action of DR, it is conceivable that effects on proteins and protein metabolism can be of primary importance since proteins are involved in all life maintenance processes. We have, therefore, focused our approach on proteins and protein metabolism in investigating the antiaging mechanisms of DR.

EFFECT ON PROTEIN AND ITS METABOLISM

Potentially harmful altered proteins increase in cells and tissues of aged animals. We have reported that an increased percentage of heat-labile aminoacyl-tRNA synthetases of the liver, brain, and kidney in old mice was reduced to the level of younger (11-month-old) animals by two months of DR initiated at the age of 23.5 months.[10,11] It is worth noting that mild oxidation *in vitro* can mimic the age-related heat labilization of the enzymes *in vivo*, suggesting that the alteration might be caused by reactive oxygen species (ROS).[12] It was then hypothesized that protein turnover is decreased in the old, extending the dwelling time of damaged proteins, and that DR may reverse this process. In fact, half-lives of proteins introduced into hepatocytes and pulse-labeled proteins in the primary culture of old mice were prolonged with age[13] and shortened to that of young animals by DR.[14] In a more recent study the half-life of the degradation of oxidatively modified lysozymes introduced into the hepatocytes was also extended in old cells (Takahashi *et al.*, in preparation).

EFFECT ON PROTEASOMES

It has been demonstrated that altered or damaged proteins[15] and proteins in general[16] are degraded by proteasomes, multifunctional cytoplasmic protease complexes consisting of catalytic core subunits in one form (sedimentation coefficient of 20 S), and with additional regulatory subunits in the other (26 S).[17] To study whether oxidized protein was degraded by proteasomes in hepatocytes in primary cultures isolated from young and old mice, we examined the effects of proteasome inhibitor or the lysosome inhibitor on the degradation. While ammonium chloride that inhibits lysosomal proteases, cathepsins, did not affect the degradation kinetics, Z-Leu-Leu-Nva-H, a specific proteasome inhibitor, inhibited the degradation of oxidized lysozyme by 80% in both young and old cells (Kumiyama *et al.*, in preparation). Thus, age-related decline of protein turnover is likely to be due to change in the proteasomal degradation system. To confirm and extend the results of these studies, we measured the activity of proteasomes in rat liver extracts after separation of 20 S and 26 S forms on glycerol gradients using fluorogenic peptides as substrates.[18] Peptidase activities in proteasomes of the liver were found decreased as a function of age in mice and rats, being consistent with the observation in cultured cells mentioned above. It appeared that both 20 S and 26 S forms are affected similarly. Other investigators also reported age-associated decline of proteasome activities.[19,20] Interestingly, the quantity of proteasomes did not appear to change with age, indicating that molecular activity of the enzyme is reduced with age. It is, therefore, conceivable that chemical or structural alterations, the nature of which is unclear, may occur in proteasomes.

Three and half months of DR initiated at the age of 26.5 months significantly up-regulated the proteasome activity for fluorogenic peptidylglutamyl peptide hydrolysis in rat livers without appreciable change in the amount (Kumiyama *et al.*, in preparation). The finding suggests that DR can promote turnover of the proteasome itself, replacing impaired forms with newly synthesized intact molecules, and thus increase degradation of altered proteins.

EFFECT ON MITOCHONDRIAL PROTEIN OXIDATION

Deterioration of mitochondria, the major source and target of ROS, is implicated in aging and a variety of age-related diseases.[21–23] Particularly, a vicious cycle of oxidative stress in this organelle constitutes the basis of the mitochondria theory of aging.[24,25] As a matter of course, the effect of DR on mitochondria has been a focus of interest because DR is thought to reduce the rate of metabolism with oxygen consumption and therefore ROS generation from the electron transport system in this organelle. In fact, lifelong DR attenuates mitochondrial formation of superoxide and hydrogen peroxide that increase with age and oxidative damage to lipid and protein.[26,27] It was not clear, however, whether late-onset DR can reduce oxidative damage to these molecules. We demonstrated that the regimen of 3.5 months of DR initiated at the age of 26.5 months in rat, as described above, significantly reduced age-associated increase (about 55% compared with 10-month-old animals) in the oxidation of mitochondrial proteins of the liver, as measured by carbonyl content in Western blot.[28] The extent of oxidation in DR rats was similar to that found in younger counterparts (FIG. 1). The mechanism for the decrease in mitochondrial protein carbonyls by the short-term DR in aged animals is not clear. One mechanism, however, is likely to be reduction of ROS generation from the organelle,[26,29] while up-regulation of antioxidant enzymes does not appear to be responsible.[26] Additionally, increased mitochondrial protein degradation by ATP-dependent proteases[30,31] and/or mitochondria turnover as a whole could be candidates. Contrary to our findings, the mitochondrial protein carbonyl level in the skeletal muscle was reported not to change by shorter-term (6 weeks) caloric restriction in aged mouse.[32] It was noted

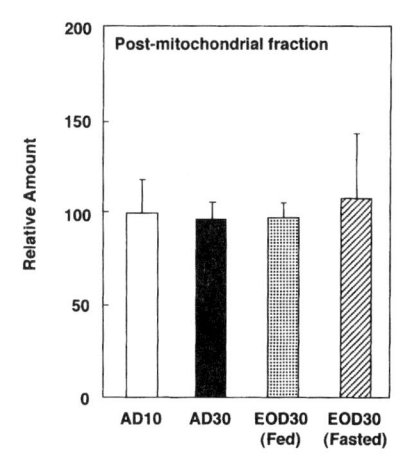

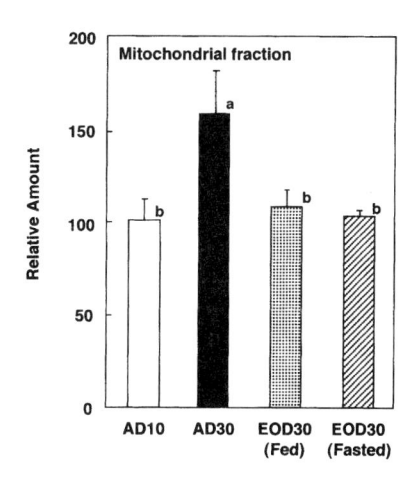

FIGURE 1. Relative amount of protein carbonyl in postmitochondrial and mitochondrial fractions from the livers of rats fed *ad libitum* or every other day initiated at old age. Values normalized to the young as 100% represent the means ± SE for four rats in each group. AD10: ad libitum, 10 months old; AD30: ad libitum, 30 months old; EOD30: every other day (EOD) feeding initiated at 26.5 months of age for 3.5 months, 30 months old. a: Significantly different from AD10; b: significantly different from AD30 ($P < 0.05$). (Data from Ref. 28.)

in our experiments that the increase with age and the decrease by DR were not significant in postmitochondrial cytoplasmic proteins (see FIG. 1). Cytoplasmic protein carbonyl is reported to increase remarkably (5- to 7-fold greater than the young levels) in various brain areas of aged (30-month-old) rats, but it was reduced by lifelong DR.[33] It should, however, be mentioned that the level of the carbonyl was much higher (4 to 7 nmoles/mg protein) in the aged than other published results for aged rodent brains.[26,34] Sohal *et al.* also reported that an age-associated increase in cytoplasmic protein carbonyls was attenuated in the brain, heart, and kidney by lifelong DR of mouse.[26]

EFFECT ON APOLIPOPROTEIN IN RESPONSE TO FASTING

Regulation of triglyceride metabolism constitutes an important part of energy utilization as well as of the morbidity of degenerative vascular diseases such as arteriosclerosis.[35] Storage and mobilization of triglycerides are dependent on plasma lipoproteins. We have studied the effect of fasting on lipoprotein metabolism in young and aged mice to investigate possible impairment of lipid mobilization with age. Fasting for a few days resulted in a remarkable increase in the plasma level of apolipoprotein A-IV (apoA-IV) in young animals (6-month-old), while it was marginal in the old (25-month-old) (Araki and Goto, in preparation). The amount of mRNA for apoA-IV in the liver largely paralleled these changes. The plasma level of apoA-IV (data not shown) and induction of apoA-IV mRNA by fasting in 25-month-old mice were up-regulated, albeit not significantly, by three months of prior

TABLE 1. Effects of age, dietary restriction, and fasting on the relative amount of hepatic apoA-IV and apoC-III mRNAs per unit amount of total RNA[a]

	apoA-IV mRNA		apoC-III mRNA	
	F(0)	F(3)	F(0)	F(2)
Young	1.00	52.3 ± 11.3	1.00	0.75 ± 0.05
Old	1.62 ± 0.75	1.95 ± 0.61[b]	1.57 ± 0.23[c]	1.43 ± 0.26[d]
Old-DR	0.97 ± 0.16	9.64 ± 1.73	1.01 ± 0.22[e]	0.89 ± 0.08[e]

[a]The values are relative intensity of radioactive signals on Northern blot for each mRNA relative to young unfasted (F(0)) levels. Young: 6 months old, Old: 25 months old, Old-DR: 25 months old (after 3 months of dietary restriction). F(0): fasting day 0; F(2): fasting day 2; F(3): fasting day 3.
[b]Young vs. Old, $P<0.001$
[c]Young vs. Old, $P<0.05$
[d]Old vs. Old, $P<0.01$
[e]Old vs. Old-DR, $P<0.05$

DR (TABLE 1). ApoC-III mRNA was present in larger amounts in the liver of aged mice than that in young counterparts but was reduced to the level of young animals by the DR. Physiological functions of plasma apoA-IV are not fully understood, but it has been established that it plays an important role in reverse cholesterol transport. In addition, it is suggested that apoA-IV is involved in the regulation of triglyceride transport. In view of the reports that apoC-III is an inhibitor of lipoprotein lipase (LPL)[36] and that apoA-IV modulates LPL activity in the presence of apoC-II,[37] the late onset DR can be beneficial for efficient mobilization of triglyceride and in preventing development of vascular disorders.

CONCLUSIONS

Taking our available findings regarding late-onset DR and those of other investigators together, the regimen appears to be beneficial, in that proteins with lost and/or reduced functions in old animals are replaced by functionally active molecules due to improved protein turnover in DR. This may possibly constitute an important feature of the mechanism of the antiaging effects of DR.

In view of recent reports on DNA array analysis of gene expression for the effect of aging and DR in rodents[38,39] and primates,[40] even late onset short-term regimens in mouse can reproduce a large part of the changes seen in animals subjected to life-long DR.[41] Notably, genes of which expression is "rejuvenated" include those suggestive of improved maintenance of quality of proteins, for example, chaperons and proteasome subunits. These findings are in line with previous results showing potentially beneficial effects of life-long as well as adult-onset DR. It would obviously be interesting to search for means mimicking such potentially beneficial regulation of gene expression as observed in DR initiated late in life. Among those may be moderate regular exercise that confers oxidative stress resistance,[42] pharmacological treatment that up-regulates antioxidant enzymes by deprenyl,[43] and the idea of hormetic intervention.[1,44,45]

REFERENCES

1. MASORO, E.J. 2000. Mini-review caloric restriction and aging: an update. Exp. Gerontol. **35**: 299–305.
2. YU, B.P. 1996. Aging and oxidative stress: modulation by dietary restriction. Free Radic. Biol. Med. **21**: 5651–5668.
3. WEINDRUCH, R. 1996. Caloric restriction and aging. Sci. Am. **274**: 46–52.
4. WEINDRUCH, R. & R.L. WALFORD. 1982. Dietary restriction in mice beginning at 1 year of age: effect on life-span and spontaneous cancer incidence. Science **215**:1415–1418.
5. MARTIN, G.M., S.N. AUSTAD & T.E. JOHNSON. 1998. Genetic analysis of ageing: role of oxidative damage and environmental stresses. Nat. Genet. **13**: 25–34.
6. SOHAL, R.S. & R. WEINDRUCH. 1996. Oxidative stress, caloric restriction, and aging. Science **273**: 59–63.
7. LANE, M.A., D.J. BAER, W.V. RUMLER, et al. 1996. Calorie restriction lowers body temperature in rhesus monkeys, consistent with a postulated anti-aging mechanism in rodents. Proc. Natl. Acad. Sci. USA **93**: 4159–4164.
8. MASORO, E.J. 1998. Hormesis and the antiaging action of dietary restriction. Exp. Gerontol. **33**: 61–66.
9. MASORO, E.J., R.J.M. MCCATER, M.S. KATZ, et al. 1992. Dietary restriction alters characteristics of glucose fuel use. J. Gerontol. **47**: B202–B208.
10. TAKAHASHI, R. & S. GOTO. 1987. Influence of dietary restriction on the accumulation of heat-labile aminoacyl tRNA synthetases in senescent mice. Arch. Biochem. Biophys. **257**: 200–206.
11. GOTO, S., A. ISHIGAMI & R. TAKAHASHI. 1991. Effect of age and dietary restriction on accumulation of altered proteins and degradation of proteins in mouse. *In* Liver and Aging-1990. K. Kitani, Ed.: 137–147. Elsevier. Amsterdam.
12. TAKAHASHI, R. & S. GOTO. 1990. Alteration of aminoacyl-tRNA synthetase with age: heat-labilization of the enzyme by oxidative damage. Arch. Biochem. Biophys. **277**: 228–233.
13. ISHIGAMI, A. & S. GOTO. 1990. Age-related change in the degradation rate of ovalbumin microinjected into mouse liver parenchymal cells. Arch. Biochem. Biophys. **277**: 189–195.
14. ISHIGAMI, A. & S. GOTO. 1990. Effect of dietary restriction on the degradation of proteins in senescent mouse liver parenchymal cells in culture. Arch. Biochem. Biophys. **283**: 362–366.
15. GRUNE, T., T. REINHECKEL & K.J. DAVIES. 1997. Degradation of oxidized proteins in mammalian cells. FASEB J. **11**: 526–534.
16. ROCK, K.L., C. GRAMM, L. ROTHSTEIN, et al. 1994. Inhibitors of the proteasome block the degradation of most cell proteins and the generation of peptides presented on MHC class I molecules. Cell **78**: 761–771.
17. COUX, O., K. TANAKA & A.L. GOLDBERG. 1996. Structure and functions of the 20S and 26S proteasomes. Annu. Rev. Biochem. **65**: 801–847.
18. HAYASHI, T. & S. GOTO. 1998. Age-related changes in the 20S and 26S proteasome activities in the liver of male F344 rats. Mech. Ageing Dev. **102**: 55–66.
19. SHIBATANI, T., M. NAZIR & W.F. WARD. 1996. Alteration of rat liver 20S proteasome activities by age and food restriction. J. Gerontol. **51**: B316–322.
20. CONCONI, M., L.I. SZWEDA, R.L. LEVINE, et al. 1996. Age-related decline of rat liver multicatalytic proteinase activity and protection from oxidative inactivation by heat-shock protein 90. Arch. Biochem. Biophys. **331**: 232–240.
21. BARJA, G. 1999. Mitochondrial oxygen radical generation and leak: sites of production in states 4 and 3, organ specificity, and relation to aging and longevity. J. Bioenerg. Biomembr. **31**: 347–366.
22. WALLACE, D.C. 1999. Mitochondrial diseases in man and mouse. Science **283**: 1482–1488.
23. RAHA, S. & B.H. ROBINSON. 2000. Mitochondria, oxygen free radicals, disease and ageing. Trends Biochem. Sci. **25**: 502–508.

24. HARMAN, D. 1972. The biological clock: the mitochondria. J. Am. Geriatr. Soc. **20:** 145–147.
25. LINNANE, A.W., S. MARZUKI, T. OZAWA, et al. 1989. Mitochondrial DNA mutations as an important contributor to ageing and degenerative diseases. Lancet **1:** 642–645.
26. SOHAL, R.S., H.-H. KU, S. AGARWAL, et al. 1994. Oxidative damage, mitochondrial oxidant generation and antioxidant defenses during aging and in response to food restriction in the mouse. Mech. Ageing Dev. **74:** 121–133.
27. SOHAL, R.S. & R. WEINDRUCH. 1996. Oxidative stress, caloric restriction, and aging. Science **273:** 59–63.
28. NAGAI, M., R. TAKAHASHI & S. GOTO. 2000. Dietary restriction initiated late in life can reduce mitochondrial protein carbonyls in rat livers: Western blot studies. Biogerontol. **1:** 321–328.
29. GREDILLA, R., G. BARJA & M. LOPEZ-TORRES. 2001. Effect of short-term caloric restriction on H_2O_2 production and oxidative DNA damage in rat liver mitochondria and location of the free radical source. J. Bioenerg. Biomembr. **33:** 279–287
30. MARCILLAT, O., Y. ZHANG, W. LIN, et al. 1988. Mitochondria contain a proteolytic system which can recognize and degrade oxidatively denatured proteins. Biochem. J. **254:** 677–683.
31. LANGER, T. & W. NEUPERT. 1996. Regulated protein degradation in mitochondria. Experientia **52:** 1069–1076.
32. LASS, A., B.H. SOHAL, R. WEINDRUCH, et al. 1998. Caloric restriction prevents age-associated accrual of oxidative damage to mouse skeletal muscle mitochondria. Free Radic. Biol. Med. **25:** 1089–1097.
33. AKSENOVA, M.V., M.Y. AKSENOV, J.M. CARNE, et al. 1998. Protein oxidation and enzyme activity decline in old brown Norway rats are reduced by dietary restriction. Mech. Ageing Dev. **100:** 157–168.
34. GOTO, S. & A. NAKAMURA. 1997. Age-associated, oxidatively modified proteins: a critical evaluation. Age **20:** 81–89.
35. SPRECHER, D.L. 1998. Triglycerides as a risk factor for coronary artery disease. Am. J. Cardiol. **82:** 49U–56U.
36. WANG, C.S., W.J. MCCONATHY, H.U. KLOER, et al. 1985. Modulation of lipoprotein lipase activity by apolipoproteins. Effect of apolipoprotein C-III. J. Clin. Invest. **75:** 384–390.
37. GOLDBERG, I.J., C.A. SCHERALDI, L.K. YACOUB, et al. 1990. Lipoprotein ApoC-II activation of lipoprotein lipase. Modulation by apolipoprotein A-IV. J. Biol. Chem. **265:** 4266–4272.
38. LEE, C.K., R.G. KLOPP, R. WEINDRUCH, et al. 1999. Gene expression profile of aging and its retardation by caloric restriction. Science **285:** 1390–1393.
39. LEE, C.K., R. WEINDRUCH & T.A. PROLLA. 2000. Gene-expression profile of the ageing brain in mice. Nat. Genet. **25:** 294–297.
40. KAYO, T., D.B. ALLISON, R. WEINDRUCH, et al. 2001. Influences of aging and caloric restriction on the transcriptional profile of skeletal muscle from rhesus monkeys. Proc. Natl. Acad. Sci. USA **98:** 5093–5098.
41. CAO, S.X., J.M. DHAHBI, P.L. MOTE, et al. 2001. Genomic profiling of short- and long-term caloric restriction effects in the liver of aging mice. Proc. Natl. Acad. Sci. USA **98:** 10630–10635.
42. RADAK, Z., A.W. TAYLOR, H. OHNO, et al. 2001. Adaptation to exercise-induced oxidative stress: from muscle to brain. Exerc. Immunol. Rev. **7:** 90–107.
43. KITANI, K., S. KANAI, G.O. IVY, et al. 1999. Pharmacological modifications of endogenous antioxidant enzymes with special reference to the effects of deprenyl: a possible antioxidant strategy. Mech. Ageing Dev. **111:** 211–221.
44. MINOIS, N. 2000. Longevity and aging: beneficial effects of exposure to mild stress. Biogerontology **1:** 15–29
45. JOHNSON, T.E., E. CASTRO, S.H. CATRO, et al. 2001. Relationship between increased longevity and stress resistance as assessed through gerontogene mutations in *C. elegans*. Exp. Gerontol. **36:** 1609–1617.

Pigments in Aging: An Overview

EDUARDO A. PORTA

*Department of Pathology, University of Hawaii,
School of Medicine, Honolulu, Hawaii 96822, USA*

ABSTRACT: Although during the normal aging process there are numerous pigmentary changes, the best recognized are those of melanin and lipofuscin. Melanin may increase (e.g., age spots, senile lentigo, or melanosis coli) or decrease (e.g., graying of hair or ocular melanin) with age, while lipofuscin (also called age pigment) always increases with age. In fact, the time-dependent accumulation of lipofuscin in lysosomes of postmitotic cells and some stable cells is the most consistent and phylogenetically constant morphologic change of aging. This pigment displays a typical autofluorescence (Ex: ~440; Em: ~600 nm), sudanophilia, argyrophilia, PAS positiveness, and acid fastness. Advances on its biogenesis, composition, evolution, and lysosomal degradation have been hampered by the persistent confusion between lipofuscin and the large family of ceroid pigments found in a variety of pathological conditions, as evidenced by the frequent use of the hybrid term *lipofuscin/ceroid* by investigators mainly working with *in vitro* systems of disputable relevance to *in vivo* lipofuscinogenesis. While lipofuscin and ceroid pigments may share some of their physicochemical properties at one moment or another in their evolutions, these pigments have different tissue distribution, rates of accumulation, origin of their precursors, and lectin binding affinities. Although it is widely believed that lipofuscin is a marker of oxidative stress, and that it can be, therefore, modified by antioxidants and prooxidants, these assumptions are mainly based on *in vitro* experiments and are not generally supported by *in vivo* studies. Another common misconception is the belief that lipofuscin can be extracted from tissues by lipid solvents and measured spectrofluorometrically. These and other disturbing problems are reviewed and discussed in this presentation.

KEYWORDS: ceroidogenesis; lipid peroxidation; lectin histochemistry

INTRODUCTION

Although during the aging process there are numerous quantitative pigmentary changes, the best recognized are those occurring in the normal endogenous pigments, melanin and lipofuscin. In humans, melanin is normally found in the skin, retina, iris, and certain areas of the nervous system, while lipofuscin is particularly found in postmitotic cells (i.e., neurons and cardiac myocytes) and in some stable cells (i.e., hepatocytes and glial cells). At least in postmitotic cells the amount of lipofuscin always increases with age, and it is, therefore, considered the best marker

---

Address for correspondence: Eduardo A. Porta, M.D., Department of Pathology, University of Hawaii, School of Medicine, 1960 East-West Road, Honolulu, HI 96822. Voice: 808-956-8845; fax: 808-956-5506.

portae@jabsom.biomed.hawaii.edu

of cellular aging, and also properly called *age pigment*.[1] On the other hand, melanin may increase or decrease with age. Because of its external visibility, the best known decrease of melanin with advancing age is the graying of the hair, which occurs in all individuals irrespective of gender and race.[2] It is now generally believed that the graying of the hair is due to a genetically regulated exhaustion and marked reduction in melanogenically active melanocytes in the hair bulb.[2,3] The age-related reduction in the amount of melanin is not limited to the hair bulb but is also observed in the epidermis, in the retinal pigment epithelial cells, and in certain areas of the central nervous system.[4–6] The declines in human neuromelanin content of the substantia nigra and locus caeruleus during advanced age were first reported by Gellersted[7] and by Scharrer.[8] From 60 to 90 years of age a gradual decline was quantitatively demonstrated by Mann *et al.*,[9] particularly in the substantia nigra. An increase in melanin is found in the so-called senile lentigo, which commonly occurs on exposed surfaces of the skin in about one third of individuals past middle age. The lesion is multiple (i.e., lentigines or "aging spots") and histologically characterized by linear melanocytic hyperplasia associated with hyperkeratosis, parakeratosis, and fringelike elongation of the hyperpigmented rete ridges. Another increase in melanin is observed in melanosis coli, but rather than a strictly age-dependent lesion, this condition is due to the prolonged use of anthranoid laxatives.[10] It is commonly found in elderly subjects simply because constipation is frequent among old people. The brownish-black pigmentation of the colon results from the accumulation of a granular pigment in the phagosomes of macrophages of the colonic lamina propia. The pigment of melanosis coli should be categorized as a melanized ceroid rather than as a simple melanin.[11]

Although lipofuscin is the most consistent and phylogenetically constant cellular morphologic change of the normal aging process, advances on its biogenesis, composition, evolution, and lysosomal degradation have been hampered by the persistent confusion between this important age pigment and the large family of ceroid pigments found in a variety of pathological conditions. The confusion is in part due to the fact that both pigments display a golden-yellow autofluorescence, and at one moment or another of their evolutions both types of pigments have somewhat similar histochemical properties, such as sudanophilia, PAS-positiveness, and acid fastness. There are, however, a number of differences between these pigments that permit their proper identification. Because lipofuscin is the most characteristic morphologic manifestation of the aging process, it is important to present first a comparative historical framework of lipofuscin and ceroid pigments as well as a brief overview of the most notable differences between these two types of pigments. Finally, because it is widely, but unfoundedly, believed, that lipofuscin is a proven marker of oxidative stress, this persistent notion will be discussed.

HISTORICAL FRAMEWORK

The pigment presently called lipofuscin was first described in isolated nerve cells by the Dutch histologist Hannover in 1842,[12] and four decades later Koneff[13] noted that the amount of this neuronal pigment correlated with the age of the individuals. In 1900, Rosin and Fenyvessy[14] described its sudanophilia. The typical autofluorescence of lipofuscin in cardiac myocytes was first reported by Stübel[15] in 1911, and in 1915 Zivery[16] described its acid fastness. Although in 1912 Hueck[17] first used the term lipofuscin for the age pigment, the term was in fact given by Borst who first used it in his lectures but only used it in published form in 1922.[18] Lipofuscin granules were first isolated and analyzed biochemically in 1955 by Heidenreich and Siebert,[19] and in 1960, Essner and Novikoff[20] found that lipofuscin accumulates in lysosomes. Although from the historical point of view the term lipofuscin denotes the age-dependent pigment that invariably accumulates in long-lived cells of all animal species, it is unfortunate to see that it is also frequently used for the ceroid pigments formed in pathological conditions.

The first description of a pigment occurring in a disease entity was most probably that of von Recklinghausen,[21] who in 1983 observed the presence of an iron-free brownish pigment in tissues of patients dying from hemochromatosis. He termed this pigment *hemofuscin* to differentiate it from the most abundant iron-containing hemosiderin. At about the same time, and also in subsequent years, similar pigments commonly referred to as lipofuscin or simply brown pigment, were recorded in the gastrointestinal tract of patients dying with a variety of diseases usually associated with malabsorption.[22–24] The tissue accumulation of ceroid in vitamin E deficiency was first observed in rats by Martin and Moore.[25] The term *ceroid*, meaning wax-like, was introduced by Lillie *et al.*[26] to describe the pigment accumulating in cirrhotic livers of rats fed diets low in choline and protein. The list of diseases associated with the accumulation of ceroid has lengthened in recent years and includes diverse types of malnutrition, genetic deffects, trauma, infections, irradiation, hormonal imbalances, toxins and drugs, hiperoxia, hypoxia, atheromatosis, and intravenous fat emulsions.

MAIN DIFFERENCES BETWEEN LIPOFUSCIN AND CEROID PIGMENTS

Although the physical and histochemical characteristics of lipofuscin and ceroid pigments are often quite similar, there are, however, as listed in TABLE 1, important differences between these pigments, such as universality, intrinsicality, and time dependence, typically of lipofuscin, but not of ceroid pigments. At least in human postmitotic cells, lipofuscin starts being detected during infancy (3–4 months in neurons, and late infancy in cardiac myocytes), whereas the onset of formation of ceroid pigments may occur at any age, depending of the determinant pathogenic factors. The *in vivo* deleteriousness of lipofuscin was never convincingly demonstrated, but the accumulation of ceroids is sometimes even fatal. Their rates of accumulation are quite different and so are their tissues distributions, mode of formation, and predominant origin of the precursors. In the case of ceroid formation due to vitamin E deficiency, the tissue distribution is different from that of lipofuscin in the uterus, extraocular muscles, inferior olivary nucleus, thoracic spinal cord, intestinal villi, and liver (TABLE 2).

Although, with the exception of the ceroid pigment, which accumulates in the diverse types of Batten's disease, little is known about the chemical composition of other types of ceroid pigments. Nevertheless, important quantitative differences in the content of dolichols, proteins, and saccharides have been found between isolated human neurolipofuscin and ceroid pigments isolated from brains of patients with

TABLE 1. Differences between lipofuscin and most ceroid pigments *in vivo*

	Lipofuscin	Ceroids
Universality	Yes	No
Intrinsicality	Yes	No
Time Dependence	Yes	No
Initial occurrence	Infancy	Any time
Deleteriousness	Never demonstrated	Frequent
Accumulation rate	Very slow	Usually rapid
Tissue distribution	Only intracellular	Intra- and extracellular
Mode of formation	Mainly autophagy	Mainly heterophagy
Origin of precursors	Mainly intracellular	Mainly extracellular

TABLE 2. Differential tissue distribution between lipofuscin (age pigment) and the ceroid pigment associated with vitamin E deficiency

	Lipofuscin	Ceroid
Uterus		
(myocytes)	–	+++
Extraocular muscles		
(myocytes)	–	+++
Inferior olivary nucleus		
(Neurons)	+++	–
Thoracic spinal cord		
(neurons)	+++	–
Intestinal villi		
(histiocytes)	–	+++
Liver		
(hepatocytes)	+++	+
(Kupffer cells)	–	+++

Batten's disease.[26,27] Because the chemical analysis of lipofuscin and ceroid pigments involves the laborious procedures of isolation and does not permit determination of the location of substances in different cells of a tissue or organ, pathologists generally prefer the *in situ* location of substances by histochemical means.[28] We have explored by lectin histochemistry possible saccharide differences between *in situ* lipofuscin and diverse ceroid pigments.[29] The lectin reactivities were determined in neurons and cardiac myocytes of old human subjects (74–85 years) and rats (>30 months), in the ceroid pigment of human aortic atheromas, as well as in the ceroid pigments that accumulate in the uteri of vitamin E–deficient rats, in the livers of choline-deficient rats, and in the crushed epididymal fat pad of rats. Although in the human specimens the neurolipofuscin and the ceroid in atheromas both contain mannose, sialic acid, and *N*-acetyl-D-galactosamine, the atheromas also contain α-

D-fucose and lactose. In the rat specimens, the saccharides of neurolipofuscin differ from those of the diverse ceroid pigments studied, and differences were also found between the different ceroids.

IS LIPOFUSCIN A PROVEN MARKER OF OXIDATIVE STRESS?

Although in the past there were uncertainties about the origin of the precursors in the formation of lipofuscin, it is now well established that lipofuscin, which exclusively accumulates in lysosomes, is the end product of the physiological decay or natural turnover of all cell constituents. However, still unresolved are two important questions: Why is lipofuscin not totally degraded in the lysosomes, and why does this end product become autofluorescent. Of all the hypotheses advanced to answer these two questions, the most favored is the peroxidative stress theory originated by Tappel,[30] who proposed that free radical reactions cause damage and polymerization of lipids and proteins into autofluorescent undergradable residues. Furthermore, the well-known autofluorescent and histochemical similarities between lipofuscin and the ceroid pigments, due to vitamin E deficiency, as well as the demonstration that reactive oxygen species are constantly generated in normal cells[31] has made this theory very appealing. Although many investigators, have embraced the peroxidative theory, the evidence in its favor is totally indirect and mainly based on *in vitro* findings of questionable significance.[32] The cornerstone of this theory was a key paper published in 1969 by Chio *et al.*[33] in which lipid peroxidation was induced in isolated subcellular organelles by shaking in oxygen. Uncorrected fluorescent spectra from these reactions were considered similar to previously uncorrected spectra of lipofuscin, and it was therefore suggested that the fluorescent materials of lipofuscin were products of lipid peroxidation. This was followed by another paper by the same group of investigators[34] in which the fluorescent reaction products of malonaldehyde and several amino acids were considered similar to the fluorophores of lipofuscin extracts. The conclusion of these studies was that lipofuscin was a lipid peroxidation product and that its autofluorescence was due to the formation of an imino-conjugated Schiff base linkage. A few years later, Tappel's group contended that the relative fluorescence of the organic solvent–extracted material from tissue homogenates could be used to measure the amounts of lipofuscin in the corresponding tissues.[35] This peroxidative stress theory had many inconsistencies. For example, while the imino-conjugated Schiff base fluorescent product has an excitation maxima at 360 nm, and emission maxima at 430 nm, the excitation maxima of lipofuscin is 420 nm and emission maxima is 600 nm.[36] Eldred *et al.*[37] were the first to develop a thin chromatographic system capable of resolving at least 10 distinct and well-defined fluorescent bands from the chloroform-methanol–extracted lipofuscin fluorophores when viewed under UV light. Using this system, Eldred[38] later found that when the lipofuscin of the human retinal pigment epithelium (RPE) was extracted via Folch's procedure, a golden-yellow fluorescence was seen in the chloroform phase when viewed with transmitted light, and an intense dark orange-yellow color when viewed under UV light. When the chromatograms were seen under transmitted light, no bands were seen, but when illuminated with UV light, several brown, greenish, and yellow bands were observed. Similar extractions and chromatographic analysis were performed with the imino-conjugated Schiff base formed *in vitro*, as Chio and Tappel have done before, but it was found that the chloroform phase was clear and colorless when viewed under white light. Under UV light, the chloroform phase exhibited a bright blue color fluorescence, and the polar phase exhibited a bright yellow fluorescence. Upon chromatography under UV light, only blue fluorophores were present. Finally, the same extractions were made with the *in vitro*–synthesized polymerization product of malonaldehyde. When the reaction product was extracted as before and viewed under white light, a dark color was seen in the chloroform phase, and a yellow substance in the polar phase. Viewed under UV light the polar phase emitted a bright green fluorescence, and the chloroform phase a very dull olive green fluorescence. Upon chromatography of the chloroform phase, the fluorescence was associated with a bright band migrating close to the solvent front. Clearly, the solubility and fluorescent emission properties, as well as the chromatographic mobilities of lipofuscin are quite different from those of the two *in vitro*–formed products.

With regard to the organic solvent extraction and spectroscopic method of Fletcher *et al.*[35] for the alleged measurement of lipofuscin, it became quite obvious in recent years that it is totally inadequate to quantify this pigment. No correlation was ever found between the amounts or concentrations of organic solvent fluorescent materials and the amounts of *in situ* morphometrically determined lipofuscin, as shown by Bieri *et al.*[39] in rat tissues, by Donato and Sohal[40] in houseflies, by Beatty *et al.*[41] in Rhesus monkeys, and by Sheehy[42] in the crayfish.

THE ALLEGED ROLE OF DIETARY AMOUNTS OF VITAMIN E AND THE TYPE OF DIETARY FAT ON LIPOFUSCINOGENESIS

Given the apparent physicochemical similarities between lipofuscin and ceroid pigments, and the role of oxidative stress in ceroidogenesis, it seems almost natural to infer that lipofuscinogenesis can also be modified by antioxidants and prooxidants. In fact, some investigators have concluded that either the administration of supplementary amounts of vitamin E to mice and rats[43–45] or the type of dietary lipids in rats[46] influenced lipofuscinogenesis. On the other hand, Sato and coworkers[47] reported that neither the various amounts of dietary corn oil nor the dietary presence or absence of vitamin E modified the amounts of lipofuscin in the cerebellar Purkinje cells of rats.

In our studies on the effect of the type of dietary fats (saturated vs. unsaturated) at two levels of dietary vitamin E (2 or 200 mg%), the results showed that lipofuscin significantly increases with time in the cortical neurons, cerebellar Purkinje cells, and cardiac myocytes but not significantly in the hepatocytes.[48–50] These age-dependent lipofuscin modalities were not influenced by the dietary treatments. In order to determine whether the different diets could influence the lipoperoxidative indices, and whether these indices correlate with the amounts of lipofuscin in the rats killed at 3, 6, 12, 18, and 24 months, we determined the levels of thiobarbituric acid reactants (i.e., malonaldehyde) and the presence of diene conjugates in the brain, heart, and liver. In the group of rats fed the diets with only 2 mg% of vitamin E and unsaturated fat, the levels of malonaldehyde were generally higher than in the other groups fed diets high in vitamin E (200 mg%) and saturated fat. The diene conjugation analysis showed the presence of these dienes in the liver and brain of rats fed diets with unsaturated fat, particularly in those with 2 mg% of vitamin E. However, no conjugate dienes were found in the heart of rats at any of the periods studied, despite the fact that cardiac lipofuscin increased with age. Neither in the liver nor in the brain did the lipid peroxidation indices correlate with the incremental amounts of lipofuscin.

Although the peroxidative stress theory of lipofuscinogenesis is appealing (and we might be premature to reject it), it has not been yet convincingly demonstrated that lipofuscin is a proven marker of oxidative stress or that dietary antioxidants and prooxidants may significantly modify the age-dependent pigment.

REFERENCES

1. PORTA, E.A. 1991. Advances in age pigment research. Arch. Gerontol. Geriatr. **12:** 303–320.
2. TOBIN, D.J. & R. PAUS. 2001. Review: Graying: gerontobiology of the hair follicle pigmentary unit. Exp. Gerontol. **36:** 29–54.
3. ORFANOS, A. 1970. Das weisse Haar alterer Menschen. Ark. Klin. Exp. Dermatol. **236:** 368–384.
4. QUEVEDO, W.C., G. SZABO & J. VIRKS. 1969. Influence of age and UV on the population of dopa-positive melanocytes in human skin. J. Invest. Dermatol. **52:** 287–290.
5. FEENEY, L. 1981. Lipofuscin and melanin of human retinal pigment epithelium. Invest. Ophthalmol. Vis. Sci. **17:** 583–600.
6. BARDEN, H. 1981. The biology and chemistry of neuromelanin. *In* Age Pigments. R.S. Sohal, Ed.: 155–180. Elsevier/North Holland Biomedical Press. Amsterdam.
7. GELLERSTEDT, N. 1933. Zur Kenntnis der Hirnveränderungen bei der nomalen Altersinvolution. Upsala Läk.-Fören. Förh. **38:** 193–408.
8. SCHARRER, E. 1935. Uber das Pigment in Anphibiengehirn. Zool. Anz. **109:** 304–307.
9. MANN, D.M.A., P.O. YATES & C.M. BARTON. 1977. Variations in melanin content with age in the human substantia nigra. Biochem. Exp. Biol. **36:** 137–139.
10. BOCKUS, H.J., J.H. WILLARD & J. BANK. 1933. Melanosis coli. The etiologic significance of the anthracene laxatives; a report of forty-one cases. JAMA **101:** 1–6.
11. BENAVIDES, S.H., P.E. MORGANTE, A.J. MONSERRAT, *et al.* 1997. The pigment of melanosis coli: a lectin histochemical study. Gastrointest. Endosc. **46:** 131–138.
12. HANNOVER, A. 1842. Mikroskopiske undersögelser af nervesystemet. Kgl. Danbske Vidensk. Kabernes Selkobs Naturv. Math. Afh. Copenhagen **10:** 1–112.
13. KONEFF, H. 1886. Beiträge zur Kenntniss der Nervenzellen den pertipheren Ganglien. Mitt. Naturforsch. Gesellsch. Bern. **44:** 13–14.
14. ROSIN, H. & B. FENYVESSY. 1900. Über das Lipochrom der Nervenzellen. Virchows Arch. Path. Anat. **162:** 534–540.
15. STÜBEL, H. 1911. Die Fluoreszenz tierischer Gewebe im ultravioletten Litch. Pflüger's Arch. **142:** 1–20.
16. ZIVERY, A. 1915. Sul comportamento delle sostanze del sistema nervoso centrale dopo l'autolisi. Arch. Zellforsch. **13:** 119–144.
17. HUECK, W. 1912. Pigmentstudiem. Beitrag. Path. Anat. **54:** 68–232.
18. BORST, M. 1922. Pathologische Histologie. Vogel. Leipzig.
19. HEINDEREICH, O. & G. SIEBERT. 1955. Untersuchungen an isolierten, unverändertem Lipofuscin aus Herzmuskulatur. Virchows Arch. Path. Anat. **327:** 112–126.
20. ESSNER, E. & A.B. NOVIKOFF. 1960. Human hepatocellular pigments and lysosomes. J. Ultrastruct. Res. **3:** 374–391.
21. VON RECKLINGHAUSEN, F. 1883. Handbuck der Allgem Pathologie des Kreisilanfs und der Ernahrung. Deut. Chir. I und II.
22. BLASCHKO, A. 1893. Mitteilung uber eine Erkrankung der Sympathischen Geflechte der Darmward . Virchows Arch. **94:** 136–147.
23. PAPPENHEIMER, A.M. & J. VICTOR. 1946. "Ceroid" pigment in human tissues. Am. J. Pathol. **22:** 395–412.

24. Fox, B. 1967. Lipofuscinosis of the gastrointestinal tract in man. J. Clin. Pathol. **22:** 806–813.
25. MARTIN, A.J.P & T. MOORE. 1936. Changes in the uterus and kidneys of rats kept on a vitamin E-free diet. J. Soc. Chem. Ind. **55:** 236.
26. HOOGHWINKEL, G.J.M., A.J. BLAAUBER, L. NOVAK, et al. 1986. On the composition of autofluorescent accumulation products: ceroid and lipofuscin. *In* Enzymes of Lipid Metabolism. L. Freysz et al., Eds. **2:** 827–831. Plenum. New York.
27. HALL, N.A., B.D. LAKE, D.N. PALMER, et al. 1990. Glycoconjugates in storage cytosomes from ceroid-lipofuscinosis (Batten's disease) and in lipofuscin from old-age brain. *In* Lipofuscin and Ceroid Pigments. E.A. Porta, Ed.: 225–241. Plenum. New York.
28. PORTA, E.A. & A.J. MONSERRAT. 1999. Revisión sobre el valor y aplicación de lectinohistoquímica en pathología. Patología (Mex) **37:** 41–58.
29. MONSERRAT, A.J., S.H. BENAVIDES, A. BERRA, et al. 1995. Lectin histochemistry of lipofuscin and certain ceroid pigments. Histochemistry **103:** 435–445.
30. TAPPEL, A.L. 1973. Lipid peroxidation damage to cell membranes. Fed. Proc. Fed. Am. Soc. Exp. Biol. **32:** 1870–1874.
31. CHANCE, B.H. SIES & A. BOVERIS. 1979. Hydroperoxide metabolism in mammalian organs. Physiol. Rev. **59:** 527–605.
32. BRUNK, T.U. & R.S. SOHAL. 1990. Mechanisms of lipofuscin formation. *In* Membrane Lipid Oxidation. C. Vigo-Pelfrey, Ed. **II:** 191–201. CRC Press. Boca Raton.
33. CHIO, K.S., U. REISS, B. FLETCHER, et al. 1969. Peroxidation of subcellular organelles: formation of lipofuscin-like fluorescent pigments. Science **166:** 1535–1536.
34. CHIO, K.S. & A.L. TAPPEL. 1969. Synthesis and characterization of the fluorescent products derived from malonaldehyde and amino acids. Biochemistry **8:** 2821–2827.
35. FLETCHER, B.L., C.J. DILLARD & A.L. TAPPEL. 1973. Measurement of fluorescent lipid peroxidation products in biological systems and tissues. Anal. Biochem. **5:** 1–9.
36. ELDRED G.E. & M.L. KATZ. 1989. The autofluorescent products of lipid peroxidation may not be lipofuscin-like. Free Radic. Biol. Med. **7:** 157–163.
37. ELDRED, G.E., et al. 1982. Lipofuscin: resolution of discrepant fluorescent data. Science **216:** 757–759.
38. ELDRED, G.E. 1987. Questioning the nature of the fluorophores in age pigments. *In* Advances in Age Pigments Research. E. Aloj-Totaro, et al., Eds.: 23–36. Pergamon Press. Oxford.
39. BIERI, J.G., T.J. TOLLIVER, W.G. ROBISON & T. KUWABARA. 1980. Lipofuscin in vitamin E deficiency and the possible role of retinal. Lipids **15:** 10–13.
40. DONATO, H. & R.S. SOHAL. 1978. Age-related changes in lipofuscin associated fluorescent substances in the adult male housefly, *Musca domestica*. Exp. Gerontol. **13:** 171–179.
41. BEATTY, C.H., et al. 1982. Aged *Rhesus* skeletal muscle: histochemistry and lipofuscin content. Age **5:** 1–9.
42. SHEEHY, M.R.J. 1996. Quantitative comparison of in situ lipofuscin concentration with autofluorescent intensity in the crustacean brain. Exp. Gerontol. **31:** 421–432.
43. NANDY, K. 1982. Neuronal lipofuscin and its significance. *In* Geriatrics. D. Platt, Ed. **1:** 257–262. Springer-Verlag. Berlin.
44. CONSTANTINIDIS, P., M. HARKEY & D. MCLAURY. 1986. Prevention of lipofuscin development in neurons by antioxidants. Virchows Arch. Pathol. Anat. **409:** 583–593.
45. MONJI, K., et al. 1994. The effect of dietary vitamin E on lipofuscin accumulation with age in the rat brain. Brain Res. **634:** 62–68.
46. BRIZZEE, K.R., D.E. EDDY & D. HARMAN. 1984. Free radical theory of aging: effect of dietary lipids on lipofuscin accumulation in the hippocampus of rats. Age **7:** 9–15.
47. SATO, T., et al. 1988. Morphometrical and biochemical analysis on autofluorescent granules in various tissues and cells of the rats under several nutritional conditions. Mech. Ageing Dev. **43:** 229–238.
48. PORTA, E.A., et al. 1980. Effects of the type of dietary fat at two levels of vitamin E in Wistar male rats during development and aging. II. Biochemical and morphometric parameters of the brain. Mech. Ageing Dev. **13:** 319–355.

49. PORTA, E.A., *et al.* 1981. Effects of the type of dietary fat at two levels of vitamin E in Wistar male rats during development and agin. III. Biochemical and morphometric parameters of the liver. Mech. Ageing Dev. **15:** 297–335.
50. PORTA, E.A., *et al.* 1982. Effects of the type of dietary fat at two levels of vitamin E in Wistar male rats during development and aging. IV. Biochemical and morphometric parameters of the heart. Mech. Ageing Dev. **18:** 159–199.

Aging and the Role of Reactive Nitrogen Species

BARRY DREW AND CHRISTIAAN LEEUWENBURGH

Biochemistry of Aging Laboratory, Box 118206, College of Health and Human Performance, College of Medicine, Center for Exercise Science, University of Florida, Gainesville, Florida 32611, USA

ABSTRACT: The role of reactive oxygen species and its effects on aging has received considerable attention in the past 47 years since Dr. Denham Harman first proposed the "free radical theory of aging." Though not completely understood due to the incalculable number of pathways involved, the number of manuscripts that facilitate the understanding of the underlying effects of reactive radical species on the oxidative stress on lipids, proteins, and DNA and its contribution to the aging process increases nearly exponentially each year. More recently, the role of reactive nitrogen species, such as nitric oxide and its by-products—nitrate (NO_3^-), nitrite (NO_2^-), peroxynitrite ($ONOO^-$), and 3-nitrotyrosine—have been shown to have a direct role in cellular signaling, vasodilation, and immune response. Nitric oxide is produced within cells by the actions of a group of enzymes called nitric oxide synthases. Presently, there are three distinct isoforms of nitric oxide synthase: neuronal (nNOS or NOS-1), inducible (iNOS or NOS-2), and endothelial (eNOS or NOS-3), and several subtypes. While nitric oxide ($NO^•$) is a relative unreactive radical, it is able to form other reactive intermediates, which could have an effect on protein function and on the function of the entire organism. These reactive intermediates can trigger nitrosative damage on biomolecules, which in turn may lead to age-related diseases due to structural alteration of proteins, inhibition of enzymatic activity, and interferences of the regulatory function. This paper will critically review the evidence of nitration and the important role it plays with aging. Furthermore, it will summarize the physiological role of nitration as well as the mechanisms leading to proteolytic degradation of nitrated proteins within biological tissues.

KEYWORDS: nitric oxide; apoptosis; oxidants; protein nitration; denitrase

INTRODUCTION

The role of nitric oxide (NO) has received considerable attention during the past 15 years. Because of its harmful effects on the environment from automobile exhaust, short half-life, and relatively unknown therapeutic benefits, it did not receive much attention from a biological perspective until the 1980s. However in 1987, NO

Address for correspondence: Christiaan Leeuwenburgh, Ph.D., University of Florida, Biochemistry of Aging Laboratory, 25 FLG, Stadium Road, P.O. Box 118206, Gainesville, FL 32611. Voice: 352-392-9575, ext. 1356; fax: 352-392-0316.

cleeuwen@ufl.edu; web page: http://grove.ufl.edu/~cleeuwen/

was discovered to be produced in biological tissue by nitric oxide synthase (NOS). NOS acts as a catalyst to convert L-arginine to nitric oxide and L-citrulline. In 1977, Murad et al.[1] revealed that NO has the ability to dilate blood vessels and relax smooth muscle tissue. In 1992, *Science* magazine chose NO as "molecule of the year.[2]" Six years later, three pharmacologists were awarded the Nobel Prize in Physiology and Medicine[3] for their discoveries pertaining to NO as a signaling molecule in the cardiovascular system. These discoveries led to the importance NO plays in cellular signaling, vasodilation, and immune response.

NO in an uncharged lipophilic molecule that contains a single unpaired electron (NO•),[4] which causes it to be reactive with other molecules, such as oxygen, glutathione, and superoxide radicals. Therefore, nitric oxide could function as an electron donor (oxidant) or an electron acceptor (antioxidant). After NO is produced by NOS, it diffuses across cellular membranes and into adjacent cells. It binds to soluble gaunylate cyclase covalently to convert guanosine 5′-triphosphate to cyclic guanosine 3′,5′-monophosphate (cGMP). The subsequent increase in cGMP level alters the activity of several main target proteins:[5] cGMP-dependent protein kinase,[6] cGMP-regulated phosphodiesterase,[7,8] and cGMP-gated ion channels.[9]

AGING AND THE NITRIC OXIDE SYNTHASE ISOENZYME

Aging is a natural and inevitable part of the life process that is characterized by a gradual and general decline in physiological functions that ultimately lead to morbidity and mortality. The process of aging is not completely understood due to the seemingly endless number of biological mechanisms and pathways. However, considerable progress has been made to understand and explain the effects of oxidants (reactive oxygen and reactive nitrogen species) on the oxidative stress on lipids, proteins, and DNA and how this contributes to the aging process.[10–14]

Some of the conditions associated with aging are neurodegenerative diseases such as Alzheimer's disease, cardiovascular disease, cancer, stroke, and a decline in the immunoresponse to pathogens,[15–18] which have been shown to be directly related to the amount or incidence of nitric oxide available for biomolecular modification.[5,19–34] Therefore, alterations in nitric oxide production could have a profound effect on normal aging and disease conditions. Examples of both aging and disease conditions will be presented. Often it is difficult to distinguish between the two (i.e., arteriosclerosis), and few studies have examined NOS activity and their by-products with normal aging.

NO is produced within cells by the actions of a group of enzymes called nitric oxide synthases. Presently, there are three distinct isoforms of nitric oxide synthase: neuronal (nNOS or NOS-1), inducible (iNOS or NOS-2), and endothelial (eNOS or NOS-3), with several additional subtypes (nNOSμ and mtNOS) of the aforementioned isoforms. All three isoforms bind calmodulin, but iNOS carries a permanently bound molecule of calmodulin that allows this isoform to function at low cytoplasmic Ca^{2+} levels.[4] Both nNOS and eNOS are expressed constitutively and are Ca^{2+} dependant, whereas iNOS is independent of the Ca^{2+} concentration.

While each isoform varies in its tissue specificity, different NOSs occur at multiple locations within the body. It appears that several isoforms can be found in the same tissue but may have different functions. For example, nNOS is found in a variety of neurons in both the central and peripheral nervous system, but eNOS is expressed in some neurons.[35] While eNOS can be stimulated by shear stress in the vascular endothelium,[36] iNOS may occur in normal epithelium such as the lung.[35] In a recent study by Grange et al.,[37] nNOS and eNOS knockout mice were studied to see which isoform contributes to a decrease in smooth muscle myosin regulatory light chain (smRLC) phosphorylation in contracting fast-twitch muscle. From their studies, they suggest that NO derived from nNOS contributes to vascular smooth muscle cell relaxation during skeletal muscle contraction; however, that vascular regulation overall requires eNOS.[37]

Neuronal NOS regulates synaptic transmission and is found in the cytoplasm of neurons in the nervous system tissues, skeletal muscle, and in lung epithelium. nNOS plays a direct role in the physiological activity of contracting skeletal muscle. While nNOS and eNOS may be activated during repetitive muscle contractions,[38,39] nNOS is probably the predominant NO producer during contractile activity.[40] Aging in the brain is characterized by a loss of activity in neuronal cells, which leads to a loss of memory and a reduction in learning capacity. Since NO is an important neurotransmitter in the central nervous system (CNS), Cheng et al.[41] examined the changes in nNOS from isolated cerebellum of Wistar rats aged 2 to 24 months to see if there was a correspondence between nNOS levels and the lowering of activity in the CNS during aging. In rats aged 6 months, there is an increase of NOS activity, which returned to the level of 2-month-old rats and/or 12-month-old rats, and further decreased in the 24-month group.[41] While this reduction in activity could be attributed to a decrease in the number of cells in brain tissue, it does show a correlation between nNOS expression in the cerebellum region and the aging process.

Endothelial NOS, which is the only isoform of the three to be membrane associated, produces NO that is responsible for the regulation of blood pressure. eNOS is located primarily in endothelial tissue, cardiac myocytes, and hippocampal pyramidal cells.[4,42] Furthermore, eNOS is widely available in very vascular tissues, such as the kidney, spleen, and liver. eNOS is associated with skeletal muscle mitochondria and acts to limit oxidative metabolism by the production and influence of NO on electron transport.[13,39] NO production from eNOS regulates platelet aggregation, vasorelaxation, and production of vascular smooth muscle cells.[4] In addition, it also mediates sexual function in males (penile erection) by diffusing NO to smooth muscle tissue. This release stimulates the enzyme guanylyl cyclase to elevate cGMP levels that, in turn, trigger a reduction of cytoplasmic Ca^{2+} and the subsequent relaxation of the corpora cavernosa.[43] The tautness and duration of the erection is dependant on the balance among the levels of NO synthesized in the penile nerves, the compliance of the smooth muscle, and the release of contractile factors.[43] In the heart, in vivo studies using NO donor or eNOS knockout mice have demonstrated that NO inhibits neutrophil-mediated injury by inhibiting neutrophil adhesion to the endothelial cells and preserves endothelial function, resulting in myocardial protection.[44–47] eNOS-dependant NO synthesis regulates arterial pressure and is defective in human essential hypertension.[48,49] Hence, a deficiency in the production of NO may therefore provide a plausible mechanism linking cardiovascular disease in humans.

iNOS is located in macrophages and liver cells and is induced by endotoxin and by inflammatory cytokines, such as interleukin-1 or tumor necrosis factor α.[5,50,51] Because it is independent of Ca^{2+} concentrations, it is produced in higher amounts and for longer periods of time. High amounts of NO are released by iNOS in response to inflammatory stimuli, where it is involved in host-defense against pathogens. Excess NO production, often involving iNOS may occur in certain diseases and has been hypothesized as a major contributor in the disease pathway[35] and also may play a significant role with aging. Hence, many groups[52–58] are currently studying physiological or synthetic agents that inhibit cytokine-induced iNOS expression at the transcriptional level.[5] For example, nitrones are used in the aging brain to attenuate iNOS activity[59–61] and may explain the increase in the life span of animals receiving radical spin-trap compounds. One of the characteristics seen in stroke victims is the increased activity of myocardial iNOS. High levels of nitric oxide and peroxynitrite (formed from nitric oxide) produced by iNOS is particularly neurotoxic.[61] Alpha-phenyl-N-tert-butyl nitrone (PBN) inhibits iNOS production by inhibiting the induction of cytokines.[60] Therefore, it appears that nitrones show promise in inhibiting cytokine-induced iNOS expression at the transcriptional level by mediating proinflammatory conditions in the brain.

NOS has been primarily investigated in endothelial cells, but recent experiments have been performed that indicate that NOS in the mitochondria (mtNOS) produce NO. Recently, NO was detected using electron paramagnetic resonance with spin-trapping techniques. Giulivi *et al.* isolated nitric oxide synthase from Percoll-purified rat liver mitochondria.[62] Several different mitochondrial preparations, such as toluene-permeabilized mitochondria, mitochondrial homogenates, and a crude preparation of NOS, were incubated with the spin trap N-methyl-D-glucamine-dithiocarbamate-Fe II, which produced a signal ascribed to the NO$^\bullet$ spin adduct. It has been suggested that mitochondrial NOS and NO production may not only have an important role as a cellular transmitter, messenger, or regulator, but that it is also an active player in oxidative metabolism.[63,64] In addition, mtNOS stimulation has been shown to induce mitochondrial cytochrome *c* release and increase lipid peroxidation (LPO), which, in turn, may mediate Ca^{2+}-induced apoptosis.[65]

In summary, the production of NO can result from an immunoresponse against macrophage activation of tumoral cells, from induction of iNOS in tumoral cells themselves, or from the vasodilation (eNOS) of blood vessel cells (endothelial and smooth muscle cells) by proinflammatory cytokines. Cytokines could also effect the production of nitric oxide by neuronal NOS, which may be inhibited by antioxidants and/or antiinflammatory compounds. Alterations of the levels of mtNOS and nitric oxide production could also have an influence on mitochondrial metabolism and oxidant production. Therefore, with aging, a variety of events, such as sickness, disease or injury, exposure to toxins, or physical activity levels could influence the levels of NOS and the production of nitric oxide.

BRIEF CHEMISTRY OF PROTEIN NITRATION

Nitric oxide itself is a relatively unreactive radical and cannot nitrate proteins irreversibly. However, it is able to form other reactive intermediates that could have an effect on protein function and on the function of the entire organism. For example, the reaction between NO$^\bullet$ and $O_2^{\bullet-}$ produces a very reactive oxidant, peroxynitrite (ONOO$^-$). Peroxynitrate reacts with tyrosine in proteins to form 3-nitrotyrosine (FIG. 1). However, besides nitration by peroxynitrate, other chemical reactions can

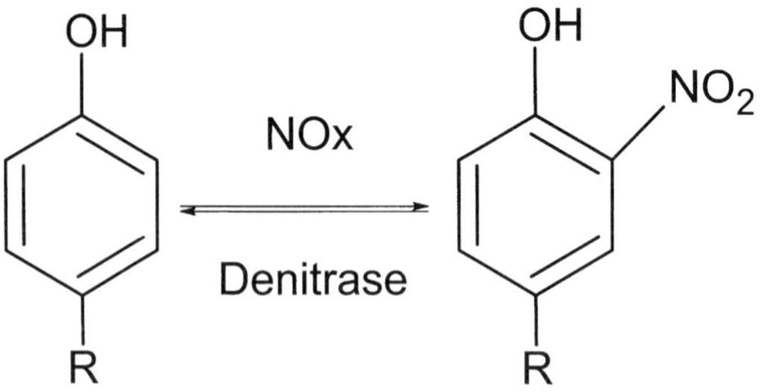

FIGURE 1. The interaction of nitric oxide (NO•) with superoxide yields peroxynitrite (ONOO−). Protonated peroxynitrite rapidly decomposes to generate several other NO$_x$, including the nitronium ion (NO$_2^+$) and nitrogen dioxide (NO$_2$•). Physiological combinations of nitrite, hypochlorous acid, and myeloperoxidase can also generate NO$_x$ species, which can nitrate tyrosines to form 3-nitrotyrosines. Specific denitrases may be able to remove molecular structures containing nitrogen from tyrosine residues (see text).

generate specific reactive nitrogen species, which could form 3-nitrotyrosine. Nitryl-chloride (NO$_2$Cl) a gas formed from the reaction of hypochlorous acid and nitrite (NO$_2^-$)—a major decomposition product of NO—can generate the nitrogen dioxide radical (NO$_2$•). This very reactive oxidant is also able to oxidize tyrosine to 3-nitrotyrosine.[66–68] Moreover, NO$_2^-$ at physiological or pathological levels is a substrate for the mammalian peroxidases myeloperoxidase and lactoperoxidase and forms NO$_2$• via peroxidase-catalyzed oxidation of NO$_2^-$. This provides an additional pathway contributing to cytotoxicity or host defense associated with increased NO production and an alternative pathway for the formation of 3-nitrotyrosine.[69]

PHYSIOLOGICAL RELEVANCE OF PROTEIN NITRATION

Modification of tyrosine residues in receptor molecules has been shown to impair signaling pathways.[70–74] For example, a specific modification, such as nitration of a tyrosine residue would compromise one of the most important mechanisms of cellular regulation, the cyclic interconversion between the phosphorylated and unphosphorylated form of tyrosine.[75] This possibility is underscored by the demonstration that nitration of tyrosine residues in model substrates prevents the phosphorylation of these residues by protein tyrosine kinases.[70–72,76,77] It is postulated that the nitration of tyrosine residues is an irreversible process and may lock the enzyme into a relatively inactive form. However, it appears that specific systems may be in place for the removal of potential unwanted nitrogen dioxide groups (see later section and Fig. 1).

The physiological importance of nitration has become more apparent in its effects on neurotransmission, vasodilation, and immunology. Growing attention is being given to endothelial function in hypertension and to the possibility that an inadequate NO-mediated vasodilation may have a direct impact on sexual function. Blood pressure is controlled by the release of NO by the vascular endothelium—inhibiting the production of NO can cause elevated levels.[78] The erection of the penis during sexual excitation is controlled by the release of NO. Relaxation of these vessels causes blood to pool in the blood sinuses producing an erection. The popular prescription drug sildenafil citrate (Viagra®) inhibits the breakdown of NO by acting on the nitric oxide-cyclic GMP pathway that mediates penile erection and thus enhances its effect.[79] Recent evidence shows that there is significant nitration (3-nitrotyrosine) and induction of iNOS in the normal aging rat penis.[43] These findings could lead to targeted interventions to reduce iNOS activity and may point to possible site-specific nitration of a tyrosine residue on signaling proteins. Therefore, nitration intermediates can induce a number of covalent modifications in various signaling proteins that lead to functional or structural changes.

A specific protein that could become nitrated in a given tissue (i.e., brain or penis) could be the platelet-derived growth factor (PDGF) receptor. This receptor has five known tyrosine autophosphorylation sites. Mutations or modifications in specific tyrosine residues in the receptor—for example, tyrosines 1009 and 1021—prevent the binding and activation of phospholipase C-gamma (PLC-gamma), an important signaling protein. If PLC-gamma does not bind to the tyrosine residues, then the inositol phospholipid signaling pathway is not activated.[80] Other important receptors, such as the insulin receptor also contains key tyrosine residue for phosphorylation and may become inactivated due to nitration. Thus, a site-specific modification of a single amino acid by an oxidant could result in the decline of a protein's activity and a specific tissue this protein is abundant in. Hence, the role of reactive nitrogen species on biological aging is of great importance, and more research needs to be carried out in order to better understand if reactive nitrogen species play a role with age and what interventions can inhibit or reverse the aging process.

There are many other physiological effects of reactive nitrogen species. For example, the free radical gas nitric oxide has been shown to have a wide variety of biological effects, including the ability to act as an inhibitor of mitochondrial electron transport.[81] Nitric oxide binds reversibly to cytochrome oxidase and can completely inhibit mitochondrial oxygen consumption.[81] Another example concerns mitochondrial aconitase, a key enzyme in the citric acid cycle, which is a major target of superoxide and peroxynitrite mediated disruption of the [4Fe-4S] prosthetic group. This results in significant losses of aconitase activity.[82] Interestingly, aconitase activity declines as a function of age both in skeletal and heart muscle[83–85] Therefore, this may be a mechanism by which enzyme function declines with age. However, even postmitotic cells are continuously repaired, and cellular components are entirely replaced, making it unclear what the physiological effects are during the aging process.

Trounce et al.[86] isolated intact skeletal muscle mitochondria from 29 subjects aged 16–92 years. State-3 (activated) mitochondrial respiration rates using several substrates were assayed and showed a negative correlation between respiration rate and age with all substrates tested. In addition, respiratory enzyme activities assayed in muscle homogenate also declined. They suggested that a substantial fall in mitochondrial oxidative capacity in aging muscle might contribute to reduced exercise capacity in elderly people. However, no direct evidence of a decrease in bioenergetics (i.e., ATP production) was presented, and the role of nitric oxide has not been investigated. Others have found very similar findings in the decline of respiratory function in skeletal muscle and liver of aged animals.[87–89] Furthermore, nitric oxide, some of its intermediates, and/or by-products may promote the induction of apoptosis with time. Apoptosis may therefore be involved in aging where it could serve to eliminate nonfunctional, harmful, abnormal, or misplaced cells, especially in advanced age.[90–93] The death of cells in the heart and skeletal muscle fibers could therefore explain a decline in function.

REVERSIBILITY OF NITRATION

As mentioned earlier, the mechanisms for oxidative cellular damage during aging are poorly understood. However, oxidative damage on biomolecules leads to age-related diseases due to structural alteration of proteins, inhibition of enzymatic activity, and interferences of the regulatory function. Specifically, one of the mechanisms that plays a direct role in cellular signaling and cytotoxic host defense mechanisms may also directly contribute to a mechanism for aging, due to the nitration of intracellular proteins. This could contribute to a variety of disease states, such as cardiovascular disease, and to neurodegenerative diseases,[94–97] in which 3-nitrotyrosine has been detected. However, few studies have investigated whether 3-nitrotyrosine nitration is reversible and if specific proteolytic mechanisms are in place for the removal of covalently bound reactive intermediates.

In general, the level of oxidized or nitrated proteins in a tissue reflects the balance between the relative rates of protein oxidation and clearance. For example, lens or collagen proteins turn over extremely slowly and thus should accumulate products of oxidative and nitrosative damage over time. Protein turnover and repair in skeletal muscle is also relatively slow compared to more mitotically active tissues. Oxidized and nitrated proteins may accumulate in muscle tissues due to the slower repair capacity.[98] The production of reactive oxygen and reactive nitrogen species in old compared to young animals may be of key importance because it is likely to increase the rate at which proteins are damaged.

Starke-Reed, Stadtman, and coworkers[99,100] have performed several studies addressing how proteins are oxidized and subsequently, proteolytically degraded and how these systems may change with age. They found that with age there is less efficient removal of oxidized proteins through proteolytic cleavage, which may cause the accumulation of protein carbonyls with aging.[99,100] Several proteolytic enzymes responsible for degrading oxidized proteins decline with age in tissues.[99,100] These proteases rapidly degrade oxidized enzymes but do not affect native nonoxidized enzymes. Several multicatalytic proteases provide major intracellular pathways for protein degradation.[101–105]

Ischiropoulos *et al.* established that a nitrated protein (tyrosine hydroxylase) is selectively degraded *in vivo* by chymotrypsin.[106] In addition, it was found that protein nitration enhances susceptibility to proteolytic degradation by the proteasome.[106] In their experiments, peroxynitrite was used in the nitration of tyrosine hydroxylase and detected by immunoprecipitation with a monoclonal antityrosine hydroxylase antibody. After the first two hours, there was no detectable change in the amount of nitrated protein; however, there was a significant decrease (~50%) in the antinitrotyrosine immunoreactivity after four hours. Hence, it is apparent that the chymotrypsin activity may be critical for the induction of accelerated proteolytic degradation of nitrated proteins *in vivo* and provides a model for studying the structural basis for the removal of oxidatively modified proteins.[106] It is therefore feasible that specific systems for the removal of nitrating species exist to reduce the toxicity of reactive nitrogen species. One indication of this possibility is provided by the studies performed by Murad *et al.*[107] As mentioned earlier, it is postulated that the nitration of tyrosine residues is an irreversible process. However, in a study by Murad *et al.*,[107] they identified a possible "nitrotyrosine denitrase" that reversed protein nitration (FIG. 1). In their study,[107] they examined tissues (spleen, lung, liver, and kidney) from rats treated with lipopolysacharide—a cytokine, which increases nitric oxide and superoxide production—to see what effect it had on the modification of nitrated bovine serum albumin (BSA). It was concluded that homogenates (containing the "denitrase enzymes") from rat spleen and lung could modify 3-nitrotyrosine-containing BSA; however, no activity was observed in homogenates from rat liver and kidney, suggesting that there may also be some tissue specificity for the apparent denitrase activity.[107] We show (see next section) that 3-nitrotyrosine in liver tissues tends to increase with age, which may be partly explained by the lack of activity of denitrase. Hence, the presence of a denitrase within human tissues could have an acute and significant chronic effect on cell signaling pathways.

3-NITROTYROSINE IN PROTEINS AND TISSUES OF AGING ANIMALS

Caloric restriction has widely been investigated and in almost every species studied, it has been found to impede the aging process. One of the postulated mechanisms is that a reduction in reactive oxygen species (and hence peroxynitrate production) can lower the chronic constant oxidative stress with age and therefore attenuates protein oxidation, DNA damage, and lipid peroxidation.[11–14] Thus, during the aging process, protein oxidation is increased in a wide variety of human and animal tissues. However, the exact pathways for oxidative cellular damage are poorly understood because the reactive metabolites are very short-lived and difficult to detect directly *in vivo*.

We have determined 3-nitrotyrosine levels in liver homogenate of young, mid-aged, and old mice and young and old rats (FIG. 2). We found that 3-nitrotyrosine tended to increase with age in the liver of both old mice and rats. In addition, caloric restriction in the mice lowered the levels of 3-nitrotyrosine. However, the results from an isotope-dilution gas chromatography mass spectrometry study[10] suggest that proteins oxidized by reactive nitrogen species do not accumulate significantly with normal aging in the skeletal muscle, heart, and liver of rats, though there was an apparent increase of 3-nitrotyrosine in the liver of old rats. Though the results were somewhat surprising, it did suggest that reactive nitrogen species damage proteins during biological aging; however, the accumulation of these proteins may have been prevented by removal mechanisms. Thus, proteolytic degradation of intracellular proteins may account for the relatively constant level of protein oxidation products seen in these tissues. The study on mice was performed on a small number of animals. Consequently, additional investigations are needed to better quantify the effects of reactive nitrogen species on the oxidation of proteins; however, it does appear that caloric restriction plays an integral role in the reduction of nitrosative stress. In addition, these findings are suggestive that nitrosative stress has a greater

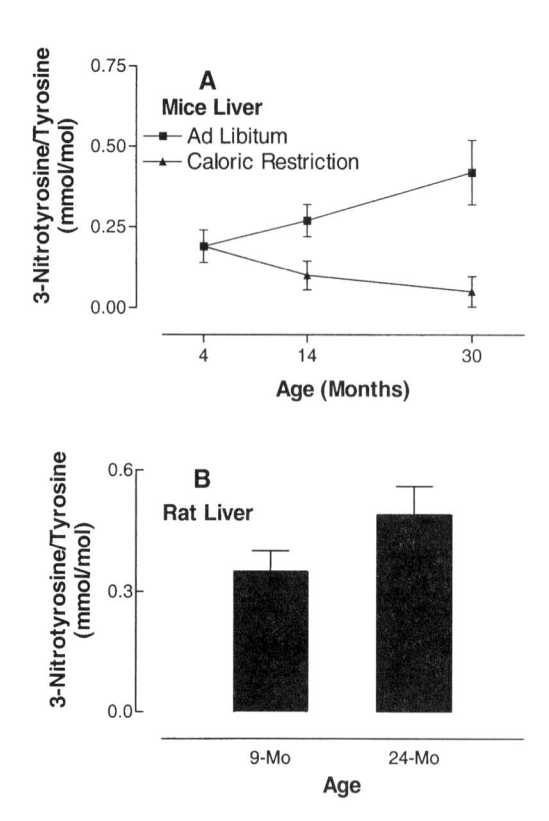

FIGURE 2. Effect of age on the levels of 3-nitrotyrosine in (A) the liver of young, mid-aged, and old mice on an ad libitum or caloric-restricted (CR) diet, and (B) the liver of young and old rats.[10] Ad libitum and caloric-restricted mice were sacrificed at 4 months ($n = 5$), 14 months ($n = 9$; ad libitum $n = 4$, CR $n = 5$), and 28–30 months of age ($n = 9$; ad libitum $n = 5$, CR $n = 4$). Rats were sacrificed at 9 months (young; $n = 5$) and 24 months of age (old; $n = 6$).

impact on some tissues over others, possibly due to the availability of a "denitrase" enzyme.

A study by Weindruch *et al.* showed that caloric restriction lowers oxidative and nitrosative damage in aging primates.[108] They were able to quantify the age-dependant accumulation of oxidative damage in mammalian skeletal muscle as well as characterize its attenuation by caloric restriction.[108] Using immunogold light microscopy (LM), an age-dependant decrease of 3-nitrotyrosine in skeletal muscle was observed, whereas no change was observed using immunogold electron microscopy (EM). However, the authors[108] mention that these differences could be explained by the increased sensitivity due to the enhanced preservation of the tissue with immunogold EM as well as inconsistencies in software analysis using immunogold LM. Additionally, it appeared that caloric restriction reduced the level of nitration by 20% using both techniques. The authors go on to suggest that if an age-dependant increase in oxidative damage is pivotal for the sarcopenia in mammalian skeletal muscle, the target of oxidative stress is more crucial than the subcellular site of free radical production.[108] These findings are in agreement with an earlier report from Leeuwenburgh et al.[10] who also did not find increases in 3-nitrotyrosine in rat skeletal muscle homogenate with age.

Others have looked at subcellular modifications of reactive nitrogen species in aged skeletal muscle. A study by Viner et al. stated that the level of nitration of the SERCA2a isoform of calcium-ATPase in sarcoplasmic reticulum vesicles isolated from rat skeletal muscle increases with age; there are approximately one and four nitrotyrosine residues per young and old Ca-ATPase, respectively.[109] In addition, nitration was undetectable in a closely related form of the protein,[110] which strongly suggests that certain calcium-ATPases are selectively modified by reactive nitrogen species. *In vitro* studies suggest that this level of protein oxidation may alter the function of SERCA2a *in vivo*.[110] These observations raise the possibility that specific proteins accumulate oxidative damage during aging. Therefore, it is plausible that increases in nitric oxide and/or superoxide production with age in, for example, the mitochondria discussed previously could become deleterious to mitochondrial respiratory enzymes and critical cellular components.

OTHER INDICATORS OF THE LEVELS OF REACTIVE NITROGEN SPECIES AND AGING

Many of the studies on the effect of NO on aging have shown that there is a decrease in the level of basal secretion with increased age. Because of the short half-life and low levels of NO in tissues and biological fluids, estimations of NO are based mostly on measurements of nitrite and nitrate—end products of NO metabolism. Nitrite and nitrate are either partly formed by auto-oxidation of nitric oxide with oxygen and/or derived from the diet (see next section). In a recent study on age-associated changes in NO metabolites in humans, Toprakci et al. found that NO release declines with age in healthy people, with the most pronounced decrease between 46 and 60 years of age.[111] Consequently, this reduction in NO synthesis with age could help in explaining the onset of vascular disease with increasing age due to the decline in endothelium-dependant vasodilation.

Nitrite (NO_2^-) can be formed from nitrate (NO_3^-) by a chemical process called reduction. Nitrate is relatively harmless unless it is reduced to nitrite. The vast majority (80–90%) of the nitrate most people consume comes from vegetables; however, because very little of the nitrate in vegetables is converted to nitrite, any health problem is unlikely. While meat products account for very little of nitrate in the diet (<10%), it does account for 60 to 90% of the nitrite consumed. Nitrites are unstable and can combine readily with other compounds in the digestive tract to form carcinogenic nitrosamines. In an earlier study by Witter et al.,[112] the distribution of ^{13}N-labeled nitrate in humans and rats was observed. The radiolabeled nitrate rapidly distributed in the bloodstream throughout the body. The radioactivity accumulated almost linearly with time in a small region of the abdomen, which was probably due to the swallowing of salivary nitrate.[112] Nitrite salts are the predominant preservatives used in cured or processed meats. Based on early results of a major new study, eating lots of preserved meats, such as salami, bacon, cured ham, and hot dogs could increase the risk of bowel cancer by 50%.[113] Hence it appears that there is a strong correlation between dietary nitrite consumption and the mechanisms of such diseases as vascular disease and cancer. Finally, besides dietary consumption of nitrates and nitrites, there are other sources for intake of harmful nitrites into biological tissues and fluids. Municipal drinking water, though not as severe a problem since the passage in 1972 of the Clean Water Act, used to be a huge source of nitrite exposure in humans. For this reason, the U.S. Environmental Protection Agency has set a maximum contaminant level, requiring that the maximum nitrate concentration content not exceed 1 part per million in public drinking water supplies. However, private sources of water, such as wells in rural areas, are still susceptible to high levels of nitrate and nitrite. Smoking is another source of nitration for biological tissues. Tobacco contains specific carcinogenic nitrosamines, which are derived from nicotine. These compounds may be among the causative agents for the various cancers (lung, oral cavity, esophagus, bladder, and pancreas) that are associated with tobacco usage.[114] Therefore, exogenous levels of nitrate and nitrite could significantly affect mean and maximum life span potential. In addition, when investigating the levels of nitrite and nitrate with age in blood or urine, dietary and environmental influences could play a major role in the cumulative levels.

ACKNOWLEDGMENTS

We thank Sharon Phaneuf and Amie Dirks for their valuable comments and critical reading of the manuscript. This research was supported by grants from the Society of Geriatric Cardiology, the National Institutes of Health, and the National Institute on Aging (AG17994-01).

REFERENCES

1. ARNOLD, W.P., C.K. MITTAL, S. KATSUKI & F. MURAD. 1977. Nitric oxide activates guanylate cyclase and increases guanosine 3':5'-cyclic monophosphate levels in various tissue preparations. Proc. Natl. Acad. Sci. USA **74:** 3203–3207.
2. KOSHLAND, D. E., JR. 1992. The molecule of the year. Science **258:** 1861.
3. RABELINK, A.J. 1998. [Nobel prize in Medicine and Physiology 1998 for the discovery of the role of nitric oxide as a signalling molecule]. Ned. Tijdschr. Geneeskd. **142:** 2828–2830.
4. SMUTZER, G. 2001. Research Tools for Nitric Oxide. The Scientist **15:** 23–24, 28.
5. BECK, K.F., W. EBERHARDT, S. FRANK, et al. 1999. Inducible NO synthase: role in cellular signalling. J. Exp. Biol. **202:** 645–653.
6. LOHMANN, S.M., A.B. VAANDRAGER, A. SMOLENSKI, et al. 1997. Distinct and specific functions of cGMP-dependent protein kinases. Trends Biochem. Sci. **22:** 307–312.
7. DEGERMAN, E., P. BELFRAGE & V.C. MANGANIELLO. 1997. Structure, localization, and regulation of cGMP-inhibited phosphodiesterase (PDE3). J. Biol. Chem. **272:** 6823–6826.
8. HOUSLAY, M.D. & G. MILLIGAN. 1997. Tailoring cAMP-signalling responses through isoform multiplicity. Trends Biochem. Sci. **22:** 217–224.
9. ZAGOTTA, W.N. & S.A. SIEGELBAUM. 1996. Structure and function of cyclic nucleotide-gated channels. Annu. Rev. Neurosci. **19:** 235–263.
10. LEEUWENBURGH, C., P. HANSEN, A. SHAISH, et al. 1998. Markers of protein oxidation by hydroxyl radical and reactive nitrogen species in tissues of aging rats. Am. J. Physiol. **274:** R453–461.

11. AMES, B.N., M.K. SHIGENAGA & T.M. HAGEN. 1993. Oxidants, antioxidants, and the degenerative diseases of aging. Proc. Natl. Acad. Sci. USA **90:** 7915–7922.
12. BARJA, G. 2000. The flux of free radical attack through mitochondrial DNA is related to aging rate. Aging (Milano) **12:** 342–355.
13. POLLACK, M. & C. LEEUWENBURGH. 1999. Molecular mechanisms of oxidative stress and aging: free radicals, aging, antioxidants, and disease. *In* Handbook of Oxidants and Antioxidants in Exercise. C.K. Sen, L. Packer & O. Hänninen, Eds.: Chapter 30: 881–926. Elsevier. Amsterdam & New York.
14. SOHAL, R.S. & W.C. ORR. 1992. Relationship between antioxidants, prooxidants, and the aging process. Ann. N. Y. Acad. Sci. **663:** 74–84.
15. BEAL, M.F. 1995. Aging, energy, and oxidative stress in neurodegenerative diseases. Ann. Neurol. **38:** 357–366.
16. AMES, B.N. 1995. Understanding the causes of aging and cancer. Microbiologia **11:** 305–308.
17. BUNKER, V.W. 1992. Free radicals, antioxidants and ageing. Med. Lab. Sci. **49:** 299–312.
18. CUTLER, R.G. 1991. Antioxidants and aging. Am. J. Clin. Nutr. **53:** 373S–379S.
19. LAKE-BAKAAR, G., D. SORBI & V. MAZZOCCOLI. 2001. Nitric oxide and chronic HCV and HIV infections. Dig. Dis. Sci. **46:** 1072–1076.
20. FLOYD, R.A. 1999. Antioxidants, oxidative stress, and degenerative neurological disorders. Proc. Soc. Exp. Biol. Med. **222:** 236–245.
21. RADAELLI, A., L. MIRCOLI, I. MORI, *et al.* 1998. Nitric oxide dependent vasodilation in young spontaneously hypertensive rats. Hypertension **32:** 735–739.
22. FERRARI, R., T. BACHETTI, L. AGNOLETTI, *et al.* 1998. Endothelial function and dysfunction in heart failure. Eur. Heart J. **19** (Suppl G)**:** G41–47.
23. KHADOUR, F.H., R.H. KAO, S. PARK, *et al.* 1997. Age-dependent augmentation of cardiac endothelial NOS in a genetic rat model of heart failure. Am. J. Physiol. **273:** H1223–1230.
24. MASSI, D., A. FRANCHI, I. SARDI, *et al.* 2001. Inducible nitric oxide synthase expression in benign and malignant cutaneous melanocytic lesions. J. Pathol. **194:** 194–200.
25. CHEON, K.T., K.H. CHOI, H.B. LEE, *et al.* 2000. Gene polymorphisms of endothelial nitric oxide synthase and angiotensin—converting enzyme in patients with lung cancer. Lung **178:** 351–360.
26. KOMAI, H., Y. NAITO, Y. AIMI & H. KIMURA. 2001. Nitric oxide synthase expression in lungs of pulmonary hypertensive patients with heart disease. Cardiovasc. Pathol. **10:** 29–32.
27. KONOPKA, T.E., J.E. BARKER, T.L. BAMFORD, *et al.* 2001. Nitric oxide synthase II gene disruption: implications for tumor growth and vascular endothelial growth factor production. Cancer Res. **61:** 3182–3187.
28. PAYNE, C.M., C. BERNSTEIN, H. BERNSTEIN, *et al.* 1999. Reactive nitrogen species in colon carcinogenesis. Antioxid. Redox Signal **1:** 449–467.
29. CHISTIAKOV, D.A., O.E. VORON'KO, K.V. SAVOST'IANOV & L.O. MINUSHKINA. 2000. [Polymorphic markers of endothelial NO-synthase and angiotensin II vascular receptor genes and predisposition to ischemic heart disease]. Genetika **36:** 1707–1711.
30. MITSUKE, Y., J.D. LEE, H. SHIMIZU, *et al.* 2001. Nitric oxide synthase activity in peripheral polymorphonuclear leukocytes in patients with chronic congestive heart failure. Am. J. Cardiol. **87:** 183–187.
31. SHI, Y., K.A. PRITCHARD, JR., P. HOLMAN, *et al.* 2000. Chronic myocardial hypoxia increases nitric oxide synthase and decreases caveolin-3. Free Radic. Biol. Med. **29:** 695–703.
32. HENEKA, M.T. & D.L. FEINSTEIN. 2001. Expression and function of inducible nitric oxide synthase in neurons. J. Neuroimmunol. **114:** 8–18.
33. PAULUS, W.J. 2001. The role of nitric oxide in the failing heart. Heart Fail. Rev. **6:** 105–118.
34. LIU, Z.Q., S.M. WILDHIRT & H.H. ZHOU. 1999. Specificity of inducible nitric-oxide synthase inhibitors: prospects for their clinical therapy. Zhongguo Yao Li Xue Bao **20:** 1052–1056.

35. HALLIWELL, B. & J.M.C. GUTTERIDGE. 1999. Free radicals in biology and medicine. Oxford University Press. Oxford, England.
36. UEMATSU, M., Y. OHARA, J.P. NAVAS, et al. 1995. Regulation of endothelial cell nitric oxide synthase mRNA expression by shear stress. Am. J. Physiol. **269:** C1371–1378.
37. GRANGE, R.W., E. ISOTANI, K.S. LAU, et al. 2001. Nitric oxide contributes to vascular smooth muscle relaxation in contracting fast-twitch muscles. Physiol. Genomics **5:** 35–44.
38. KOBZIK, L., M.B. REID, D.S. BREDT & J.S. STAMLER. 1994. Nitric oxide in skeletal muscle. Nature **372:** 546–548.
39. KOBZIK, L., B. STRINGER, J.L. BALLIGAND, et al. 1995. Endothelial type nitric oxide synthase in skeletal muscle fibers: mitochondrial relationships. Biochem. Biophys. Res. Commun. **211:** 375–381.
40. HIRSCHFIELD, W., M.R. MOODY, W.E. O'BRIEN, et al. 2000. Nitric oxide release and contractile properties of skeletal muscles from mice deficient in type III NOS. Am. J. Physiol. Regul. Integr. Comp. Physiol. **278:** R95–R100.
41. YU, W., S. JUANG, J. LEE, et al. 2000. Decrease of neuronal nitric oxide synthase in the cerebellum of aged rats. Neurosci. Lett. **291:** 37–40.
42. DINERMAN, J.L., T.M. DAWSON, M.J. SCHELL, et al. 1994. Endothelial nitric oxide synthase localized to hippocampal pyramidal cells: implications for synaptic plasticity. Proc. Natl. Acad. Sci. USA **91:** 4214–4218.
43. FERRINI, M., T.R. MAGEE, D. VERNET, et al. 2001. Aging-related expression of inducible nitric oxide synthase and markers of tissue damage in the rat penis. Biol. Reprod. **64:** 974–982.
44. KANNO, S., P.C. LEE, Y. ZHANG, et al. 2000. Attenuation of myocardial ischemia/reperfusion injury by superinduction of inducible nitric oxide synthase. Circulation **101:** 2742–2748.
45. LEFER, D.J., K. NAKANISHI, W.E. JOHNSTON & J. VINTEN-JOHANSEN. 1993. Antineutrophil and myocardial protecting actions of a novel nitric oxide donor after acute myocardial ischemia and reperfusion of dogs. Circulation **88:** 2337–2350.
46. WEYRICH, A.S., X.L. MA & A.M. LEFER. 1992. The role of L-arginine in ameliorating reperfusion injury after myocardial ischemia in the cat. Circulation **86:** 279–288.
47. JONES, S.P., W.G. GIROD, A.J. PALAZZO, et al. 1999. Myocardial ischemia-reperfusion injury is exacerbated in absence of endothelial cell nitric oxide synthase. Am. J. Physiol. **276:** H1567–1573.
48. DUPLAIN, H., R. BURCELIN, C. SARTORI, et al. 2001. Insulin resistance, hyperlipidemia, and hypertension in mice lacking endothelial nitric oxide synthase. Circulation **104:** 342–345.
49. FORTE, P., M. COPLAND, L.M. SMITH, et al. 1997. Basal nitric oxide synthesis in essential hypertension. Lancet **349:** 837–842.
50. MONCADA, S., R.M. PALMER & E.A. HIGGS. 1991. Nitric oxide: physiology, pathophysiology, and pharmacology. Pharmacol. Rev. **43:** 109–142.
51. NATHAN, C. & Q.W. XIE. 1994. Regulation of biosynthesis of nitric oxide. J. Biol. Chem. **269:** 13725–13728.
52. PFEILSCHIFTER, J., W. EBERHARDT, R. HUMMEL, et al. 1996. Therapeutic strategies for the inhibition of inducible nitric oxide synthase—potential for a novel class of anti-inflammatory agents. Cell Biol. Int. **20:** 51–58.
53. ANDERSSON, A.K., M. FLODSTROM & S. SANDLER. 2001. Cytokine-induced inhibition of insulin release from mouse pancreatic beta-cells deficient in inducible nitric oxide synthase. Biochem. Biophys. Res. Commun. **281:** 396–403.
54. KATSUYAMA, K., M. SHICHIRI, H. KATO, et al. 1999. Differential inhibitory actions by glucocorticoid and aspirin on cytokine-induced nitric oxide production in vascular smooth muscle cells. Endocrinology **140:** 2183–2190.
55. PANAS, D., F.H. KHADOUR, C. SZABO & R. SCHULZ. 1998. Proinflammatory cytokines depress cardiac efficiency by a nitric oxide-dependent mechanism. Am. J. Physiol. **275:** H1016–1023.
56. PENG, H.B., M. SPIECKER & J.K. LIAO. 1998. Inducible nitric oxide: an autoregulatory feedback inhibitor of vascular inflammation. J. Immunol. **161:** 1970–1976.

57. WRIGHT, K., S.G. WARD, G. KOLIOS & J. WESTWICK. 1997. Activation of phosphatidylinositol 3-kinase by interleukin-13. An inhibitory signal for inducible nitric-oxide synthase expression in epithelial cell line HT-29. J. Biol. Chem. **272:** 12626–12633.
58. GANSTER, R.W., B.S. TAYLOR, L. SHAO & D.A. GELLER. 2001. Complex regulation of human inducible nitric oxide synthase gene transcription by Stat 1 and NF-kappa B. Proc. Natl. Acad. Sci. USA **98:** 8638–8643.
59. FLOYD, R.A. 1997. Protective action of nitrone-based free radical traps against oxidative damage to the central nervous system. Adv. Pharmacol. **38:** 361–378.
60. FLOYD, R.A., K. HENSLEY, F. JAFFERY, et al. 1999. Increased oxidative stress brought on by pro-inflammatory cytokines in neurodegenerative processes and the protective role of nitrone-based free radical traps. Life Sci. **65:** 1893–1899.
61. FLOYD, R.A. & K. HENSLEY. 2000. Nitrone inhibition of age-associated oxidative damage. Ann. N. Y. Acad. Sci. **899:** 222–237.
62. GIULIVI, C., J.J. PODEROSO & A. BOVERIS. 1998. Production of nitric oxide by mitochondria. J. Biol. Chem. **273:** 11038–11043.
63. TATOYAN, A. & C. GIULIVI. 1998. Purification and characterization of a nitric-oxide synthase from rat liver mitochondria. J. Biol. Chem. **273:** 11044–11048.
64. SARKELA, T.M., J. BERTHIAUME, S. ELFERING, et al. 2001. The modulation of oxygen radical production by nitric oxide in mitochondria. J. Biol. Chem. **276:** 6945–6949.
65. GHAFOURIFAR, P., U. SCHENK, S.D. KLEIN & C. RICHTER. 1999. Mitochondrial nitric-oxide synthase stimulation causes cytochrome c release from isolated mitochondria. Evidence for intramitochondrial peroxynitrite formation. J. Biol. Chem. **274:** 31185–31188.
66. VAN DER VLIET, A., J.P. EISERICH, H. KAUR, et al. 1996. Nitrotyrosine as biomarker for reactive nitrogen species. Methods Enzymol. **269:** 175–184.
67. EISERICH, J.P., C.E. CROSS, A.D. JONES, et al. 1996. Formation of nitrating and chlorinating species by reaction of nitrite with hypochlorous acid. A novel mechanism for nitric oxide-mediated protein modification. J. Biol. Chem. **271:** 19199–19208.
68. CROWLEY, J.R., K. YARASHESKI, C. LEEUWENBURGH, et al. 1998. Isotope dilution mass spectrometric quantification of 3-nitrotyrosine in proteins and tissues is facilitated by reduction to 3-aminotyrosine. Anal. Biochem. **259:** 127–135.
69. VAN DER VLIET, A., J.P. EISERICH, B. HALLIWELL & C.E. CROSS. 1997. Formation of reactive nitrogen species during peroxidase-catalyzed oxidation of nitrite. A potential additional mechanism of nitric oxide-dependent toxicity. J. Biol. Chem. **272:** 7617–7625.
70. MACMILLAN-CROW, L.A., J.S. GREENDORFER, S.M. VICKERS & J.A. THOMPSON. 2000. Tyrosine nitration of c-SRC tyrosine kinase in human pancreatic ductal adenocarcinoma. Arch. Biochem. Biophys. **377:** 350–356.
71. TAKAKURA, K., J.S. BECKMAN, L.A. MACMILLAN-CROW & J.P. CROW. 1999. Rapid and irreversible inactivation of protein tyrosine phosphatases PTP1B, CD45, and LAR by peroxynitrite. Arch. Biochem. Biophys. **369:** 197–207.
72. DI STASI, A.M., C. MALLOZZI, G. MACCHIA, et al. 1999. Peroxynitrite induces tryosine nitration and modulates tyrosine phosphorylation of synaptic proteins. J. Neurochem. **73:** 727–735.
73. SQUIER, T.C. & D.J. BIGELOW. 2000. Protein oxidation and age-dependent alterations in calcium homeostasis. Front. Biosci. **5:** D504–526.
74. MARTIN, B.L., D. WU, S. JAKES & D.J. GRAVES. 1990. Chemical influences on the specificity of tyrosine phosphorylation. J. Biol. Chem. **265:** 7108–7111.
75. HUNTER, T. 1995. Protein kinases and phosphatases: the yin and yang of protein phosphorylation and signaling. Cell **80:** 225–236.
76. GOW, A.J., D. DURAN, S. MALCOLM & H. ISCHIROPOULOS. 1996. Effects of peroxynitrite-induced protein modifications on tyrosine phosphorylation and degradation. FEBS Lett. **385:** 63–66.
77. KONG, S.K., M.B. YIM, E.R. STADTMAN & P.B. CHOCK. 1996. Peroxynitrite disables the tyrosine phosphorylation regulatory mechanism: Lymphocyte-specific tyrosine kinase fails to phosphorylate nitrated cdc2(6-20)NH2 peptide. Proc. Natl. Acad. Sci. USA **93:** 3377–3382.

78. FANG, T.C., C.C. WU & W.C. HUANG. 2001. Inhibition of nitric oxide synthesis accentuates blood pressure elevation in hyperinsulinemic rats. J. Hypertens. **19:** 1255–1262.
79. BOOLELL, M., M.J. ALLEN, S.A. BALLARD, et al. 1996. Sildenafil: an orally active type 5 cyclic GMP-specific phosphodiesterase inhibitor for the treatment of penile erectile dysfunction. Int. J. Impot. Res. **8:** 47–52.
80. ALBERTS, B. 1994. Molecular biology of the cell. Garland Publications. New York.
81. BROWN, G.C. & C.E. COOPER. 1994. Nanomolar concentrations of nitric oxide reversibly inhibit synaptosomal respiration by competing with oxygen at cytochrome oxidase. FEBS Lett. **356:** 295–298.
82. HAUSLADEN, A. & I. FRIDOVICH. 1994. Superoxide and peroxynitrite inactivate aconitases, but nitric oxide does not. J. Biol. Chem. **269:** 29405–29408.
83. HANSFORD, R.G. & F. CASTRO. 1982. Age-linked changes in the activity of enzymes of the tricarboxylate cycle and lipid oxidation, and of carnitine content, in muscles of the rat. Mech. Ageing Dev. **19:** 191–200.
84. YAN, L.J., R.L. LEVINE & R.S. SOHAL. 1997. Oxidative damage during aging targets mitochondrial aconitase. Proc. Natl. Acad. Sci. USA **94:** 11168–11172.
85. VITORICA, J., J. CANO, J. SATRUSTEGUI & A. MACHADO. 1981. Comparison between developmental and senescent changes in enzyme activities linked to energy metabolism in rat heart. Mech. Ageing Dev. **16:** 105–116.
86. TROUNCE, I., E. BYRNE & S. MARZUKI. 1989. Decline in skeletal muscle mitochondrial respiratory chain function: possible factor in ageing. Lancet **1:** 637–639.
87. YEN, T.C., Y.S. CHEN, K.L. KING, et al. 1989. Liver mitochondrial respiratory functions decline with age. Biochem. Biophys. Res. Commun. **165:** 944–1003.
88. BYRNE, E., X. DENNETT & I. TROUNCE. 1991. Oxidative energy failure in post-mitotic cells: a major factor in senescence. Rev. Neurol. **147:** 532–535.
89. CARDELLACH, F., J. GALOFRE, R. CUSSO & A. URBANO-MARQUEZ. 1989. Decline in skeletal muscle mitochondrial respiration chain function with ageing. Lancet **2:** 44–45.
90. WARNER, H.R. 1999. Apoptosis: a two-edged sword in aging. Ann. N. Y. Acad. Sci. **887:** 1–11.
91. WARNER, H.R., R.J. HODES & K. POCINKI. 1997. What does cell death have to do with aging? J. Am. Geriatr. Soc. **45:** 1140–1146.
92. WARNER, H.R. 1997. Aging and regulation of apoptosis. Curr. Top. Cell. Regul. **35:** 107–121.
93. PHANEUF, S. & C. LEEUWENBURGH. 2001. Apoptosis and exercise. Med. Sci. Sports Exercise **33:** 393–396.
94. BECKMANN, J.S., Y.Z. YE, P.G. ANDERSON, et al. 1994. Extensive nitration of protein tyrosines in human atherosclerosis detected by immunohistochemistry. Biol. Chem. Hoppe-Seyler **375:** 81–88.
95. BRUIJN, L.I., M.F. BEAL, M.W. BECHER, et al. 1997. Elevated free nitrotyrosine levels, but not protein-bound nitrotyrosine or hydroxyl radicals, throughout amyotrophic lateral sclerosis (ALS)-like disease implicate tyrosine nitration as an aberrant in vivo property of one familial ALS-linked superoxide dismutase 1 mutant. Proc. Natl. Acad. Sci. USA **94:** 7606–7611.
96. LEEUWENBURGH, C., M.M. HARDY, S.L. HAZEN, et al. 1997. Reactive nitrogen intermediates promote low density lipoprotein oxidation in human atherosclerotic intima. J. Biol. Chem. **272:** 1433–1436.
97. SMITH, M.A., P.L. RICHEY HARRIS, L.M. SAYRE, et al. 1997. Widespread peroxynitrite-mediated damage in Alzheimer's disease. J. Neurosci. **17:** 2653–2657.
98. WEINDRUCH, R. 1995. Interventions based on the possibility that oxidative stress contributes to sarcopenia. J. Gerontol. A Biol. Sci. Med. Sci. **50** (Spec No)**:** 157–161.
99. STARKE-REED, P.E. & C.N. OLIVER. 1989. Protein oxidation and proteolysis during aging and oxidative stress. Arch. Biochem. Biophys. **275:** 559–567.
100. STADTMAN, E. R. 1992. Protein oxidation and aging. Science **257:** 1220–1224.
101. MARCILLAT, O., Y. ZHANG, S.W. LIN & K.J. DAVIES. 1988. Mitochondria contain a proteolytic system which can recognize and degrade oxidatively-denatured proteins. Biochem. J. **254:** 677–683.

102. PACIFICI, R.E. & K.J. DAVIES. 1990. Protein degradation as an index of oxidative stress. Methods Enzymol. **186:** 485–502.
103. DAVIES, K.J. 1987. Protein damage and degradation by oxygen radicals. I. General aspects. J. Biol. Chem. **262:** 9895–9901.
104. GIULIVI, C. & K.J. DAVIES. 1994. Dityrosine: a marker for oxidatively modified proteins and selective proteolysis. Methods Enzymol. **233:** 363–371.
105. GIULIVI, C. & K.J. DAVIES. 1993. Dityrosine and tyrosine oxidation products are endogenous markers for the selective proteolysis of oxidatively modified red blood cell hemoglobin by (the 19 S) proteasome. J. Biol. Chem. **268:** 8752–8759.
106. SOUZA, J.M., I. CHOI, Q. CHEN, et al. 2000. Proteolytic degradation of tyrosine nitrated proteins. Arch. Biochem. Biophys. **380:** 360–366.
107. KAMISAKI, Y., K. WADA, K. BIAN, et al. 1998. An activity in rat tissues that modifies nitrotyrosine-containing proteins. Proc. Natl. Acad. Sci. USA **95:** 11584–11589.
108. ZAINAL, T.A., T.D. OBERLEY, D.B. ALLISON, et al. 2000. Caloric restriction of rhesus monkeys lowers oxidative damage in skeletal muscle. FASEB J. **14:** 1825–1826.
109. VINER, R.I., D.A. FERRINGTON, A.F. HUHMER, et al. 1996. Accumulation of nitrotyrosine on the SERCA2a isoform of SR Ca-ATPase of rat skeletal muscle during aging: a peroxynitrite-mediated process? FEBS Lett. **379:** 286–290.
110. VINER, R.I., A.F. HUHMER, D.J. BIGELOW & C. SCHONEICH. 1996. The oxidative inactivation of sarcoplasmic reticulum Ca(2+)-ATPase by peroxynitrite. Free Radic. Res. **24:** 243–259.
111. TOPRAKCI, M., D. OZMEN, I. MUTAF, et al. 2000. Age-associated changes in nitric oxide metabolites nitrite and nitrate. Int. J. Clin. Lab. Res. **30:** 83–85.
112. WITTER, J.P., S.J. GATLEY & E. BALISH. 1979. Distribution of nitrogen-13 from labeled nitrate (13No3-) in humans and rats. Science **204:** 411–413.
113. NORAT, T. & E. RIBOLI. 2001. Meat consumption and colorectal cancer: a review of epidemiologic evidence. Nutr. Rev. **59:** 37–47.
114. HECHT, S.S., C.B. CHEN, R.M. ORNAF, et al. 1978. Chemical studies on tobacco smoke LVI. Tobacco specific nitrosamines: origins, carcinogenicity and metabolism. IARC Sci. Publ. **19:** 395–413.

Exercise-induced Modulation of Antioxidant Defense

LI LI JI

Department of Kinesiology, Interdisciplinary Nutritional Science, and Institute on Aging, University of Wisconsin-Madison, Madison, Wisconsin 53706, USA

ABSTRACT: Maintaining mobility is a critical element for the quality of life. Skeletal muscle, the primary organ for locomotion, undergoes age-associated deterioration in size, structure, and function. Recent research suggests that oxidative stress is an important etiology for sarcopenia. The level of oxidative stress imposed on aging muscle is influenced by two fundamental biological processes: the increased generation of reactive oxygen species (ROS) and age-associated changes in antioxidant defense. It appears that despite increased ROS production, aging muscle has a decreased gene expression of antioxidant enzymes possibly due to a diminished ability for cell signaling. A major benefit of nonexhaustive exercise is to induce a mild oxidative stress that stimulates the expression of certain antioxidant enzymes. This is mediated by the activation of redox-sensitive signaling pathways. For example, gene expression of muscle mitochondrial (Mn) superoxide dismutase is enhanced after an acute bout of exercise preceded by an elevated level of NF-κB and AP-1 binding. An increase in *de novo* protein synthesis of an antioxidant enzyme usually requires repeated bouts of exercise. Aging does not abolish but seems to attenuate training adaptations of antioxidant enzymes. Thus, for senescent muscle, training should be assisted with supplementation of exogenous antioxidants to research the optimal level of defense.

KEYWORDS: mobility; skeletal muscle; oxidative stress; sarcopenia; reactive oxygen species

Living an active lifestyle and at least maintaining mobility is essential for quality of life during old age. Skeletal muscle health is a key factor in this regard. Unfortunately, skeletal muscle undergoes loss of mass and functionality during aging; this is known as *sarcopenia*.[1] Recent research suggests that an important etiological mechanism for sarcopenia is increased ROS generation and oxidative stress.[2,3]

The benefits of endurance exercise in health and disease prevention in the elderly are well established.[4] Recent evidence suggests that resistance exercise (weight lifting) is an effective way to maintain muscle mass during old age.[5,6] However, it has been shown over the past two decades that heavy exercise increases free radical gen-

---

Address for correspondence: Li Li Ji, Ph.D., 2000 Observatory Drive, Madison, WI 53706. Voice: 608-262-7250; fax: 608-262-1656.
ji@soemadison.wisc.edu

eration and the risk of oxidative damage to skeletal muscle.[7] These risks are aggregated in aging muscle due to the following reasons: (a) The rate of ROS production in skeletal muscle is increased at old age.[8,9] Both mitochondrial and extramitochondrial sources of ROS contribute to this increment. (b) Aged muscle generates more ROS during heavy exercise than its younger counterpart, even though workload is reduced so that young and old muscles exercise at the save relative workload (i.e., same percentage of their respective VO_{2max}).[9] (c) Aged muscles are more susceptible to damage caused by eccentric (lengthening) contraction, which is an integral part of heavy dynamic exercise.[10] (d) Increased muscle damage can provoke inflammatory response and further oxidative stress and dysfunction.[11–13] (e) Finally, repair and regenerative capacity of muscle fibers are decreased with age.[14] All of the aforementioned side effects of exercise pose a question to us: Should we recommend participation in exercise to the aged population?

Answering this question requires a multifaceted approach, which is beyond the scope of this review. The purpose of this article is to address a focal point of this complicated issue by emphasizing that exercise not only increases free radical generation but also modulates cellular antioxidant defense systems. Our working hypothesis is that exercise can induce antioxidant adaptation, thereby reducing oxidative stress and damage in aging skeletal muscle.

ANTIOXIDANT DEFENSE IS WEAKENED AT OLD AGE

According to the free radical theory of aging postulated by Harmon,[15] the aging process is the deleterious and irreversible changes produced by free radicals throughout the life span. The theory simultaneously predicts that the ability of the cell to resist or prevent oxidative stress is a key determinant of longevity.[16] Two basic observations are relevant. First, in skeletal muscle enzymatic and nonenzymatic antioxidant defense capacity is relatively low compared to other organs and tissues because oxidative processes take place at a slow rate in resting muscle cells and so does the rate of ROS generation.[17] Second, aging seems to influence a muscle's antioxidant profiles differently than other tissues.[7] Endogenous antioxidant defenses in most tissues are weakened at old age, possibly due to decreased cell proliferation and protein synthesis, whereas aged skeletal muscle showed increased antioxidant enzyme activities.[18] However, the increased enzyme activity does not seem to be the result of enhanced *de novo* protein synthesis.

For all the enzymes investigated, such as superoxide dismutase (SOD), glutathione peroxidase (GPX), and catalase, the increased enzyme activity did not parallel enzyme protein content, suggesting posttranslational modification (activation) of the existing enzyme molecules.[19,20] Furthermore, mRNA abundance for CuZn-SOD, MnSOD, and GPX was found unchanged or decreased with age in all types of muscles examined.[19,20] Interestingly, binding of nuclear factor κB (NF-κB) to corresponding oligonucleotide sequences present in the MnSOD gene was decreased in both type 1 and 2 fibers, whereas activator protein 1 (AP-1) binding was decreased in type 2 muscle fibers.[20] In the signaling process of MnSOD gene expression, NF-κB and AP-1 play an important role.[21,22] Both NF-κB and AP-1 binding sites are present in the promoter of the mammalian MnSOD gene, and oxidative stress has been shown to activate their bindings.[23,24] A decrease in the binding of these nuclear factors in spite of increased ROS generation observed in aged muscle suggests that molecular signaling of antioxidant gene expression may be impaired due to aging. Considering the fact that senescent skeletal muscles demonstrate augmented levels of lipid peroxidation, protein oxidation, and DNA damage,[17] it can be concluded that the compensatory increases in antioxidant enzyme activity observed in aged muscle are insufficient to counter the increased ROS generation. This could result in mDNA deletion, increased apoptosis, and energy deficiency, leading to sarcopenia.[1]

EXERCISE MODULATES ANTIOXIDANT DEFENSE CAPACITY BY ACTIVATING CELL SIGNALING

Several strategies have been employed to enhance endogenous antioxidant levels such as dietary restriction, transgenic animal models, dietary antioxidant supplementation, and use of pharmaceutical antioxidant mimetics.[16] None of the above strategies to this date has been shown to successfully boost antioxidant defense in skeletal muscle. In a recent review, Finkel and Holbrook[16] elegantly stated that the best strategy to enhance endogenous antioxidant levels may actually be oxidative stress itself, based on the classical physiological concept of *hormesis*. Hormesis is a Greek word referring to a sublethal dose of toxin that can increase the tolerance of the organism to withstand higher doses of toxins. Exercise at high intensity is a form of oxidative stress due to the generation of ROS that exceeds the defense capacity in skeletal muscle.[25,26] However, it has been consistently observed that individuals undergoing exercise training have high levels of antioxidant enzymes and certain nonenzymatic antioxidants in muscle and demonstrate greater resistance to exercise-induced or -imposed oxidative stress.[17,27] Presumably, these adaptations result from cumulative effects of repeated exercise bouts on the gene expression of antioxidant enzymes. The question arises as to how exercise could trigger cellular mechanisms to increase antioxidant defense, that is, signal transduction.

Mammalian cells are endowed with several signaling pathways that can be activated by oxidative stress. Those include NF-κB, heat-shock transcriptional factor 1 (HSF-1), and P53 pathways, as well as mitogen-activated protein kinase (MAPK) and PI(3)K/Art that regulate the first three pathways through phosphorylation.[16] Recent evidence suggests that a single bout of muscular contraction, especially eccentric contraction, can activate the MAPK pathway in human skeletal muscle.[28–30] Sixty minutes after an acute bout of one-leg cycling, the activity of MAPK-activated protein kinase 2 was increased by 300%.[31] Furthermore, extracellular signal-regulated kinase (ERK) and p38 MAPK activity was increased in rat slow- and fast-twitch skeletal muscle after electrically stimulated contraction.[32] Also, Nader and Esser[33] showed that immediately after an acute bout of treadmill running, ERK and p38 were activated in rat soleus and tibialis muscles. Activation of various kinases involved in the MAPK pathway can lead to the sequential phosphorylation of a series of proteins, resulting in increased expression of c-Jun, a subunit of the transcription factor AP-1.[34] Alternatively, it may phosphorylate downstream kinases, such as the p90 ribosomal S6 kinase (p90rsk), whose activity was found to increase up to 25-fold in human muscle after exercise.[31] Although the cause of exercise-activated MAPK pathway has not been identified, and so far no data has linked MAPK to antioxidant

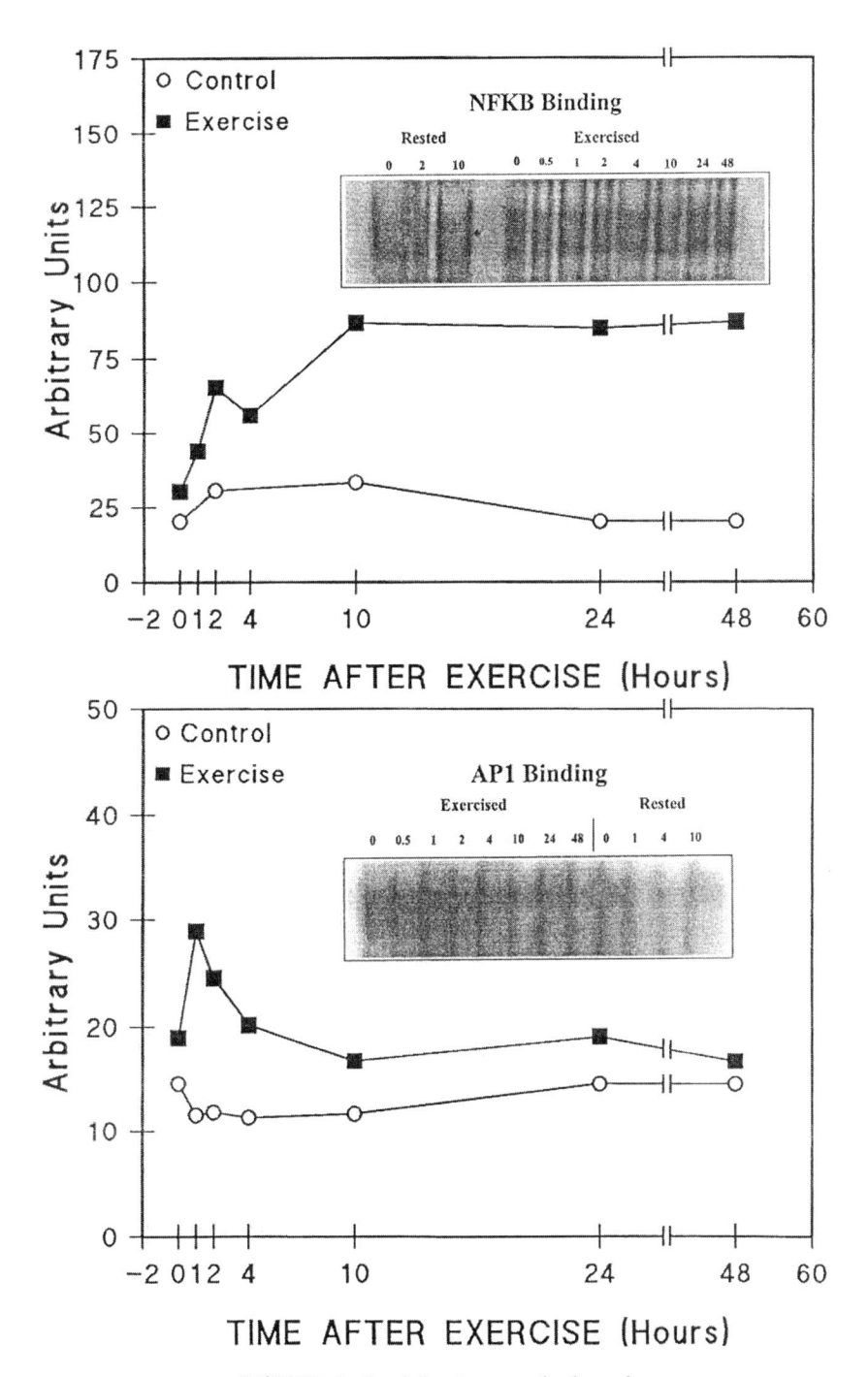

FIGURE 1. *See following page for legend.*

gene expression, oxidative stress is a well-established mechanism for increasing AP-1 binding to target genes, including antioxidant enzymes.[35] Furthermore, activation of the kinases involved in the AP-1 pathway may phosphorylate enzymes having critical roles in other oxidative stress-sensitive signaling pathways.[16]

Mechanisms of NF-κB–induced signaling in response to oxidative stress is well defined.[36,37] ROS have been shown to activate several kinases that phosphorylate serine residues 32 and 36, or 19 and 23 on the inhibitory subunit (I-κB) of NF-κB, causing its ubiquitination and release from the NF-κB complex. The p50 and p65 dimer subsequently translocates into the nucleus and binds to the κB domain of the target gene promoter, leading to transcriptional activation. Cellular redox status influences NF-κB activation profoundly.[38] Although ROS and other prooxidant cytokines, such as TNF-α, initiate I-κB dissociation, binding of activated and translocated p50 and p65 dimers to the DNA sequence requires a reduced cellular milieu with possible participation of GPX and thioredoxin.[35]

Several antioxidant enzymes contain NF-κB and AP-1–binding sites in their gene promoter region, such as MnSOD and γ-glumatylcysteine synthetase (GCS).[36] Therefore, they are potential targets for exercise-activated up-regulation via the NF-κB signaling pathway. Hollander et al.[39] investigated the time course after an acute bout of treadmill running on MnSOD gene expression in rat skeletal muscle. In both type 2a (DVL) and 2b (SVL), NF-κB, binding was significantly increased approximately two hours after the acute exercise bout and remained elevated during the following 48 h (FIG. 1). AP-1 binding in these two muscle types was also dramatically increased by acute exercise, reaching a peak at 30 min but returning to resting levels within a few hours. mRNA abundance for MnSOD in DVL was increased in the exercised rats, whereas an increases in MnSOD protein level was observed in SVL only after 48 h (FIG. 2). These data suggest that an acute bout of exercise may represent a sufficiently large oxidative stress to activate MnSOD gene transcription via NF-κB signaling. Several intermediary steps leading to increased mRNA levels remain to be delineated.

Despite the increased MnSOD mRNA abundance, only a small increase in the MnSOD protein content was observed, with no change in enzyme activity in type 2a or type 1 muscle during the 48-hour postexercise period. These findings were consistent with previous reported data.[40,41] Substantial up-regulation of MnSOD may require sustained and cumulative stimulation on these redox-sensitive pathways, which conceivably occurs during chronic exercise training.[42–44] It is also possible that the intracellular environment in the trained muscle is more protective against

---

FIGURE 1. Electromobility shift assay showing NF-kB (*top panel*) and AP-1 (*lower panel*) binding in rat vastus lateralis muscle using nuclear extracts with multiple runs. Assay reaction contained 20 μg of nuclear extract protein, 1x gel shift reaction buffer, 0.5 μg poly [dI-dC], and ≈0.1 ng of ^{32}P-labeled probe (50,000 cpm), with a total volume of 30 μL. Each point represents pooled samples from six animals.

FIGURE 2. Relative abundance of MnSOD mRNA (*top panel*) and enzyme protein content (*lower panel*) in rat vastus lateralis muscle. Each data point represents the mean (±SEM) from six animals, derived from autoradiographic signals. Relative abundance of mRNA was normalized with the 18S signal of the same sample as a reference. $^*P<0.05$; $^+P<0.01$, exercise vs. control.

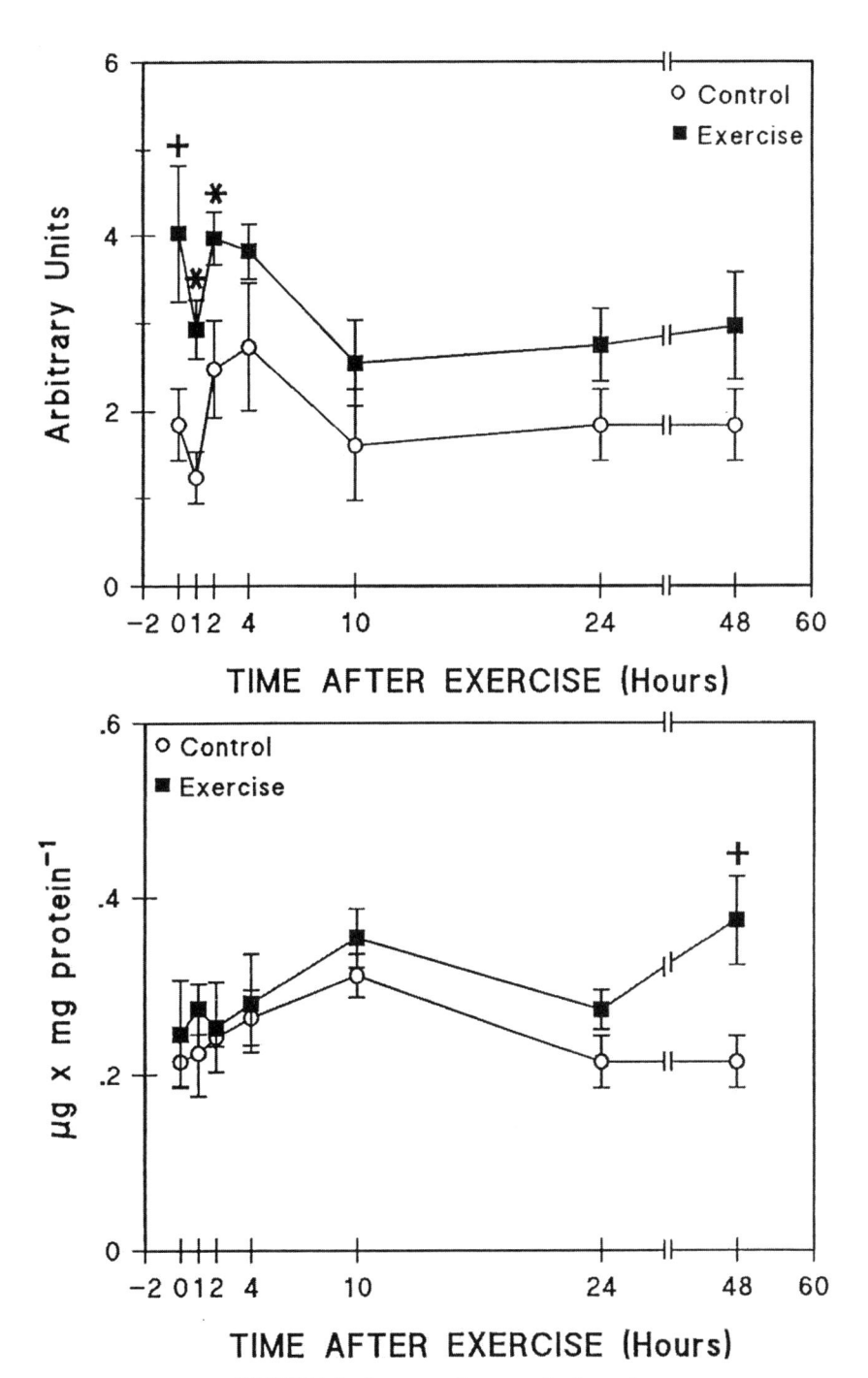

FIGURE 2. *See preceding page for legend.*

rapid degradation of MnSOD mRNA following transcriptional activation, and thus more conducive to protein synthesis.

EXERCISE TRAINING INCREASES THE EFFICACY OF ANTIOXIDANT SUPPLEMENTATION

While exercise training and antioxidant supplementation may independently increase endogenous antioxidant reserve and protect against oxidative injury, the combination of the two regimens may provide additional benefit. This is because (a) endurance training improves muscle (skeletal and myocardial) microperfusion status, due to the adaptation of angiogenesis that facilitates the transport and incorporation of certain antioxidants into the tissues,[45] and (b) key enzymes controlling the biosynthesis of some antioxidants may be activated or induced by acute and/or chronic exercise.[46] A good example to illustrate this potential benefit of exercise is glutathione (GSH) homeostasis in heart ischemia-reperfusion (I-R).

GSH is a major nonenzymatic antioxidant and has been reported to play an important role in protecting the skeletal muscle from exercise-induced oxidative injury and fatigue.[47] In the heart GSH serves as a critical antioxidant, as the levels of antioxidant enzymes and vitamin E are relatively low compared to myocardial oxidative potential.[48] The role of GSH is clearly demonstrated in the antioxidant protection against myocardial I-R injury.[49,50] Depletion of endogenous GSH has been shown to intensify oxidative damage induced by I-R.[51–53] However, supplementation of exogenous GSH by intraperitoneal or intravenous injection has demonstrated a limited and controversial effect on increasing tissue GSH levels and improving functional performance in a postischemic heart.[54] A major obstacle is that high plasma GSH concentration, resulting from exogenous supplementation can pose a strong feedback inhibition on the rate-limiting enzyme GCS and impair operation of the γ-glutamyl cycle.[55] Oral GSH ingestion, on the other hand, has been advocated as a more effective method to increase tissue GSH.[56] Since previous studies in our laboratory and those of others have shown that endurance training could increase γ-glutamyl transpeptidase (GGT) and GCS activity in the myocardium and skeletal muscle,[57–59] we hypothesized that this important adaptation may facilitate GSH cross-membrane transport and resynthesis, resulting in increased GSH levels in the cardiomyocytes for better protection against I-R.

To test this hypothesis, an open-chest *in situ* rat heart model was employed, wherein the main coronary artery was surgically occluded for 45 min followed by a 30-min reperfusion or sham operation.[60] Prior to surgery rats were either trained by running on a treadmill employing a progressive workload for 10 weeks or remained sedentary. Half of each group of rats was fed a GSH-supplemented diet at the dose of 5 g/kg during the final 17 days of training. The other half group received a control diet. The results showed that GSH supplementation alone only had marginal improvement on cardiovascular function and did not change myocardial antioxidant capacity or susceptibility to I-R injury. GSH-supplemented and -trained (T/GSH) rats demonstrated 18% ($P < 0.05$) higher left ventricle peak systolic pressure (LVSP) and 29% ($P < 0.05$) greater postischemic contractility (+dP/dt), compared to controls (FIG. 3). T/GSH hearts had 15% ($P < 0.05$) higher GSH reserve and 32% higher GSH:GSSG ratio ($P < 0.05$) than untrained controls after I-R. I-R–induced myocar-

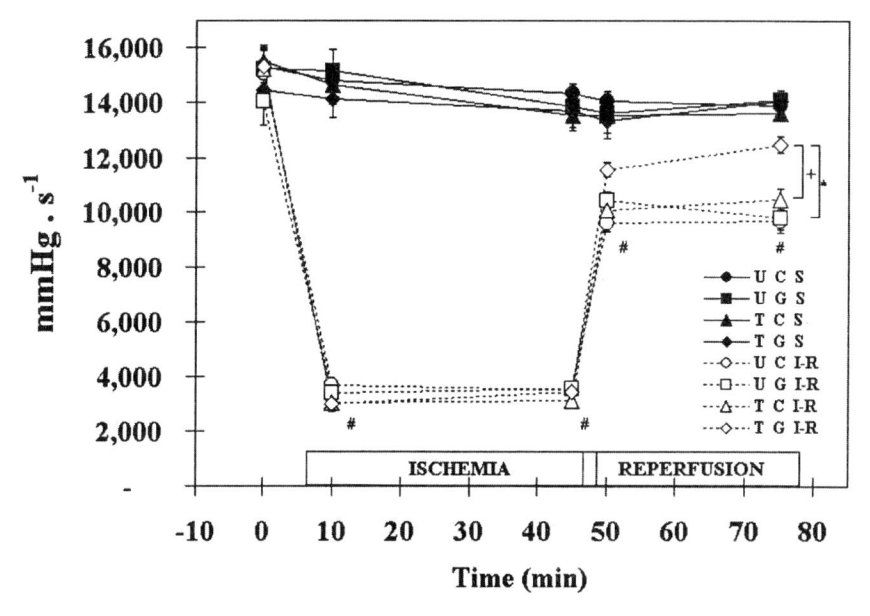

FIGURE 3. Response of left ventricle contractility (+dP/dt) to ischemia-reperfusion (I-R) and sham surgery (S) in trained (T) and untrained (U) rats fed either a control (C) or GSH-supplemented diet (G). #$P<0.01$, I-R vs. sham in a given time point. *$P<0.05$, T/G vs. U/G or U/C; +$P<0.05$, T/G vs. T/C.

dial lipid peroxidation (measured by MDA content) and lesions (measured LDH release to plasma) were significantly reduced with T/GSH-S treatment. Although myocardial antioxidant enzymes SOD and GPX, and glutathione reductase (GR) activities were increased with training in both dietary groups, training alone had limited protection against I-R–induced functional deterioration, lipid peroxidation, or lesions. Hepatic GCS activity and myocardial GGT activity were elevated in the trained rats.[60] Moreover, GSH contents in the liver and plasma were increased in T/GSH-S rats in response to ischemic insult. These data indicate that training enhances the efficacy of GSH supplementation due to adaptation of myocardial and hepatic enzymes in the γ-glutamyl cycle.

CONCLUSION

Skeletal muscle is a remarkably adaptive tissue that is capable of changing its morphological, physiological, and biochemical properties in response to various perturbations. The adaptations are accomplished by various signal transduction pathways that relay external stimuli to changes in intracellular enzyme activity and/or gene expression. Exercise-induced oxidative stress serves as an important signal to stimulate muscle adaptation of antioxidant systems via activation of the redox-sensitive signaling pathways. While an acute bout of muscular contraction is sufficient to activate these pathways, up-regulation of enzyme protein synthesis requires cumulative effects from repeated bouts of exercise, that is, exercise training. Training adaptation also allows the cell to incorporate higher levels of exogenous antioxidants in forms of dietary supplementation. Despite higher antioxidant enzyme activities, aged muscle demonstrates lower messenger RNA levels and weakened transcription factor binding to relevant sequences on antioxidant genes. Whether or not exercise would be effective in reversing the age-related decline in antioxidant adaptation requires further research.

REFERENCES

1. MORLEY, J.E., R.N. BAUMGARTNER, R. ROUBENOFF & K.S. NAIR. 2001. Sarcopenia. J. Lab. Clin. Med. **137:** 231–243.
2. WEINDRUCH, R. 1995. Interventions based on the possibility that oxidative stress contributes to sarcopenia. J. Gerontol. **50:** 157–161.
3. LEE., C, L.E. ASPNES, S.S. CHUNG, et al. 1997. Influences of caloric restriction on age-related skeletal muscle fiber characteristics and miochondrial changes in rats and mice. Ann. N. Y. Acad. Sci. **854:** 182–191.
4. FRIES, J.F. 1996. Physical activity, the compression of morbidity, and the health of the elderly. J. R. Soc. Med. **89:** 64–68.
5. TRAPPE, S., D. WILLIAMSON, M. GODARD, et al. 2000. Effect of resistance training on single muscle fiber contractile function in older men. J. Appl. Physiol. **89:** 143–152.
6. BALAGOPAL, P., J.G. SCHEMKE, P. ADES, et al. 2001. Age effect on transcript levels and synthesis rate of muscle MHC and response to resistance exercise. Am. J. Physiol. **280:** E203–208.
7. JI, L.L., C. LEEUWENBURGH, S. LEICHTWEIS, et al. 1998. Oxidative Stress and Aging: Role of Exercise and its Influences on Antioxidant Sythems. Ann. N. Y. Acad. Sci. **854:** 102–117.
8. MEYDANI, M. & W.J. EVANS. 1993. Free radicals, exercise, and aging. In Free Radicals in Aging. B.P. Yu, Ed. 183–204. CRC Press. Boca Raton, Florida.
9. BEJMA, J. & L.L. JI. 1999. Aging and acute exercise enhances free radical generation and oxidative damage in skeletal muscle. J. Appl. Physiol. **87:** 465–470.
10. ZERBA, E., T.E. KOMOROWSKI & J.A. FAULKNER. 1990. Free radical injury to skeletal muscle of young, adult, and old mice. Am. J. Physiol. **258:** C429–C435.
11. PEDERSEN, B.M. & L. HOFFMAN-GOETZ. 2000. Exercise and immune system: regulation, integration and adaptation. Physiol. Rev. **80:** 1055–1081.
12. CANNON, J.G. & J.B. BLUMBERG. 1994. Acute phase immune responses in exercise. In Exercise and Oxygen Toxicity. C.K. Sen, L. Packer & O. Hanninen, Eds.: 447–479. Elsevier Science. New York.
13. PIZZA, F.X., I.J. HERNANDEZ & J.G. TIDBALL. 1998. Nitric oxide synthase inhibition reduces muscle inflammation and necrosis in modified muscle use. J. Leukocyte Biol. **64:** 427–433.
14. NAVARRO, A., J.M. LOPEZ-CEPERO & M.J.S. DEL PINO. 2001. Skeletal muscle and aging. Front. Biosci. **6:** 26–44.
15. HARMAN, D. Aging: a theory based on free radical and radiation chemistry. 1956. J. Gerontol. **11:** 298–300.
16. FINKEL, T. & N. HOLBROOK. 2000. Nature **408:** 239–247.
17. JI, L.L. 1995. Exercise and free radical generation: role of cellular antioxidant systems. In Exercise and Sport Science Review. J. Holloszy, Ed. 135–166. Williams & Wilkins Co. Baltimore, Maryland.
18. JI, L.L., D. DILLON & E. WU. 1990. Alteration of antioxidant enzymes with aging in rat skeletal muscle and liver. Am. J. Physiol. **258:** R918–R923.
19. OH-ISHI, S., T. KIZAKI, H. YAMASHITA, et al. 1996. Alteration of superoxide dismutase iso-enzyme activity, content, and mRNA expression with aging in rat skeletal muscle. Mech. Ageing Dev. **84:** 65–76.

20. HOLLANDER, J., J. BEJMA, T. OOKAWARA, et al. 2000. Superoxide dismutase gene expression in skeletal muscle: fiber-specific effect of age. Mech. Ageing Dev. **116:** 33–45.
21. MEYER, M., R. SCHRECK & P.A. BAEUERLE. 1993. Hydrogen peroxide and antioxidants have opposite effects on activation of NF-κB and AP-1 in intact cells: AP-1 as secondary antioxidant-response factor. EMBO J. **12:** 2005–2015.
22. SCHRECK, R. & P.A. BAEUERLE. 1991. The role of oxygen radical as a second messenger. Trends Cell Biol. **1:** 39–42.
23. HO, Y.S., A.J. HOWARD & J.D. CRAPO. 1991. Molecular structure of a functional rat gene for manganese-containing superoxide dismutase. Am. J. Respir. Cell. Mol. Biol. **4:** 278–286.
24. WARNER, B.B., L. STUART, S. GEBB & J.R. WISPE. 1996. Redox regulation of manganese superoxide dismutase. Am. J. Physiol. **271:** L150–L158.
25. MCARDLE, A., D. PATTWELL, A. VASILAKI, et al. 2001. Contractile activity-induced oxidative stress: cellular origin and adaptive responses. Am. J. Physiol. Cell Physiol. **280:** C621–627.
26. MCARDLE, A. & M.J. JACKSON. 2000. Exercise, oxidative stress and ageing. J. Anat. **197:** 539–541.
27. SEN, C.K. 1995. Oxidants and antioxidants in exercise. J. Appl. Physiol. **79:** 675–686.
28. ARONSON, D., M.A. VIOLAN, S.D. DUFRESNE, et al. 1997. Exercise stimulates the mitogen-activated protein kinase pathway in human skeletal muscle. J. Clin. Invest. **99:** 1251–1257.
29. BOPPART, M.D., D. ARONSON, L. GIBSON, et al. 1999. Eccentric exercise markedly increases c-Jun NH$_2$-terminal kinase activity in human skeletal muscle. J. Appl. Physiol. **87:** 1668–1673.
30. WIDEGREN, U., X.J. JIANG, A. KROOK, et al. 1998. Divergent effects of exercise on metabolic and mitogenic signaling pathways in human skeletal muscle. FASEB J. **12:** 1379–1389.
31. KROOK, A., U. WIDEGREN, X.J. JIANG, et al. 2000. Effects of exercise on mitogen- and stress-activated kinase signal transduction in human skeletal muscle. Am. J. Physiol. **279:** R1716–1721.
32. WRETMAN, C., U. WIDEGREN, A. LIONIKAS, et al. 2000. Differential activation of mitogen-activated protein kinase signalling pathways by isometric contractions in isolated slow- and fast-twitch rat skeletal muscle. Acta Physiol. Scand. **170:** 45–99.
33. NADER, G.A. & K.A. ESSER. 2001. Intracellular signaling specificity in skeletal muscle in response to different modes of exercise. J. Appl. Physiol. **90:** 1936–1942.
34. PULVERER, B.J., J.M. KYRIAKIS, J. AVRUCH, et al. 1991. Phosphorylation of c-Jun mediated MAP kinases. Nature **353:** 670–674.
35. MEYER, M., H.L. PAHL & P.A. BAEUERLE. 1994. Regulation of the transcription factors NF-kB and AP-1 by redox changes. Chem.-Biol. Interactions **91:** 91–100.
36. ALLEN, R.G. & M. TRESINI. Oxidative stress and gene regulation. 2000. Free Radic. Biol. Med. **28:** 463–499.
37. FLOHE, L., R. BRIGELIUS-FLOHE, C. SLIOU, et al. 1997. Redox regulation of NF-kappaB activation. Free Radic. Biol. Med. **22:** 1115–1126.
38. SEN, C.K. & L. PACKER. 1996. Antioxidant and redox regulation of gene transcription. FASEB J. **10:** 709–720.
39. HOLLANDER, J., R. FIEBIG, M. GORE, et al. 2001. Superoxide dismutase gene expression is activated by a single bout of exercise in rat skeletal muscle. Pflugers Arch. **442:** 426–434.
40. OH-ISHI, S., T. KIZAKI, J. NAGASAWA, et al. 1997. Effects of endurance training on superoxide dismutase activity, content, and mRNA expression in rat muscle. Clin. Exp. Pharm. Phys. **24:** 326–332.
41. OH-ISHI, S., T. KIZAKI, T. OOKAWARA, et al. 1997. The effect of exhaustive exercise on the antioxidant enzyme system in skeletal muscle from calcium-deficient rats. Pflugers Arch.- Eur. J. Physiol. **435:** 767–774.
42. GORE, M., R. FIEBIG, J. HOLLANDER & L.L. JI. 1998. Endurance training alters antioxidant enzymes gene expression in rat skeletal muscle. Can. J. Physiol. Pharmacol. **76:** 1139–1145.

43. HOLLANDER, J., R. FIEBIG, M. GORE, et al. 1999. Superoxide dismutase gene expression: fiber-specific adaptation to endurance training. Am. J. Physiol. **277:** R856–R862.
44. LEEUWENBURGH, C., J. HOLLANDER, S. LEICHTWEIS, et al. 1997. Adaptations of glutathione antioxidant system to endurance training are tissue and muscle fiber specific. Am. J. Physiol. **272:** R363–R369.
45. GUSTAFSSON, T. & W.E. KRAUS. 2001. Exercise-induced angiogenesis-related growth and transcription factors in skeletal muscle, and their modification in muscle pathology. Front. Biosci. **6:** D75–89.
46. JI, L.L. & C. LEEUWENBURGH. 1995. Exercise and Glutathione. In Pharmocology in Exercise and Sports. S. Somani, Ed: 97–123. CRC Press. Boca Raton, Florida.
47. SEN, C.K. & L. PACKER. 2000. Thiol homeostasis and supplements in physical exercise. Am. J. Clin. Nutr. **72**(suppl): 653–669.
48. JI, L.L. 1999. Oxidative stress in the heart. In Handbook of Oxidants and Antioxidants in Exercise. C.K. Sen, L. Packer & O. Hanninen, Eds.: 689–712. Elsevier Science Publisher. Armsterdam, Netherland.
49. CECONI, C., S. CURELLO, A. CARGNONI, et al. 1988. The role of glutathione status in the protection against ischaemic and reperfusion damage: effects of N-acetyl cysteine. J. Mol. Cell. Cardiol. **20:** 5–13.
50. LESNEFSKY, E.J., I.M. DAUBER & L.D. HORWITZ. 1991. Myocardial sulfhydryl pool alterations occur during reperfusion after brief and prolonged myocardial ischemia in vivo. Circ. Res. **68:** 605–613.
51. BLAUSTEIN, A., S.M. DENEKE, R.I. STOLZ, et al. 1989. Myocardial glutathione depletion impairs recovery after short periods of ischemia. Circulation **80:** 1449–1457.
52. WERNS, S.W., J.C. FANTONE, A. VENTURA & B.R. LUCCHESI. 1992. Myocardial glutathione depletion impairs recovery of isolated blood-perfused hearts after global ischaemia. J. Mol. Cell. Cardiol. **24:** 1215–1220.
53. LEICHTWEIS, S. & L.L. JI. 2001. Glutathione depletion intensifies ischemia-reperfusion induced cardiac dysfunction and oxidative stress. Acta Physiol. Scand. **172:** 1–10.
54. TSAN, M.F., J.E. WHITE & C.L. ROSANO. 1989. Modulation of endothelial GSH concentrations: effect of exogenous GSH and GSH monoethyl ester. J. Appl. Physiol. **66:** 1029–1034.
55. DENEKE, S.M. & B.L. FANBURG. 1989. Regulation of cellular glutathione. Am. J. Physiol. **257:** L163–L173.
56. HAGEN, T.M., G.T. WIERZBICKA, A.H. SILLAU, et al. 1990. Bioavailability of dietary glutathione: effect on plasma concentration. Am. J. Physiol. **259:** G524–G529.
57. LEICHTWEIS, S.B., C. LEEUWENBURGH, D.J. PARMELEE, et al. 1997. Rigorous swim training impairs mitochondrial function in post-ischaemic rat heart. Acta Physiol. Scand. **160:** 139–148.
58. SEN, C.K., E. MARIN, M. KRETZSCHMAR & O. HANNINEN. 1992. Skeletal muscle and liver glutathione homeostasis in response to training, exercise and immobilization. J. Appl. Physiol. **73:** 1265.
59. MARIN, E., M. KRETZSCHMAR, J. AROKOSKI, et al. 1993. Enzymes of glutathione synthesis in dog skeletal muscle and their response to training. Acta Physiol. Scand. **147:** 369.
60. RAMIRES, P. & L.L. JI. 2001. Glutathione supplementation and training increases myocardial resistance to ischemia-reperfusion in vivo. Am. J. Physiol. **281:** H679–H688.

The Role of Apoptosis in the Normal Aging Brain, Skeletal Muscle, and Heart

MICHAEL POLLACK, SHARON PHANEUF, AMIE DIRKS, AND CHRISTIAAN LEEUWENBURGH

Biochemistry of Aging Laboratory, Box 118206, College of Health and Human Performance, College of Medicine, Center for Exercise Science, University of Florida, Gainesville, Florida 32611, USA

ABSTRACT: During aging, there is a significant loss of some postmitotic cells, for example, cardiac and skeletal myocytes. Mitochondrial damage and dysfunction with age may trigger increased apoptosis, and this may explain this increase in cell loss. However, it is still unknown if apoptosis plays an important role in normal aging. *In vitro* it has been shown that several mitochondrial proteins can influence apoptosis, depending on factors such as the mitochondrial membrane potential and cellular redox status. It remains possible that mitochondrial dysfunction due to chronic oxidative stress with age is a cause of apoptosis *in vivo*. This cell loss may be due to mitochondrial-triggered apoptosis caused by age-associated increases in oxidant production or increased activation of mitochondrial permeability transition pores. Results from our laboratory and others are reviewed that relate to apoptosis in the normal aging of the brain cortex, heart, and skeletal muscle. Particular attention is paid to the role of cytochrome *c* release from mitochondria and alterations in the pro- and anti-apoptotic proteins, Bax and Bcl-2, respectively. Our results demonstrate that a tissue-specific adaptation of the Bcl-2/Bax ratio occurs with age and may directly influence the release of cytochrome *c*.

KEYWORDS: death domains; apoptosis; oxidants; nitric oxide; postmitotic tissues; cardiac myocytes; skeletal muscle; brain cortex

INTRODUCTION

Aging is characterized by a progressive deterioration in physiological functions and metabolic processes. During the normal aging of both humans and animals, some postmitotic tissues (e.g., heart, skeletal muscle, and brain) have been associated with a decrease in the total number of cells.[1–6] Therefore, a reduction in the total number of viable cells may lead to an accelerated decline in function in the heart, brain, and skeletal muscle. In addition to cell loss via necrosis, apoptosis may be a major factor contributing to the loss of postmitotic cells with age. In this paper, we examine whether apoptosis is a potential mechanism for cell loss with age and the

---

Address for correspondence: Christiaan Leeuwenburgh, Ph.D., University of Florida, Biochemistry of Aging Laboratory, 25 FLG, Stadium Road, P.O. Box 118206, Gainesville, FL 32611. Voice: 352-392-9575, ext. 1356; fax: 352-392-0316.
cleeuwen@ufl.edu; web page: http://grove.ufl.edu/~cleeuwen/

role that mitochondria may play in influencing the apoptotic process in postmitotic tissues.

The term *apoptosis* is used to describe programmed cell death, a type of cell death involved in cellular development that is distinct from necrosis. It is generally assumed that apoptotic cells die by design, whereas necrotic cells die by accident and lethal injury.[7] Researchers became interested in apoptosis after it was demonstrated in the nematode *Caenorhabditis elegans*, followed by the identification of homologous death genes in other organisms.[8] While necrotic cells swell, apoptotic cells typically shrink and detach from surrounding parenchymal cells. Concurrently, the cell volume decreases and the chromatin condenses at the edge of the nucleus.

One classic case of the role of apoptosis in development is the elimination of tissues, transitory organs, and phylogenetic vestiges. For example, the pronephros and mesonephros are eliminated by apoptosis in higher vertebrates. Anuran tails and gills undergo apoptosis as tadpoles change into frogs. Moreover, the roundworm *Caenorhabditis elegans* eliminates exactly 131 of its initial 1090 cells as it develops into an adult.[9] Another classic example concerns programmed cell death in tissue remodeling. As vertebrate limb buds develop, for example, in chick, duck, and humans, webbing between digits in the hind limbs is removed by apoptosis.[9] In these cases, aging is under strict genetic control and therefore is truly *programmed* cell death. However, senescent aging may largely be due to "wear and tear" mechanisms, which may lead to apoptosis. These "wear and tear" processes include oxygen radicals, mitochondrial DNA damage, and the formation of glycooxidation products. Nevertheless, a programmed mechanism that triggers apoptosis may become activated with age in postmitotic tissues. Future studies will need to distinguish between these two possibilities.

Apoptosis can be divided into three nondistinct phases: an induction phase, an effector phase, and a degradation phase. The induction phase depends on death-inducing signals to stimulate apoptotic signal-transduction cascades. Some of these death-inducing signals include reactive oxygen and nitrogen intermediates, TNF-α, ceramide (a sphingolipid), overactivation of Ca^{2+} pathways, and alterations in the Bcl-2 family proteins, such as Bax and Bad.[10–14] In phase two, the effector phase, the cell becomes committed to death by the action of a key regulator, that is, death domain activation from the cell surface, nuclear activators (such as p53), or activation of mitochondrial-induced pathways (release of cytochrome *c* and/or apoptosis-inducing factors, AIF). The final phase, a degradation phase, involves both cytoplasmic and nuclear events. In the cytoplasm, a complex cascade of protein-cleaving enzymes called caspases (cysteine proteases) is activated. In the nucleus, the nuclear envelope breaks down, endonucleases are activated causing DNA fragmentation, and the chromatin condenses. In addition, mitochondrial factors, such as AIF, can migrate to the nucleus and cause large-scale DNA fragmentation. Last, the cell is fragmented into apoptotic bodies and phagocytosed by surrounding cells or macrophages.[7,15]

Aberrant regulation of apoptosis contributes to well-known pathologies, such as neurodegenerative diseases, autoimmune diseases, cancer, and viral infections.[16] Despite the tremendous interest in apoptosis research, few studies have attempted to determine if apoptosis plays a role in normal aging in postmitotic tissues. There is evidence that apoptosis occurs with normal aging in postmitotic tissues, but the mechanisms remain unknown. If the mechanisms underlying the increase in apoptosis with age could be identified, it might help explain the loss of function with age. Also, such information may lead to specific therapeutic interventions that could attenuate this cell loss.

APOPTOSIS AND MITOCHONDRIAL CONTROL

Recent evidence in cell culture indicates that mitochondria exhibit major functional and structural changes that regulate apoptosis. First, the mitochondrial inner-transmembrane potential ($\Delta\Psi_m$) collapses prior to classical morphological signs of apoptosis. Second, studies using cell-free systems and isolated mitochondria suggest that specific mitochondrial proteins are released (cytochrome c and AIF) for the activation of endonucleases and caspases that cleave substrates at Asp-Xxx bonds (i.e., after aspartic acid residues).[17,18] Third, drugs, such as cyclosporin, which stabilize mitochondrial membranes, have been shown to inhibit apoptosis.[19–21] Fourth, the antiapoptotic protein Bcl-2 blocks the release of the intermembrane mitochondrial protein cytochrome c, thus often blocking apoptosis as well.[19–21]

These observations indicate that the mitochondria can serve as key regulators of apoptosis via the cytochrome c–mediated pathway (see FIG. 1). Many cells activate apoptosis via the cytochrome c pathway, but they may also use mitochondrial pathways involving other unknown molecules that reside in the mitochondrial intermembrane space.[18] Cells may also activate apoptosis through mitochondrial-independent ways, for example, death domain activation on the cell surface. Cytochrome c in its holo form (that is, with its heme group attached) associates with apoptotis protease-activating factor 1 (Apaf-1), caspase-9, and ATP to form a complex called an *apoptosome*. When the apoptosome is formed, it can proteolytically activate caspase-9, which leads to the activation of the caspase cascade (caspase-3, caspase-6) and the degradation phase of apoptosis.[22,23] To further complicate the matter, several endogenous cytosolic caspase inhibitors are present, such as XIAP, c-IAP1, and c-IAP2, which can inhibit activation of the caspase cascade.[24,25] These caspase inhibitors (IAPs, inhibitors of apoptosis proteins) may play a significant role in aging in postmitotic tissues, preventing excessive loss of irreplaceble cells in muscle and brain tissues. This possibility is currently under investigation in our laboratory. In addition, the mitochondria may release de-repressor proteins of endogenous caspase inhibitors, such as the newly discovered mitochondrial protein Smac/DIABLO.[26,27]

Another key protein released from mitochondria is AIF.[17] Various apoptotic signals, such as radicals, staurosporin, c-myc, etoposide, or ceramide can lead to mitochondrial release of this proapoptotic protein. AIF is normally confined to mitochondria and colocalizes with heat shock protein-60 (hsp-60). On induction of apoptosis, AIF (but not hsp-60) translocates to the nucleus, resulting in chromatin condensation and large-scale DNA fragmentation.[17] Thus, AIF translocation to the nucleus indicates that AIF is a caspase-independent mitochondrial death effector responsible for partial chromatinolysis.

The Bcl-2 family of proteins are able to regulate apoptosis by controlling the release of cytochrome c. In mammals, the antiapoptotic members of this family include Bcl-2, Bcl-X_L, Mcl-1, A1/Bfl-1, and Bcl-W. The proapoptotic members are Bax, Bcl-X_S, Bak, Bad, Bik, Bim, Bid, Hrk, and Bok. Homologues have been found in birds, frogs, *Caenorhabditis elegans*, and human herpes viruses.[11,28] Still unclear

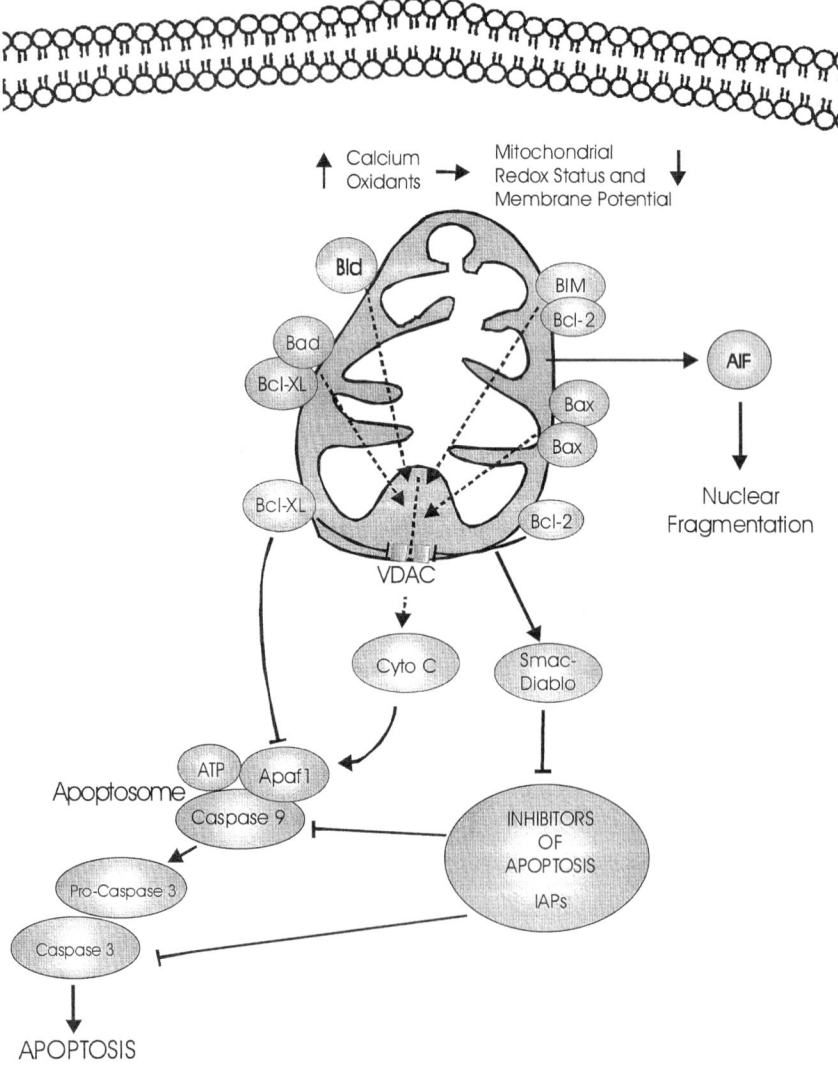

FIGURE 1. Mitochondrial-mediated pathway. Mitochondrial dysfunction could be caused by factors, such as oxidants, increases in Ca^{2+} levels, a decline in redox status, (i.e., glutathione, ATP, NADH), and collapse of mitochondrial membrane potential ($\Delta\Psi_m$). Mitochondrial proteins, such as Bcl-2, Bcl-X_L, Bid, and Bax, and their specific ratios ("check point proteins" for cell death) can influence mitochondrial outer membrane channel, the voltage-dependent anion channel (VDAC), which leads to the release of cytochrome c from the mitochondria. Cytochrome c release could lead to the formation of the "apoptosome" (Apaf-1, caspase-9, dATP), resulting in apoptosis. Other proteins released from the mitochondria, such as apoptosis-inducing factor (AIF) located in the mitochondrial intermembrane space are caspase independent and translocate to the nucleus, causing large-scale DNA fragmentation. Smac-Diablo can be released simultaneously with cytochrome c and functions to inhibit inhibitors of apoptosis proteins (IAPs). Signals and proteins responsible for apoptosis may vary remarkably among cell types and may also originate from the extracellular milieu and the nucleus.

are the exact alterations in the expression of these pro- or antiapoptotic proteins with age and their effects on cytochrome c release.

Bcl-2 family members may undergo a conformational change, inserting themselves into the outer mitochondrial membrane and forming channels. Alternatively, Bcl-2 family members may interact with other proteins to form channels. In this scenario, proteins in the Bcl-2 family interact with mitochondrial membrane proteins to form a channel large enough for intermembrane proteins to pass through (FIG. 1). Channel proteins include the voltage-dependent anion channel (VDAC) and the adenine nucleotide transporter. Since VDAC is known to bind to and be regulated by Bcl-2 type proteins, it is a likely candidate for such a role.[29] VDAC is an attractive candidate because it is known to be a subunit of the mitochondrial permeability transition pore (PTP). The opening of the permeability transition pore results in a loss of membrane potential, organellar swelling, and cytochrome c release.[30] Interestingly, these pores possess several redox-sensitive sites, including one in equilibrium with mitochondrial matrix glutathione and one directly activated by oxidants.[31] Glutathione is increased in skeletal muscle with age[32] and may therefore play an important role in preventing the activation of the permeability transition pore.

Nevertheless, the permeability transition pore cannot be the only target of Bcl-2–type proteins because cytochrome c release can occur in the absence of membrane potential loss, which normally precipitates the permeability transition pore.[33] In summary, alterations of Bcl-2 family proteins during the aging process may be critical in determining when a cell will undergo apoptosis. We will discuss the tissue-specific alterations of these proteins in the brain, skeletal muscle, and the heart in a later section.

REACTIVE OXYGEN AND NITROGEN INTERMEDIATES IN AGING AND APOPTOSIS

The free radical theory of aging proposed by Dr. Harman links senescence to damage inflicted by superoxide-derived radicals and other reactive intermediates generated primarily during mitochondrial respiration.[34–36] Indeed, it was found that one important source of reactive oxygen and nitrogen intermediates is mitochondria.[37–41] Another related theory of aging, the mitochondrial theory of aging, proposes that aging is the result of accumulated free radical damage to mitochondrial DNA (mtDNA). The accumulation of errors in mtDNA results in errors in the polypeptides encoded by mtDNA, leading to dysfunctional proteins in mitochondrial respiratory chain complexes. If a complex is defective, more radicals could be produced, leading to a cycle of increasing mtDNA damage, radical generation, and possibly apoptosis.[42–45] Since aging is characterized by a chronic production of radical intermediates in all tissues,[42,46–48] the consequences, an increase in mtDNA damage,[45,49] may promote the induction of apoptosis with time. Apoptosis may therefore be involved in aging, where it could serve to eliminate nonfunctional, harmful, abnormal, or misplaced cells, especially in advanced age.[10,12–14]

Oxidants can indirectly induce apoptosis by changing cellular redox potentials, depleting reduced glutathione, reducing ATP levels, and decreasing reduced equivalents, such as NADH and NADPH.[31,50–52] These changes can facilitate the formation of permeability transition pores, leading to the subsequent release of cytochrome c. Reactive oxygen and nitrogen species, such as hydrogen peroxide, peroxynitrite, and nitric oxide (NO•), a free radical gas, have been shown to induce apoptosis in several cell lines. For example, Ca^{2+} and oxidants, such as hydrogen peroxide, have additive effects on megachannel permeability transition (MPT) *in vitro*[53] and may, in part, play a role in the increased susceptibility of MPT with age. Mitochondria from aged cells (lymphocytes, brain, and liver) have an increased susceptibility to MPT,[53] which is an apoptotic event that allows release of apoptogenic proteins into the cytosol. Aged cells have been associated with increased mitochondrial oxidant production[48] and elevated intracellular Ca^{2+} levels,[54,55] a favorable intracellular environment for MPT and release of apoptogenic factors.

Nitric oxide is known to be an important regulator of mitochondrial function, cell signaling, and gene expression and it also functions as the endothelial derived relaxing factor.[56] Nitric oxide may directly regulate the activity of cytochrome c oxidase and could therefore have an effect on oxidant production.[57] Nitric oxide can cause apoptosis when administered at high levels. In one study, nitric oxide from sodium nitroprusside was shown to cause hepatocyte apoptosis and hepatocellular enzyme release, which indicates cell damage.[58] Also, exogenous release of NO• from various NO• donors has been shown to trigger apoptosis of rat renal mesangial cells. In striking contrast, nitric oxide is a potent antioxidant at low concentrations and can therefore inhibit apoptosis.[59,60]

Another reactive nitrogen species with apoptotic effects is peroxynitrite. Peroxynitrite is not a radical, but an anion oxidant generated by the reaction of nitric oxide with superoxide. In one experiment, it was shown that treating HL-60 leukemia cells with increasing concentrations of peroxynitrite induced apoptosis in a time- and concentration-dependent manner.[61] However, at low levels researchers found that oxidants can stimulate cells to proliferate, and mild oxidative conditions have been shown to counteract apoptotic stimuli.

Besides the production of reactive intermediates by mitochondria, other endogenous compounds derived from oxidants are also potent mediators of apoptosis. These include fatty acid metabolites, derived from arachidonic acid by the lipoxygenase and cyclooxygenase pathways;[62–64] ceramide, a sphingolipid that can influence overexpression of p53;[65] and advanced glycation end (AGE) products, which were found to increase with age.[66–68] AGE products are produced from glycoxidation reactions, and AGE product formation is accelerated by reactive oxygen intermediates.[69]

AGING AND APOPTOSIS IN POSTMITOTIC TISSUES

Mitotic cells, such as skin cells and cells in the intestinal lining, frequently undergo apoptosis to make space for new healthy cells. Age-enhanced apoptosis, in mitotic cells may be protective mechanisms against age-associated tumorigenesis.[70] In striking contrast, mechanisms preventing apoptosis in postmitotic cells must be available, since postmitotic cell replacement does not occur. If a postmitotic cell is damaged, the possible outcomes are repair, survival in a less functional state, or apoptosis.[10,12–14] Therefore, with normal aging, a variety of factors, such as mitochondrial deterioration from oxygen radicals, products from glycooxidation, and nuclear and mitochondrial DNA damage could eventually influence apoptosis in postmitotic tissues.

TABLE 1. Summary table of changes of Western blot analysis of mitochondrial Bcl-2, Bax, Bcl-2/Bax-ratio, mitochondrial cytochrome *c* release, and caspase-3 activity in the heart, brain, and skeletal muscle of 6- and 24-month-old Fischer 344 rats

6 Months vs. 24-Months	Bcl-2	Bax	Bcl-2/Bax Ratio	Cytosolic Cytochrome *c*	Caspase-3
Heart	↓	→	↓	↑	→
Skeletal Muscle	→	↓	↑	→	→
Brain	→	↓	↑	→	→

NOTE: → no change, ↑ increase, ↓ decrease. From FIGURES 1–5 and Refs. 73 and 74.

The human heart loses a significant number of myocytes during aging by apoptotic and necrotic death. In fact, the initial ventricular myocyte population may decline by as much as 30% as the heart ages; however, it appears that apoptosis is more prevalent in the later stages of aging.[6] In one study of the aging heart of Fischer 344 rats, both necrotic and apoptotic cell death occurred.[6] Necrotic myocytes were localized and quantified by using a myosin monoclonal antibody. Increases in apoptotic myocytes, which was restricted to the left ventricular free wall, were quantified using the TUNEL (terminal deoxynucleotidyl transferase-mediated dUTP-digoxigenin nick-end labeling) assay followed by DNA laddering to confirm DNA strand breaks in myocyte nuclei.[6] This study also showed that apoptosis in the left ventricle increased by more than 200% in the 24-month-old animals compared to the 16-month-old rats, with no change in necrotic cell death, indicating an accelerated rate of apoptosis at a later age.

The underlying mechanism for apoptosis in the heart has not been investigated, but reactive intermediates from nitrogen and oxygen may contribute to oxidative mitochondrial damage. In support of this hypothesis, it should be noted that superoxide and hydrogen peroxide production increased with age in isolated mitochondria and submitochondrial particles from the hearts of mongolian gerbils.[46] Also, such factors as tumor necrosis factor (TNF), angiotensin II, and glucocorticoids are increased with age and also increase reactive oxygen species production.[71] Therefore, increased oxidative stress may play an important role in cardiovascular abnormalities, perhaps through the loss of viable cardiac myocytes.[72]

Research in our laboratory was conducted on the hearts of male Fischer 344 rats. Various assays were performed to measure markers of apoptosis and oxidative stress to determine if there was a relationship between these factors (TABLE 1). We found that cytosolic cytochrome *c* was significantly elevated in the 16- and 24-month-old animals compared to the 6-month-old animals, and this could render myocytes more vulnerable to apoptosis.[73] Also, mitochondrial Bcl-2 levels tended to decrease with age, but no alterations in mitochondrial Bax proteins were observed. Since Bcl-2 can block cytochrome *c* release, this may provide one mechanism for the increase in apoptosis in the aged heart. Nevertheless, no significant differences in caspase activity were found among the three age groups using two different caspase assays. Since apoptosis occurs within minutes to hours, it may be that caspase activity also transiently changed during this time period and that our assays were not sufficiently sensitive to distinguish between caspase activities in the young and old animals. We did find increases in the activity of several key mitochondrial antioxidant enzymes, which indicates an adaptation to age-associated chronic exposure to reactive oxygen species.[73] Barja *et al.* have shown increases in mtDNA damage in the hearts of old animals, which may suggest a link between mitochondrial deterioration and apoptosis.[45]

Only one report exists that documents an age-dependent loss of human skeletal muscle cells by apoptosis.[5] An age-dependent increase in apoptosis (as measured by TUNEL staining) of the striated human muscle fibers of the rhabdosphincter led to a dramatic decrease in the number of striated muscle cells. A direct linear correlation between the age of the specimens and decrease in volume densities of the striated muscle cells was evident. This study concluded that apoptosis represents the morphological basis for the high incidence of stress incontinence.

Studies in our laboratory have been conducted to determine how apoptosis influences age-related muscle loss. Using locomotor skeletal muscle (gastrocnemius) from 6-month and 24-month-old male Fischer 344 rats, we found a 50% increase in mono- and oligonucleosome DNA fragments in skeletal muscle of old rats compared to young animals, indicative of apoptosis and/or loss of nuclei.[74] Since skeletal muscle is multinucleated, further studies are required to determine the significance of a potential loss in nuclei and muscle fibers. We did observe very modest increases in the levels of cytosolic cytochrome c and caspase-3 activity with age; however, these changes were not significant. We did find a significant positive correlation between cytosolic cytochrome c and caspase-3 activity in the Fischer 344 rats ($r = 0.76$). Therefore, it remains possible that there is a relationship between cytochrome c and caspase-3 activity *in vivo* in skeletal muscle. In addition, it remains possible that specific inhibitors for caspases are increased with age that prevent the loss of irreplaceable skeletal muscle cells. Differences seen in heart and skeletal muscle in regulating apoptosis may stem from the chronic oxidative stress the heart is exposed to as compared to skeletal muscle in aging rats.

Recent research, based on new stereological techniques to estimate neuron number, has revealed that during normal aging there is no significant age-related decline in hippocampal and neocortical neurons. However, some age-related decline does occur in the hilus of the dentate gyrus and the subiculum.[75] In other studies, morphological characteristics of apoptosis, such as cell shrinkage and chromatin condensation were found, but only in approximately 2% of the nigral dopaminergic neurons studied.[2] In addition, the mitochondria of these cells were shrunken, and there were signs of oxidative stress even in neurons devoid of apoptotic features.[76]

Research in our laboratory has focused on detecting apoptosis and apoptotic markers in brain cortex from young (6-month) and old (24-month) male Fischer 344 rats. Our studies are some of the first to systematically determine if apoptosis plays a role in the normal aging brain. We measured markers of apoptosis, such as cytosolic cytochrome c levels and caspase activation, as well as levels of mitochondrial Bcl-2 family proteins. First, we determined if superoxide production was increased in isolated mitochondria from the brain cortices of the old rats. Indeed, superoxide production was significantly increased in the old Fischer 344 rats (FIG. 2). This finding supports our hypothesis that oxidants may influence the induction of mitochondrial-mediated apoptosis in the brain.

We found no changes in the levels of cytochrome c (FIG. 3) in the cytosol or in caspase-3 activity (FIG. 4) between the young and old animals. However, Western blotting for Bax and Bcl-2 proteins from brain cortex mitochondria did show age-related alterations (FIG. 5), which could partly explain the attenuation of cytochrome

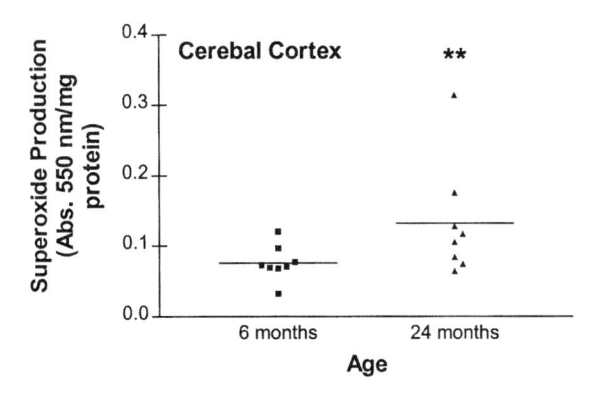

FIGURE 2. Oxidant production was determined by cytochrome c reduction in the mitochondria from cerebral cortices of 6-month-old ($n = 8$) and 24-month-old ($n = 8$) male Fischer 344 rats. Cerebral cortices were homogenized in isolation buffer on ice and centrifuged at 4000 rpm for 16 minutes at 4°C. The supernatant was then centrifuged at 13,700 rpm for 11 min at 4°C, and the resulting mitochondrial pellet was resuspended in isolation buffer. The change in absorbance was measured at 550 nm at 37°C using a spectrophotometric plate reader from Molecular Devices (Sunnyvale, CA). Protein concentration was analyzed using the Bradford assay, and results are expressed as absorbance units/mg protein. There was a significant increase in superoxide production in the mitochondria isolated from the cortices of the old animals compared to the young animals ($P<0.039$).

c release and caspase activation. Bcl-2 levels tended to increase in the old animals relative to the young animals. This finding is supported by another study, which found that Bcl-2 was up-regulated in the hippocampus and cerebellum of aged (24 mo) Fischer 344 rats.[77] Interestingly, Bcl-2 was also found to significantly increase with age in 20 human postmortem brains. The brains were from normally aged individuals, none of whom died of CNS-related or psychiatric illnesses.[78] By contrast, Western blotting for Bax showed a significant decrease in Bax levels in the older samples ($P<0.05$). An increased Bcl-2/Bax ratio would inhibit cytochrome c release and activation of caspase-3, resulting in decreased apoptosis. Perhaps the increased Bcl-2/Bax ratio results from an adaptive defense to the increased superoxide production in the cortex of the older rats.

Last, using a cell-death detection ELISA (FIG. 6), we found no increase in apoptosis with age. This assay quantifies cytosolic mono- and oligonucleosomes using monoclonal antibodies directed against DNA-associated histones. The increased superoxide production in the brain cortex of the older rats may have induced apoptosis above background levels in a small number of the cells. However, this miniscule amount of apoptotic death may not have been detectable for two reasons: (1) the few apoptotic cells in the old animals did not provide a sufficient signal, or (2) recent apoptotic cells were recognized and effectively removed by macrophages or neighboring cells. Alternatively, the increased superoxide production in the brain cortex of the older rats may not have been enough to induce a significant amount of apoptosis above normal levels. This is in agreement with the literature, which suggests that neurodegenerative disorders are characterized by extensive neuron death but that normal aging and apoptosis in neurons are less well defined and not often document-

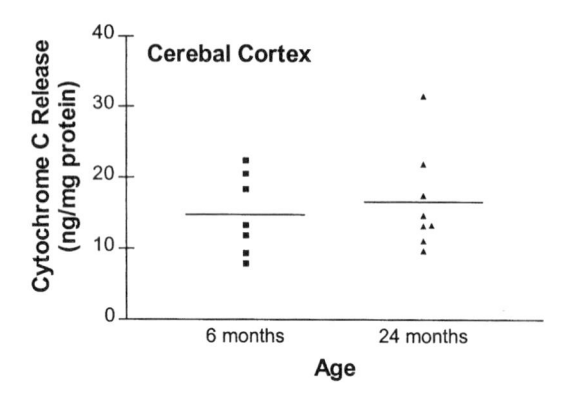

FIGURE 3. Cytosolic cytochrome *c* levels were analyzed in the brains of the young and old rats using a cytochrome *c* **ELISA kit** (R&D Systems, Minneapolis, MN). The cytosol was used to measure the levels of cytochrome *c*, and the levels were normalized to mg protein. Cytochrome *c* levels in cytosol of brain cortices are not significantly different in the old vs. the young animals.

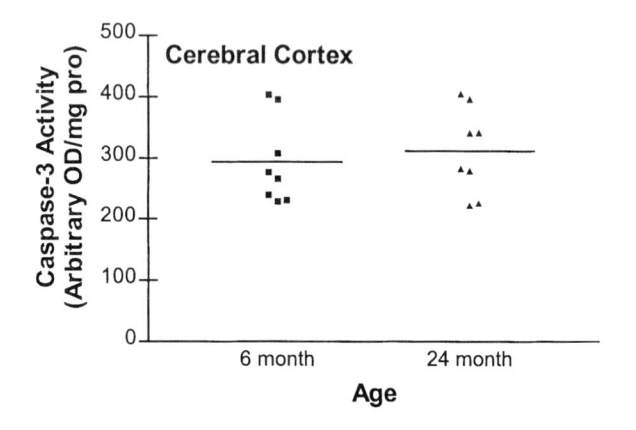

FIGURE 4. Cytosolic caspase-3 activity in the brain was determined using a fluorogenic peptide (Ac-DEVD-AMC; Pharmingen, San Diego) **for caspase-3.** Caspase activity was performed on isolated cytosolic fractions. Briefly, 1 mL of assay buffer per sample was prepared (20 mM HEPES and 10% glycerol with total volume of 100 mL in distilled H_2O, pH 7.5). We added 2 µL 1 M DTT and 14 µL Ac-DEVD-AMC (1 mg suspended in 1 mL DMSO) to assay buffer. Then 50 µL of brain cortex cytosol was added from each sample, vortexed, and incubated for 1 hour at 37°C. Fluorescence was determined with an excitation wavelength of 380 nm and an emission wavelength of 440 nm. As a positive control, 100 ng of purified active caspase-3 (Pharmingen, San Diego) was used in place of sample. We found no difference in cytosolic caspase-3 activity in the old animals compared to the young animals.

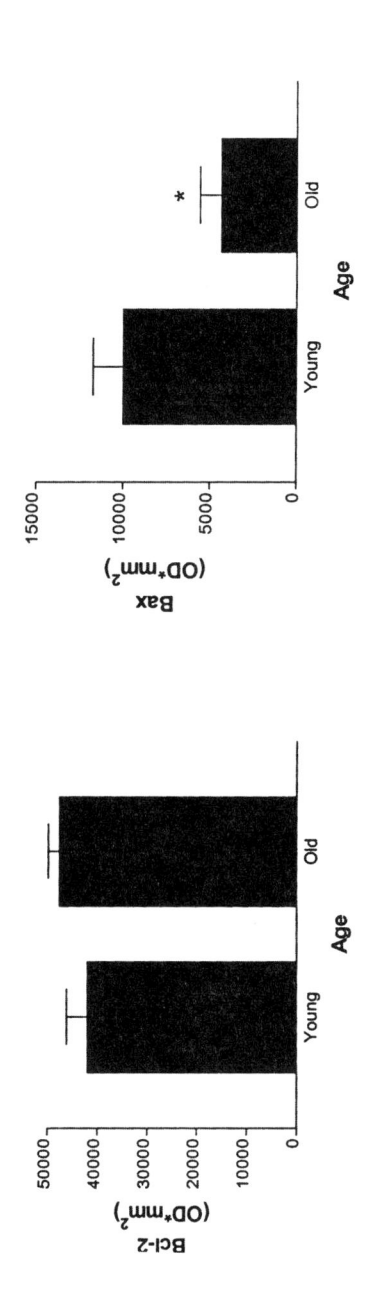

FIGURE 5. The effect of age on mitochondrial Bcl-2 and Bax levels in brain cortices of male Fischer F344 rats. For Western analysis, the proteins were separated on precast 4–12% polyacrylamide gels (BMA, Rockland). Western blots were performed using 15 μg of protein per well. Proteins were transferred onto a nitrocellulose membrane (Bio-Rad Laboratories) and blocked overnight using a solution of 0.05% Tween, 5.0% milk, and the primary polyclonal antibodies Bcl-2 or Bax (Santa Cruz Biotechnology, Santa Cruz). Bcl-2 was diluted 1:100, and Bax was diluted 1:200. Membranes were then incubated for 90 minutes in anti-rabbit IgG secondary antibody, diluted 1:1000. Values presented are means ± SEM as arbitrary optical density (OD) units/mg protein. For Bcl-2, OD for the young samples was 42020 ± 4087, $n = 3$; the OD for the old samples was 47610 ± 2244, $n = 5$; $P = 0.25$. For Bax, OD for the young samples was 10010 ± 1709, $n = 4$; the OD for the old samples was 4345 ± 1246, $n = 4$; *$P = 0.036$.

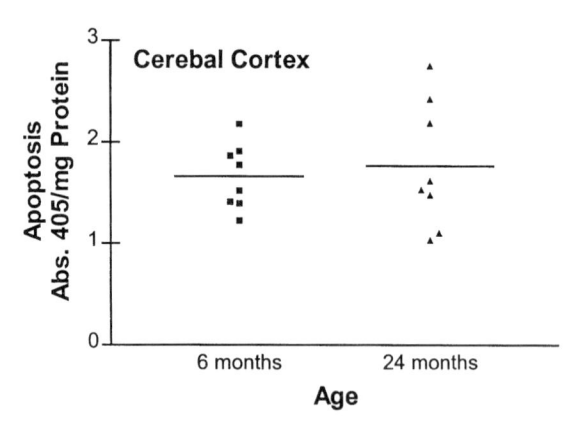

FIGURE 6. DNA fragmentation was quantified by determination cytosolic mononucleosomes and oligonucleosomes using an ELISA kit (Roche Molecular Biochemicals, Germany). This kit quantifies cytosolic mono- and oligonucleosome-bound DNA using monoclonal antibodies directed against DNA-associated histones. Brain cortex cytosol was used directly as an antigen source in the sandwich enzyme immunoassay. Double absorbancies were read at 405 nm and 490 nm, and all samples were run in duplicate. The ELISA showed no significant difference in cell death between the young and old animals.

ed.[75] Adaptive responses as documented in our study may prevent cell loss in the aging brain. It appears that structural changes in neurons may be the primary neurobiological alterations to impair function in normal aging and differ from those in neurodegenerative disorders such as Alzheimer's disease.[75]

In summary, our aging studies demonstrate that these three postmitotic tissues show different alterations in pro- and antiapoptotic proteins with aging (TABLE 1). In cardiac myocytes, the increased release in cytochrome c may be directly due to a decrease in the Bcl-2/Bax ratio. In striking contrast, the brain (cortex) and skeletal muscle (gastrocnemius) showed an increase in the Bcl-2/Bax ratio, which may explain the decrease in cytochrome c release and increased resistance to apoptosis. These results show that *in vivo* studies on the role of apoptosis in normal aging animals will be challenging, specifically in postmitotic tissues. Also, the use of innovative models, such as accelerated aging models (e.g., senescence-accelerated mice) and transgenic mice models may provide more conclusive results[79,80] on the *in vivo* role mitochondria play in controlling apoptosis.

ACKNOWLEDGMENTS

This research was supported by grants from the Society of Geriatric Cardiology and the National Institute on Aging (AG17994-01 and AG 10485-08). We would like to thank Phuong Nguyen for the graphical assistance.

REFERENCES

1. ADAMS, V., S. GIELEN, R. HAMBRECHT & G. SCHULER. 2001. Apoptosis in skeletal muscle. Front. Biosci. **6:** D1–D11.
2. ANGLADE, P., S. VYAS, E.C. HIRSCH & Y. AGID. 1997. Apoptosis in dopaminergic neurons of the human substantia nigra during normal aging. Histol. Histopathol. **12:** 603–610.
3. ANVERSA, P., B. HILER, R. RICCI, et al. 1986. Myocyte cell loss and myocyte hypertrophy in the aging rat heart. J. Am. Coll. Cardiol. **8:** 1441–1448.
4. ANVERSA, P., et al. 1990. Myocyte cell loss and myocyte cellular hyperplasia in the hypertrophied aging rat heart. Circ. Res. **67:** 871–885.
5. STRASSER, H., et al. 2000. Age dependent apoptosis and loss of rhabdosphincter cells. J. Urol. **164:** 1781–1785.
6. KAJSTURA, J., et al. 1996. Necrotic and apoptotic myocyte cell death in the aging heart of Fischer 344 rats. Am. J. Physiol. **271:** H1215–228.
7. KERR, J.F., A.H. WYLLIE & A.R. CURRIE. 1972. Apoptosis: a basic biological phenomenon with wide-ranging implications in tissue kinetics. Br. J. Cancer **26:** 239–257.
8. SULSTON, J.E. & H.R. HORVITZ. 1977. Post-embryonic cell lineages of the nematode, *Caenorhabditis elegans.* Dev. Biol. **56:** 110–156.
9. DUKE, R.C., D.M. OJCIUS & J.D. YOUNG. 1996. Cell suicide in health and disease. Sci. Am. **275:** 80–87.
10. PHANEUF, S. & C. LEEUWENBURGH. 2001. Apoptosis and exercise. Med. Sci. Sports Exercise **33:** 393–396.
11. GREEN, D.R. & J.C. REED. 1998. Mitochondria and apoptosis. Science **281:** 1309–1312.
12. WARNER, H.R. Aging and regulation of apoptosis. Curr. Top. Cell. Regul. **35:** 107–121.
13. WARNER, H.R., R.J. HODES & K. POCINKI. 1997. What does cell death have to do with aging? J. Am. Geriatr. Soc. **45:** 1140–1146.
14. WARNER, H.R. 1999. Apoptosis: a two-edged sword in aging. Ann. N. Y. Acad. Sci. **887:** 1–11.
15. SUSIN, S.A., N. ZAMZAMI & G. KROEMER. 1998. Mitochondria as regulators of apoptosis: doubt no more. Biochim. Biophys. Acta **1366:** 151–165.
16. CARSON, D.A. & J.M. RIBEIRO. 1993. Apoptosis and disease. Lancet **341:** 1251–1254.
17. DAUGAS, E., et al. 2000. Mitochondrio-nuclear translocation of AIF in apoptosis and necrosis. FASEB J. **14:** 729–739.
18. PATTERSON, S.D., et al. 2000. Mass spectrometric identification of proteins released from mitochondria undergoing permeability transition. Cell Death Differ. **7:** 137–144.
19. GREEN, D. & G. KROEMER. 1998. The central executioners of apoptosis: caspases or mitochondria? Trends Cell Biol. **8:** 267–271.
20. KLUCK, R.M., E. BOSSY-WETZEL, D.R. GREEN & D.D. NEWMEYER. 1997. The release of cytochrome c from mitochondria: a primary site for Bcl-2 regulation of apoptosis. Science **275:** 1132–1136.
21. GREEN, D.R. & J.C. REED. 1998. Mitochondria and apoptosis. Science **281:** 1309–1312.
22. GREEN, D. & G. KROEMER. 1998. The central executioners of apoptosis: caspases or mitochondria? Trends Cell Biol. **8:** 267–271.
23. LI, P., et al. 1997. Cytochrome c and dATP-dependent formation of Apaf-1/caspase-9 complex initiates an apoptotic protease cascade. Cell **91:** 479–489.
24. BRAUN, J.S., E.I. TUOMANEN & J.L. CLEVELAND. 1999. Neuroprotection by caspase inhibitors. Expert Opin. Investig. Drugs **8:** 1599–1610.
25. HAY, B.A. 2000. Understanding IAP function and regulation: a view from Drosophila. Cell Death Differ. **7:** 1045–1056.
26. MACKENZIE, A. & E. LACASSE. 2000. Inhibition of IAP's protection by Diablo/Smac: new therapeutic opportunities? Cell Death Differ. **7:** 866–867.
27. LIU, Z., et al. 2000. Structural basis for binding of Smac/DIABLO to the XIAP BIR3 domain. Nature **408:** 1004–1008.
28. JURGENSMEIER, J.M., et al. 1997. Bax- and Bak-induced cell death in the fission yeast *Schizosaccharomyces pombe.* Mol. Biol. Cell **8:** 325–339.

29. SHIMIZU, S., M. NARITA & Y. TSUJIMOTO. 1999. Bcl-2 family proteins regulate the release of apoptogenic cytochrome c by the mitochondrial channel VDAC. Nature **399:** 483–487.
30. HENGARTNER, M.O. 2000. The biochemistry of apoptosis. Nature **407:** 770–776.
31. COSTANTINI, P., B.V. CHERNYAK, V. PETRONILLI & P. BERNARDI. 1996. Modulation of the mitochondrial permeability transition pore by pyridine nucleotides and dithiol oxidation at two separate sites. J. Biol. Chem. **271:** 6746–6751.
32. LEEUWENBURGH, C., R. FIEBIG, R. CHANDWANEY & L.L. JI. 1994. Aging and exercise training in skeletal muscle: responses of glutathione and antioxidant enzyme systems. Am. J. Physiol. **267:** R439–445.
33. GROSS, A., J.M. MCDONNELL & S.J. KORSMEYER. 1999. BCL-2 family members and the mitochondria in apoptosis. Genes & Dev **13:** 1899–911.
34. HARMAN, D. 1992. Free radical theory of aging. Mutat. Res. **275:** 257–266.
35. HARMAN, D. 1994. Free-radical theory of aging. Increasing the functional life span. Ann. N. Y. Acad. Sci. **717:** 1–15.
36. HARMAN, D. 1992. Free radical theory of aging: history. Exs **62:** 1–10.
37. CADENAS, E., J.J. PODEROSO, F. ANTUNES & A. BOVERIS. 2000. Analysis of the pathways of nitric oxide utilization in mitochondria. Free Radical Res. **33:** 747–756.
38. GIULIVI, C., J.J. PODEROSO & A. BOVERIS. 198. Production of nitric oxide by mitochondria. J. Biol. Chem. **273:** 11038–11043.
39. LEEUWENBURGH, C. & J. HEINECKE. 2001. Oxidative stress and antioxidants in exercise. Curr. Med. Chem. **8:** 829–838.
40. CADENAS, E. & K.J. DAVIES. 2000. Mitochondrial free radical generation, oxidative stress, and aging. Free. Radic. Biol. Med. **29:** 222–230.
41. BOVERIS, A., L.E. COSTA, J.J. PODEROSO, et al. 2000. Regulation of mitochondrial respiration by oxygen and nitric oxide. Ann. N. Y. Acad. Sci. **899:** 121–135.
42. SASTRE, J., F.V. PALLARDO & J. VINA. 2000. Mitochondrial oxidative stress plays a key role in aging and apoptosis. IUBMB Life **49:** 427–435.
43. BECKMAN, K.B. & B.N. AMES. 1998. Mitochondrial aging: open questions. Ann. N. Y. Acad. Sci. **854:** 118–127.
44. BECKMAN, K.B. & B.N. AMES. 1999. Endogenous oxidative damage of mtDNA. Mutat. Res. **424:** 51–58.
45. BARJA, G. & A. HERRERO. 2000. Oxidative damage to mitochondrial DNA is inversely related to maximum life span in the heart and brain of mammals. FASEB J. **14:** 312–318.
46. SOHAL, R.S., S. AGARWAL & B.H. SOHAL. 1995. Oxidative stress and aging in the Mongolian gerbil (*Meriones unguiculatus*). Mech. Ageing Dev. **81:** 15–25.
47. SOHAL, R.S. & W.C. ORR. 1992. Relationship between antioxidants, prooxidants, and the aging process. Ann. N. Y. Acad. Sci. **663:** 74–84.
48. POLLACK, M. & C. LEEUWENBURGH. 1999. Molecular mechanisms of oxidative stress and aging: Free radicals, aging, antioxidants, and disease. *In* Handbook of Oxidants and Antioxidants in Exercise. C.K. Sen, L. Packer & O. Hanninen, Eds.: 881–926. Elsevier. Amsterdam.
49. BARJA, G. 2000. The flux of free radical attack through mitochondrial DNA is related to aging rate. Aging (Milano) **12:** 342–355.
50. ZORATTI, M. & I. SZABO. 1995. The mitochondrial permeability transition. Biochim. Biophys. Acta **1241:** 139–176.
51. BERNARDI, P. 1996. The permeability transition pore. Control points of a cyclosporin A- sensitive mitochondrial channel involved in cell death. Biochim. Biophys. Acta **1275:** 5–9.
52. BERNARDI, P. & V. PETRONILLI. 1996. The permeability transition pore as a mitochondrial calcium release channel: a critical appraisal. J. Bioenerg. Biomembr. **28:** 131–138.
53. MATHER, M. & H. ROTTENBERG. 2000. Aging enhances the activation of the permeability transition pore in mitochondria. Biochem. Biophys. Res. Commun. **273:** 603–608.
54. SQUIER, T.C. & D.J. BIGELOW. 2000. Protein oxidation and age-dependent alterations in calcium homeostasis. Front. Biosci. **5:** D504–526.
55. NITAHARA, J.A. et al. 1998. Intracellular calcium, DNase activity and myocyte apoptosis in aging Fischer 344 rats. J. Mol. Cell. Cardiol. **30:** 519–535.

56. BECK, K.F. et al. 1999. Inducible NO synthase: role in cellular signalling. J. Exp. Biol. **202:** 645–653.
57. BOVERIS, A. & E. CADENAS. 2000. Mitochondrial production of hydrogen peroxide regulation by nitric oxide and the role of ubisemiquinone. IUBMB Life **50:** 245–250.
58. WANG, J.H., H.P. REDMOND, Q.D. WU & D. BOUCHIER-HAYES. 1998. Nitric oxide mediates hepatocyte injury. Am. J. Physiol. **275:** G1117–1126.
59. MISSO, N.L., C.D. PEACOCK, D.N. WATKINS & P.J. THOMPSON. 2000. Nitrite generation and antioxidant effects during neutrophil apoptosis. Free Radic. Biol. Med. **28:** 934–943.
60. SAUGSTAD, O.D. 2000. Does nitric oxide prevent oxidative mediated lung injury? Acta Paediatr. **89:** 905–907.
61. LIN, K.T., J.Y. XUE, M. NOMEN, B. SPUR & P.Y. WONG. 1995. Peroxynitrite-induced apoptosis in HL-60 cells. J. Biol. Chem. **270:** 16487–16490.
62. CAO, Y., A.T. PEARMAN, G.A. ZIMMERMAN, et al. 2000. Intracellular unesterified arachidonic acid signals apoptosis. Proc. Natl. Acad. Sci. USA **97:** 11280–11285.
63. DASH, P.K., S.A. MACH & A.N. MOORE. 2000. Regional expression and role of cyclooxygenase-2 following experimental traumatic brain injury. J. Neurotrauma **17:** 69–81.
64. KATZ, E. et al. 2001. B cell receptor-stimulated mitochondrial phospholipase A(2) activation and resultant disruption of mitochondrial membrane potential correlate with the induction of apoptosis in WEHI-231 B cells. J. Immunol. **166:** 137–147.
65. POLYAK, K., Y. XIA, J.L. ZWEIER, et al. 1997. A model for p53-induced apoptosis [see comments]. Nature **389:** 300–305.
66. KASPER, M. et al. 2000. Induction of apoptosis by glyoxal in human embryonic lung epithelial cell line L132. Am. J. Respir. Cell. Mol. Biol. **23:** 485–491.
67. KIKUCHI, S., et al. 1999. Neurotoxicity of methylglyoxal and 3-deoxyglucosone on cultured cortical neurons: synergism between glycation and oxidative stress, possibly involved in neurodegenerative diseases. J. Neurosci. Res. **57:** 280–289.
68. NIWA, H., et al. 1998. Accelerated formation of N epsilon-(carboxymethyl) lysine, an advanced glycation end product, by glyoxal and 3-deoxyglucosone in cultured rat sensory neurons. Biochem. Biophys. Res. Commun. **248:** 93–97.
69. BAYNES, J.W. & S.R. THORPE. 2000. Glycoxidation and lipoxidation in atherogenesis. Free Radic. Biol. Med. **28:** 1708–1716.
70. HIGAMI, Y. & I. SHIMOKAWA. 2000. Apoptosis in the aging process. Cell Tissue Res. **301:** 125–132.
71. NAKAMURA, K. et al. 1998. Inhibitory effects of antioxidants on neonatal rat cardiac myocyte hypertrophy induced by tumor necrosis factor-alpha and angiotensin II. Circulation **98:** 794–799.
72. KAJSTURA, J., et al. 1996. Apoptotic and necrotic myocyte cell deaths are independent contributing variables of infarct size in rats. Lab. Invest. **74:** 86–107.
73. PHANEUF, S. & C. LEEUWENBURGH. 2002. Cytochrome c release from mitochondria in the aging heart: a possible mechanism for apoptosis with age. Am. J. Physiol. Regul. Integr. Comp. Physiol. **282:** R423–430.
74. DIRKS, A. & C. LEEUWENBURGH. 2002. Apoptosis in skeletal muscle with aging. Am. J. Physiol. Regul. Integr. Comp. Physiol. **282:** R519–527.
75. MORRISON, J.H. & P.R. HOF. 1997. Life and death of neurons in the aging brain. Science **278:** 412–419.
76. RUBERG, M., et al. 1997. Neuronal death caused by apoptosis in Parkinson disease. Rev. Neurol. (Paris) **153:** 499–508.
77. KAUFMANN, J.A., P.C. BICKFORD & G. TAGLIALATELA. 2001. Oxidative-stress-dependent up-regulation of Bcl-2 expression in the central nervous system of aged Fisher-344 rats. J. Neurochem. **76:** 1099–1108.
78. JARSKOG, L.F. & J.H. GILMORE. 2000. Developmental expression of Bcl-2 protein in human cortex. Brain Res. Dev. Brain Res. **119:** 225–230.
79. KUMAR, V.B., M.W. FRANKO, S.A. FARR, et al. 2000. Identification of age-dependent changes in expression of senescence- accelerated mouse (SAMP8) hippocampal proteins by expression array analysis. Biochem. Biophys. Res. Commun. **272:** 657–661.
80. TAKAHASHI, Y., O.M. KURO & F. ISHIKAWA. 2000. Aging mechanisms. Proc. Natl. Acad. Sci. USA **97:** 12407–12408.

Generation of Reactive Oxygen and Nitrogen Species in Contracting Skeletal Muscle

Potential Impact on Aging

MICHAEL B. REID AND WILLIAM J. DURHAM

*Department of Medicine, Baylor College of Medicine,
One Baylor Plaza, Houston, Texas 77030, USA*

ABSTRACT: Since the early 1980s biologists have recognized that skeletal muscle generates free radicals. Of particular interest are two closely related redox cascades—reactive oxygen species (ROS) and nitric oxide (NO) derivatives. The ROS cascade is initiated by superoxide anion radicals derived from the mitochondrial electron transport chain, the membrane-associated NAD(P)H oxidase complex, or other sources. NO is produced by two NO synthase isoforms constitutively expressed by muscle fibers. ROS and NO derivatives are produced continually and are detectable in both the cytosolic and extracellular compartments. Production increases during strenuous exercise. Both ROS and NO modulate contractile function. Under basal conditions, low levels of ROS enhance force production. Excessive ROS accumulation inhibits force, for example, during fatiguing exercise. NO inhibits skeletal muscle contraction, an effect that is partially mediated by cyclic GMP as a second messenger. With aging, redox modulation of muscle contraction may be altered by changes in the rates of ROS and NO production, the levels of endogenous antioxidants that buffer ROS and NO, and the sensitivities of regulatory proteins to ROS and NO action. The impact of aging on contractile regulation depends on the relative magnitude of these changes and their net effects on ROS and NO activities at the cellular level.

WHY READ THIS ARTICLE?

Since the early 1980s biologists have recognized that skeletal muscle generates free radicals. Of particular interest are two closely related redox cascades: reactive oxygen species (ROS) and nitric oxide (NO) derivatives. ROS and NO derivatives are continually synthesized by skeletal muscle fibers via processes that tick along slowly under resting conditions and are markedly accelerated during strenuous exercise. The biological activities of muscle-derived ROS and NO are buffered by a panel of antioxidant pathways within skeletal muscle cells. ROS and NO derivatives that escape buffering act as signaling molecules and modulators of cellular function.

Address for correspondence: Michael B. Reid, Ph.D., Pulmonary Medicine, Suite 520B, Baylor College of Medicine, One Baylor Plaza, Houston, TX 77030. Voice: 713-798-7224; fax: 713-798-3619.

reid@bcm.tmc.edu

Ann. N.Y. Acad. Sci. 959: 108–116 (2002). © 2002 New York Academy of Sciences.

Accordingly, muscle-derived ROS and NO acutely influence contractile regulation, altering force production and muscle endurance; they also exert chronic effects on muscle gene expression.

A growing body of evidence indicates that aging exaggerates the effects of muscle-derived oxidants. This change may reflect the combined effects of accelerated ROS production, declining antioxidant activity, and increased sensitivity of regulatory proteins to oxidative modification. As a result, redox-sensitive processes within the cell are altered, including contractile function and gene expression. These alterations appear to contribute to losses of strength and muscle mass that occur in aged individuals.

The present article briefly outlines the scientific bases for these concepts. This is not an exhaustive review. Rather, we have attempted to describe the essential ideas, depicted in FIGURE 1, for individuals who seek an introduction to the topic. Those who desire more detailed information are referred to the reference list, which comprises key papers in the field and authoritative reviews on specific areas of interest.

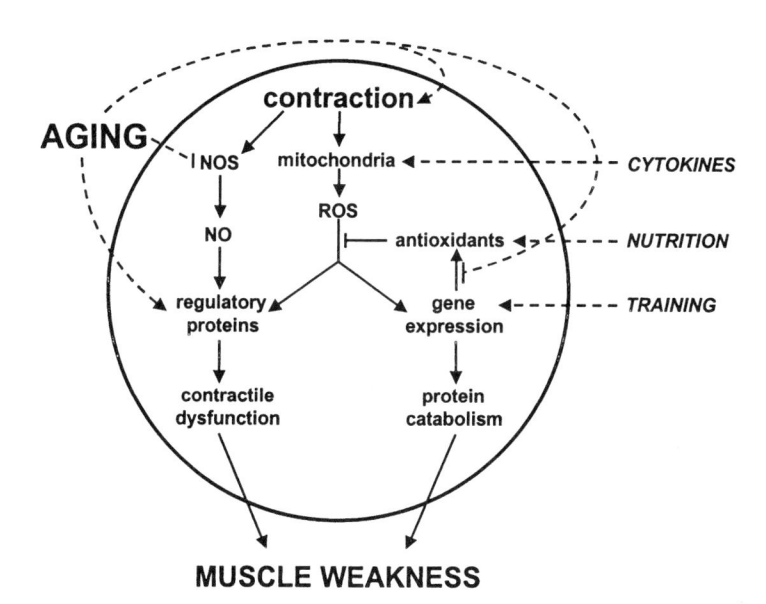

FIGURE 1. Effects of aging on pathways regulated by ROS and NO in contracting muscle. Intracellular pathways by which ROS and NO modulate force of contracting muscle are shown within *circle* (representing sarcolemma). Effects of aging and external factors (cytokines, nutrition, and exercise) are indicated by *dashed lines*. Arrows denote processes that are stimulated; *blunt ends* indicate processes that are inhibited.

ROS, NO, AND CELLULAR HOMEOSTASIS

The acronym *ROS* refers to a cascade of low molecular weight oxygen derivatives that are generated by skeletal muscle at low rates under resting conditions and at higher rates during exercise.[1] Typically, the parent molecule in this cascade is the superoxide anion, a free radical generated by addition of an electron to the outer orbital of diatomic oxygen. Superoxide anions undergo electron exchange reactions to form derivatives that include singlet oxygen, hydrogen peroxide, hydroxyl radicals, and other partially reduced oxygen derivatives. All of these derivatives retain redox activity, to a greater or lesser degree, and can influence redox-sensitive processes within the cell. In most eukaryotic cells, the principal source of superoxide anions is the mitochondrial electron transport chain. Unpaired electrons are lost at several steps in the chain (ubiquinone is the primary site of this electron "leak"), and molecular oxygen functions as the electron acceptor. This pathway is estimated to account for 2–3% of mitochondrial oxygen consumption. Superoxide anions can also be generated by enzymes, for example, NAD(P)H oxidases, cyclooxygenses, lipoxygenases, and NO synthases, but the biological importance of these production sites has not been established in skeletal muscle.[2] With aging, ROS production by muscle appears to be accelerated.[3] This increase is generally attributed to an age-dependent decline in mitochondrial function characterized by slowed turnover, decreased efficiency, and increased electron displacement from the transport chain.[4-6]

NO is generated by the enzyme NO synthase (NOS), which metabolizes L-arginine to NO. Skeletal muscle fibers constitutively express two NOS isoforms, the type I or neuronal isoform (nNOS) and the type III or endothelial isoform (eNOS), and continually produce NO.[1] Analogous to the ROS cascade, NO is the parent molecule in a redox cascade of NO derivatives that retain varying degrees of biological activity. Indeed, ROS and NO derivatives are closely related molecules that can directly interact; for example, NO reacts with the superoxide anion to form peroxynitrite, a highly unstable and potentially damaging molecule. Despite similarities with the ROS cascade, aging appears to have opposite effects on NO metabolism. NOS expression declines with age in skeletal muscle and NO production appears to decrease.[7] These changes predict that NO signaling and NO-mediated processes may play a lesser role in the muscles of aged individuals.

Antioxidants and stress-related proteins within muscle cells act to limit the biological effects of ROS and NO, a process recently reviewed by Powers and Hamilton.[8] Reduced glutathione (GSH) is the most plentiful antioxidant in muscle cells, present in millimolar concentrations, and is the most important biologically. GSH inactivates a variety of oxidant species directly. GSH also buffers peroxides via the enzymatic reaction catalyzed by glutathione peroxidase. Both pathways yield the oxidized glutathione dimer (GSSG), a by-product that is recycled back to GSH via the enzyme glutathione reductase. The balance of this dynamic process is reflected by the ratio of GSH and GSSG contents, a standard marker of cellular redox status. In addition to glutathione-mediated buffering, muscle cells contain a number of other antioxidants with differing biochemical activities and differing localizations. These include the antioxidant enzymes superoxide dismutase (SOD; dismutes superoxide anions to hydrogen peroxide) and catalase (dehydrates hydrogen peroxide to water) as well as antioxidant nutrients. The latter include α-tocopherol, vitamin C, carotenoids, β-carotene and α-lipoic acid. As reviewed by Ji and associates,[9] aging does not systematically compromise antioxidant activity in skeletal muscle. Vitamin C levels appear to decline with age, but GSH regulation, SOD activity, and catalase activity are not obviously compromised. Similarly, vitamin E levels can equal or exceed the levels in normal adult muscle. It is not known whether the antioxidant levels are adequate to buffer the rise in oxidant production that occurs with aging. Stress-related proteins, that is, heat shock proteins (HSPs) also have cytoprotective effects that oppose oxidative stress-related damage. McArdle and colleagues[10] have outlined the importance of this response in skeletal muscle. HSPs function as intracellular chaperones for newly synthesized proteins, aiding in their proper localization and minimizing protein aggregation. Both antioxidant and HSP levels are increased in skeletal muscle following bouts of oxidative stress, for example, strenuous exercise. However, there is evidence to suggest that these adaptive responses may be blunted with aging.[11] Such a deficit would render muscles from aged individuals more sensitive to oxidative insults than muscles of young individuals.

REDOX SIGNALING AND MUSCLE FUNCTION

Contractile Function

Muscle-derived ROS and NO continually modulate force production on a moment-to-moment basis.[1] NO depresses skeletal muscle force, an action similar to the effects seen in smooth and cardiac muscles. The decrements in NOS expression and NO production that occur with aging are likely to diminish this effect in muscles of older individuals. ROS promote force production by skeletal muscle under basal conditions but inhibit force in conditions where ROS activity is exaggerated, for example, strenuous exercise. These biphasic effects have been modeled as a bell-shaped continuum of contractile function across a range of redox statuses (FIG. 2). Under basal conditions, normal muscle is in a relatively reduced status and falls to the left of "optimal." By contrast, the redox status of aged muscle is likely to be shifted rightward (FIG. 2). This shift reflects the increase in oxidant production and possible decrements in antioxidant capacity that occur in aged muscle.[9,12] This shift is also consistent with the observation that aged muscle is more sensitive to oxidative stimuli than normal adult muscle.[13,14]

ROS are thought to depress force by altering the function of one or more redox-sensitive regulatory proteins in skeletal muscle. There are two schools of thought on the proteins responsible. Studies in intact muscle fibers have shown that exogenous ROS can markedly depress force without altering calcium regulation.[15,16] These findings argue that the proteins most sensitive to oxidative modification are located downstream of the calcium signal, for example, actin, myosin, troponin, or other myofibrillar proteins.[2] As reviewed by Schöneich and associates,[17] there is a separate body of research that implicates the calcium-dependent ATPase of the sarcoplasmic reticulum (SERCA). Data from aged rats indicate that the type 2a SERCA isoform exhibits marked dysfunction that is linked to extensive oxidative modification. The molecule contains fewer reduced cysteine moities and an increased number of nitrotyrosine residues. These observations suggest that peroxynitrite contributes to oxidative damage of SERCA in aged muscle.

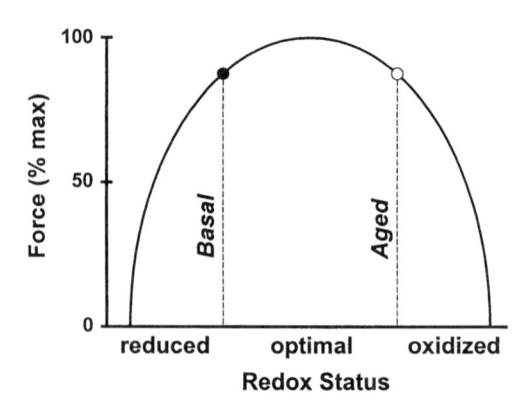

FIGURE 2. Redox sensitivity of muscle force production. *Curve* depicts biphasic response of force as muscle redox status is altered. *Closed circle* is proposed status of healthy adult muscle under basal conditions. *Open circle* is proposed status of aged muscle. Model adapted from Reid et al.[38]

Gene Expression

ROS and NO exert complex effects on gene transcription and protein expression by eukayotic cells.[18] Adaptation of skeletal muscle involves at least two major systems that are sensitive to redox regulation. By far, the most extensively studied response is the capacity of oxidative stimuli to induce cytoprotective proteins. As reviewed by Ji and colleagues,[9] aging is associated with increased tissue levels of antioxidants. These include the major antioxidant enzymes (SOD, catalase, and glutathione peroxidase) and key regulators of glutathione metabolism (e.g., glutathione S-transferase and glutathione reductase). The authors identified muscle-derived ROS as a potential stimulus for antioxidant adaptation. They further speculated that antioxidant adaptation is regulated at both the translational and posttranslational levels, a model supported by the recent work of Hollander, et al.[19] HSP regulation is a related target for oxidative signaling in skeletal muscle. ROS exposure can influence expression of HSP 25, HSP 72, and other members of the HSP family.[11,20] Spiers and associates[11] have emphasized the importance of redox control in HSP gene expression and have suggested that aging-related muscle dysfunction may represent failure to adapt to oxidative stress.

The second process affected by oxidative signaling is the regulation of muscle protein content. A rise in sarcoplasmic ROS levels has been shown to activate redox-sensitive kinases and nuclear factor-κB (NF-κB), one of several transcription factors that exhibit oxidative activation.[21,22] In turn, persistent activation of NF-κB leads to progressive loss of muscle protein.[23] It is tempting to speculate that the increased oxidant levels measured in aging muscle[12] represent a chronic stimulus for NF-κB–mediated signaling and that this pathway contributes to the sarcopenia of aging. However, this remains only an attractive hypothesis and is yet to be tested.

PERTURBING THE SYSTEM: EFFECTS OF EXTERNAL FACTORS

Nutrition

Anorexia and malnutrition are common elements of the aging process. Nutritional interventions are therefore advocated to slow or reverse the progression of aging-related sarcopenia.[24,25] The primary goal has been to increase amino acid availability and thereby facilitate resynthesis of muscle protein. To the extent that ROS and NO contribute to aging-related losses, Weindruch[26] has reasoned that increased intake of antioxidant nutrients might also be beneficial. This concept has not been tested systematically. In principle, however, oxidative signaling could be blunted in muscle cells by increasing the availability of antioxidant nutrients: for example, reduced thiols, vitamins E and C, β-carotene, carotenoids, and α-lipoic acid. Nutritional antioxidants may also enhance NO signaling in biological systems,[27] potentially restoring age-related losses. Antioxidant supplementation is not likely to affect function in the basal state since muscles of aged individuals are not overtly deficient in antioxidant nutrients.[9] However, supplements may be important for aged individuals who are physically active or chronically ill. Exercise and inflammation increase the oxidant burden in muscle, and aged muscle may be especially susceptible to the loss of nutritional antioxidants.[9]

Cytokines

Loss of muscle function with aging has long been linked to circulating cytokines that stimulate contractile dysfunction and muscle catabolism.[28–32] Potential mediators include interleukin 1 (IL-1), interleukin 6 (IL-6), and tumor necrosis factor-α (TNF-α). These cytokines are elevated in the circulation of elderly individuals.[33] Basal levels are further elevated by inflammatory disease and are transiently increased following strenuous exercise.[34] IL-1, IL-6, and TNF-α each stimulate cellular ROS production and induce loss of muscle function. The signaling events that regulate this process are best understood for TNF-α, the prototypical regulator of this biology. As recently reviewed,[35] binding of TNF-α to sarcolemmal receptors stimulates ROS production by muscle mitochondria. TNF-α–stimulated ROS stimulate two series of events that have additive effects on muscle performance. Within hours after TNF-α exposure, ROS can disrupt contractile regulation and weaken the muscle. With longer exposure, ROS act via NF-κB to up-regulate the ubiquitin/proteasome pathway, accelerate protein breakdown, and diminish muscle mass. Given their likely clinical importance, catabolic cytokines are major targets for therapeutic development. Interventions to inhibit cytokine effects on muscle are in the early stages of clinical testing.[30] If proven safe and effective, such compounds would be a potential treatment for muscle loss in the elderly.

Training

Exercise is among the most effective interventions for loss of function in aging muscle. A well-designed strength training program can safely increase muscle mass, muscle strength, and the functional capacity of elderly individuals.[25,36] By definition, the exercise bouts that are used for training will transiently elevate tissue ROS and NO levels. In young adults, such training evokes adaptive responses in skeletal muscle fibers. These include an increase in antioxidant enzyme activity that renders the muscle more resistant to oxidative stress.[37] HSP levels are also up-regulated in trained muscle,[10,20] which further contributes to cytoprotection. Concerns have been raised that aging may limit the capacity of muscle to adapt in this manner.[11] However, most reports suggest otherwise. The increases in antioxidant enzyme activities and HSP expression levels that occur in muscles after training are generally similar between adults and aged individuals.[9] In addition to antioxidant and HSP up-regulation, which blunts ROS activity, exercise training also decreases circulating TNF-α levels in the elderly,[33] thereby diminishing the stimulus for ROS production. These adaptive responses are expected to oppose the action of ROS, decreasing the activity of oxidant-activated pathways and improving muscle function.

CONCLUSION

The loss of muscle function that occurs with aging is likely mediated, at least in part, by muscle-derived ROS and NO and by the signaling cascades they regulate. It appears that ROS production during muscle contraction is exaggerated due to the loss of mitochondrial regulation that occurs with aging. It is also likely that proteins in aged skeletal muscle are more susceptible to oxidative modification, rendering muscle fibers more sensitive to oxidant effects. Redox homeostasis of the aging myocyte is further disrupted by humoral factors, including increased exposure to catabolic cytokines. As our understanding of this biology matures, targeted interventions are being developed that may lessen or reverse the deleterious effects of aging on skeletal muscle.

ACKNOWLEDGMENTS

Our work in this area has been supported by National Institutes of Health Grants HL45721 and HL59878; Dr. Durham is supported by National Institutes of Health Training Grant (HL07676).

REFERENCES

1. REID, M.B. 2001. Nitric oxide, reactive oxygen species, and skeletal muscle contraction. Med. Sci. Sports Exercise **33:** 371–376.
2. REID, M.B. 2001. Redox modulation of skeletal muscle contraction: what we know and what we don't. J. Appl. Physiol. **90:** 724–731.
3. FIELDING, R.A. & M. MEYDANI. 1997. Exercise, free radical generation, and aging. Aging **9:** 12–18.
4. WALLACE, D.C. 2001. A mitochondrial paradigm for degenerative diseases and ageing. Novartis Found. Symp. **235:** 247–263.
5. PESCE, V., A. CORMIO, F. FRACASSO, et al. 2001. Age-related mitochondrial genotypic and phenotypic alterations in human skeletal muscle. Free Radic. Biol. Med. **30:** 1223–1233.
6. NAVARRO, A., J.M. LOPEZ-CEPERO & M.J. SANCHEZ DEL PINO. 2001. Skeletal muscle and aging. Front. Biosci. **6:** d26–d44.

7. RICHMONDS, C.R., K. BOONYAPISIT, L.L. KUSNER, et al. 1999. Nitric oxide synthase in aging rat skeletal muscle. Mech. Ageing Dev. **109:** 177–189.
8. POWERS, S.K. & K. HAMILTON. 1999. Antioxidants and exercise. Clin. Sports Med. **18:** 525–536.
9. JI, L.L., C. LEEUWENBURGH, S. LEICHTWEIS, et al. 1998. Oxidative stress and aging; role of exercise and its influences on antioxidant systems. Ann. N. Y. Acad. Sci. **854:** 102–117.
10. MCARDLE, A. & M.J. JACKSON. 2000. Exercise, oxidative stress, and ageing. J. Anat. **197:** 539–541.
11. SPIERS, S., F. MCARDLE & M.J. JACKSON. 2000. Aging-related muscle dysfunction: failure of adaptation to oxidative stress? Ann. N. Y. Acad. Sci. **908:** 341–343.
12. BEJIMA, J. & L.L. JI. 1999. Aging and acute exercise enhance free radical generation in rat skeletal muscle. J. Appl. Physiol. **87:** 465–470.
13. LAWLER, J.M., C.C. CLINE, Z. HU, et al. 1997. Effect of oxidant challenge on contractile function of the aging rat diaphragm. Am. J. Physiol. **272:** E201–E207.
14. RICHMONDS, C.R. & H.J. KAMINSKI. 2000. Nitric oxide myotoxicity is age related. Mech. Ageing Dev. **113:** 183–191.
15. ANDRADE, F.H., M.B. REID, D.G. ALLEN, et al. 1998. Effect of hydrogen peroxide and dithiothreitol on contractile function of single skeletal muscle fibres from mouse. J. Physiol. **509:** 565–575.
16. ANDRADE, F.H., M.B. REID & H. WESTERBLAD. 2001. Contractile response to low peroxide concentrations: myofibrillar calcium sensitivity as a likely target for redox modulation of skeletal muscle function. FASEB J. **15:** 309–311.
17. SCHONEICH, C., R.I. VINER, D.A. FERRINGTON, et al. 1999. Age-related chemical modification of the skeletal muscle sarcoplasmic reticulum Ca-ATPase of the rat. Mech. Ageing Dev. **107:** 221–231.
18. SEN, C.K. & L. PACKER. 1996. Antioxidant and redox regulation of gene transcription. FASEB J. **10:** 1–12.
19. HOLLANDER, J., J. BEJIMA, T. OOKAWARA, et al. 2000. Superoxide dismutase gene expression in skeletal muscle: fiber-specific effect of age. Mech. Ageing Dev. **116:** 33–45.
20. NAITO, H., S.K. POWERS, H.A. DEMIREL, et al. 2001. Exercise training increases heat shock protein in skeletal muscles of old rats. Med. Sci. Sports Exercise **33:** 729–734.
21. LI, Y.-P., R.J. SCHWARTZ, I.D. WADDELL, et al. 1998. Skeletal muscle myocytes undergo protein loss and reactive oxygen-mediated NF-κB activation in response to tumor necrosis factor-α. FASEB J. **12:** 871–880.
22. LI, Y.-P., C.M. ATKINS, J.D. SWEATT, et al. 1999. Mitochondria mediate tumor necrosis factor-α/NF-κB signaling in skeletal muscle myotubes. Antiox. Redox Signal. **1:** 97–104.
23. LI, Y.-P. & M.B. REID. 2000. NF-κB mediates the protein loss induced by TNF-α in differentiated skeletal muscle myotubes. Am. J. Physiol. **279:** R1165–R1170.
24. PARISE, G. & K.E. YARASHESKI. 2000. The utility of resistance exercise training and amino acid supplementation for reversing age-associated decrements in muscle protein mass and function. Curr. Opin. Clin. Nutr. Metab. Care **3:** 489–495.
25. HEBUTERNE, X., S. BERMON & S.M. SCHNEIDER. 2001. Ageing and muscle: the effects of malnutrition, re-nutrition, and physical exercise. Curr. Opin. Clin. Nutr. Metab. Care **4:** 295–300.
26. WEINDRUCH, R. 1995. Interventions based on the possibility that oxidative stress contributes to sarcopenia. J. Gerontol. A Biol. Sci. Med. Sci. **50:** 157–161.
27. CARR, A. & B. FREI. 2000. The role of natural antioxidants in preserving the biological activity of endothelium-derived nitric oxide. Free Radic. Biol. Med. **28:** 1806–1814.
28. CANNON, J.G. 1998. Intrinsic and extrinsic factors in muscle aging. Ann. N. Y. Acad. Sci. **854:** 72–77.
29. CANNON, J.G. 1995. Cytokines in aging and muscle homeostasis. J. Gerontol. A Biol. Sci. Med. Sci. **50:** 120–123.
30. KOTLER, D.P. 2000. Cachexia. Ann. Intern. Med. **133:** 622–634.
31. MACKINNON, L.T. 1998. Future directions in exercise and immunology: regulation and integration. Int. J. Sports Med. **19:** S205–S209.

32. PAHOR, M. & S. KRITCHEVSKY. 1998. Research hypotheses on muscle wasting, aging, loss of function and disability. J. Nutr. Health Aging **2:** 97–100.
33. GRIEWE, J.S., B. CHENG, D.C. RUBIN, *et al.* 2001. Resistance exercise decreases skeletal muscle tumor necrosis factor alpha in frail elderly humans. FASEB J. **15:** 475–482.
34. ARGILES, J.M. & F.J. LOPEZ-SORIANO. 1998. Catabolic proinflammatory cytokines. Curr. Opin. Clin. Nutr. Metab. Care **1:** 245–251.
35. REID, M.B. & Y.-P. LI. 2001. Cytokines and oxidative signaling in skeletal muscle. Acta Physiol. Scand. **171:** 225–232.
36. ROTH, S.M., R.F. FERRELL & B.F. HURLEY. 2000. Strength training for the prevention and treatment of sarcopenia. J. Nutr. Health Aging **4:** 143–155.
37. POWERS, S.K., L.L. JI & C. LEEUWENBURGH. 1999. Exercise training-induced alterations in skeletal muscle antioxidant capacity: a brief review. Med. Sci. Sports Exercise **31:** 987–997.
38. REID, M.B., F.A. KHAWLI & M.R. MOODY. 1993. Reactive oxygen in skeletal muscle: III. Contractility of unfatigued muscle. J. Appl. Physiol. **75:** 1081–1087.

Can Exercise Training Improve Immune Function in the Aged?

JEFFREY A. WOODS, THOMAS W. LOWDER, AND K. TODD KEYLOCK

Department of Kinesiology, University of Illinois at Urbana/Champaign, 906 South Goodwin Avenue, Urbana, Illinois 61801, USA

ABSTRACT: Many strategies have been used to improve immune function in the aged. Unfortunately, many of these interventions have been disappointing, impractical, costly to develop and administer, or accompanied by adverse side effects. Aside from dietary manipulation (caloric restriction without malnutrition or antioxidant supplementation), research involving behavioral preventative or restorative therapies has been lacking. Moderate exercise training has been shown to elicit beneficial outcomes in both the prevention and rehabilitation of many diseases of the elderly. It has been hypothesized that moderate levels of exercise improves, whereas strenuous exercise or overtraining suppresses, various immune function measures. Three general approaches have been implemented to study the impact of exercise on immune functioning in the elderly: (1) cross-sectional studies, (2) longitudinal studies, and (3) animal studies. In general, cross-sectional studies examining highly active elderly have demonstrated improved *in vitro* T cell responses to polyclonal stimulation when compared to sedentary elderly. This is corroborated by several animal studies that have shown improved splenic T cell responses *in vitro*. Unfortunately, human prospective studies have failed to demonstrate consistent improvements in various measures of immune function in older adults. However, it should be cautioned that these studies have included small samples followed over a short duration, measuring a limited number of *in vitro* immune parameters, with some failing to account for potential confounding influences. Although such findings have the potential to be of substantial public health importance, very few systematic studies have been conducted.

KEYWORDS: immune function; exercise; training; aging; elderly; physical activity

INTRODUCTION

The enormous healthcare costs associated with supporting a rapidly growing aged population and the overall concern for the well-being of older persons makes research on aging of vital interest to everyone. Several measures of immunity are altered with aging,[1] and this is believed to be a contributing factor in the increased incidence of respiratory, neoplastic, and arthritic diseases[2,3] and higher mortality rates

Address for correspondence: Jeffrey A. Woods, Department of Kinesiology, University of Illinois at Urbana/Champaign, 906 South Goodwin Avenue, Urbana, IL 61801. Voice: 217-244-8815; fax: 217-244-7322.
   woods1@uiuc.edu

from bacterial and viral infections.[4] The realization of dysregulated immune function and increased disease incidence in the elderly has been the impetus for interventions designed to improve immune function in the elderly.[5–8] Unfortunately, pharmacologic/hormonal, genetic, and tissue grafting interventions have been either disappointing, impractical, costly to develop and administer, or accompanied by adverse side effects. For example, despite early enthusiasm for dehydroepiandrosterone (DHEA) treatment in retarding the effects of aging on the immune system,[9] more recent studies have not found it to be a panacea for immunosenescence.[10,11] Two nutritional paradigms have resulted in improved T cell–mediated immune function in elderly subjects, suggesting that the aged immune system is amenable to change. It has long been known that caloric restriction without malnutrition in rodents has been found to improve T cell functions, including mitogenic proliferation and interleukin (IL)-2 production.[12] Likewise, dietary supplementation with vitamin E for four months in elderly humans can improve delayed-type hypersensitivity (DTH) responses, *in vitro* T lymphocyte function, and tetanus toxoid and hepatitis B (but not diptheria or pneumococcal) antibody response to vaccination.[13] Aside from dietary manipulation, research involving behavioral preventative or restorative therapies has been lacking.

Alternatively, moderate aerobic exercise training has been shown to elicit beneficial outcomes in both the prevention and rehabilitation of many diseases of the elderly.[14] With respect to immune function, it has been hypothesized that moderate levels of exercise improves, whereas strenuous exercise or overtraining suppresses, various immune function measures. This theoretical model has been called the "inverted J hypothesis" due to the shape of the immune function (Y axis) versus exercise intensity (X axis) curve.[15] The extent to which moderate exercise training or lifelong physical activity influences dysregulated immune function in the elderly is unclear. Despite this, exercise is currently being used by elderly populations to enhance muscle functioning and combat diseases, such as osteoporosis, diabetes, and heart disease. Three general approaches have been implemented to study exercise and immune function in aged populations: (1) human cross-sectional studies comparing master's athletes with sedentary elderly, (2) human longitudinal studies in which exercise training commenced in old age, and (3) animal studies. Several other studies have examined the effects of single bouts of exercise on various immune parameters in old when compared to young subjects; they will not be reviewed.

HUMAN CROSS-SECTIONAL STUDIES

Cross-sectional studies have examined the relationship between a physically active lifestyle and aging in terms of *in vitro* NK cell activity (NKCA), T cell function, and cytokine production. Basal killing of NK-sensitive K562 cells has been commonly used to assess NKCA in humans and yet there are conflicting reports as to whether basal NKCA is altered in older individuals.[16] Several cross-sectional exercise studies offer conflicting data in regards to basal NK cell function in older adults. Nieman *et al.* reported a 54% higher basal NKCA in elderly athletes when compared to sedentary controls.[17] This increase was seen in the absence of changes in NK cell number. In this study athletes were highly competitive females, aged 65 to 84, who had exercised at least an hour a day for a minimum of five years. By contrast, there was no difference in NKCA when Shinkai et al. examined older athletes when compared to age-matched sedentary controls.[18] The athletes in that study had run recreationally an average of about 1 hour a day, 5 days a week for over 17 years. There is obviously a big difference between recreational runners and highly competitive athletes, which may explain the discrepancy of findings between the two studies. It may be that regularly performed high intensity exercise is needed to alter NKCA. Unfortunately, none of these studies examined the effects of exercise on the known age-related suppression in sensitivity of NK cells to endogenous activators such as IL-2 or IL-12.[19]

Aging seems to affect functions of T cells the most, particularly in their ability to proliferate *in vitro* in response to polyclonal mitogens, such as concanavalin A (Con A) or phytohemmagglutinin (PHA). The cross-sectional data on the impact of exercise on this is clearer, pointing to improved T cell responses in physically active elderly when compared to sedentary controls. Shinkai et al.[18] and Nieman et al.[17] reported very similar increases (~40–50%) when comparing proliferative response to PHA in an elderly exercise group when compared to the sedentary group. Shinkai[18] studied all male subjects and found decreased proliferative response in the aged, not only to PHA, but also to pokeweed mitogen (PWM) and alloantigens. The aged exercising group had higher proliferative responsiveness to PHA (41%) and PWM (46%) than the aged sedentary group (adjusted to per cell basis). Looking at a different measure, Gueldner et al. examined T cell responsiveness in older women and found that CD25 expression in response to fixed anti-CD3 antibody was higher on T cells in the active group when compared to an inactive control group.[20] The exercise group consisted of subjects who had engaged in long-term moderate exercise in formal exercise classes. DiPietro et al. reported an increase in the percentage of peripheral blood mononuclear cells forming rosettes with sheep red blood cells (SRBC) after incubation with PHA in noncompetitive elderly cyclists when compared to sedentary controls.[21] This indicated that physically active elderly responded more vigorously to PHA with enhanced expression of CD2, the receptor responsible for SRBC binding and a molecule important in T cell costimulation. This was accompanied by alterations in signal transduction through the phosphatidylinositol pathway. Wang et al.[22] found that basal protein kinase C (PKC) activity, phorbol myristate acetate (PMA)-induced redistribution of PKC, and PHA-induced enhancement of PKC activity were reduced in cytosolic and membrane fractions in lymphocytes obtained from older adults, but the magnitude of these reductions was smaller among elderly who were physically fit, as determined by estimated maximal oxygen uptake (VO_{2max}) testing. PKC is a serine/threonine kinase important in T cell activation. Taken together, these data indicate that T cells obtained from physically active, cardiovascularly fit older adults may be better able to respond to polyclonal stimulation.

Cytokines are also affected by the aging process, most notably a decrease in production and responsiveness to IL-2. Shinkai et al.[18] confirmed this and reported that PHA-stimulated IL-2, interferon-γ, and IL-4 production in elderly runners was higher compared to an elderly sedentary group. This brings up the possibility that older individuals who exercise regularly may have improved type I cytokine responses that may ultimately contribute to improved cell-mediated immunity.

Summary

In addition to the low subject number, a major limitation with these cross-sectional studies is that inclusion of elderly athletes as a comparison group is likely not relevant in determining the effect of moderate physical activity on immune function in older individuals. Most elderly will never realistically become (or desire to become) competitive athletes. Indeed, the recent public health message is that moderate levels of exercise can result in considerable improvements in physiological/psychological functioning in the aged with concomitant reductions in disease.[14] These moderate levels of exercise are likely the ones that can be attained by the majority of elderly persons. Obviously, the major drawback of the cross-sectional approach is that other factors, including nutritional status, genetics, smoking history, and psychosocial factors (among others) exist to explain the relationship between physical activity status and high levels of immune function. However, as a starting point, it would be of interest to determine if cardiovascular fitness (e.g., VO_{2max}) and/or self-reported physical activity are associated in any way with various measures of immune function. Unfortunately, no studies have had sufficient subject numbers to adequately address this issue.

HUMAN PROSPECTIVE STUDIES

Prospective studies can definitively determine whether exercise training improves immune function in older adults. Several studies have examined the impact of either moderate aerobic exercise or resistance training on indicators of immune function in the aged.

Aerobic Exercise

Woods *et al.* examined 6 months of moderate aerobic training (60–65% of VO_{2max}, 40 min/day, 3 times/wk) or flexibility/toning control (FT-CON) on previously sedentary elderly (65.3 ± 0.8 years) adults.[23] Measures of both T lymphocyte and natural killer cell function were examined. While both groups revealed a small intervention-induced increase in *in vitro* T cell proliferation to Con A and PHA, the aerobic-trained group showed a higher percentage change over several doses of Con A. Basal NKCA versus K562 cells tended to be higher in the aerobic-trained group, while little change was evident in the FT-CON group. In another study, Fahlman *et al.* examined the effects of a 10-week endurance-training program (walking at 70% of heart rate reserve 3 d/wk) in elderly (76 ± 5 years) nuns.[24] One clear advantage to the use of this particular population was that all of the subjects lived and ate together, and had similar lifestyle and activity patterns. The short training program was without effect on basal NKCA and Con A–induced proliferation. In a 17-week randomized controlled intervention, Chin *et al.* combined very mild exercise and enriched foods in frail elderly subjects (79.2 ± 5.9 years).[25] They found no effect of enriched foods, so they combined the exercise and exercise plus enriched foods into one group. Using a DTH skin test, it was shown that exercise had only a small beneficial effect on the DTH response. In effect, the control group significantly declined, whereas the exercise group maintained their cumulative DTH responses to multiple antigens. This effect was quite small and associated with large variability. Crist *et al.* examined the effects of 20–30 minutes of chair-callisthenic exercises (three times per week for 16 wks) that were designed to improve functional aerobic capacity and neuromuscular performance in a population of ambulatory seniors (72 years old).[26] Although it was demonstrated that basal NKCA was 33% higher in trained versus untrained, these measures were only taken posttraining, and it was assumed that initial differences between subjects were equally balanced across the two treatment conditions through the randomization process and that any posttreatment differences were due to the experimental treatment. This is clearly not an ideal study design. Nieman *et al.* examined the effects of 12 weeks of walking on *in vitro* immunological responsiveness in aged (73-year-old) sedentary females.[17] Although a significant increase (12.6%) in VO_{2max} was seen following the intervention, no effect in basal NKCA or T cell proliferation to PHA was observed. They suggested that either the duration or the intensity of the exercise prescribed may not have been stimulating enough to elicit any functional immunological change in this population despite the increase in VO_{2max}.

Resistance Training

Resistance or strength training is also being recommended to elderly populations as a means of combating sarcopenia and osteoporosis.[14] Although the majority of exercise intervention studies focus on aerobic exercise as the model, there are a few studies that have examined resistance training as the mode of exercise. Rall *et al.* found that 12 weeks of progressive resistance training did not affect immune function in young (22–30 years) or healthy elderly (65–80 years) individuals.[27] Training did not induce changes in lymphocyte subsets, *in vitro* cytokine production (IL-1, IL-2, TNF-α, or IL-6), lymphocyte proliferation, or *in vivo* DTH responses to multiple antigens. There were eight and six elderly subjects in the exercise and control groups, respectively. This small number and the high variability in the measures would make detection of small differences in immune function difficult. In a later study by Bermon *et al.*, it was demonstrated that 8 weeks of strength training did not modify counts of lymphocyte subsets in previously sedentary elderly (70.1 ± 1.0 years) adults.[28] In both studies, no changes in body composition or body weight were observed, although in the Rall study strength increases were seen in all groups, the variability in strength increases were very high. The inconsistent increases in strength, accompanied by the fact that subjects failed to alter body composition, indicate that the intervention was probably too short to induce significant physiological changes that may have affected immune function measures in these populations. Moreover, Flynn *et al.* examined the effects of 10 weeks of lower-body resistance training in elderly (67–84 years) women. They found no significant changes in lymphocyte subsets or proliferation or basal NKCA.[29]

Summary

Despite the suggestive results from cross-sectional studies, data from the few prospective studies that have been published appear not to support a role for moderate aerobic or resistance exercise training in imparting a substantial beneficial effect on various measures of immune function in the elderly. However, the studies that have been performed have been very short in duration (most <12 wks) and limited in statistical power due to small sample number. Moreover, some have used poor designs and have failed to control or account for influential covariates or seasonal variations in immune function. Although they are difficult and costly to administer, there exists a clear-cut need for long-term (>12 months) exercise-intervention studies in older adults to definitively determine if moderate exercise training can improve immune function in the elderly. It cannot be assumed that changes in immune function in response to exercise training, if they occur, take place within the same time frame as improvements in VO_{2max} or strength.

Clinical Relevance of Exercise Training–induced Changes in Immune Function

A limitation of most exercise-immune studies is the use of *in vitro* responses of peripheral blood cells to assess global immune functioning. Unfortunately, most of these measures lack clinical disease correlates. One measure that has demonstrated clinical significance is the DTH response. The DTH response has long been used as an overall indicator of the robustness of cell-mediated immunity,[30] and its clinical significance is evidenced by studies demonstrating an association between low DTH response and subsequent mortality.[31,32] Although several exercise studies have examined DTH responses, the variability associated with this measure is high, making studies with small sample numbers difficult to interpret. Arguably, the most clinically relevant measure would be the response to a defined antigenic challenge. Unfortunately, there are no published studies on measures such as antibody response to influenza vaccination in elderly exercisers versus sedentary controls. Two studies have demonstrated a decrease in upper respiratory tract infection (URTI) rates in active elderly subjects when compared to sedentary controls.[17,33] However, these studies have been small with respect to epidemiological standards, and the identification of URTI was based on self-report and not clinical diagnosis.

ANIMAL STUDIES

Animal models allow for a more direct examination of the host's overall immunological response to exercise in tissues that are unavailable in human models (e.g., spleen, heart, brain, and bone marrow). Additionally, investigators can control virtually every aspect of the study, including housing, diet, exercise, room temperature, and light cycle. Ultimately, these models allow for the testing of physiological significance of exercise training–induced changes in immune function using relevant disease models. The majority of studies involving exercise, aging, and immune function involve the use of rodents (various mouse or rat strains), although larger animals are sometimes used.

In one of the first papers to measure the effects of exercise on the aged immune system, Pahlavani *et al.* found that six months of twice-a-day swimming (one hour each session) resulted in an age-related decrease in mitogen-induced splenic lymphocyte proliferation in male Fischer 344 rats.[34] They found that the age-related decline in proliferation and IL-2 production was less in the exercised rats, but this was due to lower levels in the young exercised rats and not due to any exercise-related protective effect. In a later study using less stressful treadmill training for 16 weeks,

Nasrullah and Mazzeo showed that exercise enhanced splenocyte proliferation and IL-2 production in response to Con A in aged (27-month-old) Fischer 344 rats, while a decreased splenic proliferation and a reduction in IL-2 production were seen in young and middle-aged rats.[35] Further, the authors demonstrated that increased activity levels had little effect on splenic NKCA. This mode of exercise differs greatly from swim training, in that volume and intensity of the stimulus (exercise) can be controlled to a greater degree, and the effects of the water (i.e., a fear of drowning) is eliminated. Barnes *et al.* followed with a study examining the same strain of rats, also using treadmill running as the exercise stimulus.[36] These investigators concluded that while 10 weeks of endurance training (75% of maximal capacity) resulted in significant increases in VO_{2max} and reductions in the respiratory exchange ratios in both young and aged rats, exercise training did not significantly alter the antibody response to keyhole limpet hemocyanin (KLH), an antigenic protein that is a T cell–dependent antigen.

In a study involving exercise in conjunction with caloric restriction, Utsuyama *et al.* suggested that lifelong (19 months) physical exercise in addition to dietary restriction might retard certain immunological functions that are shown to decrease with age.[37] They found that 5 of 13 rats (exercised voluntarily by means of a wheel in their cages and fed 80% of the ad libitum–fed group) exhibited a highly proliferative response of T cells to mitogens and that this contributed to higher levels of proliferation when compared to the calorically restricted groups alone. It is worth noting that in this study, rats had to run on an exercise wheel in order to receive food and that they learned to perform this exercise throughout the experiment (a period lasting 21 months). Based on previous studies showing that mature mice that are able to explore a T-shaped maze more quickly have an above-average longevity, De la Fuente *et al.* divided 70-week-old female outbred Swiss mice into "fast" or "slow" groups.[38] Upon sacrifice (6 ± 1 week later), it was shown that the "fast" mice had a better *in vitro* immune function than the "slow" mice based on measurements made on macrophages, lymphocytes, and NK cells. These studies bring up the possibility that heterogeneity likely exists in subjects' alteration of immune responses to exercise training and that this heterogeneity needs to be accounted for when analyzing exercise and aging studies.

In a study by Lu *et al.*, exercise training in the form of treadmill running (18–22 m/min, 45 min/day, 5 day/wk for 16 wks) significantly increased *in vitro* peritoneal macrophage tumor cytolysis in young and aged mice, although the effect was larger in young mice.[39] This effect could be abrogated by the inducible nitric oxide synthase inhibitor monomethyl-L-arginine. The latter finding suggested that exercise training increased the ability of IFN-γ and LPS-stimulated macrophages to produce nitric oxide and that this was indeed the mechanism that was responsible for the increase in cytolytic activity. A strength of this study was the documentation of an intracellular mechanism responsible for exercise training–induced changes in *in vitro* tumor killing.

Summary

Many of the limitations of human immune studies can be reduced or eliminated through the use of animal models. For example, although an exercise protocol may alter activity levels in a human population, activity outside of the researcher's control, such as a subject who participates in a supervised exercise program of moderate intensity but works off-peak (shift) hours in a physically laborious occupation, may confound the data because of increased activity levels, as well as adversely affected sleeping cycles. Housing conditions may act as a further confounding variable (e.g., human subjects living alone may have a more structured lifestyle than someone who is caring for children or a dependent). Furthermore, most human studies in exercise immunology are limited to sampling of blood that contains a small fraction of the body's leukocyte pool and may not reflect sites important in *in vivo* immune functioning. The animal data regarding exercise and immune function in the aged suggests that exercise-trained animals may manifest improved T cell–mediated immune functions when compared to sedentary controls. Although testable, the physiological significance of these observations is not known.

Potential Mechanisms for an Association Between Exercise and Immune Function

The aging process does not affect the immune system uniformly, and there is a high degree of individual variability that may be associated with confounding factors. There are several factors that have not been adequately accounted for in previous studies of exercise and immune function, including diet, substance abuse, smoking status, psychological stress, underlying disease, recent illness or vaccination, medication usage (including hormone supplements), seasonal/diurnal/assay variation, body composition, and socioeconomic status. These factors have the potential to either confound data interpretation or contribute to an interaction between exercise and immune function, or both. For example, people who are physically active may adopt other healthy behaviors (e.g., not smoking and eating a healthy diet). However, the role these factors play in explaining improved immune function in the physically active elderly is unknown. Likewise, a myriad of physiological mechanisms exist that could potentially explain how exercise training might affect immune function, including changes in neuroendocrine status,[40] altered hematopoiesis,[41] leukocyte apoptosis,[42] muscle damage,[43] metabolic changes including increased protein synthesis[44] or improved glucose utilization,[45] and changes in antioxidant defenses,[46] to name a few. Some of the above factors may lead to alterations in the makeup of leukocyte subsets in such tissues as blood or spleen. Given that the aged manifest higher numbers of memory T cells, at the expense of naive T cells, and that this likely contributes to age dysregulation in T cell immune function,[47,48] it will be important to examine various subsets of leukocytes in future exercise studies to determine if functional changes are associated with cell subset shifts in the samples obtained. However, testing of the contribution of mechanisms such as these seems premature until we know whether or not exercise-induced changes can be accounted for by other lifestyle variables.

CONCLUSIONS

The limited preliminary evidence from cross-sectional human, prospective human, and animal studies suggests that exercise-trained or physically active elderly subjects have higher *in vitro* measures of immune function and, perhaps, lower incidence rates and severity of URTIs when compared to sedentary controls. Although such findings have the potential to be of substantial public health importance, very few cross-sectional or randomized prospective trials of exercise and immune function have been conducted to date in the elderly. These studies can be characterized as comprising small samples followed over a short duration, measuring a limited number of *in vitro* immune parameters whose clinical significance is unknown, and failing to account for potential confounding influences. There is clearly a need for definitive human prospective and animal studies examining the physiological relevance of exercise training–induced changes in immune function with regard to disease models.

REFERENCES

1. MILLER, R.A. 1994. Immune System (Chapter 21). *In* Handbook of Physiology (Section 11: Aging) E. J. Masoro, Ed.: Oxford University Press. Oxford, UK.
2. ERSHLER, W.B. 1993. The influence of an aging immune system on cancer incidence and progression. J. Gerontol. Biol. Sci. **48:** B3–B7.
3. MACKINODAN, T., S.J. JAMES, T. INAMIZU & M-P. CHANG. 1984. Immunologic basis for susceptibility to infection in the aged. Gerontology **30:** 279–289.
4. YOSHIKAWA, T.T. 1983. Geriatric infectious diseases: an emerging problem. J. Am. Geriatr. Soc. **31:** 34–45.
5. FAGIOLO, U.A. AMADORI & F. BORGHESAN. 1990. Immune dysfunction in the elderly: Effect of thymic hormone administration on several in vivo and in vitro immune function parameters. Aging **2:** 347–350.
6. HIRAKOWA, K. & M. UTSUYAMA. 1989. Combined grafting of bone marrow and thymus, and sequential multiple thymus graftings in various strains of mice. The effect on immune function and life span. Mech. Ageing Dev. **49:** 49–56.
7. JAZWINSKI, S.M. 1996. Longevity, genes, and aging. Science **273:** 54–58.
8. YU, B.P. 1994. Putative Interventions (Chapter 23) *In* Handbook of Physiology (Section 11: Aging) E. J. Masoro, Ed.: Oxford University Press. Oxford, UK.
9. WEKSLER, M.E. 1993. Immune senescence and adrenal steroids: immune dysregulation and the action of dehydroepiandrosterone (DHEA) in old animals. Eur. J. Clin. Pharmacol. **45:** S21–23.
10. MILLER R.A. & C. CHRISP. 1999. Lifelong treatment with oral DHEA sulfate does not preserve immune function, prevent disease, or improve survival in genetically heterogeneous mice. J. Am. Geriatr. Soc. **47:** 960–966.
11. SIRRS, S.M. & R.A. BEBB. 1999. DHEA: panacea or snake oil? Can. Fam. Physician **45:**1723–1728.
12. GROSSMAN, A., L. MAGGIO-PRICE, J.C. JINNEMAN, *et al.* 1990. The effect of long-term caloric restriction on function of T-cell subsets in old mice. Cell. Immunol. **131:** 194–204.
13. MEYDANI, S.N., M. MEYDANI, J.B. BLUMBERG, *et al.* 1997. Vitamin E supplementation and in vivo immune response in healthy elderly subjects. A randomized controlled trial. JAMA **277:** 1380-1386.
14. MAZZEO, R.S., P. CAVANAUGH, W.J. EVANS, *et al.* 1998. Exercise and physical activity for older adults. American College of Sports Medicine Position Stand. Med. Sci. Sports Exercise **30:** 992–1008.
15. HOFFMAN-GOETZ, L. & B.K. PEDERSEN. 1994. Exercise and the immune system: a model of the stress response? Immunol. Today **15:** 382–387.
16. WOODS, J.A., J.K. EVANS, B.W. WOLTERS, *et al.* 1998. Effects of maximal exercise on natural killer (NK) cell activity and responsiveness to interferon-α in the young and old. J. Gerontol. Biol. Sci. **53:** B430–B437.
17. NIEMAN, D.C., D.A. HENSON, G. GUSEWITCH, *et al.* 1993. Physical activity and immune function in elderly women. Med. Sci. Sports Exercise **25:** 823–831.

18. SHINKAI, S., H. KOHNO, K. KIMURA, et al. 1995. Physical activity and immune senescence in men. Med. Sci. Sports Exercise **27:** 1516–1526.
19. KUTZA, J. & D.M. MURASKO. 1994. Effects of aging on natural killer cell activity and activation by interleukin-2 and IFN-α. Cell. Immunol. **155:** 195–204.
20. GUELDNER, S.H., L.W. POON, M. LAVIA, et al. 1997. Long term exercise patterns and immune function in healthy older women. Mech. Ageing Dev. **93:** 215–222.
21. DIPEITRO, R., R.A. RANA, A. SCISCIO, et al. 1996. Age- and training-related events in active T subpopulation. Mech. Ageing Dev. **90:** 103–109.
22. WANG, H.Y., T.R. BASHORE, Z.V. TRAN & E. FRIEDMAN. 2000. Age-related decreases in lymphocyte protein kinase C activity and translocation are reduced by aerobic fitness. J. Gerontol. Biol. Sci. **55A:** B545–B551.
23. WOODS, J.A., M.A. CEDDIA, B.W. WOLTERS, et al. 1999. Effects of 6 months of moderate aerobic exercise training on immune function in the elderly. Mech. Ageing Dev. **109:** 1–19.
24. FAHLMAN, M.D., M.G. BOARDLEY, W.A. FLYNN, et al. 2000. Effects of endurance training on selected parameters of immune function in elderly women. Gerontology **46:** 97–104.
25. CHIN A PAW, M.J.M., N. DEJONG, E.G.M. PALLAST, et al. 2000. Immunity in frail elderly: a randomized controlled trial of exercise and enriched foods. Med. Sci. Sports Exercise **32:** 2005–2011.
26. CRIST, D.M., L.T. MACKINNON, R.F. THOMPSON, et al. 1989. Physical exercise increases natural cellular-mediated tumor cytotoxicity in elderly women. Gerontology **35:** 66–71.
27. RALL, L.C., R. ROUBENOFF, J.G. CANNON, et al. 1996. Effects of progressive resistance training on immune response in aging and chronic inflammation. Med. Sci. Sports Exercise **28:** 1356–1365.
28. BERMON, S., P. PHILIP, P. FERRARI, et al. 1999. Effects of a short-term strength training programme on lymphocyte subsets at rest in elderly humans. Eur. J. Appl. Physiol. **79:** 336–340.
29. FLYNN, M.G., M. FAHLMAN, W.A. BRAUN, et al. 1999. Effects of resistance training on selected indexes of immune function in elderly women. J. Appl. Physiol. **86:** 1905–1913.
30. PICKER, L.J. & M.H. SIEGELMAN. 1999. Lymphoid tissues and organs. In Fundamental Immunology, 4th ed. W.E. Paul, Ed.: 479–531. Lippencott-Raven. Philadelphia, PA.
31. CHRISTOU, N.V., J. TELLADO-RODRIGUEZ, L. CHARTRAND, et al. 1989. Estimating mortality risk in preoperative patients using immunologic, nutritional, and acute-phase response variables. Ann. Surg. **210:** 69–77.
32. WAYNE, S.J., R.L. RHYNE, P.J. GARRY & J.S. GOODWIN. 1990. Cell-mediated immunity as a predictor of morbidity and mortality in subjects over 60. J. Gerontol. Med. Sci. **45:** M45–M48.
33. KOSTKA, T., S.E. BERTHOUZE, J. LACOUR, et al. 2000. The symptomatology of upper respiratory tract infections and exercise in elderly people. Med. Sci. Sports Exercise **32:** 46–51.
34. PAHLAVANI, M.A., T.H. CHEUNG, J.A. CHESKY & A. RICHARDSON. 1988. Influence of exercise on the immune function of rats of various ages. J. Appl. Physiol. **64:** 1997–2001.
35. NASRULLAH, I. & R.S. MAZZEO. 1992. Age-related immunosenescence in Fischer 344 rats: influence of exercise training. J. Appl. Physiol. **73:** 1932–1938.
36. BARNES, C.A., M.J. FORSTER, M. FLESHNER, et al. 1991. Neurobiol. Aging **12:** 47–53.
37. UTSUYAMA, M., M. ICHIKAWA, A. KONNO-SHIRAKAWA, Y. FUJITA & K. HIROKAWA. 1996. Retardation of the age-associated decline of immune functions in aging rats under dietary restriction and daily physical exercise. Mech. Ageing Dev. **91:** 219–228.
38. DE LA FUENTE, M., M. MINANO, V.M. VICTOR, et al. 1998. Relation between exploratory activity and immune function in aged mice: a preliminary study. Mech. Ageing & Dev. **102:** 263–277.
39. LU, Q., M.A. CEDDIA, E.A. PRICE, et al. 1999. Chronic exercise increases macrophage-mediated tumor cytolysis in young and old mice. Am. J. Physiol. **276:** R482–R489.
40. VIRU, A. 1992. Plasma hormones and physical exercise. Int. J. Sports Med. **13:** 201–209.
41. SZYGULA, Z. 1990. Erythrocytic system under the influence of physical exercise and training. Sports Med. **10:** 181-197.

42. AZENABOR, A.A. & L. HOFFMAN-GOETZ. 1999. Intrathymic and intrasplenic oxidative stress mediates thymocyte and splenocyte damage in acutely exercised mice. J. Appl. Physiol. **86:** 1823-1827.
43. NORTHOFF, H., A. BERG & C. WEINSTOCK. 1998. Similarities and differences of the immune response to exercise and trauma: the IFN-γ concept. Can. J. Physiol. Pharmacol. **76:** 497–504.
44. EVANS, W.J., R. ROUBENOFF & A. SHEVITZ. 1998. Exercise and the treatment of wasting: aging and human immunodeficiency virus infection. Semin. Oncol. **25:** 112–122.
45. MORIGUCHI, S., M. KATO, K. SAKAI, S. YAMAMOTO & E. SHIMIZU. 1998. Exercise training restores decreased cellular immune functions in obese Zucker rats. J. Appl. Physiol. **84:** 311–317.
46. JI, L.L. 1995. Exercise and oxidative stress: role of the cellular antioxidant systems. Exerc. Sport Sci. Rev. **23:** 135–166.
47. ERNST, D.N., O. WEIGLE & M.V. HOBBS. 1995. Aging and lymphokine gene expression by T cell subsets. Nutr. Rev. **53:** S18–S26.
48. MILLER, R.A. 1999. Aging and Immune Function (Chapter 28). *In* Fundamental Immunology, 4th ed. W.E. Paul, Ed.: Lippencott-Raven. Philadelphia, PA.

Fruit Polyphenolics and Brain Aging

Nutritional Interventions Targeting Age-related Neuronal and Behavioral Deficits

RACHEL L. GALLI,[a,b] BARBARA SHUKITT-HALE,[a] KURESH A. YOUDIM,[a] AND JAMES A. JOSEPH[a]

[a]*USDA-ARS, HNRCA at Tufts University, Boston, Massachusetts 02111, USA*

[b]*Department of Psychology, Simmons College, Boston, Massachusetts 02215, USA*

ABSTRACT: Nutritional interventions, in this case, increasing dietary intake of fruits and vegetables, can retard and even reverse age-related declines in brain function and in cognitive and motor performance in rats. Our lab has shown that as Fischer 344 rats age their brains are increasingly vulnerable to oxidative stress. Dietary supplementation with fruit or vegetable extracts high in antioxidants (e.g., blueberry, BB, spinach, respectively) can decrease this vulnerability to oxidative stress as assessed *in vivo* by examining reductions in neuronal signaling and behavioral deficits and *in vitro* via H_2O_2-induced decrements in striatal synaptosomal calcium buffering. Examinations have also revealed that BB supplementations are effective in antagonizing other age-related changes in brain and behavior, as well as decreasing indices of inflammation and oxidative stress in gastrocnemius and quadriceps muscles. In ongoing studies we are attempting to determine the most effective BB polyphenolic components. To date, the anthocyanins show the most efficacy in penetrating the cell membrane and in providing antioxidant protection. In sum, our results indicate that increasing dietary intake of fruits and vegetables high in antioxidant activity may be an important component of a healthy living strategy designed to maximize neuronal and cognitive functioning into old age.

KEYWORDS: dietary supplementation; diet; memory; learning; phytochemicals; phytonutrients; free radicals; oxidative stress; inflammation; behavior; cognitive behavior; blueberry; signal transduction; calcium flux; rats

As humans age they become increasingly likely to display age-related deficits in cognitive and motor performance, even when there is no underlying disease. One strategy to maximize the healthy life span and to retard and/or reverse the impairments associated with normal aging is through nutritional interventions. Research has demonstrated that diets rich in fruits and vegetables are effective at reducing the

---

Address for correspondence: Rachel L. Galli, Ph.D., Neuroscience Laboratory, USDA-ARS, HNRCA at Tufts University, 711 Washington St., Boston, MA 02111. Voice: 617-521-2607; fax: 617-556-3222.

rachel.galli@simmons.edu

rates of certain types of cancer and cardiovascular disease.[1] Our lab has examined the effects of dietary supplementation with fruits and vegetables on the neuronal and behavioral decrements seen with aging. To date, supplementing a rat's diet with a fruit or vegetable (e.g., blueberry, strawberry, spinach) has slowed and, in some cases, even reversed deficits in brain function, motor performance, and learning and memory in old animals.[2-5]

The brain uses a proportionally large amount of the body's oxygen supply, and with age its endogenous capacity to fight oxidative stress decreases.[6] The free radical theory of aging purports that as the balance between prooxidants and antioxidants shifts in favor of the prooxidants, damage to the brain results in decrements in neuronal and behavioral functioning.[7,8] We have shown that the fruits and vegetables that are most effective at ameliorating age-related deficits (e.g., signal transduction, motor performance, and cognitive behavior)[2-4] are those highest in antioxidant capacity.[9] However, cumulatively the multiple polyphenolic compounds present in fruits and vegetables have been shown to have additional effects, including antiinflamatory, antiallergic, antiviral, and antiproliferative, which suggests that their impact on central nervous system (CNS) function and on behavioral parameters may stem from a combination of factors.[1,10-13]

A number of neuronal mechanisms and behavioral measures have been shown by us and others to be affected by age in Fischer 344 (F344) rats.[5,14-20] Significant decrements occur in neuronal signal transduction, as measured by striatal dopamine release and GTPase activity as well as calcium clearance from striatal synaptosomes and measures of neuronal membrane fluidity, which appear to be age and oxidative stress dependent.[2,3,4,21-24] Age-related changes in CNS function are also evident in altered psychomotor and cognitive behaviors. Motor performance tests of balance, coordination, strength, and stamina clearly illustrate age-related declines starting at 12 months and continuing through 22 months.[18,19] A cognitive task assessing spatial learning and memory, the Morris water maze, has also characterized deficits associated with normal aging,[18,19] changes that parallel decrements in similar abilities in humans.[25,26] Age-sensitive neuronal and behavioral measures such as these can be expected to be affected by nutritional interventions seeking to retard or reverse the effects of brain aging.

Dietary supplementation with strawberry extract (STB) or spinach extract (SPC) from 6 to 15 months of age (Male F344 rats, source: NIA colony) prevented the onset of age-related deficits in signal transduction as measured by oxotremorine-enhanced dopamine (OX-enhanced DA) release and carbachol-stimulated GTPase coupling/uncoupling in isolated striatal slices, as compared to animals fed a control diet.[2,3] Additionally, aged animals fed a STB-, SPC-, or blueberry extract (BB)–supplemented diet for 8 weeks (19–21 months) demonstrated similar antiaging effects. In fact, the BB diet *reversed* the age-related deficits in OX-enhanced DA release.[3,4]

Efficient regulation of calcium flux and homeostasis is critical for signal transduction and optimal neuronal functioning. Fruit-supplemented diets high in polyphenolics were shown to have an antiaging effect on striatal Ca^{2+} uptake and recovery after depolarization in striatal synaptosomes.[2,3] The BB diet was especially effective, reversing the age-related decrement in Ca^{2+} recovery in the presence of hydrogen peroxide (H_2O_2)–induced oxidative stress, as compared to control groups. In addition, the BB diet improved cerebellar membrane fluidity, as measured by significantly reduced anistropy, compared to aged subjects maintained on a control diet.[4]

Behavioral measures showed some of the strongest antiaging effects of the fruit polyphenolic–supplemented diet. On three psychomotor tasks, the rod walk and accelerating roto-rod, which assess balance, coordination, and resistance to fatigue, and the inclined screen, which measures strength, stamina, and balance, the BB diet significantly improved the performance of old animals.[3,4]

In addition, a measure of cognitive performance was improved by all three fruit- and vegetable-supplemented diets. The Morris water maze (MWM) is a spatial learning task that measures acquisition, working memory, reference memory, the ability to shift set, and spatial learning strategies.[18,27] The maze is a featureless circular pool of room temperature water (1 m diameter) containing a 10-cm-diameter movable platform hidden just below the surface of the water. Rats swim well and use distal cues to learn to navigate to the hidden platform. This age-sensitive paradigm is a well-accepted measure of hippocampally based learning and memory. Dietary supplementation with either STB, SPC, or BB for eight weeks antagonized the age-related impairments in MWM performance.[3,4]

As might be suggested by the robust behavioral results, the physiological effects of polyphenolic dietary supplementation is not limited to the CNS. In the periphery, we have found that a BB diet decreases markers of inflammation and oxidative stress in the gastrocnemius and quadriceps muscles (in preparation) and have also shown BB supplementation to significantly increase red blood cell (RBC) membrane fluidity.[4]

Ongoing studies seek to characterize which polyphenolic compounds present in BB and other fruits and vegetables may contribute to the significant antiaging effects described above. Initial studies have determined that anthocyanins and hydroxycinnamic acids (HCA) isolated from blueberries are able to ameliorate *in vitro* H_2O_2-induced oxidative stress, with the anthocyanins significantly protecting RBCs against reactive oxygen species even at low doses.[28] Following a 24-hour fast, F344 rats were anesthetized and either anthocyanin or HCA, extracted from blueberry skin or flesh, respectively, were administered by stomach intubation. RBC susceptibility to H_2O_2-mediated oxidative stress was assessed by dichlorofluorescein assay at 0-, 1-, 6-, and 24-hours postgavage. While the total concentration of plasma anthocyanin and HCA fell off rapidly from 1 hour on, significant protection from reactive oxygen species was seen at 6 and 24 hours. Other experiments have shown that berry anthocyanins penetrate a variety of cell types and that incorporation into the cell's cytosol protects against H_2O_2-induced oxidative stress and loss of cell function.[29] Further studies will investigate the protective effects of a variety of polyphenolic compounds in order to clarify the complete profile of phytonutrients found in fruits and vegetables with antiaging effects.

Diets supplemented with fruits and vegetables rich in color and correspondingly high in anthocyanins and other polyphenolic phytonutrients with antioxidant and additional bioactive properties antagonize the effects of aging in our animal model. The amounts of BB, STB, and SPC added to the diets were matched for antioxidant capacity[2,3,9] and are roughly equivalent to a daily one cup portion for humans. In sum, research from our lab and others suggests that increasing dietary intake of fruits and vegetables high in antioxidant activity may be an important component of a healthy living strategy designed to maximize neuronal and cognitive functioning into old age.

REFERENCES

1. HOLLMAN, P.C. & M.B. KATAN. 1999. Health effects and bioavailability of dietary flavonols. Free Radical Res. **31:** S75–S80.
2. JOSEPH, J.A., B. SHUKITT-HALE, N.A. DENISOVA, *et al.* 1998. Long-term dietary strawberry, spinach, or vitamin E supplementation retards the onset of age-related neuronal signal-transduction and cognitive behavioral deficits. J. Neurosci. **18:** 8047–8055.
3. JOSEPH, J.A., B. SHUKITT-HALE, N.A. DENISOVA, *et al.* 1999. Reversals of age-related declines in neuronal signal transduction, cognitive and motor behavioral deficits with diets supplemented with blueberry, spinach or strawberry dietary supplementation. J. Neurosci. **19:** 8114–8121.
4. YOUDIM, K.A., B. SHUKITT-HALE, A. MARTIN, *et al.* 2000. Short-term dietary supplementation of blueberry polyphenolics: beneficial effects on aging brain performance and peripheral tissue function. Nutr. Neurosci. **3:** 383–397.
5. BICKFORD, P.C. 1993. Motor learning deficits in aged rats are correlated with loss of cerebellar noradrenergic function. Brain Res. **620:** 133–138.
6. SOKOLOFF, L., G.G. FITZGERALD & E.E. KAUFMAN. 1977. Determinants of the availability of nutrients to the brain. *In* Nutrition and the Brain. J.R. Wurtman & J.J. Wurtman, Eds.: 87–139. Raven Press. New York.
7. AMES, B.N., M.K. SHIGENAGA & T.M. HAGEN. 1993. Oxidants, antioxidants, and the degenerative disease of aging. Proc. Natl. Acad. Sci. USA **90:** 7915–7922.
8. HARMAN, D. 1994. Free-radical theory of aging. Increasing the functional life span. Ann. N.Y. Acad. Sci. **717:** 1–15.
9. WANG, H., G. CAO & R.L. PRIOR. 1996. Total antioxidant capacity of fruits. J. Agric. Food Chem. **44:** 701–705.
10. MIDDLETON, E., JR. 1998. Effect of plant flavonoids on immune and inflammatory cell function. Adv. Exp. Med. Biol. **439:** 175–182.
11. EASTWOOD, M.A. 1999. Interaction of dietary antioxidants in vivo: how fruit and vegetables prevent disease? Q.J.M. **92:** 527–530.
12. GERRITSEN, M.E. 1998. Flavonoid inhibitors of cytokine induced gene expression. *In* Flavonoids in the Living System. J. Manthey & B. Buslig, Eds.: 183–190. Plenum Press. New York.
13. FOTSIS, T., M.S. PEPPER, E. AKTAS, *et al.* 1997. Flavonoids, dietary-derived inhibitors of cell proliferation and in vitro angiogenesis. Cancer Res. **57:** 2916–2921.
14. JOSEPH, J.A. R.E. BERGER, B.T. ENGEL & G.S. ROTH. 1978. Age-related changes in the nigrostriatum: a behavioral and biochemical analysis. J. Gerontol. **33:** 643–649.
15. JOSEPH, J.A., M.A. KOWATCH, T. MAKI & G.S. ROTH. 1990. Selective cross activation/inhibition of second messenger systems and the reduction of age-related deficits in the muscarinic control of dopamine release from perfused rat striata. Brain Res. **537:** 40–48.
16. JOSEPH, J.A., R.T. BARTUS, D.E. CLODY, *et al.* 1983. Psychomotor performance in the senescent rodent: reduction of deficits via striatal dopamine receptor up-regulation. Neruobiol. Aging **4:** 313–319.
17. INGRAM, D.K., M. JUCKER & E. SPANGLER. 1994. Behavioral manifestations of aging. *In* Pathobiology of the Aging Rat. U. Mohr, D.L. Cungworth & C.C. Capen, Eds.: 149–170. ILSI. Washington.
18. SHUKITT-HALE, B., G. MOUZAKIS & J.A. JOSEPH. 1998. Psychomotor and spatial memory performance in aging male Fischer 344 rats. Exp. Gerontol. **33:** 615–624.
19. SHUKITT-HALE, B. 1999. The effects of aging and oxidative stress on psychomotor and cognitive behavior. Age **22:** 9–17.
20. CANTUTI-CASTELVETRI, I., B. SHUKITT-HALE & J.A. JOSEPH. 2000. Neurobehavioral aspects of antioxidants and aging. Int. J. Dev. Neurosci. **18:** 367–381.
21. JOSEPH, J.A., J.G. STRAIN, N.D. JIMENEZ & D. FISHER. 1997. Oxidant injury in PC12 cells—a possible model of calcium deregulation in aging. I. Selectivity of protection against oxidative stress. J. Neurochem. **69:** 1252–1258.
22. DENISOVA, N.A., S.A. ERAT, J.F. KELLY & G.S. ROTH. 1998. Differential effect of aging on cholesterol modulation of carbachol stimulated Low-Km GTPase in striatal synaptosomes. Exp. Gerontol. **33:** 249–265.

23. DENISOVA, N.A., D. FISHER, M. PROVOST & J.A. JOSEPH. 1999. The role of glutathione, membrane sphingomyelin, and its metabolites in oxidative stress-induced calcium 'dysregulation' in PC12 cells. Free Radic. Biol. Med. **27:** 1292–1301.
24. JOSEPH, J.A., B. SHUKITT-HALE, J. MCEWEN & B. RABIN. 1999. Magnesium activation of GTP hydrolysis or incubation in S-Adenosyl-1-methionine reverses 56Fe-induced decrements in oxotremorine-enhancement of K+ evoked striatal dopamine release. Radiat. Res. **152:** 637–641.
25. MUIR, J.L. 1997. Acetylcholine, aging, and Alzheimer's disease. Pharmacol. Biochem. Behav. **56:** 687–696.
26. WEST, R.L. 1996. An application of pre-frontal cortex function theory to cognitive aging. Psych. Bull. **120:** 272–292.
27. MORRIS, R. 1984. Developments of a water maze procedure for studying spatial learning in the rat. J. Neurosci. Methods **11:** 47–60.
28. YOUDIM, K.A., B. SHUKITT-HALE, S. MACKINNON, *et al.* 2000. Polyphenolics enhance red blood cell resistance to oxidative stress: in vitro and in vivo. Biochim. Biophys. Acta **1523:** 117–122.
29. YOUDIM, K.A., A. MARTIN & J.A. JOSEPH. 2000. Incorporation of the elderberry anthocyanins by endothelial cells increases protection against oxidative stress. Free Radic. Biol. Med. **29:** 51–60.

Delaying Brain Mitochondrial Decay and Aging with Mitochondrial Antioxidants and Metabolites

JIANKANG LIU,[a] HANI ATAMNA,[a] HIROHIKO KURATSUNE,[b] AND BRUCE N. AMES[a]

[a]*Division of Biochemistry and Molecular Biology, University of California, Berkeley, California 94720, USA and Children's Hospital Oakland Research Institute, Oakland, California 94609, USA*

[b]*Department of Hematology and Oncology, Osaka University, Osaka 565-0871, Japan*

ABSTRACT: Mitochondria decay with age due to the oxidation of lipids, proteins, RNA, and DNA. Some of this decay can be reversed in aged animals by feeding them the mitochondrial metabolites acetylcarnitine and lipoic acid. In this review, we summarize our recent studies on the effects of these mitochondrial metabolites and mitochondrial antioxidants (α-phenyl-*N-t*-butyl nitrone and *N-t*-butyl hydroxylamine) on the age-associated mitochondrial decay of the brain of old rats, neuronal cells, and human diploid fibroblast cells. In feeding studies in old rats, these mitochondrial metabolites and antioxidants improve the age-associated decline of ambulatory activity and memory, partially restore mitochondrial structure and function, inhibit the age-associated increase of oxidative damage to lipids, proteins, and nucleic acids, elevate the levels of antioxidants, and restore the activity and substrate binding affinity of a key mitochondrial enzyme, carnitine acetyltrasferase. These mitochondrial metabolites and antioxidants protect neuronal cells from neurotoxin- and oxidant-induced toxicity and oxidative damage; delay the normal senescence of human diploid fibroblast cells, and inhibit oxidant-induced acceleration of senescence. These results suggest a plausible mechanism: with age, increased oxidative damage to proteins and lipid membranes, particularly in mitochondria, causes a deformation of structure of enzymes, with a consequent decrease of enzyme activity as well as substrate binding affinity for their substrates; an increased level of substrate restores the velocity of the reaction and restores mitochondrial function, thus delaying mitochondrial decay and aging. This loss of activity due to coenzyme or substrate binding appears to be true for a number of other enzymes as well, including mitochondrial complex III and IV.

KEYWORDS: acetyl-L-carnitine; aging; brain; *N-t*-butyl hydroxylamine; lipoic acid; memory; mitochondria; neurotoxicity; oxidative damage; α-phenyl-*N-t*-butyl nitrone

Address for correspondence: Professor Bruce Ames, Children's Hospital Oakland Research Institute, 5700 Martin Luther King Jr. Way, Oakland, CA 94609. Voice: 510-450-7625; fax: 510-597-7128.

bnames@uclink4.berkeley.edu

INTRODUCTION

Aging is characterized by a general decline in physiological functions that affects many tissues and increases the risk of death. The role of mitochondria in the process of the age-dependent deterioration of tissues has become the focus of many studies with the gradually accepted idea that mitochondrial decay is a major contributor to aging.[1-10] The age-dependent changes in mitochondria are characterized by a high rate of generation of oxidants, a decline in the activity of electron transport complexes, and a decrease in amount and fatty acid composition of cardiolipin, an essential phospholipid for normal function of mitochondria. During ATP production by oxidative phosphorylation, electrons from NADH or succinate in the mitochondrial matrix are transferred through the electron transport chain (complexes I through IV) and reduce molecular oxygen to water. In this process, about 2% of the electrons leak and reduce O_2 to $O^{\bullet-}_2$ radical and H_2O_2. The leakage of oxidants from the electron transport chain appears unavoidable, and mitochondria are considered the main endogenous source for the formation of the superoxide radical. As the source of these toxic oxidants, mitochondria are also their potential victims. Their proximity to the oxidants they produce, combined with their exceedingly intricate structure and the combination of continuous formation of $O^{\bullet-}_2$, as well as a limited antioxidant capacity of mitochondria, make them vulnerable to oxidative damage. For example, mitochondria lack catalase, the ability to synthesize GSH, the ability to transport GSSG out of the matrix, and chelators for heavy metals, all of which act as elements to decrease oxidant production.[1-16] Mitochondrial decay is also a contributor to acceleration of aging in the senescence-accelerated mouse[17-19] and in stress.[20,21]

Compared with young rats, old rats have a lower mitochondrial potential, cardiolipin level, respiratory control ratio, and cellular oxygen uptake and antioxidants, and have higher oxidants, neuronal RNA oxidation, and mutagenic aldehydes from lipid peroxidation.[22-28] Heart mitochondria in old rats had significantly lower cardiolipin content, reduced activities of cytochrome *c* oxidase and adenine nucleotide translocase, and slower rates of phosphate and pyruvate transport, palmitoylcarnitine-supported respiration, and the exchange reactions of carnitine–carnitine and carnitine–palmitoylcarnitine.[29-34] In addition, old rats show a decline of ambulatory activity and memory.[27,35-40] Feeding old rats acetylcarnitine and/or lipoic acid restores mitochondrial function, lowers oxidants, inhibits oxidative damage to lipids, proteins, and nucleic acids, enhances ambulatory activity, and improves memory, thus reversing mitochondrial decay.[22-28,31-34,36-38,41-44] Creatine, another mitochondrial metabolite, shows neuroprotective effects in a transgenic mouse model of Huntington's disease. Creatine may exert these neuroprotective effects by increasing phosphocreatine levels or by stabilizing the mitochondrial permeability transition.[45] Clinical trials in old people with creatine showed that creatine improves exercise performance, has a beneficial effect on reducing muscle fatigue,[46-49] and increases the anaerobic power and work capacity of both young and old sedentary persons during maximal pedaling tasks.[50]

In this review, we summarize some of our recent studies on the effects of the mitochondrial metabolites acetyl-L-carnitine (ALCAR) and lipoic acid (LA) and of mitochondrial antioxidants (α-phenyl-*N-t*-butyl nitrone [PBN] and *N-t*-butyl hydroxylamine, also including LA) on age-associated mitochondrial decay in the brain of old rats, neuronal cells, and human diploid fibroblast cells.

LIPOIC ACID COUNTERACTS THE EFFECT OF OXIDANTS AND NEUROTOXINS ON HT4 AND HT22 NEURONAL CELL LINES

Lipoic acid plays a fundamental role in mitochondrial metabolism. Biologically, it exists in proteins, where it is linked covalently to a lysyl residue as a lipoamide. The mitochondrial E3 enzyme, dihydrolipoyl dehydrogenase, reduces lipoate to dihydrolipoate at the expense of NADH. Lipoate is also a substrate for the NADPH-dependent enzyme glutathione reductase.[51–53] In recent years, lipoic acid has gained considerable attention as an antioxidant.[52,54,55] The reduced form of lipoic acid, dihydrolipoic acid, reacts with oxidants such as superoxide radicals, hydroxyl radicals, hypochlorous acid, peroxyl radicals, and singlet oxygen. It also protects membranes by reducing oxidized vitamin C and glutathione, which may in turn recycle vitamin E. Administration of alpha-lipoic acid is beneficial to a number of oxidative stress models such as diabetes, cataract, HIV activation, neurodegeneration, and radiation injury in animals. Furthermore, lipoic acid functions as a redox regulator of proteins such as myoglobin, prolactin, thioredoxin, and NF-kappa B transcription factor.[51,54,56] Lipoic acid has neuroprotective effects in neuronal cells.[57–61] One possible mechanism for the antioxidant effect of lipoic acid is its metal chelating activity.[62] Lipoic acid can increase ambulatory activity, improve memory in aged animals, and partially restore age-associated mitochondrial decay in liver and heart.[24,63,64] Lipoic acid is used to treat or prevent peripheral neuropathy and cardiac autonomic neuropathy, insulin resistance in type II diabetes, retinopathy and cataract, glaucoma, HIV/AIDS, cancer, liver disease, Wilson's disease, cardiovascular disease, and lactic acidosis caused by inborn errors of metabolism. It has also been used for treating Alzheimer-type dementia.[65]

The glutamate receptors mediate excitatory neurotransmission in the brain and are important in memory acquisition and learning and implicated in some neurodegenerative disorders.[66–68] This receptor family is classified in three groups: the N-methyl-D-aspartate (NMDA), alpha-amino-3-hydroxy-5-methyl-4-isoxazolepropionate (AMPA)-kainate, and metabotropic receptors. Excessive activation of the NMDA receptor leads to a large influx of calcium into neurons and subsequent generation of oxidants and oxidative stress by the stimulation of phospholipase A_2.[20,69,70] Increased intracellular calcium may cause mitochondrial dysfunction, which can result in localized oxidant formation within mitochondria and an inability to handle free calcium.[66,71]

Intact mitochondrial function appears to be essential for neuronal resistance to excitotoxic insults. It is believed that the reduced levels of ATP that accompany abnormal mitochondrial function are insufficient to drive the ion pumps that maintain neuronal membrane polarization. With depolarization of the neuronal membrane, the magnesium that normally blocks the NMDA receptor ion channel is extruded, and ambient extracellular levels of glutamate may become lethal via NMDA receptor mechanism. On the basis of this mechanism, it seems likely that compounds such as lipoic acid, which could enhance mitochondrial function, scavenge free radicals, or increase the levels of the antioxidants glutathione (GSH) and ascorbate, might be useful neuroprotective agents. Therefore, we have examined the effects of lipoic acid on neurotoxin- or oxidant-induced toxicity in HT4 cells and HT22 cells. The HT4 cell line was constructed by McKay *et al.* in 1989, and was derived from mouse neuronal tissue. Morimoto and Koshland have shown that HT4 cells possess

NMDA receptors.[72] The HT22 cell line is a subclone of HT4. HT22 (the immortalized mouse cell line) lacks ionotropic glutamate receptors and responds to oxidative glutamate toxicity with a form of programmed cell death that is distinct from classical apoptosis.[73–75]

Dose-dependent cell injury in HT4 and HT22 cells is caused by glutamate (an excitotoxin), thapsigargin (an apoptosis-inducing agent), hydrogen peroxide (a typical oxidant), homocysteic acid (a cysteine uptake inhibitor), diethyl maleate (a proxidant which depletes intracellular glutathione), apomorphine (a memory-impairing agent), SIN-1 (a generator of peroxynitrate), and 6-hydroxydopamine (an oxidant generator in brain).

FIGURE 1 shows a morphologic picture of the toxicity of glutamate and thapsigargin in HT4 cells, suggesting that glutamate, like thapsigargin, induces apoptosis in neuronal cells.

FIGURE 2 shows the dose-dependent toxicity of glutamate and SIN-1 in HT4 cells. The TD50 in HT22 was twice that in HT4 (data not shown), possibly due to the lack of ionotropic glutamate receptors in HT22 cells.

Lipoic acid appears to have an antiapoptotic effect because it prevents the cells from glutamate-induced toxicity. FIGURE 3 shows the dose-dependent protective effect of lipoic acid on cell viability in HT22 cells. Lipoic acid displayed its protective effect from 10 µM up to 1 mM under the conditions studied. FIGURE 4 shows the protective effect of lipoic acid on cell death induced by glutamate, evaluated by trypan blue exclusion assay, confirming the results of the viability assay by MTT.

FIGURE 5 gives a morphological picture of the toxicity of 6-hydroxydopamine (6-OHDA) and the protective effect of lipoic acid in HT22 cells, and FIGURE 6 shows the toxicity of homocysteic acid and the protective effect of lipoic acid also in HT22 cells. These results suggest that lipoic acid can prevent neuronal cells from a variety of neurotoxins.

FIGURE 7 depicts the glutamate-induced generation of oxidants and the inhibition by lipoic acid of both the spontaneous and glutamate-induced oxidants in HT4 cells, measured by the fluorescence of the oxidation of $2',7'$-dichlorodihydrofluorescein diacetate (DCFH).

FIGURE 8 shows that glutamate induces a decrease of GSH in HT4 cells and lipoic acid increases the level of GSH and also inhibits the glutamate-induced GSH decrease.

FIGURE 9 shows that all forms of lipoic acid, including the natural form R-, the unnatural form S-, and R,S-lipoic acid as well as its reduced form, dihydrolipoic acid, have similar protective effects whether in a short-term (24 h) or a long-term (72 h) treatment.[76,77] This result is similar to that obtained by Wolz and Krieglstein in primary cultures of neurons from chick embryo telencephalons and also an *in vivo* study in rats using subcutaneous injection,[57,58] but different from that in an *ex vivo* study with isolated rat hepatocytes.[24]

Lipoic acid effectively protects against most neurotoxin-induced toxicity by inhibiting generation of oxidants and elevating antioxidant GSH level, thus preventing loss in viability and cell death. These results, together with previous studies,[57–61] suggest that lipoic acid is an effective neuroprotective agent for ameliorating toxin-induced and age-associated neurodegeneration.

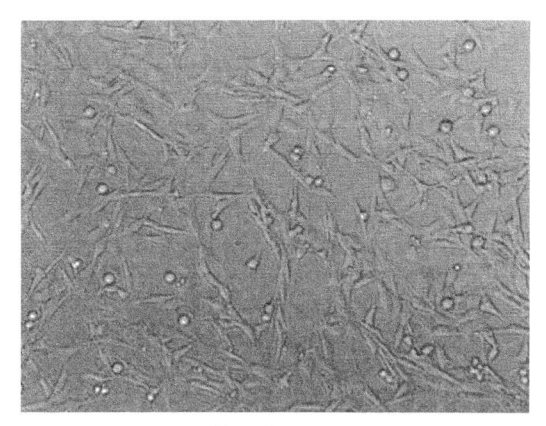

Control

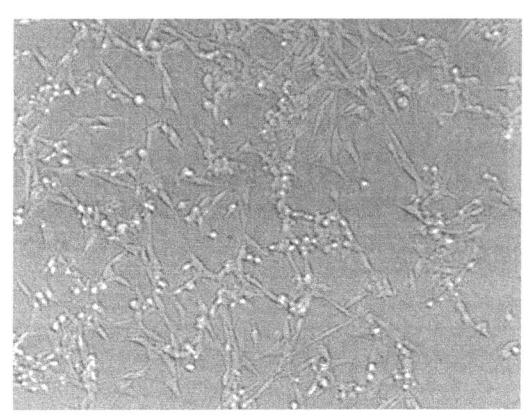

Glutamate 0.625 mM

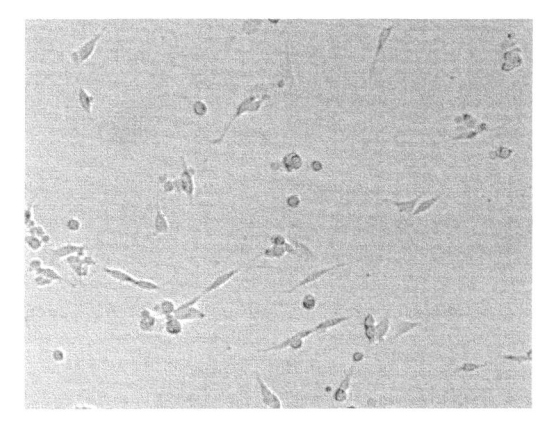

Glutamate 1.25 mM

FIGURE 1. Morphologic observation of the toxicity of glutamate and thapsigargin in HT4 cells. Cells were seeded at 3000 per well in a 96-well plate and treated with glutamate or thapsigargin for 24 h and observed under the microscope.

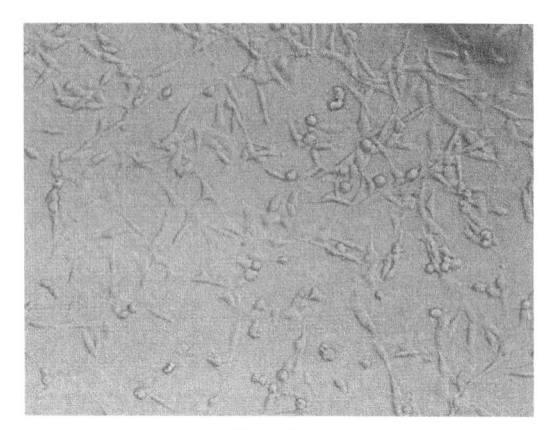

Control

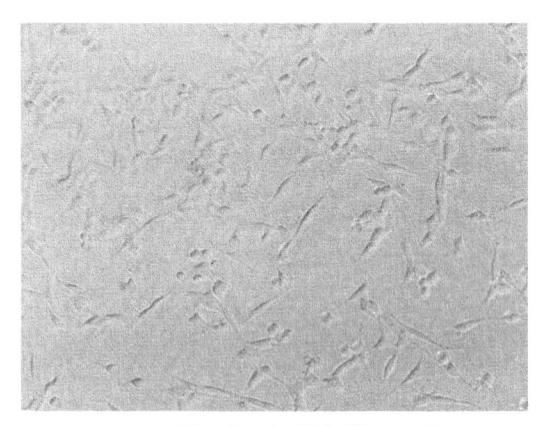

Thapsigargin 62.5 nM

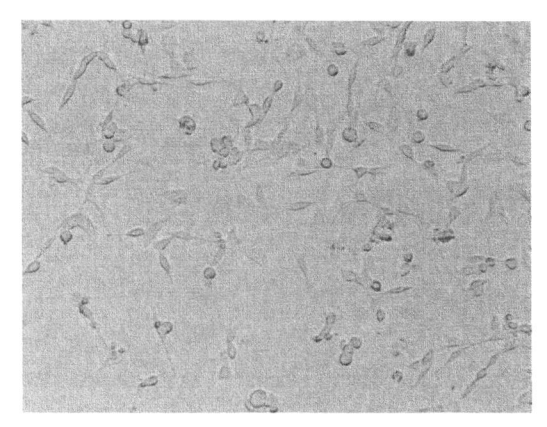

Thapsigargin 125 nM

FIGURE 1. *Continued.*

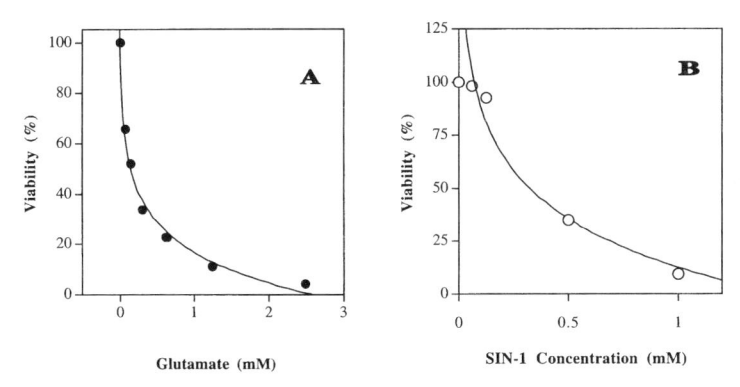

FIGURE 2. Dose-dependent toxicity of glutamate (A) and SIN-1 (B) in HT4 cells. HT4 cells were treated with toxins for 24 h, and the cell viability was evaluated by MTT assay.

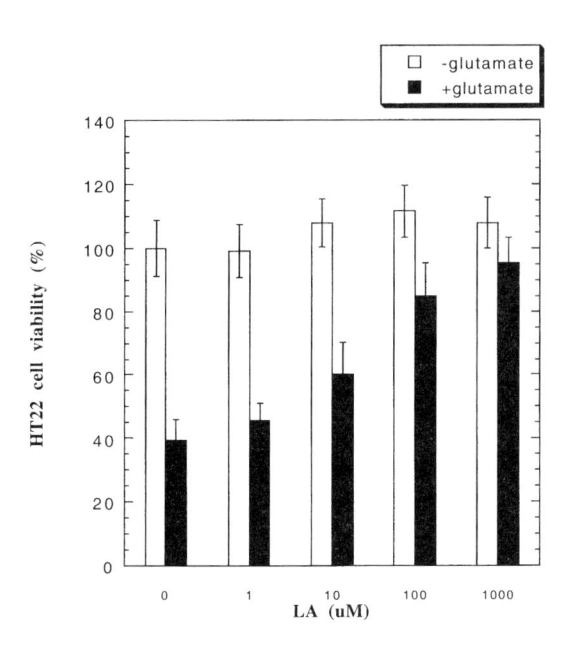

FIGURE 3. Dose-dependent protective effect of lipoic acid (LA) on glutamate-induced toxicity in HT22 cells (kindly provided by Dr. D. Schubert at the Salk Institute for Biological Studies at La Jolla, CA). Cells were seeded at 3000 per well in a 96-well plate for one day, treated with lipoic acid for 24 h, and then challenged with 2 mM glutamate for 24 h. The cell viability was evaluated by MTT assay.

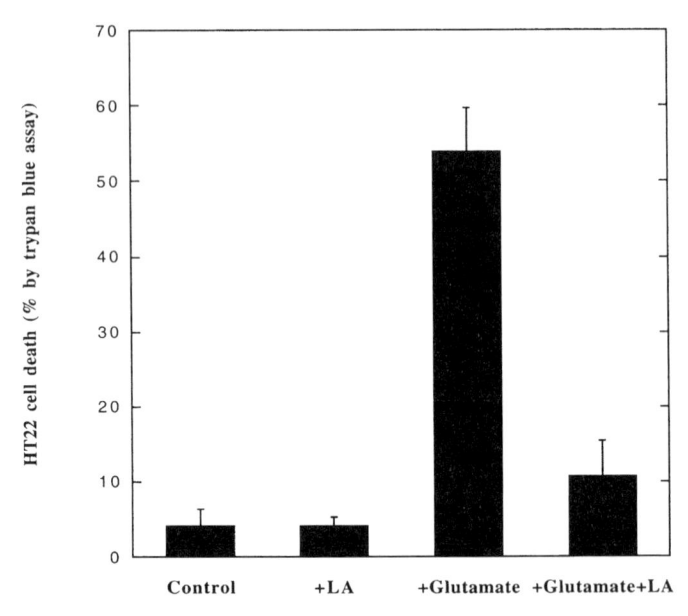

FIGURE 4. Glutamate-induced cell death and the protective effect of lipoic acid (LA) in HT22 cells. Cells were seeded at 20,000 per well in a 24-well plate for one day, treated with 100 μM lipoic acid for 24 h, and then challenged with 2 mM glutamate for 24 h in the presence or absence of LA. Cell death was evaluated by trypan blue assay.

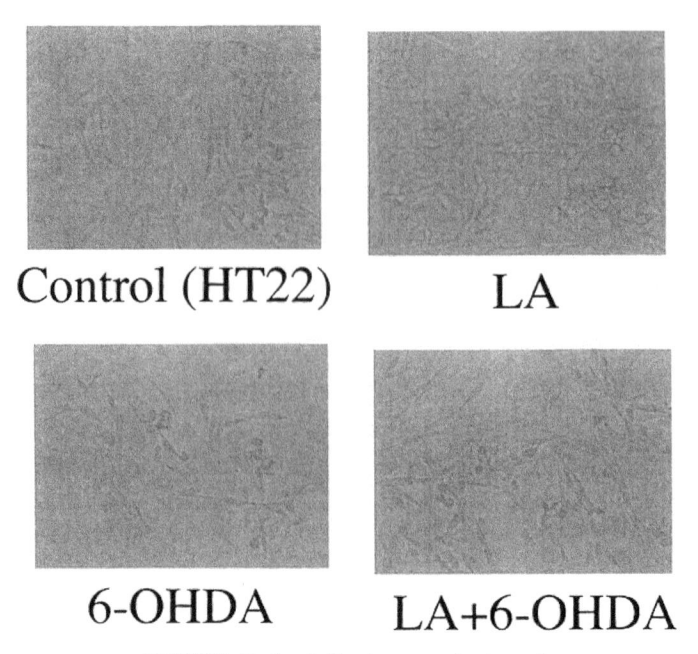

FIGURE 5. *See following page for legend.*

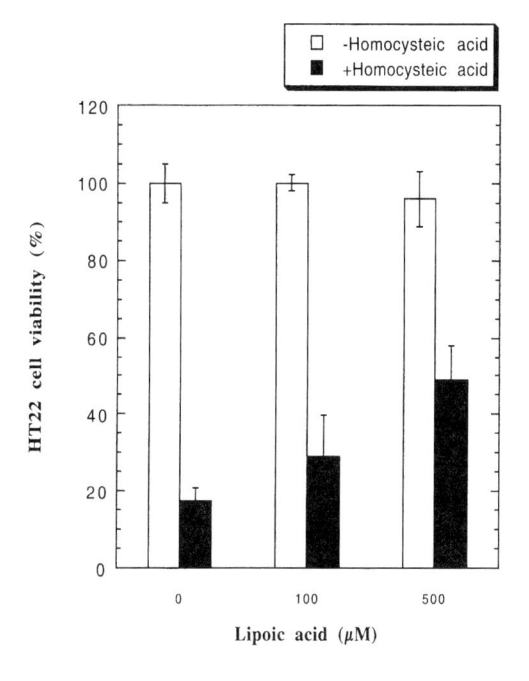

FIGURE 6. Homocysteic acid–induced toxicity and the protective effect of lipoic acid in HT22 cells. Cells were seeded 3000 per well in a 96-well plate for one day, treated with lipoic acid for 24 h, and then challenged with homocysteic acid (1 mM) for 24 h. The cell viability was evaluated by MTT assay.

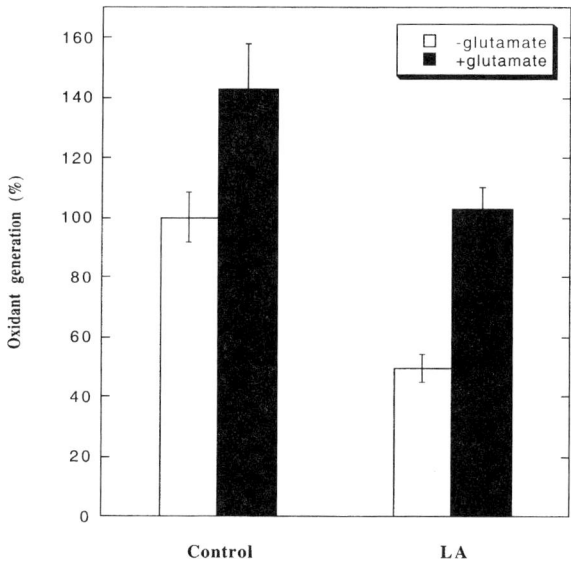

FIGURE 7. Glutamate-induced generation of oxidants and the protective effect of lipoic acid (LA). HT4 cells were pretreated with lipoic acid, 500 µM, and then challenged with 5 mM glutamate for 2 h. The oxidant generation was measured by the fluorescence of the oxidation of 2′,7′-dichlorodihydrofluorescein diacetate (DCFH) using a fluorescence spectrometer.

FIGURE 5. Morphologic picture of the toxicity of 6-hydroxydopamine (6-OHDA) and the protective effect of lipoic acid (LA) in HT22 cells. Cells were seeded at 20,000 per well in a 24-well plate for one day, treated with 100 µM lipoic acid for 24 h, then challenged with 6-OHDA (100 µM) for 24 h, and observed under the microscope.

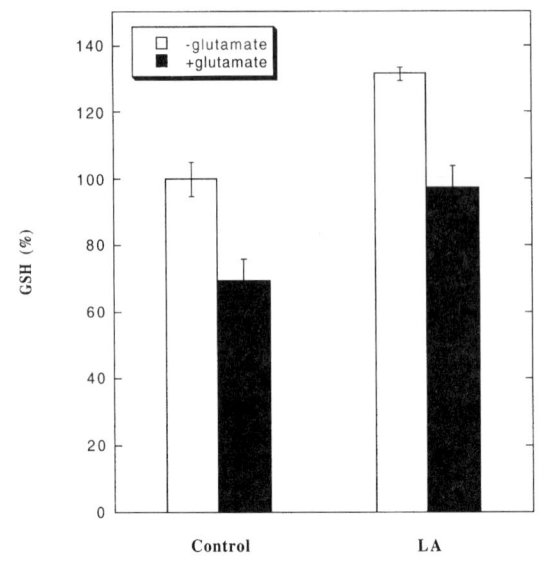

FIGURE 8. Glutamate-induced reduction of GSH and the protective effect of lipoic acid (LA). HT4 cells were pretreated with lipoic acid, 100 μM, and then challenged with 1 mM glutamate for 24 h. The GSH levels was measured with the DTNB assay using a microplate spectrometer.

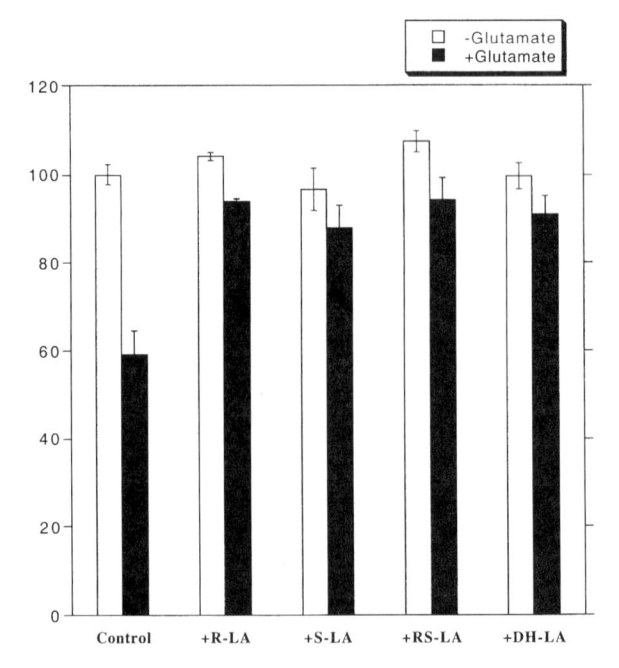

FIGURE 9. Comparison of the protective effects of R-lipoic acid (R-LA), S-lipoic acid (S-LA), RS-lipoic acid (RS-LA), and dihydrolipoic acid (DHLA) on glutamate-induced toxicity in HT22 cells. Cells were seeded at 3000 per well in a 96-well plate for one day, treated with lipoic acid (100 μM) for 24 h, and then challenged with 2 mM glutamate for 24 h. The cell viability was evaluated by the MTT assay.

LIPOIC ACID PROTECTS HUMAN DIPLOID FIBROBLAST CELLS FROM OXIDANT-INDUCED SENESCENCE AND MITOCHONDRIAL MORPHOLOGIC CHANGE

Human diploid fibroblast cells have been used as an *in vitro* model for studying the mechanism of aging. Unlike immortalized cells, the normal primary human diploid fibroblast cells gradually reach a senescent state, where the cells can no longer replicate and have altered morphology. When young cells were treated with sublethal concentrations of H_2O_2, the majority of the cells displayed a phenotype resembling senescence, including loss in the ability to respond to a variety of growth factors to replicate, reduced activity of cell cycle–related enzymes ornithine decarboxylase and thymidine kinase, and enlarged cell size, suggesting that oxidants can cause senescence.[78–80]

FIGURE 10 shows that LA treatment can prevent the human diploid fibroblast IMR-90 cells from oxidant-induced senescence. LA inhibits the H_2O_2-induced decline of population doubling, suggesting that LA has an antiaging effect.

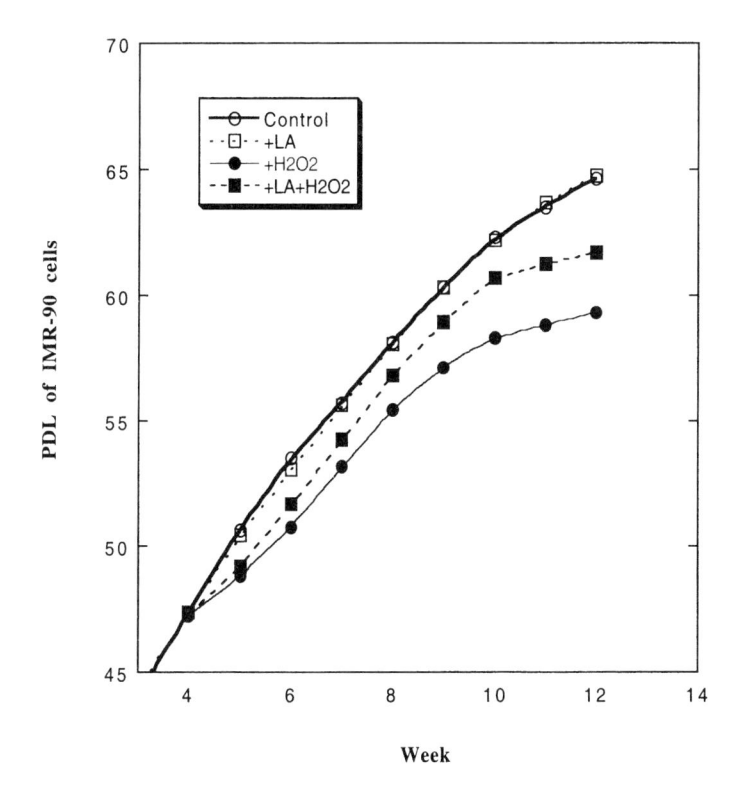

FIGURE 10. Hydrogen peroxide–induced acceleration of senescence and the protective effect of lipoic acid (LA) in IMR-90 cells. IMR-90 cells were treated with 1 µM lipoic acid continuously, and the cells were challenged with 200 µM H_2O_2 once at the fourth week.

Massive changes in the morphology of mitochondria occur during apoptosis, necrosis, and aging. Mitochondrial morphology can be studied with nonyl acridine orange (NAO), a cardiolipin-specific fluorescent label, and by flow cytometry.[81–83] When preloaded with NAO and then treated with hydrogen peroxide, cells showed an increment in the fluorescence emitted from NAO, when compared to controls (FIG. 11). We refer to this finding as hyperstaining of mitochondria because nonspecific mitochondrial toxins do not induce hyperstaining of mitochondria. Age-related hyperstaining of mitochondria is observed as human lung fibroblast senescence and in white blood cells isolated from old rats compared to young rats.[84,85] Hyperstaining of mitochondria as measured by NAO is a marker that indicates exposure of cells to conditions of stress.[81] LA was found to prevent H_2O_2-induced mitochondrial morphologic change (FIG. 11), suggesting that LA has its antiaging effect by protecting mitochondrial structure, integrity, and function.

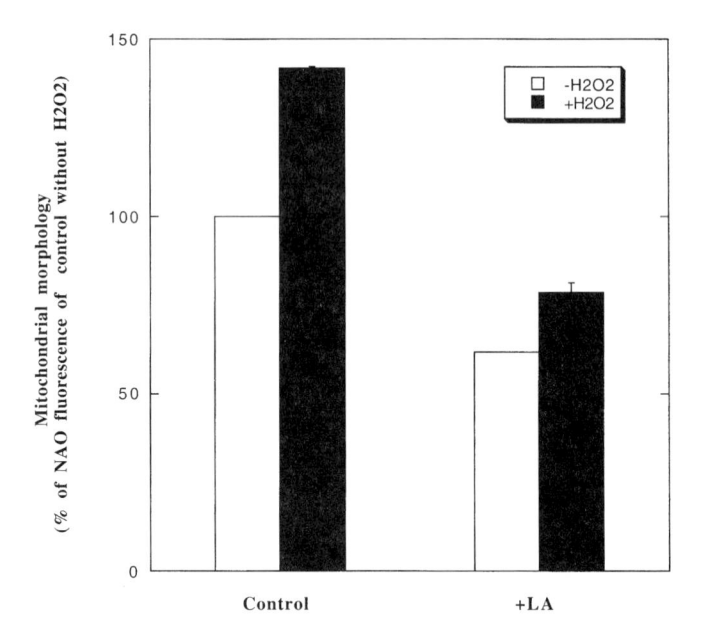

FIGURE 11. Hydrogen peroxide–induced mitochondrial morphologic change and the protective effects of lipoic acid (LA) in IMR-90 cells. Two million cells/mL in DMEM-Hepes were exposed to hydrogen peroxide (200 μM) at 37°C for 20 min. The cells were then washed and resuspended into the same medium, but supplemented with 1 μM NAO and incubated at 37°C for 10 min. Excess NAO was removed, and the cells were suspended into 500 μL Hanks' buffer and then analyzed by the flow cytometer, as described in Atamna et al.[81]

ACETYL-L-CARNITINE REVERSES AGE-ASSOCIATED MITOCHONDRIAL DECAY IN RATS: A DOSE-RESPONSE STUDY

L-Carnitine has been described as a conditionally essential nutrient for humans. L-Carnitine is a betaine required for the transport of long-chain fatty acids into the mitochondria for fuel. It also facilitates the removal from the mitochondria of the excess short- and medium-chain fatty acids that accumulate during metabolism.[86,87] L-Carnitine, and its acetyl derivative, ALCAR, affect other cellular functions, including maintenance of key proteins and lipids of the mitochondria at sufficient levels and proper membrane orientation, for maximum energy production.[86,88] ALCAR, like L-carnitine, is present in high concentration in the brain as well as muscle, and provides acetyl-equivalents for the production of the neurotransmitter acetylcholine.[89–91] Experimental data have demonstrated an age-associated decrease of tissue levels of L-carnitine in animals, including humans, and an associated decrease in the integrity of the mitochondrial membrane.[92–94]

ALCAR is more widely used than L-carnitine in animal research and clinical trials to gain metabolic benefits to the brain, heart, liver, and other organs. In aging or in conditions of disease, ALCAR is better absorbed and more efficiently crosses the blood–brain barrier, as compared to L-carnitine.[95] In animals, the effect most studied is improvement of age-associated cognitive dysfunction, including tests of Morris water maze for spatial memory,[96] active avoidance learning,[42] discrimination learning,[37] radial maze,[97] and long-term memory performance in the split-stem T-maze.[98] These tests show that ALCAR improves the age-associated decline of learning and memory in old animals. Long-term ALCAR feeding decreases mortality, does not interfere with food and water intake, and increases longevity.[99] ALCAR affects physical activity in different ways, depending on the experiment. Hagen et al.[22] found that ALCAR increases ambulatory activity in old rats, suggesting that ALCAR increases metabolic activity; Onofrj et al.[100] found that ALCAR-treated rats show heightened arousal, while Blokland et al.[101] found that ALCAR-treated old rats defecate more, make fewer crossings, and spend more time in the corner squares in an open-field test; they interpreted this in terms of an enhanced emotional reactivity of old rats treated with ALCAR.

ALCAR improves nerve regeneration in rats[102] and protects neurons from the toxicity of mitochondrial uncouplers or inhibitors.[103] Feeding old rats ALCAR restores levels of this metabolite to those found in tissues of young rats.[93] Paradies et al. fed old rats ALCAR and studied the effects on heart mitochondrial function: they showed that ALCAR feeding increases cardiolipin content, elevates activities of cytochrome c oxidase and adenine nucleotide translocase, and increases the rates of phosphate and pyruvate transport, palmitoylcarnitine-supported respiration, and carnitine–carnitine and carnitine–palmitoylcarnitine exchange reactions.[31–34,43,44] ALCAR also attenuates neurological damage after brain ischemia and reperfusion in canines,[104] elevates levels of glutathione and GABA in the brain of mice,[88] increases the activities of NADH-cytochrome c oxidoreductase, succinate cytochrome c oxidoreductase and cytochrome c oxidase in synaptosomes isolated from spf mice, an animal model to study the neuropathology of congenital ornithine transcarbamylase deficiency.[105] ALCAR seems also to possess antiapoptotic property.[106]

Clinical trials with ALCAR showed some improvements in Alzheimer disease or dementia-associated cognitive dysfunction[107–113] and cognitively impaired alcoholics.[114] Some of these studies showed that ALCAR can delay progression to dementia and improve memory, visuospatial capacity, vocabulary recall, cooperation, sociability, and attention, and alleviate depression. One of the mechanisms for improvement of cognition is that ALCAR helps the brain maintain a constant supply of energy by boosting the levels of phospholipid precursors for membrane synthesis.[113] ALCAR treatment in old rats delays progression in hearing loss, and reduces age-associated mtDNA deletions and presbyacusis by upregulating mitochondrial function and improving energy-producing capabilities.[115]

Kuratsune *et al.* showed that patients with chronic fatigue syndrome have a deficiency of serum acylcarnitine, and ALCAR supplementation improves daily activity and reduces symptoms.[116,117] They investigated brain uptake in rhesus monkeys of acetylcarnitine labeled in different positions by positron emission tomography and found a high uptake of [2–11C]acetyl-L-carnitine into the brain, suggesting that endogenous serum acetyl-L-carnitine has some role in conveying an acetyl moiety into the brain, especially under an energy crisis.[118]

It has been suggested that ALCAR has antioxidant activity, which is unexpected from its structure, and could be due to mitochondrial improvements or metal chelation. Tesco *et al.*[119] showed that ALCAR protects human diploid fibroblasts from xanthine oxidase-induced damage. Di Giacomo *et al.*[120] showed that ALCAR inhibits lipid peroxidation and xanthine oxidase activity in rat skeletal muscle. Kaur *et al.*[121] found that ALCAR reduces lipid peroxidation and lipofuscin concentration in aged rat brain. ALCAR was also shown to inhibit oxidant-induced DNA single-strand breaks.[122] Schinetti *et al.*[123] and Geremia *et al.*[124] demonstrated *in vitro* that ALCAR might possesses a direct antioxidant activity. Related compounds, such as L-propionyl carnitine and L-carnitine have been shown to have antioxidant activity by chelating metals.[125] They inhibit the age-associated increase in lipid peroxidation[126] or toxin-induced lipid peroxidation,[127] elevate antioxidants in aged rats,[126] and reduce oxidant-induced DNA single-strand breaks.[122] An antioxidant role of L-propionyl carnitine has also been implicated in ischemia-reperfusion injury.[128] Arduino[129,130] has suggested that carnitine and its acyl esters have a primary antioxidant activity (inhibiting free radical generation, scavenging the initiating free radicals, and terminating the radical propagation reactions), and also work as secondary antioxidants (repairing oxidized polyunsaturated fatty acids esterified in membrane phospholipids).

A previous study showed that feeding old rats ALCAR converted the mitochondria of liver to a more youthful state, both structurally and functionally, and increased ambulatory activity in the old rats, but caused an increase in oxidants.[22] The increased oxidants have now been found to be a side effect of the very high dose used. We carried out a dose-response study on the effects of lower doses of ALCAR on rat brain function, mitochondrial morphological change, and oxidative stress in old rats.[93] ALCAR was administered at 0.15%, 0.5%, and 1.5% in drinking water for 4 weeks. We found that there was an age-related decrease in carnitine levels in the brain and plasma (TABLE 1), with an age-related increase in the liver. The increased level of carnitines in liver may suggest an impaired net transport of carnitine from the liver to the blood in old animals, because there is an age-dependent de-

TABLE 1. Effects of different doses on the levels of total carnitines in plasma (μM) and in brain (nmol/mg protein) in rats

	Plasma	Brain
Young	82.7 ± 8.5	0.96 ± 0.05
Old	58.7 ± 5.0#	0.74 ± 0.07#
Old + 0.15% ALCAR	103.3 ± 19.3*	1.35 ± 0.27*
Old + 0.50% ALCAR	107.3 ± 6.2***	1.13 ± 0.05**
Old + 1.50% ALCAR	106.5 ± 9.7**	1.23 ± 0.10**

NOTE: Data are mean ± SEM of five rats in each group. Statistical differences were calculated by the Student's *t* test between young and old groups. #$P < 0.05$, and by one-way ANOVA between old and treated groups. *$P < 0.05$, **$P < 0.01$, and ***$P < 0.001$, compared with old group.

TABLE 2. Effects of different doses on ambulatory activity in rats

Group	Ambulatory
Young	490 ± 36
Old	160 ± 32###
Old + 0.15% ALCAR	291 ± 10***
Old + 0.50% ALCAR	357 ± 16***
Old + 1.50% ALCAR	212 ± 12*

NOTE: Data are mean ± SEM of five rats in each group. Statistical differences were calculated by the Student's *t* test between young and old groups, ###$P < 0.001$, and by one-way ANOVA between old and treated groups. *$P < 0.05$ and ***$P < 0.001$, compared with old rat group.

crease in the plasma. All the doses of ALCAR (4 weeks) showed significantly increased levels of carnitine, dependent on dose, in the brain and plasma, without apparent changes in the liver. The high dose (1.5%) for a shorter term (2 weeks) also seems effective in elevating the carnitine levels in the brain and plasma. Administration of carnitine, as well as ALCAR, also effectively elevated the carnitine levels in the brain and plasma.[93, 131]

The lower concentrations of ALCAR (0.15% and especially 0.5%) ameliorated the age-associated decline in ambulatory activity (TABLE 2) and mitochondrial cristae loss in the dentate gyrus of the hippocampus (FIG. 12) more effectively than the 1.5% dose. The lower doses had no effect on protein oxidation, in contrast to the 1.5% dose, which caused an increase in protein carbonyls in the brain. Furthermore, lower doses (0.15%) also reduced the age-dependent increase in malondialdehyde, an end product of lipid peroxidation, more effectively than the 1.5% dose (data not shown). These results suggest (1) that oxidative stress in the brain, a side effect, only occurs at very high dose of ALCAR administration to old rats, and (2) that a lower dose of ALCAR administered to old rats can improve brain function by partially reversing the age-associated mitochondrial decay, by repairing mitochondrial structure, and by reducing oxidative stress.[93,120,121,126,129]

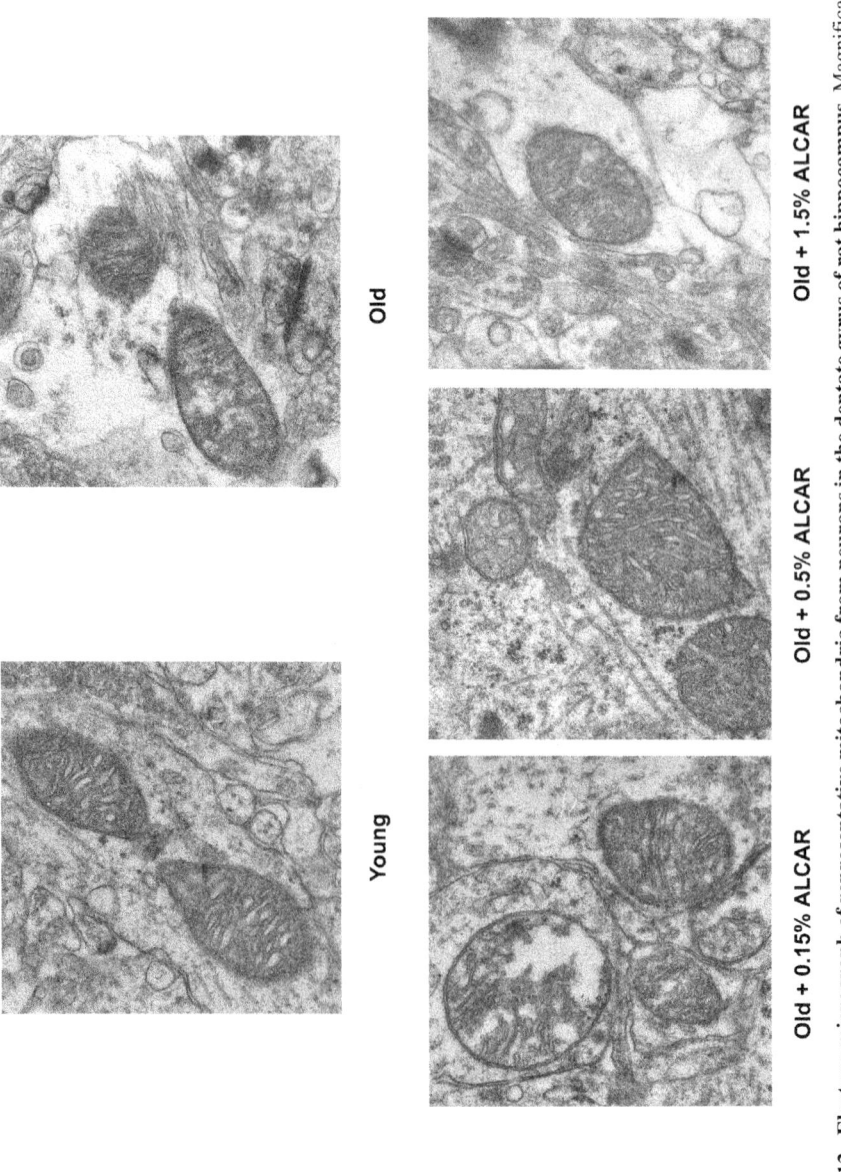

FIGURE 12. Electron micrograph of representative mitochondria from neurons in the dentate gyrus of rat hippocampus. Magnification ×27,000.

LIPOIC ACID AND ALCAR INHIBIT THE AGE-ASSOCIATED DECLINE OF COGNITIVE FUNCTION IN RATS

To extend the previous study of the effect of ALCAR and lipoic acid on mitochondrial function in the liver of old rats and brain function, and taking into account the dose-response study (93), we examined the effects of ALCAR (0.5%) and lipoic acid (0.2%) as well as their combination on memory with the Morris water maze test[132] and with the Skinner box test (fixed-interval performance in the peak procedure)[133] in young and old rats. Old rats showed an age-associated decline in spatial memory in the Morris water maze test and the treatments with ALCAR, LA, or their combination improved the age-associated spatial memory decline. FIGURE 13 shows examples of the swimming routes of young and old rats as well as old rats with treatment. FIGURE 14 shows the results of time to find target obtained from 4 consecutive days of testing with young and old rats. ALCAR, LA, or their combination improved the spatial memory by (1) reducing the time to find the hidden escape platform; (2) increasing the time at the platform position and the % time in the quadrant where the escape platform was formerly contained during the 60-s transfer (no platform) test; and (3) reducing the time to find the visible escape platform. ALCAR showed a greater effect than LA. The combination of ALCAR and lipoic acid showed a synergistic effect on reversing the decay of spatial memory in old animals (data not shown).

FIGURE 15 shows the response rate functions in the Skinner box test, which reflects the internal clock and memory, for young rats, old rats, and old rats with treatments. Clearly, old rats had a much lower response rate, and LA increased the response rate in old rats. Although ALCAR itself did not show any effect, its combination with LA had a synergistic effect on reversing the decreased response rate in old rats. FIGURE 16 shows the changes in peak rate, which reflects motivation, of young and old rats. The peak rate showed very similar changes as did the response rate. The general trend seen in FIGURE 15 and also the peak rate (data not shown) is interesting. While ALCAR does not show any effect (comparing the ALCAR group to the old controls), lipoic acid seems to slightly increase the peak rate in old rats. The combination of LA and ALCAR showed a larger and significant increase in response rate and also peak rate in old animals compared to lipoic acid alone, suggesting a synergistic action of LA and ALCAR. Other cognitive functions, such as attention and exploration, were determined by measuring the relative spreading and tail rate, which showed that a similar age-associated decline in these parameters were ameliorated by treatment with LA or its combination with ALCAR (data not shown).

The responses to light and sound signals showed a similar response (data not shown), suggesting that the remediation of the treatments is that of brain function rather than of sight or hearing.

Electron microscopic observation demonstrated that LA, or its combination with ALCAR, reversed the age-associated decay of mitochondrial structure in brain hippocampus (data not shown).

In addition, we have used even lower concentrations of ALCAR (0.2%) and LA (0.1%) as well as their combination on spatial memory with the Morris water maze test and fixed-interval performance in the peak procedure in old rats. ALCAR and

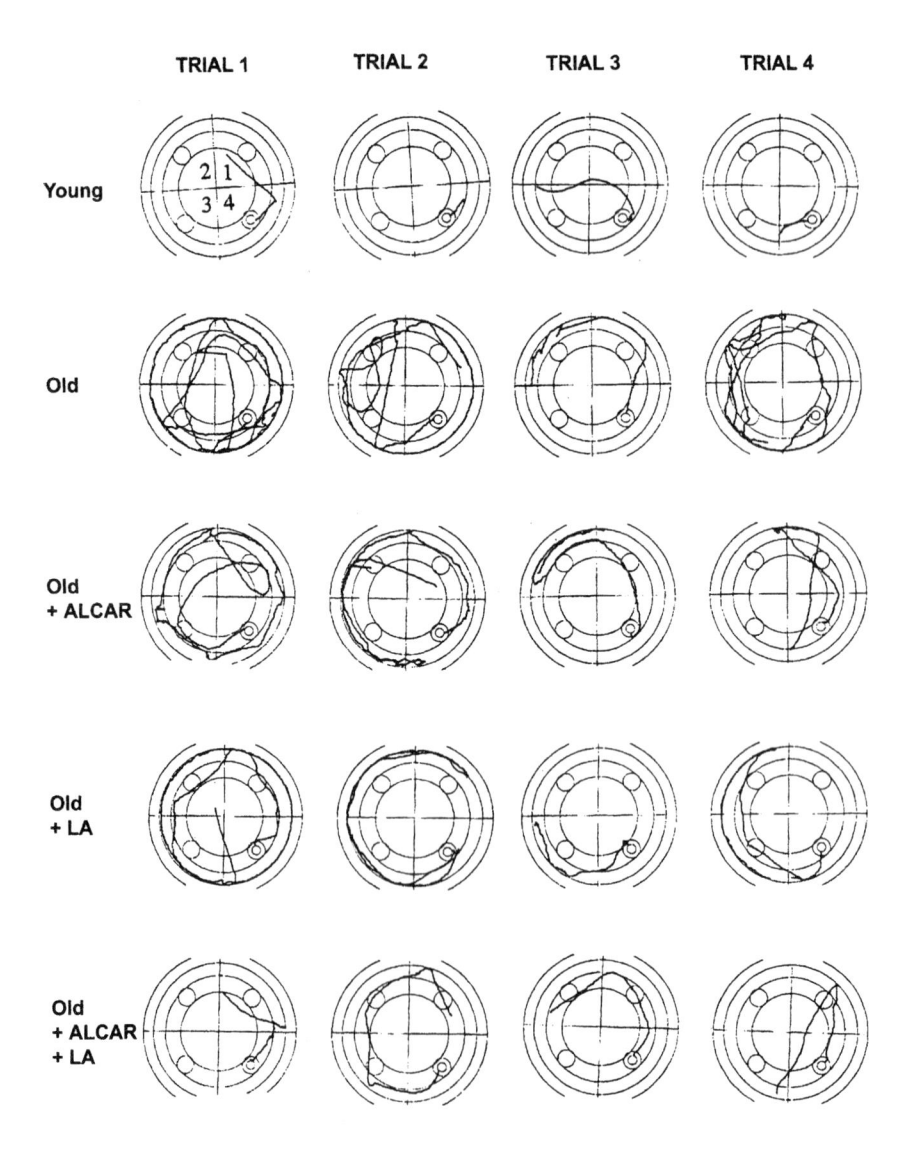

FIGURE 13. Representative paths taken on day 4 of training in Morris water maze test. The escape platform was placed at the lower right quadrant (quadrant 4). Rats were released from different points in the four trials but all the rats were released in the same order.

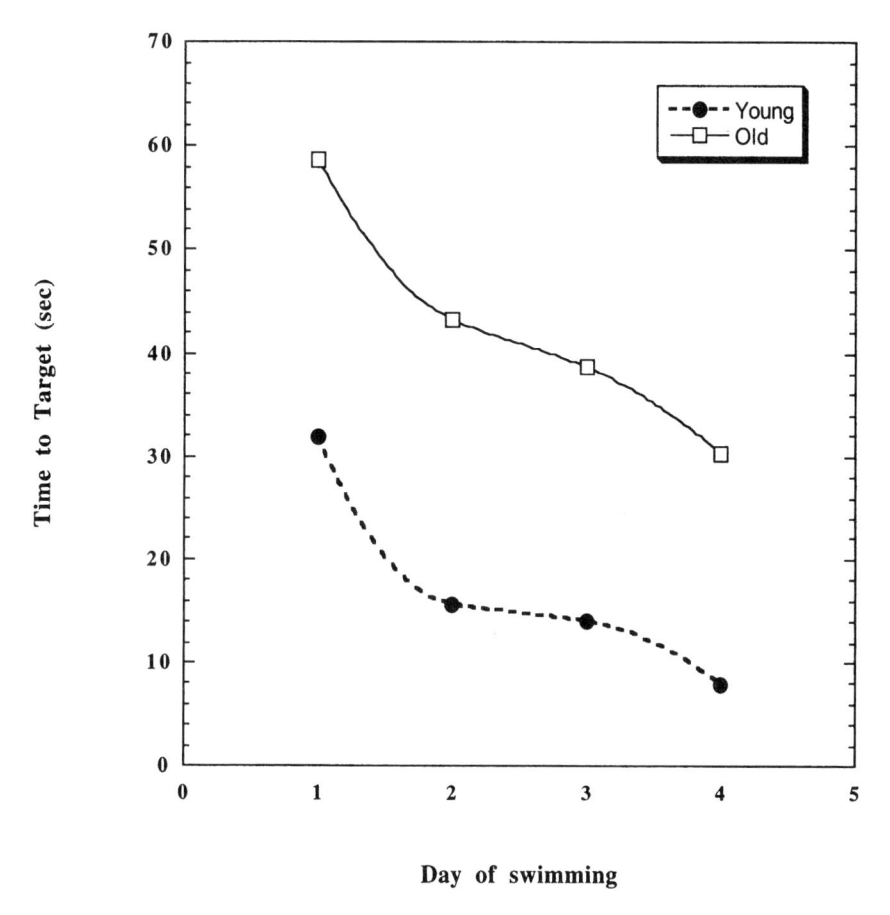

FIGURE 14. Mean escape latencies in the performance of young and old rats on days 1–4 of the training cycle in the Morris water maze.

lipoic acid at these lower doses also showed improvement on the Morris water maze and the Skinner box tests (data not shown).

In these cognitive tests, ALCAR showed a greater effect than lipoic acid in the spatial memory with the Morris water maze test, while lipoic acid showed a greater effect than ALCAR in the time discrimination task with Skinner box test. However, in both tests, the combination of ALCAR and lipoic acid showed synergistic action. These results demonstrate that ALCAR and lipoic acid can lesen age-associated memory decline in aged rats, and the combination of LA and ALCAR shows a greater effect than LA or ALCAR alone in improving memory with a synergistic action.[38,134]

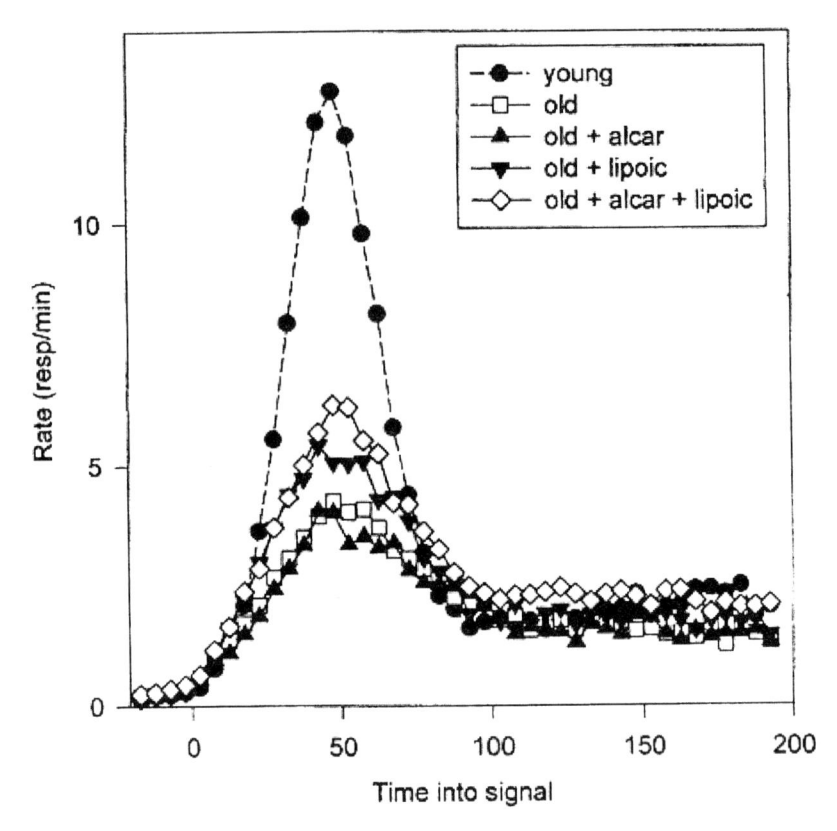

FIGURE 15. Response rate functions for the five groups of rats in the fixed-interval performance of peak procedure (Skinner box test).

IMMUNOHISTOCHEMICAL STAINING FOR OXIDATIVE DAMAGE TO PROTEIN AND NUCLEIC ACIDS IN THE BRAIN OF RATS: EFFECTS OF LA, ALCAR, OR THEIR COMBINATION

To study the mechanisms of the memory improving effect,[38] we investigated[135] the possible antioxidant effects of these mitochondrial metabolites in the brain of rats by examining oxidative biomarkers by immunohistochemical methods. Nitrotyrosine, an index of oxidative protein damage induced by reactive nitrogen species, was examined and found to increase with age in the hippocampus and cortex of rat brain. Dietary administration of ALCAR, LA, or their combination showed an inhibition of the nitrotyrosine immunostaining (data not shown).

A monoclonal antibody to oxo8dG/oxo8G (QED Bioscience, Inc., San Diego, CA) was used to study oxidative damage to nucleic acids. FIGURE 17 shows examples of the immunostaining and in the hippocampal CA_3 area in young (A) and old

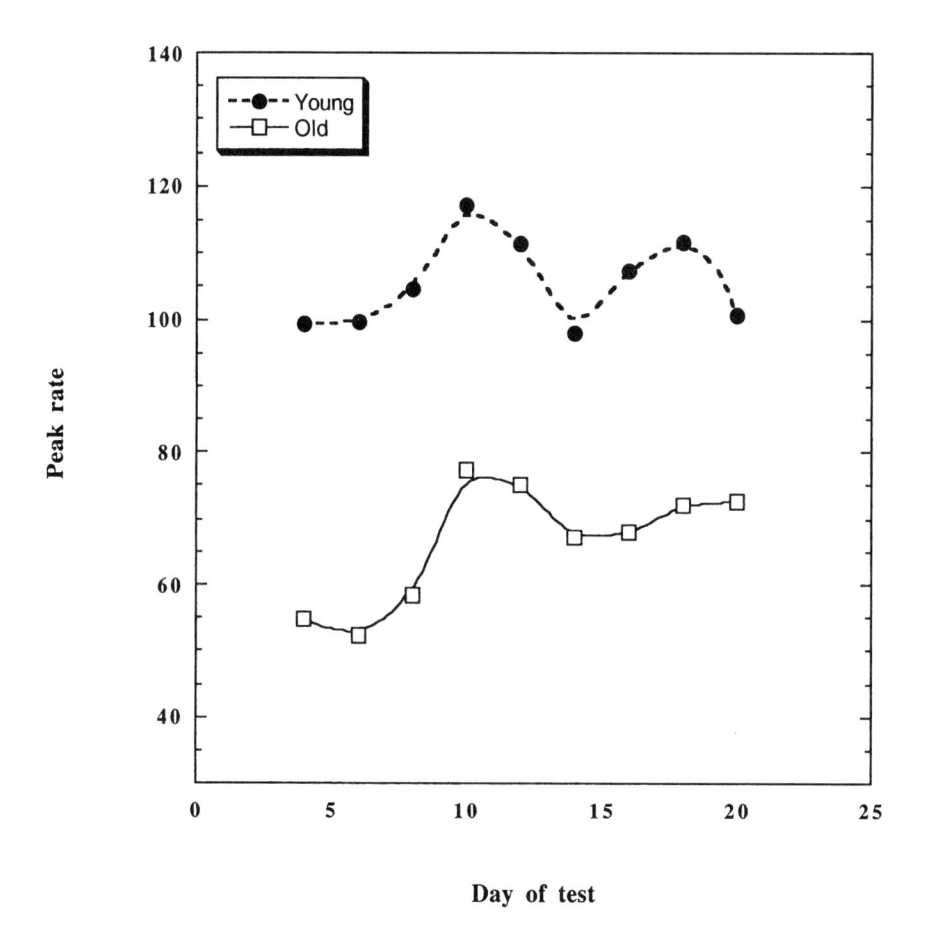

FIGURE 16. Peak rate over the 20 days of peak procedure testing of young and old rats. Each data point represents 2 days of testing.

(B) rat brain. There is a marked increase in oxidative nucleic acid damage with aging, and both ALCAR and LA inhibited the age-associated increase seen on immunostaining. In addition, the combination of ALCAR and LA showed more significant inhibition of the accumulation of oxidative nucleic acid damage (data not shown). RNase, but not DNase, reversed this increase, suggesting that RNA is the main target.[135] These results suggest that the memory-improving effects of these mitochondrial metabolites in rats may be through an antioxidant mechanism, possibly by scavenging oxidants, maintaining mitochondrial membrane integrity and mitochondrial function, or removing the accumulation of oxidative metabolic by-products in the brain.

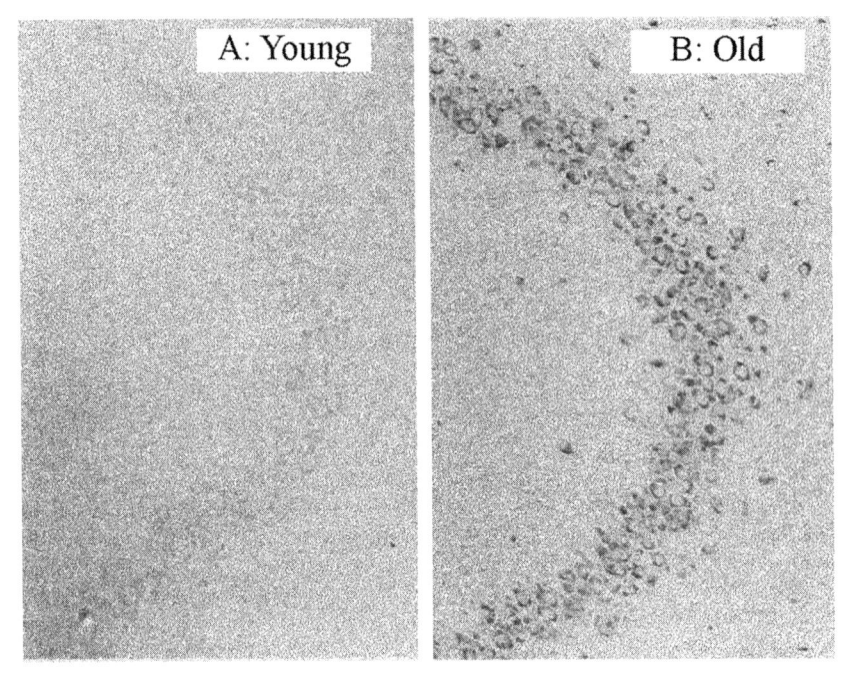

FIGURE 17. RNA oxidation in young and old rat brain hippocampal CA3 area, immunologically stained with anti-oxo8G/oxo8dG antibody.

HIGH-DOSE NUTRIENTS AMELIORATE ALTERED ENZYMES WITH POORER AFFINITY DUE TO MUTATION AND AGING: A HYPOTHESIS

High levels of vitamins have been used to successfully treat many human genetic diseases. The molecular basis for as many as one-third of the mutations in a gene causing a particular disease is an increased K_m (poorer affinity) of the enzyme for the vitamin-derived coenzyme or substrate, which in turn lowers the rate of the reaction.[136] The therapeutic vitamin regimens work by increasing intracellular coenzyme concentrations, stimulating a defective enzyme, and thereby alleviating the primary defect and curing the disease. About 50 human genetic diseases involving dysfunctional enzymes can be remedied by high levels of the vitamin component of the coenzyme. This therapeutic technique is also relevant in polymorphisms in a number of other cases where molecular evidence suggests that the mutation affects the coenzyme binding site.[136]

During aging, oxidation of proteins, and decreased fluidity of membranes due to oxidation, deforms proteins and thus decreases the affinity of many enzymes for their substrates or coenzymes. Aging also affects the K_m of many receptor proteins, including the beta-adrenergic receptor, TGF-beta receptor, dopamine receptor, acetylcholine receptor, adenylate cyclase, insulin receptor, serotonin receptor, steroid hormone receptor, retinoic acid receptor, inositol 1,4,5-trisphosphate receptor, and calmodulin.[137] Cytosol proteins also display an age-associated decline of affinity for their substrates or cofactors, such as glyceraldehyde-3-phosphate dehydrogenase and tryptophan hydroxylase.[137,138] The mitochondrial complexes III and IV show a significant increase in K_m and decrease in V_{max}.[139]

Oxidative decay is particularly acute in mitochondria.[1–3,5–7,19] Reactive aldehyde products from lipid peroxidation may be one of the causes of mitochondrial dysfunction during aging. Decreased mitochondrial cardiolipin content and change of cardiolipin composition may be one of the causes of losing mitochondrial integrity and function.[13,22,29,34] Lack of sufficient DNA repair in mitochondria and juxtaposition to the electron transport system adds to susceptibility and accumulation of mtDNA and other mitochondrial macromolecular damage. Thus, feeding high levels of several mitochondrial biochemicals, including ALCAR, LA, creatine, phopholipids, and fatty acids, may reverse some of the decay of aging and age-related cognitive impairment.[22,25,31,32,43,45,63,140,141] Dietary restriction can prolong maximum life span, eliminate aldehyde products of lipid peroxidation in mitochondria, increase membrane fluidity, decrease iron level, and attenuate the declines in genomic activity (gene expression of catalase and superoxidase dismutase), and reduce fiber loss and mitochondrial abnormality.[142,143] Dietary restriction seems to retard this deterioration of mitochondrial respiratory function by preserving enzymatic activities and function, thereby increasing mitochondrial complex activity and decreasing binding affinity to substrate.[139]

We have hypothesized that the age-associated increase of oxidative damage causes oxidation and deformation of key enzymes, with a consequent decrease in enzyme activity (V_{max}) and lessening of binding affinity (increase in K_m) for the enzyme substrate, and that an increased level of substrate (e.g., ALCAR) may restore the velocity of the reaction (or the metabolic efficiency of that enzyme), thus restoring function.[136,144] We have now found that old rats, compared with young, showed a decrease in carnitine acetyltransferase (CAT) enzyme activity and in CAT substrate

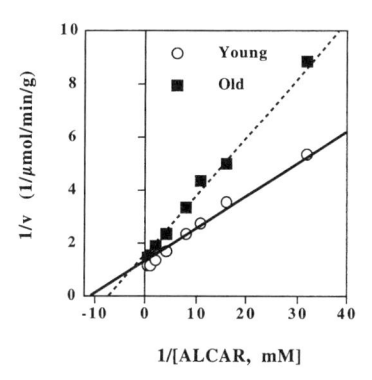

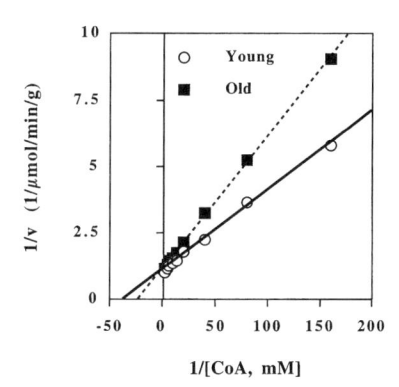

FIGURE 18. Double reciprocal plots of reaction velocity versus substrate concentrations (*left:* ALCAR; *right:* CoA) in young and old rat brain. The values are mean of 10 animals in each group.

binding affinity (K_m) (FIG. 18). The dietary administration of ALCAR, and its combination with lipoic acid, restored the enzyme activity and the binding affinity for ALCAR (data not shown). In addition, an *ex vivo* oxidation of rat brain homogenate with Fe(II) induced similar reduction of enzyme activity and binding affinity to acetylcarnitine, suggesting that the decreased enzyme activity and binding affinity in rat brain may be due to direct or indirect oxidative damage.[145] Iron and copper also accumulate with age in rat brain, as does increase in lipid peroxidation, suggesting that oxidative stress is the major contributor to brain mitochondrial decay, including the effects on key mitochondrial enzymes.[145]

INHIBITION OF OXIDANT-INDUCED SENESCENCE AND OXIDATIVE STRESS IN HUMAN FIBROBLAST CELLS AND NEURONAL CELLS BY MITOCHONDRIAL ANTIOXIDANTS, ALPHA-PHENYL-*N*-*T*-BUTYL NITRONE (PBN) AND *N*-*T*-BUTYL HYDROXYLAMINE

α-Phenyl-*N*-*t*-butyl nitrone (PBN), a widely used spin-trapping agent, has been considered a potent antioxidant.[146] PBN delays the senescence of human diploid fibroblasts in culture and inhibits senescence-associated oxidative damage to DNA.[79] In our feeding studies in old rats, PBN was as effective as lipoic acid, when in combination with ALCAR.[25] PBN protects HT4 neuronal cells from glutamate- or SIN-1 (a source of peroxynitrate)-induced toxicity (FIG. 19)[77,147] and inhibits lipid peroxidation induced by NMDA in primary hippocampus neuronal culture (FIG. 20) (Liu, McIntosh, Sapolsky, and Ames, in preparation). PBN reverses the age-related oxidative changes in the brain of old gerbils[146] and delays senescence in senescence-accelerated mice[17,148] and in normal mice.[149] *N*-*t*-butyl hydroxylamine (NtBHA) and benzaldehyde are the breakdown products of PBN.[85] NtBHA delays senescence of IMR-90 cells at concentrations as low as 10 μM compared to 200 μM of PBN to produce a similar effect, suggesting that NtBHA is the active form of PBN.[85] *N*-benzyl hydroxylamine and *N*-methyl hydroxylamine, compounds unrelated to PBN, were also effective in delaying senescence, suggesting that the active functional group is the *N*-hydroxylamine. All the hydroxylamines tested significantly decreased the endogenous production of oxidants (as measured by the fluorescence of oxidized DCFH), and increased the GSH/GSSG ratio. The acceleration of senescence induced by hydrogen peroxide is reversed by the *N*-hydroxylamines. DNA damage, as determined by the level of apurinic/apyrimidinic (AP) site,[150] also decreased significantly after treatment with *N*-hydroxylamines. The *N*-hydroxylamines appear to be acting on the mitochondria: they delay age-dependent changes in mitochondria as measured by accumulation of rhodamine-123; they prevent reduction of cytochrome c^{III} by the superoxide radical; and they reverse an age-dependent decay of mitochondrial aconitase, suggesting that they react with the superoxide radical. In human primary fibroblasts (IMR-90) cells, NtBHA delayed senescence-associated changes to mitochondria and cellular senescence that was induced by maintaining the cells under suboptimal levels of growth factors. Proteasomal activity was also higher in cells treated with NtBHA than untreated cells. Mechanistic studies using IMR-90 cells suggest that complex III and cytochrome *c* are the mitochondrial components that interact with NtBHA.[84] NtBHA offers protection against glutamate-induced toxicity in neuronal HT4 and HT22 cells (FIG. 21), but has no protection on homocysteic

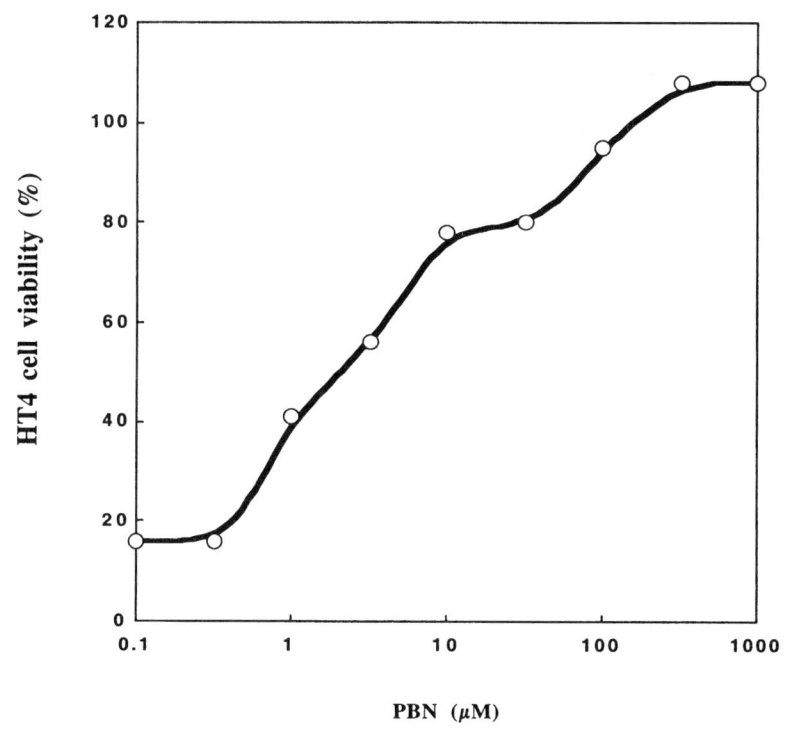

FIGURE 19. Dose-dependent protective effect of PBN on SIN-1–induced toxicity in HT4 cells. Cells were seeded at 3,000 per well in a 96-well plate for one day, treated with PBN for 24 h, and then challenged with 1 mM SIN-1 for 24 h. The cell viability was measured by MTT assay.

acid–induced toxicity, and *t*-butyl hydroxylamine has no toxicity to these neuronal cells if the concentration is lower than 500μM (Liu, Atamna, and Ames, unpublished material).

N-T-BUTYL HYDROXYLAMINE RESTORES MITOCHONDRIAL FUNCTION IN OLD RATS

Harman[151,152] has shown that several antioxidants, including hydroxylamine, 2-mercaptoethylamine, and cysteine can prolong the mean life span, inhibit spontaneous cancer, and reduce the mortality rate of female C3H mice, male AKR mice, or male LAF1 mice. In our *in vivo* study[84] the effect of NtBHA on mitochondria on young and old rats was examined. In NtBHA fed rats, the age-dependent decline in food consumption and ambulatory activity was reversed without affecting body weight. The respiratory control ratio (RCR) of mitochondria from liver was greater, indicating that mitochondria from treated rats were more coupled. NtBHA also reversed the age-dependent decline in the activity of glutamate dehydrogenase, a mitochondrial

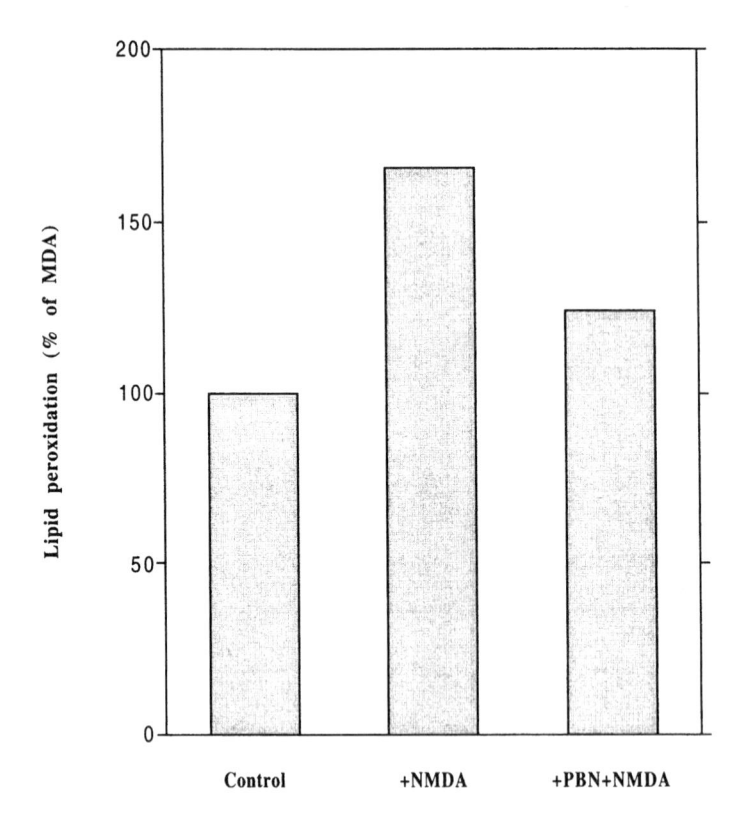

FIGURE 20. NMDA (100 μM)-induced toxicity and the protective effect of PBN (50 μM) in primary hippocampal neuronal cell culture.

enzyme, but had no effect on the cytosolic enzyme glucose-6-phosphate dehydrogenase. The age-dependent increase in proteins with thiol-mixed disulfides was significantly lower in old rats treated with NtBHA. NtBHA was effective in improving mitochondrial function only in old animals; no effect was observed in young animals. These findings suggest that NtBHA improves mitochondrial function and prevents mitochondria from age-associated oxidative decay *in vivo*.

SUMMARY

After more than 40 years, the free radical theory of aging has become one of the few most attractive hypotheses on aging.[3,153] It is generally accepted that oxidative mitochondrial decay is a major contributor to aging.[1,2,5–7,9,10,24,63] In old rats (vs. young rats) mitochondrial membrane potential, cardiolipin level, respiratory control ratio, and cellular O_2 uptake are lower; oxidants/O_2, neuron RNA oxidation, and mutagenic aldehydes from lipid peroxidation are higher; and ambulatory activity and cognition declines. However, feeding old rats ALCAR plus LA restores mitochon-

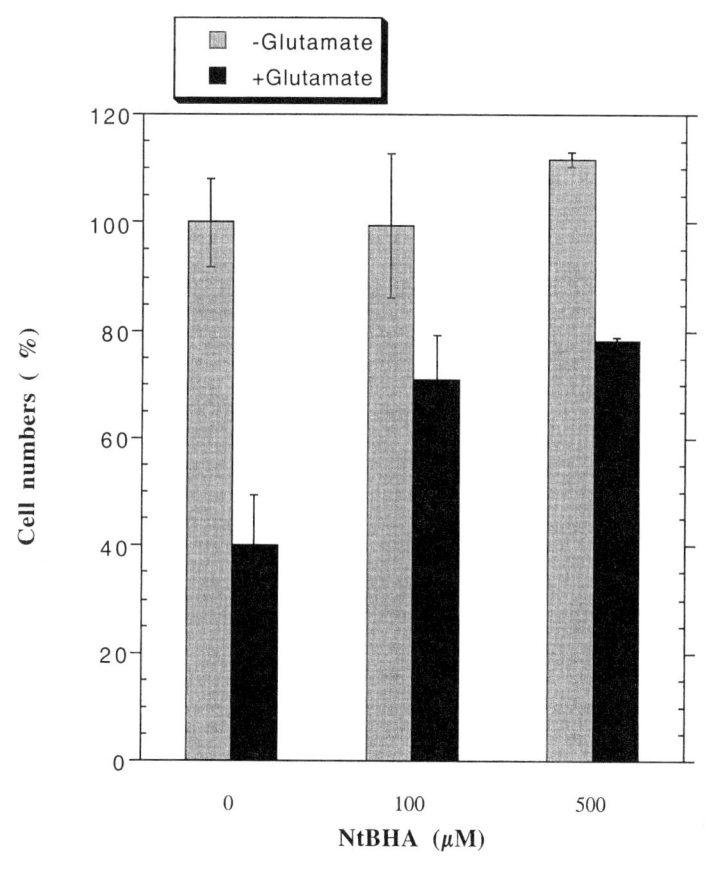

FIGURE 21. Glutamate (1 mM)-induced toxicity and the protective effect of NtBHA in HT4 cells. Cells were seeded at 20,000 per well in a 24-well plate for one day, treated with NtBHA for 24 h, and then challenged with 1 mM glutamate for 24 h. Cells were counted using the Coulter counter.

drial function; lowers oxidants, neuron RNA oxidation, and mutagenic aldehydes; elevates cardiolipin levels; improves the age-associated decline in ambulatory activity and memory; increases the level of the substrates and cofactors, thus increasing the metabolic efficiency of enzyme; and prevents mitochondria from oxidative decay and dysfunction. We have postulated[136,144] that with age, increased oxidative damage to protein and mitochondrial membranes and the loss of cardiolipin, causes a deformation of structure of enzymes, with a consequent lessening of affinity (K_m) for the enzyme substrate (e.g., acetyl carnitine). This hypothesis appears to be true for a number of enzymes, including carnitine acetyltransferase, mitochondrial complex III and IV, tryptophan hydroxylase, and several receptor proteins.[137] This hypothesis could explain why feeding mitochondrial metabolites/antioxidants restores enzyme activity and mitochondrial function, prevents age-associated diseases, and delays aging.

ACKNOWLEDGMENTS

This work was supported by grants from the National Institute on Aging (Grant AG17140), the Ellison Foundation (Grant SS0422-99), and the National Institute of Environmental Health Sciences Center (Grant P30 ES01896) to B.N.A. The authors thank A. Fischer, N. Amiri, and J. Hsu for help with the IMR-90, HT4, and HT22 cell study; L. McIntosh and R. Sapolsky, our collaborators on the primary hippocampal cell study; A. Gharib and R.T. Ingersoll, collaborators on the behavioral study; E. Head, W. Yuan, and C. W. Cotman, collaborators on the immunohistochemical study; D. Schubert for kindly providing the HT22 cells; C. Wehr for assistance in some animal work; EM Lab of the University of California at Berkeley for help in using the electron microscope; and B.V. Treadwell for critical reading of the manuscript.

REFERENCES

1. AMES, B.N., M.K. SHIGENAGA & T.M. HAGEN. 1993. Oxidants, antioxidants, and the degenerative diseases of aging. Proc. Natl. Acad. Sci. USA **90:** 7915–7922.
2. AMES, B.N., M.K. SHIGENAGA & T.M. HAGEN. 1995. Mitochondrial decay in aging. Biochim. Biophys. Acta **1271:** 165–170.
3. BECKMAN, K.B. & B.N. AMES. 1998. The free radical theory of aging matures. Physiol. Rev. **78:** 547–581.
4. HARMAN, D. 1960. The free radical theory of aging: the effect of age on serum mercaptan levels. J. Gerontol. **15:** 38–40.
5. HARMAN, D. 1972. The biologic clock: the mitochondria? J. Am. Geriatr. Soc. **20:** 145–147.
6. HARMAN, D. 1981. The aging process. Proc. Natl. Acad. Sci. USA **78:** 7124–7128.
7. SHIGENAGA, M.K., T.M. HAGEN & B.N. AMES. 1994. Oxidative damage and mitochondrial decay in aging. Proc. Natl. Acad. Sci. USA **91:** 10771–10778.
8. STADTMAN, E.R. 1992. Protein oxidation and aging. Science **257:** 1220–1224.
9. DEGREY, A.D.J. 1999. The Mitochondrial Free Radical Theory of Aging. R.G. Landers Co. Georgetown, TX.
10. TYLER, D.D. 1992. The Mitochondrion in Health and Disease. VCH Publishers. New York.
11. BEAL, M.F. 2000. Mitochondria and the pathogenesis of ALS. Brain **123:**1291–1292.
12. HALLIWELL, B. & J.M.C. GUTTERIDGE. 1999. Free Radicals in Biology and Medicine, 3rd edit. Oxford University Press. New York.
13. ROBINSON, B.H. & S. RAHA. 2001. Mitochondria, oxygen radicals, and apoptosis. Am. J. Med. Genet. **106:** 62–70.
14. KWONG, L.K. & R.S. SOHAL. 2000. Age-related changes in activities of mitochondrial electron transport complexes in various tissues of the mouse. Arch. Biochem. Biophys. **373:** 16–22.
15. SCHEFFLER, I.E. 2000. A centry of mitochondrial research: achievements and perspectives. Mitochondrion **1:** 3–31.
16. EMERIT, I. & B. CHANCE. 1992. Free radical and aging. Birkhauser Verlag. Basel.
17. EDAMATSU, R., A. MORI & L. PACKER. 1995. The spin-trap N-tert-alpha-phenyl-butylnitrone prolongs the life span of the senescence accelerated mouse. Biochem. Biophys. Res. Commun. **211:** 847–849.
18. LIU, J. & A. MORI. 1993. Age-associated changes in superoxide dismutase activity, thiobarbituric acid reactivity and reduced glutathione level in the brain and liver in senescence accelerated mice (SAM): a comparison with ddY mice. Mech. Ageing Dev. **71:** 23–30.
19. MORI, A., K. UTSUMI, J. LIU & M. HOSOKAWA. 1998. Oxidative damage in the senescence-accelerated mouse. Ann. N.Y. Acad. Sci. **854:** 239–250.

20. LIU, J. & A. MORI. 1999. Stress, aging, and brain oxidative damage. Neurochem. Res. **24:** 1479–1497.
21. LIU, J. et al.. 1996. Immobilization stress causes oxidative damage to lipid, protein, and DNA in the brain of rats. FASEB J. **10:** 1532–1538.
22. HAGEN, T.M. et al. 1998. Acetyl-L-carnitine fed to old rats partially restores mitochondrial function and ambulatory activity. Proc. Natl. Acad. Sci. USA **95:** 9562–9566.
23. HAGEN, T.M. et al. 2002. Feeding acetyl-L-carnitine combined with lipoic acid to old rats significantly improves metabolic function while decreasing oxidative stress. Proc. Natl. Acad. Sci. USA **99:** 1870–1875.
24. HAGEN, T.M., V. VINARSKY, C.M. WEHR & B.N. AMES. 2000. (R)-alpha-lipoic acid reverses the age-associated increase in susceptibility of hepatocytes to tert-butylhydroperoxide both in vitro and in vivo. Antioxid. Redox Signal **2:** 473–483.
25. HAGEN, T.M., C.M. WEHR & B.N. AMES. 1998. Mitochondrial decay in aging: reversal through supplementation of acetyl-L-carnitine and N-tert-butyl-alpha-phenyl-nitrone. Ann. N.Y. Acad. Sci. **854:** 214–223.
26. HAGEN, T.M. et al. 1997. Mitochondrial decay in hepatocytes from old rats: membrane potential declines, heterogeneity and oxidants increase. Proc. Natl. Acad. Sci. USA **94:** 3064–3069.
27. LIU, J. et al. 2001. Mitochondrial metabolites, acetyl-L-carnitine and lipoic acid, improve age-associated memory decline and inhibit brain oxidative damage in old rats. In The 2nd International Symposium on Natural Antioxidants (ISNA): Molecular Mechanisms and Health Effects. ISNA, Beijing, China, p. 101.
28. LYKKESFELDT, J., T.M. HAGEN, V. VINARSKY & B.N. AMES. 1998. Age-associated decline in ascorbic acid concentration, recycling, and biosynthesis in rat hepatocytes: reversal with (R)-alpha-lipoic acid supplementation. FASEB J. **12:** 1183–1189.
29. PARADIES, G. & F.M. RUGGIERO. 1990. Age-related changes in the activity of the pyruvate carrier and in the lipid composition in rat-heart mitochondria. Biochim. Biophys. Acta **1016:** 207–212.
30. PARADIES, G., F.M. RUGGIERO & P. DINOI. 1992. Decreased activity of the phosphate carrier and modification of lipids in cardiac mitochondria from senescent rats. Int. J. Biochem. **24:** 783–787.
31. PARADIES, G. et al.. 1994. Effect of aging and acetyl-L-carnitine on the activity of cytochrome oxidase and adenine nucleotide translocase in rat heart mitochondria. FEBS Lett. **350:** 213–215.
32. PARADIES, G. et al. 1994. The effect of aging and acetyl-L-carnitine on the function and on the lipid composition of rat heart mitochondria. Ann. N.Y. Acad. Sci. **717:** 233–243.
33. PARADIES, G. et al. 1995. Carnitine-acylcarnitine translocase activity in cardiac mitochondria from aged rats: the effect of acetyl-L-carnitine. Mech. Ageing Dev. **84:** 103–112.
34. PARADIES, G., F. M. RUGGIERO & E. QUAGLIARIELLO. 1992. Age-dependent changes in the activity of anion carriers and in the lipid composition in rat heart mitochondria. Ann. N.Y. Acad. Sci. **673:** 160–164.
35. ANDREWS, J.S. 1996. Possible confounding influence of strain, age and gender on cognitive performance in rats. Brain Res. Cogn. Brain Res. **3:** 251–267.
36. GHIRARDI, O. et al. 1992. Spatial memory in aged rats: population heterogeneity and effect of levocarnitine acetyl. J. Neurosci. Res. **31:** 375–379.
37. GHIRARDI, O., S. MILANO, M.T. RAMACCI & L. ANGELUCCI. 1988. Effect of acetyl-L-carnitine chronic treatment on discrimination models in aged rats. Physiol. Behav. **44:** 769–773.
38. LIU, J., D. KILLILEA & B.N. AMES. 2002. Age-associated mitochondrial oxidative decay: improvement of carnitine acetyltransferase substrate binding affinity and activity in brain by feeding old rats acetyl-L-carnitine and/or R-α-lipoic acid. Proc. Natl. Acad. Sci. USA **99:** 1876–1881.
39. WALLACE, J.E., E.E. KRAUTER & B.A. CAMPBELL. 1980. Motor and reflexive behavior in the aging rat. J. Gerontol. **35:** 364–370.
40. WALLACE, J.E., E.E. KRAUTER & B.A. CAMPBELL. 1980. Animal models of declining memory in the aged: short-term and spatial memory in the aged rat. J. Gerontol. **35:** 355–363.

41. DRAGO, F. et al. 1986. Behavioral effects of acetyl-L-carnitine in the male rat. Pharmacol. Biochem. Behav. **24:** 1393–1396.
42. GHIRARDI, O. et al. 1992. Active avoidance learning in old rats chronically treated with levocarnitine acetyl. Physiol. Behav. **52:** 185–187.
43. PARADIES, G., G. PETROSILLO, M.N. GADALETA & F.M. RUGGIERO. 1999. The effect of aging and acetyl-L-carnitine on the pyruvate transport and oxidation in rat heart mitochondria. FEBS Lett. **454:** 207–209.
44. PARADIES, G., F.M. RUGGIERO, M.N. GADALETA & E. QUAGLIARIELLO. 1992. The effect of aging and acetyl-L-carnitine on the activity of the phosphate carrier and on the phospholipid composition in rat heart mitochondria. Biochim. Biophys. Acta **1103:** 324–326.
45. FERRANTE, R.J. et al. 2000. Neuroprotective effects of creatine in a transgenic mouse model of Huntington's disease. J. Neurosci. **20:** 4389–4397.
46. SMITH, S.A. et al. 1998. Creatine supplementation and age influence muscle metabolism during exercise. J. Appl. Physiol. **85:** 1349–1356.
47. RAWSON, E.S. & P.M. CLARKSON. 2000. Acute creatine supplementation in older men. Int. J. Sports Med. **21:** 71–75.
48. CLARKSON, P.M. & E.S. RAWSON. 1999. Nutritional supplements to increase muscle mass. Crit. Rev. Food Sci. Nutr. **39:** 317–328.
49. RAWSON, E.S., M.L. WEHNERT & P.M. CLARKSON. 1999. Effects of 30 days of creatine ingestion in older men. Eur. J. Appl. Physiol. Occup. Physiol. **80:** 139–144.
50. WIROTH, J.B. et al. 2001. Effects of oral creatine supplementation on maximal pedalling performance in older adults. Eur. J. Appl. Physiol. **84:** 533–539.
51. BUSTAMANTE, J. et al. 1998. Alpha-lipoic acid in liver metabolism and disease. Free Radic. Biol. Med. **24:** 1023–1039.
52. FUCHS, J.L. PACKER & G. ZIMMER. 1997. Lipoic Acid in Health and Disease. Marcel Dekker. New York.
53. PACKER, L., S. ROY & C. K. SEN. 1997. Alpha-lipoic acid: a metabolic antioxidant and potential redox modulator of transcription. Adv. Pharmacol. **38:** 79–101.
54. PACKER, L., E.H. WITT & H.J. TRITSCHLER. 1995. alpha-Lipoic acid as a biological antioxidant. Free Radic. Biol. Med. **19:** 227–250.
55. SEN, C.K., S. ROY, S. KHANNA & L. PACKER. 1999. Determination of oxidized and reduced lipoic acid using high- performance liquid chromatography and coulometric detection. Methods Enzymol. **299:** 239–246.
56. PACKER, L., H.J. TRITSCHLER & K. WESSEL. 1997. Neuroprotection by the metabolic antioxidant alpha-lipoic acid. Free Radic. Biol. Med. **22:** 359–378.
57. WOLZ, P. & J. KRIEGLSTEIN. 1996. Neuroprotective effects of alpha-lipoic acid and its enantiomers demonstrated in rodent models of focal cerebral ischemia. Neuropharmacology **35:** 369–375.
58. WOLZ, P. & J. KRIEGLSTEIN. 1997. Neuroprotective activity of lipoic and dihydrolipoic acid. *In* Lipoic Acid in Health and Disease. J. Fuchs, L. Packer & G. Zimmer, Eds. : 205–225. Marcel Dekker. New York.
59. TIROSH, O., C.K. SEN, S. ROY & L. PACKER. 2000. Cellular and mitochondrial changes in glutamate-induced HT4 neuronal cell death. Neuroscience **97:** 531–541.
60. TIROSH, O. et al. 1999. Neuroprotective effects of alpha-lipoic acid and its positively charged amide analogue. Free Radic. Biol. Med. **26:** 1418–1426.
61. SEN, C. K. et al. 1998. A positively charged alpha-lipoic acid analogue with increased cellular uptake and more potent immunomodulatory activity. Biochem. Biophys. Res. Commun. **247:** 223–228.
62. OU, P., H.J. TRITSCHLER & S.P. WOLFF. 1995. Thioctic (lipoic) acid: a therapeutic metal-chelating antioxidant? Biochem. Pharmacol. **50:** 123–126.
63. HAGEN, T. M. et al. 1999. (R)-alpha-lipoic acid-supplemented old rats have improved mitochondrial function, decreased oxidative damage, and increased metabolic rate. FASEB J. **13:** 411–418.
64. SUH, J.H. et al. 2001. Oxidative stress in the aging rat heart is reversed by dietary supplementation with (R)-(alpha)-lipoic acid. FASEB J. **15:** 700–706.
65. HAGER, K. et al. 2001. Alpha-lipoic acid as a new treatment option for Azheimer type dementia. Arch. Gerontol. Geriatr. **32:** 275–282.

66. BEAL, M.F. 1992. Does impairment of energy metabolism result in excitotoxic neuronal death in neurodegenerative illnesses? Ann. Neurol. **31:**.119–130.
67. CHOI, D. 1988. Glutamate neurotoxicity and diseases of the nervous system. Neuron **1:** 623–634.
68. CHOI, D.W. 1992. Excitotoxic cell death. J. Neurobiol. **23:** 1261–1276.
69. DUMUIS, A. et al. 1988. NMDA receptors activate the arachidonic acid cascade system in striatal neurons. Nature **336:** 68–70.
70. LAFON, C.M., S. PIETRI, M. CULCAS & J. BOCKAERT. 1993. NMDA-dependent superoxide production and neurotoxicity. Nature **364:** 535–537.
71. HENNEBERRY, R.C., A. NOVELLI, J.A. COX & P.G. LYSKO. 1989. Neurotoxicity at the N-methyl-D-aspartate receptor in energy-compromised neurons. an hypothesis for cell death in aging and disease. Ann. N.Y. Acad. Sci. **568:** 225–233.
72. MORIMOTO, B.H. & D.E. KOSHLAND, JR. 1990. Excitatory amino acid uptake and N-methyl-D-aspartate-mediated secretion in a neural cell line. Proc. Natl. Acad. Sci. USA **87:** 3518–3521.
73. SAGARA, Y. & D. SCHUBERT. 1998. The activation of metabotropic glutamate receptors protects nerve cells from oxidative stress. J. Neurosci. **18:** 6662–6671.
74. MAHER, P. & J.B. DAVIS. 1996. The role of monoamine metabolism in oxidative glutamate toxicity. J. Neurosci. **16:** 6394–6401.
75. TAN, S. et al. 1998. The regulation of reactive oxygen species production during programmed cell death. J. Cell Biol. **141:** 1423–1432.
76. LIU, J., N. AMIRI, J. HSU & B.N. AMES. 2000. Lipoic acid, a mitochondrial metabolite, counteracts the effect of neurotoxins on HT4 and HT22 hippocampal cell lines. *In* The 30th Annual Meeting of the Society for Neuroscience. Society for Neuroscience, New Orleans, LA.
77. LIU, J. & B.N. AMES. 2000. Stress and brain oxidative damage: the role of monoamine transmitters, stress-related hormones, and antioxidants. Neuropsychopharmacology **23:** S53.
78. CHEN, Q. M. et al. 1998. Molecular analysis of H2O2-induced senescent-like growth arrest in normal human fibroblasts: p53 and Rb control G1 arrest but not cell replication. Biochem. J. **332:** 43–50.
79. CHEN, Q. et al. 1995. Oxidative DNA damage and senescence of human diploid fibroblast cells. Proc. Natl. Acad. Sci. USA **92:** 4337–4341.
80. CHEN, Q. & B.N. AMES. 1994. Senescence-like growth arrest induced by hydrogen peroxide in human diploid fibroblast F65 cells. Proc. Natl. Acad. Sci. USA **91:** 4130–4134.
81. ATAMNA, H., J.D. SABA & B.N. AMES. 2002. Fluorescence of N-10-nonyl-acridine orange reflects changes in morphology of mitochondria: relevance to aging and metabolic and oxidative stress. In preparation.
82. DUMAS, M. et al. 1995. Flow cytometric analysis of human epidermal cell ageing using two fluorescent mitochondrial probes. C. R. Acad. Sci. III **318:** 191–197.
83. MAFTAH, A. et al. 1994. Human epidermal cells progressively lose their cardiolipins during ageing without change in mitochondrial transmembrane potential. Mech. Ageing Dev. **77:** 83–96.
84. ATAMNA, H., C. Robinson, R. Ingersoll, et al. 2001. N-t-Butyl hydroxylamine is an antioxidant that reverses age-related changes in mitochondria in vivo and in vitro. FASEB J. **15:** 2196–2204.
85. ATAMNA, H., A. PALER-MARTINEZ & B.N. AMES. 2000. N-t-butyl hydroxylamine, a hydrolysis product of alpha-phenyl-N-t-butyl nitrone, is more potent in delaying senescence in human lung fibroblasts. J. Biol. Chem. **275:** 6741–6748.
86. BIEBER, L.L. 1988. Carnitine. Annu. Rev. Biochem. **57:** 261–283.
87. REBOUCHE, C.J. 1992. Carnitine function and requirements during the life cycle. FASEB J. **6:** 3379–3386.
88. FARIELLO, R.G., T.N. FERRARO, G.T. GOLDEN & M. DEMATTEI. 1988. Systemic acetyl-L-carnitine elevates nigral levels of glutathione and GABA. Life Sci. **43:** 289–292.
89. SHUG, A.L., M.J. SCHMIDT, G.T. GOLDEN & R.G. FARIELLO. 1982. The distribution and role of carnitine in the mammalian brain. Life Sci. **31:** 2869–2874.
90. BRESOLIN, N., L. FREDDO, L. VERGANI & C. ANGELINI. 1982. Carnitine, carnitine acyltransferases, and rat brain function. Exp. Neurol. **78:** 285–292.

91. DOLEZAL, V. & S. TUCEK. 1981. Utilization of citrate, acetylcarnitine, acetate, pyruvate and glucose for the synthesis of acetylcholine in rat brain slices. J. Neurochem. **36:** 1323–1330.
92. COSTELL, M., J.E. O'CONNOR & S. GRISOLIA. 1989. Age-dependent decrease of carnitine content in muscle of mice and humans. Biochem. Biophys. Res. Commun. **161:** 1135–1143.
93. LIU, J. *et al.* 2002. Acetyl-L-carnitine reverses age-associated mitochondrial decay in rat brain: a dose-response study. In preparation.
94. MACCARI, F. *et al.* 1990. Levels of carnitines in brain and other tissues of rats of different ages: effect of acetyl-L-carnitine administration. Exp. Gerontol. **25:** 127–134.
95. KIDD, P.M. 1999. A review of nutrients and botanicals in the integrative management of cognitive dysfunction. Altern. Med. Rev. **4:** 144–161.
96. TAGLIALATELA, G., A. CAPRIOLI, A. GIULIANI & O. GHIRARDI. 1996. Spatial memory and NGF levels in aged rats: natural variability and effects of acetyl-L-carnitine treatment. Exp. Gerontol. **31:** 577–587.
97. CAPRIOLI, A., O. GHIRARDI, M.T. RAMACCI & L. ANGELUCCI. 1990. Age-dependent deficits in radial maze performance in the rat: effect of chronic treatment with acetyl-L-carnitine. Prog. Neuropsychopharmacol. Biol. Psychiatry **14:** 359–369.
98. BARNES, C. A. *et al.*. 1990. Acetyl-L-carnitine. 2: Effects on learning and memory performance of aged rats in simple and complex mazes. Neurobiol. Aging **11:** 499–506.
99. MARKOWSKA, A.L. *et al.* 1990. Acetyl-L-carnitine. 1: Effects on mortality, pathology and sensory-motor performance in aging rats. Neurobiol Aging **11:** 491–498.
100. ONOFRJ, M., I. BODIS-WOLLNER, P. POLA & M. CALVANI. 1983. Central cholinergic effects of leveo-acetylcarnitine. Drug Exp. Clin. Res. **9:** 161–169.
101. BLOKLAND, A., W. RAAIJMAKERS, F.J. VAN DER STAAY & J. JOLLES. 1990. Differential effect of acetyl-L-carnitine on open field behavior in young and old rats. Physiol. Behav. **47:** 783–785.
102. FERNANDEZ, E. *et al.* 1989. Effects of L-carnitine, L-acetylcarnitine and gangliosides on the regeneration of the transected sciatic nerve in rats. Neurol. Res. **11:** 57–62.
103. VIRMANI, M.A. *et al.* 1995. Protective actions of L-carnitine and acetyl-L-carnitine on the neurotoxicity evoked by mitochondrial uncoupling or inhibitors. Pharmacol. Res. **32:** 383–389.
104. CALVANI, M. & E. ARRIGONI-MARTELLI. 1999. Attenuation by acetyl-L-carnitine of neurological damage and biochemical derangement following brain ischemia and reperfusion. Int. J. Tissue React. **21:** 1–6.
105. QURESHI, K., K.V. RAO & I.A. QURESHI. 1998. Differential inhibition by hyperammonemia of the electron transport chain enzymes in synaptosomes and non-synaptic mitochondria in ornithine transcarbamylase-deficient spf-mice: restoration by acetyl-L-carnitine. Neurochem. Res. **23:** 855–861.
106. DI MARZIO, L. *et al.* 1999. Acetyl-L-carnitine administration increases insulin-like growth factor 1 levels in asymptomatic HIV-1-infected subjects: correlation with its suppressive effect on lymphocyte apoptosis and ceramide generation. Clin. Immunol. **92:** 103–110.
107. LIVINGSTON, G.A., K.B. SAX, Z. MCCLENAHAN & E. AL. 1991. Acetyl-L-carnitine in dementia. Int. J. Geriatrr. Psychiatr. **6:** 853–860.
108. SPAGNOLI, A. *et al.* 1991. Long-term acetyl-L-carnitine treatment in Alzheimer's disease. Neurology **41:** 1726–1732.
109. SANO, M. *et al.* 1992. Double-blind parallel design pilot study of acetyl levocarnitine in patients with Alzheimer's disease. Arch. Neurol. **49:** 1137–1141.
110. THAL, L.J. *et al.* 1996. A 1-year multicenter placebo-controlled study of acetyl-L-carnitine in patients with Alzheimer's disease. Neurology **47:** 705–711.
111. BROOKS, J.O., III, J.A. YESAVAGE, A. CARTA & D. BRAVI. 1998. Acetyl-L-carnitine slows decline in younger patients with Alzheimer's disease: a reanalysis of a double-blind, placebo-controlled study using the trilinear approach. Int. Psychogeriatr. **10:** 193–203.
112. BONAVITA, E. 1986. Study of the efficacy and tolerability of L-acetylcarnitine therapy in the senile brain. Int. J. Clin. Pharmacol. Ther. Toxicol. **24:** 511–516.

113. PETTEGREW, J.W. et al. 1995. Clinical and neurochemical effects of acetyl-L-carnitine in Alzheimer's disease. Neurobiol. Aging **16:** 1–4.
114. TEMPESTA, E. et al. 1990. Role of acetyl-L-carnitine in the treatment of cognitive deficit in chronic alcoholism. Int. J. Clin. Pharmacol. Res. **10:** 101–107.
115. SEIDMAN, M.D. et al. 2000. Biologic activity of mitochondrial metabolites on aging and age-related hearing loss. Am. J. Otol. **21:** 161–167.
116. KURATSUNE, H. et al.. 1998. Low levels of serum acylcarnitine in chronic fatigue syndrome and chronic hepatitis type C, but not seen in other diseases. Int. J. Mol. Med. **2:** 51–56.
117. KURATSUNE, H. et al. 1994. Acylcarnitine deficiency in chronic fatigue syndrome. Clin Infect Dis **18** (Suppl 1)**:** S62–67.
118. KURATSUNE, H. et al.. 1997. High uptake of [2-11C]acetyl-L-carnitine into the brain: a PET study. Biochem. Biophys. Res. Commun. **231:** 488–493.
119. TESCO, G. et al. 1992. Protection from oxygen radical damage in human diploid fibroblasts by acetyl-L-carnitine. Dementia **3:** 58–60.
120. DI GIACOMO, C. et al. 1993. Effect of acetyl-L-carnitine on lipid peroxidation and xanthine oxidase activity in rat skeletal muscle. Neurochem. Res. **18:** 1157–1162.
121. KAUR, J., D. SHARMA & R. SINGH. 2001. Acetyl-L-carnitine enhances Na(+), K(+)-ATPase glutathione-S-transferase and multiple unit activity and reduces lipid peroxidation and lipofuscin concentration in aged rat brain regions. Neurosci. Lett. **301:** 1–4.
122. BOERRIGTER, M.E. et al. 1993. The effect of L-carnitine and acetyl-L-carnitine on the disappearance of DNA single-strand breaks in human peripheral blood lymphocytes. Carcinogenesis **14:** 2131–2136.
123. SCHINETTI, M.L., D. ROSSINI, R. GRECO & A. BERTELLI. 1987. Protective action of acetylcarnitine on NADPH-induced lipid peroxidation of cardiac microsomes. Drugs Exp. Clin. Res. **13:** 509–515.
124. GEREMIA, E. et al. 1988. Antioxidant action of acetyl-L-carnitine: in vitro study. Med. Sci. Res. **16:** 699–700.
125. REZNICK, A.Z. et al.. 1992. Antiradical effects in L-propionyl carnitine protection of the heart against ischemia-reperfusion injury: the possible role of iron chelation. Arch. Biochem. Biophys. **296:** 394–401.
126. KALAISELVI, T. & C. PANNEERSELVAM. 1998. Effect of L-carnitine on the status of liperoxidation and antioxidants in aging rats. J. Nutr. Biochem. **9:** 575–581.
127. LUO, X. et al. 1999. L-carnitine attenuates doxorubicin-induced lipid peroxidation in rats. Free Radic. Biol. Med. **26:** 1158–1165.
128. PAULSON, D.J., A.L. SHUG & J. ZHAO. 1992. Protection of the ischemic diabetic heart by L-propionylcarnitine therapy. Mol. Cell Biochem. **116:** 131–137.
129. ARDUINI, A. 1992. Carnitine and its acyl esters as secondary antioxidants? Am. Heart J. **123:** 1726–1727.
130. ARDUINI, A., et al. 1995. Is the carnitine system part of the heart antioxidant network? *In* The Carnitine System. A New Therapeutical Approach to Cardiovascular Medicine. J.W. de Jong & R. Ferrari, Eds.: 169–181. Kluwer. Amsterdam, the Netherlands.
131. AMES, B.N., J. LIU & H. ATAMNA. 2001. Delaying aging with mitochondrial micronutrients and antioxidants. *In* Miami Nature Biotechnology Winter Symposium on Cell Death and Aging. Miami, FL.
132. MORRIS, R. 1984. Developments of a water-maze procedure for studying spatial learning in the rat. J. Neurosci. Meth. **11:** 47–60.
133. GHARIB, A., S. DERBY & S. ROBERTS. 2001. Timing and the control of variation. J. Exp. Psychol. Anim. Behav. Process **27:** 165–178.
134. AMES, B.N. & J. LIU. 2001. Delaying the mitochondrial decay of aging. *In* The 9th Congress of International Association of Biomedical Gerontology, Vancouver, Canada.
135. LIU, J., E. HEAD, C.W. COTMAN & B.N. AMES. 2001. Acetyl-L-carnitine, lipoic acid, or their combination improve age-associated memory decline and inhibit brain oxidative damage in old rats: an immunohistological study. *In* The 31st Annual Meeting of the Society for Neuroscience. Society for Neuroscience, San Diego.
136. AMES, B.N., I. ELSON-SCHWAB & E. SILVER. 2002. High-dose vitamins stimulate altered enzymes with poorer coenzyme binding affinity (Km): Relevance to genetic disease and polymorphisms. Under review.

137. AMES, B.N., I. ELSON-SCHWAB & J. LIU. 2002. High-dose vitamins or substrates ameliorate altered enzymes with poorer coenzyme or substrate binding affinity (Km): Relevance to aging. In preparation.
138. HUSSAIN, A.M. & A.K. MITRA. 2000. Effect of aging on tryptophan hydroxylase in rat brain: implications on serotonin level. Drug Metab. Dispos. **28:** 1038–1042.
139. FEUERS, R.J. 1998. The effects of dietary restriction on mitochondrial dysfunction in aging. Ann. N.Y. Acad. Sci. **854:** 192–201.
140. FILBURN, C.R. 2000. Dietary supplementation with phospholipids and docosahexaenoic acid for age-related cognitive impairment. JAMA **3:** 45–55.
141. FIORE, L. & L. RAMPELLO. 1989. L-Acetylcarnitine attenuates the age-dependent decrease of NMDA-sensitive glutamate receptors in rat hippocampus. Acta Neurol. (Napoli). **11:** 346–350.
142. SOHAL, R.S. & R. WEINDRUCH. 1996. Oxidative stress, caloric restriction, and aging. Science **273:** 59–63.
143. YU, B.P. 1996. Aging and oxidative stress: modulation by dietary restriction. Free Radic. Biol. Med. **21:** 651–668.
144. AMES, B.N. 1998. Micronutrients prevent cancer and delay aging. Toxicol. Lett. **102-103:** 5–18.
145. LIU, J. et al. 2002. Memory loss in old rats is associated with brain mitochondrial decay and RNA/DNA oxidation: partial reversal by feeding acetyl-L-carnitine and/or R-α-lipoic acid. Proc. Natl. Acad. Sci. USA **99:** 2356–2361.
146. CARNEY, J.M. et al. 1991. Reversal of age-related increase in brain protein oxidation, decrease in enzyme activity, and loss in temporal and spatial memory by chronic administration of the spin-trapping compound *N-tert*-butyl-alpha-phenylnitrone. Proc. Natl. Acad. Sci. USA **88:** 3633–3636.
147. LIU, J., A. FISCHER, P.S. TIMIRAS & B.N. AMES. 1998. Stress, hormones, oxidative damage, and neurodegeneration. In The 28th Annual Meeting of the Society for Neuroscience. Society for Neuroscience. Los Angeles, CA.
148. BUTTERFIELD, D.A. et al.1997. Free radical oxidation of brain proteins in accelerated senescence and its modulation by *N-tert*-butyl-alpha-phenylnitrone. Proc. Natl. Acad. Sci. USA **94:** 674–678.
149. SAITO, K., H. YOSHIOKA & R.G. CUTLER. 1998. A spin trap, *N-tert*-butyl-alpha-phenylnitrone extends the life span of mice. Biosci. Biotechnol. Biochem. **62:** 792–794.
150. ATAMNA, H., I. CHEUNG & B.N. AMES. 2000. A method for detecting abasic sites in living cells: age-dependent changes in base excision repair. Proc. Natl. Acad. Sci. USA **97:** 686–691.
151. HARMAN, D. 1961. Prolongation of the normal lifespan and inhibition of spontaneous cancer by antioxidants. J. Gerontol. **16:** 247–254.
152. HARMAN, D. 1968. Free radical theory of aging: effect of free radical reaction inhibitors on the mortality rate of male LAF mice. J. Gerontol. **23:** 476–482.
153. HARMAN, D. 1992. Free radical theory of aging. Mutat. Res. **275:** 257–266.

Enhancing Cognitive Function across the Life Span

DONNA L. KOROL

Department of Psychology, University of Illinois, Urbana-Champaign, Champaign, Illinois 61820, USA

ABSTRACT: Glucose administration regulates many neural and behavioral processes in rodents, including learning and memory. Given the important role of glucose in brain function and the safety of glucose as a treatment, we have investigated the effects of glucose administration in humans of different ages. In previous work, we examined the effects of early-morning glucose consumption on cognitive functions in elderly individuals. In this population, glucose enhanced performance on specific measures, particularly on those tasks where mild age-related deficits appear (e.g., verbal declarative memory). Interestingly, glucose failed to enhance cognitive functions in young adults. Our recent work has examined three issues related to glucose enhancement of cognition: First, is glucose effective only in reversing impairments or can it also facilitate performance in highly functioning individuals? Second, are glucose effects dependent either on time of day or on interactions with other meals? Third, are typical breakfast foods as effective as glucose in enhancing cognitive performance? Our findings suggest that glucose can improve memory in highly functioning populations as it does in populations with deficits. However, enhancement by glucose may require sufficient levels of task difficulty and of blood glucose. In addition, like glucose, early morning consumption of cereal can improve performance on some cognitive tests. These results have important implications for the nature of glucose facilitation of memory and for the role of dietary factors in performance of many daily activities.

KEYWORDS: aging; learning and memory; enhancement; glucose

There is little doubt that good nutrition aids the development and maintenance of good cognitive functions.[1–5] What remains a key issue in research on the neurobiology of learning and memory is whether particular nutrients or diets can preferentially enhance cognition. When viewing the efficacy of dietary components or even pharmacological substances in enhancing learning and memory, one substance for which the evidence is quite robust is glucose.[6,7]

Glucose has been shown to enhance memory across a variety of contexts. In rodents, administration of glucose reverses impairments on memory tasks after phar-

---

Address for correspondence: Donna L. Korol, Department of Psychology, 603 E. Daniel Street, Champaign, IL 61820. Voice: 217- 333-3659; fax: 217-244-0673.
dkorol@uiuc.edu

macologic manipulations with cholinergic antagonists[8–10] or gamma-aminobutyric acid (GABA)[11] and opioid[12,13] agonists. Furthermore, age-related deficits in learning, memory, and sleep are reduced after glucose administration.[5,7,14] Interestingly, glucose not only reverses impairments seen with age or following drug administration, but also facilitates cognition in healthy young adult animals. Facilitation of memory by glucose is observed when glucose is given shortly before or *after* training on a variety of tasks,[16–20] suggesting that glucose modulates memory formation and not sensory-motor function or attention per se. In addition, glucose effects on learning and memory follow an inverted-U dose-response function,[14,16,21] suggesting that there is an optimal dose at which glucose is effective at modulating memory formation. That blood glucose levels following systemic glucose administration rise to levels within physiological limits[22] supports the idea that glucose contributes under normal conditions to the mechanism by which memories are formed.

This paper focuses on the following two enquiries: (1) Can glucose facilitate cognition in cognitively healthy individuals? (2) Are commonly eaten foods as effective as glucose? A common thread that will emerge from the discussion is that task difficulty or cognitive load interacts with the ability to observe enhancement by glucose. Regulation of available extracellular glucose in the brain will be discussed as a potential physiological process mediating this phenomenon.

Nearly all animals studied to date, from *Aplysia* to humans, show some changes in brain and cognition with age.[23] This deficit is often expressed as an inability to form new memories and as enhanced forgetting of recently acquired information.[24,25] The neural bases for age-related impairments in learning and memory might reflect at least two classes of changes. One is that specific brain elements or processes essential for learning and memory might be deficient, such as the loss of or change in specific neuronal populations, neurotransmitter functions, or synaptic transmission. An equally likely and not mutually exclusive idea is that these substrate mechanisms for learning and memory remain largely intact with age, but the neuroendocrine regulators that engage the mechanisms of memory storage are deficient. In this manner, the hardware necessary to make a new memory is there, but the modulators needed to activate the brain processes necessary for memory formation are deficient. Thus, aging may be a problem of the loss of regulatory events instead of, or perhaps besides, a loss of storage mechanisms.[6,26]

One candidate regulatory mechanism mediating age-related memory shifts is the release of glucose from hepatic stores following rises in circulating epinephrine.[6] Glucose metabolism is altered in old animals; these changes are especially notable in the brain.[27,28] Glucose regulation is often poor in older individuals, with severe changes corresponding to a relatively high incidence of type II diabetes with age.[29] Because of these changes, because of glucose's role as the primary fuel for normal brain function, and because glucose is a relatively safe treatment, the effectiveness of glucose administration in regulating cognitive function has been tested extensively in healthy elderly individuals.[6] In a typical experiment, participants are tested on two occasions, once after ingesting a glucose drink and once after a control drink (saccharin), the order of which is counterbalanced across all participants. Individuals are tested on a battery of tests, with matched versions for each testing session, and are monitored for blood glucose levels. Using this counterbalanced cross-over design permits analysis of within-subject differences in scores under glucose and saccharin, thereby minimizing variance and the need for large samples.

Findings across many laboratories demonstrate that glucose consumed early in the morning facilitates specific forms of cognitive function, particularly verbal declarative memory (i.e., intentional memory for words and narratives).[30–36] As seen in rats, facilitation in humans follows an inverted-U dose-response function,[37] with optimal blood levels of glucose similar to those found in rodents. Glucose appears to act on learning, memory, and retrieval of information, as the treatment is effective when given either pretraining,[31] posttraining,[38] or just prior to recall,[39] respectively. Enhancement with glucose in healthy elderly individuals is greatest on tests that reveal age-related cognitive deficits, deficits that perhaps emerge during tasks that are particularly demanding. Thus, task difficulty may play an important role in our ability to observe improvements with glucose. Consistent with this idea, patient populations with cognitive deficits such as Alzheimer's victims exhibit an enhancement by glucose[32,40] more robust and broader in extent than that seen in healthy elderly.[40] Another consistent finding across many studies is that on tests in which elderly individuals are susceptible to enhancement by glucose, young adults fail to show enhancement by glucose.[30,31]

The lack of facilitation in young adults may result from a variety of possibilities including an absence of a loss of function, leaving no room for improvement, or similarly the use of tasks that were too easy, yielding no cognitive deficit upon which to improve. We tested these ideas by examining the facilitating effects of glucose in healthy young adult college students using similar, but more complex and difficult, tests than those used in previous studies. The basic experimental design was similar to that mentioned above, with participants ($n = 18$, [13 male, 5 female], average age = 20) arriving early in the morning after an overnight fast. After baseline blood glucose was measured with a simple monitoring system (One Touch II, Lifescan, Inc.), each participant received 50 g of glucose (experimental) or 23.7 mg of saccharin (control) in 8 oz. of lemonade. Fifteen minutes following ingestion, a second blood glucose measurement was taken and cognitive testing began. Blood glucose measurements were taken throughout testing.

The battery of cognitive tests included assessment for (1) verbal logical memory from a narrative prose passage, with immediate and delayed free recall (test provided by L. Squire and J. Zouzounis); (2) attention and speed of processing with the Minnesota clerical number checking test; (3) verbal working memory using a listening span (test provided by T. Salthouse and R. Babcock); and (4) recognition memory using delayed forced-choice recognition of faces and words. In contrast to what was found in earlier studies, we found a significant 30–35% enhancement of verbal declarative memory and a trend for enhancement on the attention task (FIG. 1). Performance on the other tests failed to show enhancement by glucose, perhaps because of high variance on the listening span and near-maximal performance on the recognition memory tests.

Blood glucose responses in these students were tightly regulated. From baseline values of ~80 mg/dL (4.4 mM), blood glucose rose approximately 50 mg/dL to peak values of ~130 mg/dL (7.2 mM) 35 minutes postingestion, and then receded back to baseline (FIG. 2a). Blood values across the population tested were quite uniform across participants such that we failed to find any significant relationships between baseline blood glucose or the glycemic response and baseline performance, or between baseline values and cognitive enhancement. The glycemic response in the students in whom memory was enhanced was much smaller than that observed

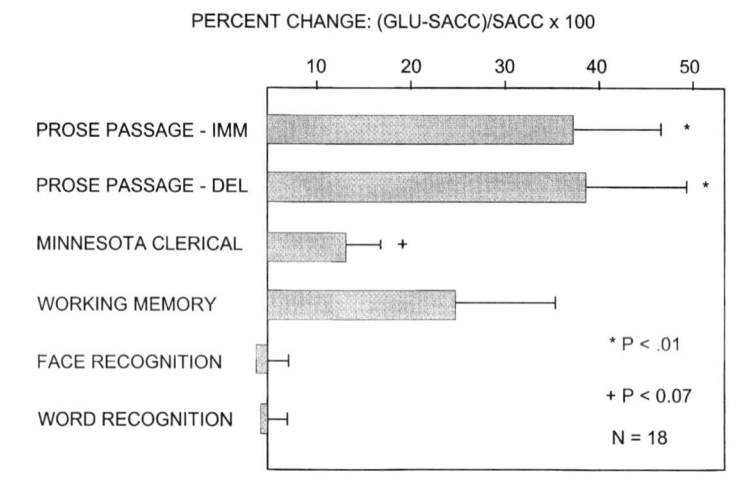

FIGURE 1. Glucose enhancement of memory in young-adult college students. Ingestion of 50 g of glucose significantly improved immediate and delayed recall of items from a narrative passage. There was a trend for improvement by glucose on a test of attention. No significant effects were found for working memory and face and word recognition. Data reflect percent differences in performance under glucose vs. saccharin using the formula: (glu score − sac score)/sac score × 100. (From Korol and Gold.[6] Reprinted with permission by the *American Journal of Clinical Nutrition*.)

previously with young adults whose baseline values and peak response to glucose were much higher (FIG. 2b). That a smaller response to a glucose load leads to better memory is well supported by findings demonstrating negative correlations between peak blood glucose response and cognitive performance in healthy young[34,41] and in healthy elderly[30,31] adults. Perhaps there are optimal blood glucose levels for glucose to enhance cognition; in effect, those individuals with exceedingly high or low changes in circulating blood glucose fall outside the effective range for cognitive enhancement. Most importantly, the results suggest that, given sufficient task difficulty, glucose ingestion can enhance performance on specific cognitive tests in individuals considered healthy cognitively.

Glucose enhancement appears to be specific to those tests on which deficits are found, and thus would enhance performance in cognitively taxing situations. In sum, across populations, task-difficulty needed to observe glucose enhancement of performance was greatest in young adults, lower in the healthy elderly, and very low in Alzheimer's patients. Thus, we can titrate task difficulty to find cognitive-enhancing effects of glucose in a variety of populations.

In extending this work to focus on more diet-related issues, one question becomes whether glucose acts through provisions of energy or acts as a specific signal for other neuronal processes. If glucose enhancement is through the supply of readily usable energy, then substituting other carbohydrates with glycemic indices similar to our glucose load should be as effective as glucose alone. To test this idea, we examined whether a commonly eaten breakfast food (i.e., ready-to-eat cereal) could substitute for glucose in its effects. Because of our extensive findings with the healthy

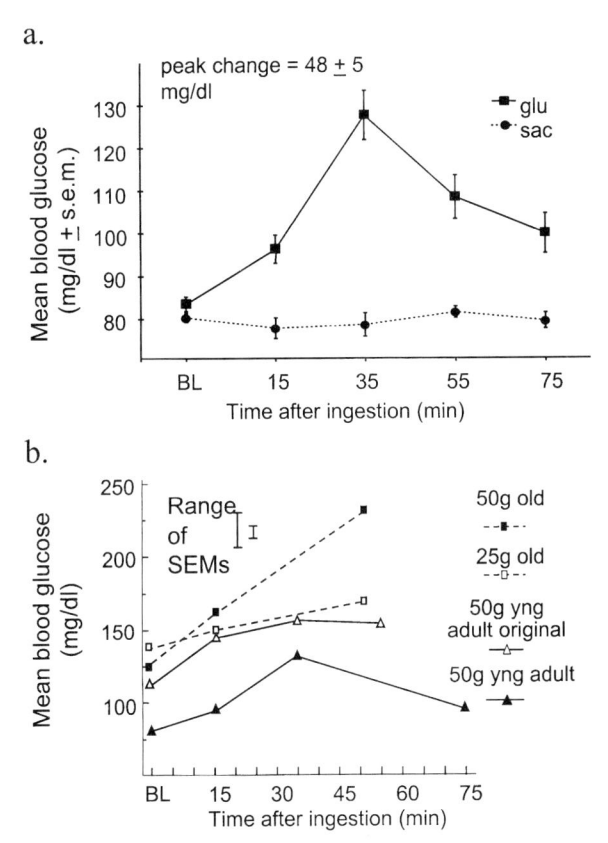

FIGURE 2. Time course and extent of blood glucose changes in different groups of individuals. (*a*) Blood glucose changes in college students tested with more difficult tests following consumption of 50 g of glucose (*solid line*) or saccharin (*dashed line*) in 8 oz of lemonade. Blood glucose levels were significantly elevated at all time points tested. (From Korol and Gold.[6] Reprinted with permission by the *American Journal of Clinical Nutrition*.) (**b**) Blood glucose changes following ingestion of different glucose loads in elderly (*open* and *solid squares*) and young (*open* and *solid triangles*) participants. Especially note the difference in the glycemic response between young adults tested originally (*open triangles*) and those tested recently (*solid triangles*).

elderly population, we chose to examine the ability of cereal to enhance a variety of cognitive processes in healthy elderly individuals ($n = 27$; 20 F, 7 M; average age = 68).

The design was similar to that used in our past experiments, with early morning provision of treatment and control meals after an overnight fast. This experiment included two treatment groups, one group in which 50 g of glucose in 8 oz of lemonade composed the experimental meal and the other in which a bowl of corn flakes and skim milk (1.7 oz of cereal, 6.7 fluid oz milk) providing 50 g of available carbohydrate composed the experimental meal. For both groups, the control treatment was 8 oz of lemonade sweetened with 23.7 mg of saccharin. The cognitive tests used with these healthy elderly subjects included immediate and delayed tests for the narrative

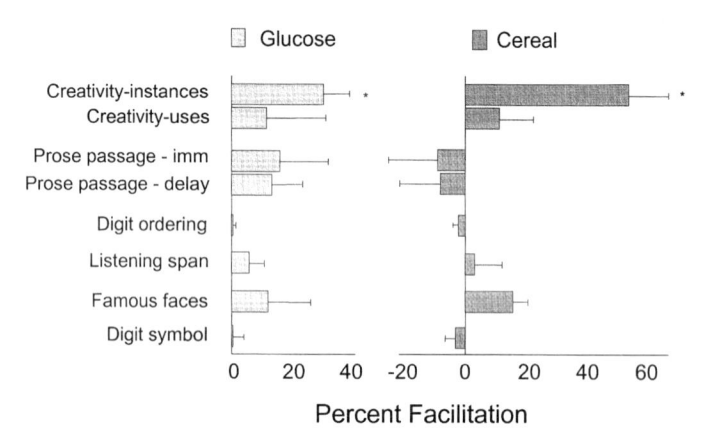

FIGURE 3. Glucose and cereal enhancement of cognition in healthy elderly adults. Ingestion of 50 g of glucose or cereal with skim milk contributing 50 g of available carbohydrate led to a robust increase in creativity measures. No other significant enhancement was seen across other cognitive tasks.

prose passage we used previously, in addition to five other tests that tap attention/speed of processing (digit symbol), verbal (listening span) and numeric (digit ordering) working memory, remote (very long-term) memory (famous faces test), and creativity or ideational fluency. For both cereal and glucose groups, there was a large and significant enhancement on the creativity test, a task that requires generation of novel items and that uses complex and relatively high levels of processing, but there was no statistically significant enhancement for any other task (FIG. 3). Interestingly, in our study with young college students, glucose increased by 40% the total number of words generated during the recall test from the prose passage, a phenomenon that may engage similar neural processes as those for the creativity test.

It was surprising that we obtained mixed results for the prose passage test and that we failed to find significant enhancement with glucose, a reliable and robust finding across many other studies. One possibility is that the population of healthy elderly used in this study was especially healthy. For example, blood glucose was more tightly regulated than it was in elderly populations tested in the past (FIGS. 2b and 4), and baseline test scores were much higher in the current elders, at times scoring 60% higher than those participants used previously (compare average baseline score on prose passage of 8 [previously] vs. 13 [currently]). Perhaps the tests were not sufficiently challenging cognitively and blood glucose rise was not sufficiently high to observe glucose enhancement.

These ideas were tested by statistical analysis of the data using control cognitive performance and glucose measures as covariates. If task difficulty is related to enhancement, then those individuals with poorer baseline performance (that is, those for which the tasks might be more difficult) would be expected to show greater enhancement following treatment. This is indeed what we found (FIG. 5a) and is supported by work with young adults showing an interaction of task difficulty with glucose enhancement of performance.[42] In contrast to the work of others[35,41,43,44] who have shown that certain measures of glucose regulation covary with perfor-

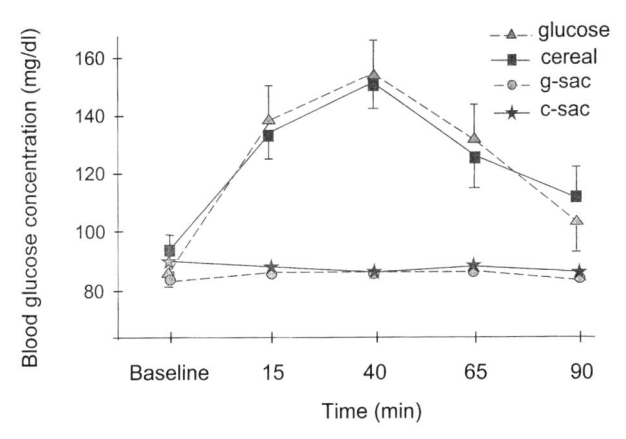

FIGURE 4. Time course and extent of blood glucose change following ingestion of 50 g of glucose, cereal with skim milk contributing 50 g of available carbohydrate, or saccharin (control) in healthy elderly adults. Glucose and cereal ingestion led to a remarkably similar increase in circulating glucose. Glucose levels were significantly elevated compared to saccharin controls at all time points measured. Notice the healthy glucose regulation in this population of elderly.

mance and enhancement in young and elderly adults, we found no relationship between glucose regulation using either baseline values, peak change in glucose, or residual levels of glucose and enhancement (FIG. 5b). Our measures of glucose regulation and cognitive performance might have been less sensitive than those used by others.

Breakfast, either as glucose or other foods providing carbohydrate, enhances some cognitive functions. Though the resultant blood glucose response was nearly identical for the cereal and glucose loads, the specific features of enhancement were somewhat different. Thus, other signals, whether psychological or physiological, are likely to play a role in cognitive enhancement, suggesting that the full nutritional context is important for developing foods that improve function. One consistency across findings is that the cognitive load demanded by the task that is also a function of the cognitive deficit brought to the task by the individual predicts the enhancing capabilities of glucose. This is likely to be a physiological property of glucose use by different brain areas and not a property of our measurement tools.

Recent evidence by Gold and colleagues shed light onto at least one mechanism through which task difficulty interacts with glucose consumption to improve cognition. They developed an elegant and sensitive technique to measure extracellular glucose in various brain regions while rats were engaged in a learning task.[45] Contrary to conventional wisdom, regional extracellular glucose levels fluctuate widely with behavior, with reductions in specific brain areas appearing soon after animals were placed in a learning situation that relied on that specific brain structure[46] (FIG. 6). Their results imply that neurons are not always saturated with glucose and that normal brain functioning may put a demand on glucose stores. Perhaps even more pertinent to the current discussion is that the severity of glucose depletion correlates with the difficulty of the task: the higher the cognitive load of the task, the greater

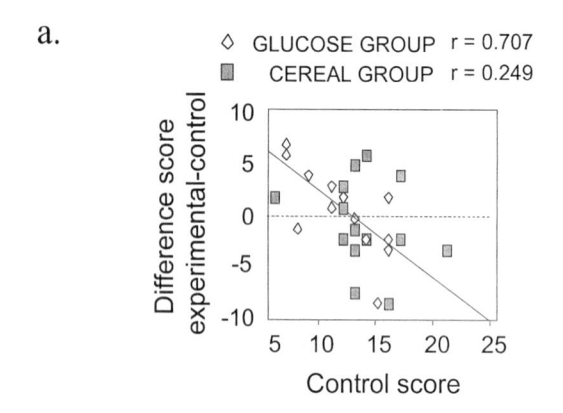

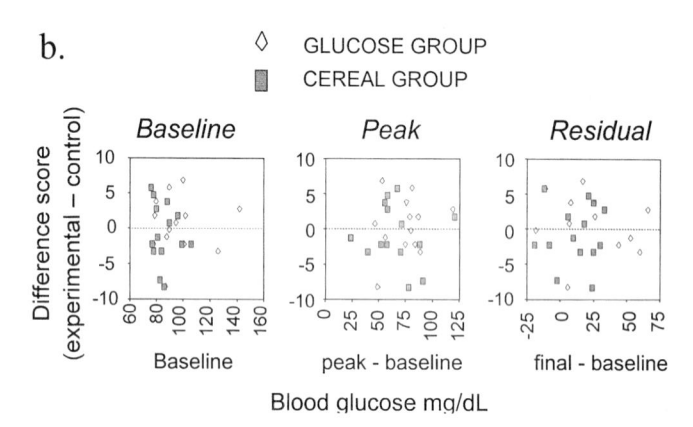

FIGURE 5. Relationships between baseline cognitive performance or blood glucose regulation and enhancement. (a) Baseline performance under saccharin (control) treatment on the verbal declarative test using the narrative passage was correlated with amount of enhancement. Specifically, those with lower baseline scores showed greater effects of glucose consumption than did those with higher scores. (b) Baseline (prior to ingestion), peak (maximal response relative to baseline), or residual (final measure relative to baseline) blood glucose measures failed to correlate with glucose enhancement of performance.

the reduction in extracellular glucose[47] (FIG. 6a). Interestingly, the decline in extracellular glucose was significantly larger and longer-lasting in old animals than it was in younger counterparts[46] (FIG. 6b).

Providing systemic glucose restores depleted brain levels of glucose in both young and old rats during maze learning and reverses age- and task-related deficits in performance of the task (FIG. 7). Regions that are highly activated may drain available stores; on less complex tasks brains of young animals may be able to sustain the supply of fuel, whereas those from old animals may have difficulty maintaining ad-

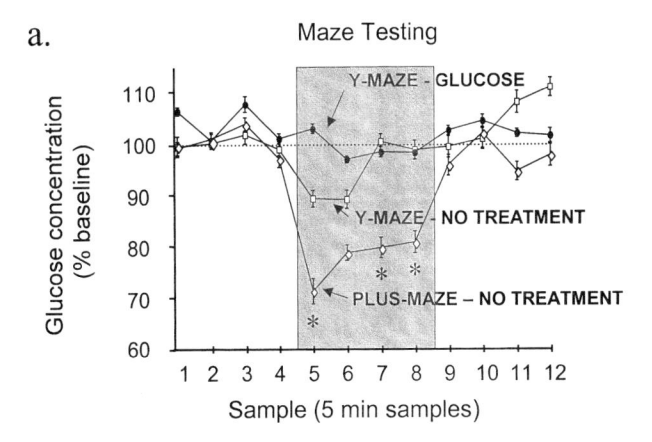

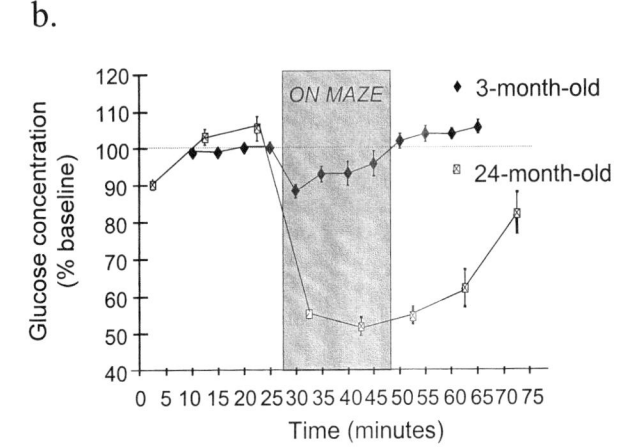

FIGURE 6. Changes in extracellular glucose concentrations sampled from the hippocampus before, during, and after maze training. Data are expressed relative to baseline values. (a) Mean extracellular glucose concentrations on two hippocampal-dependent tasks, Y-maze and plus-maze training. Note that extracellular glucose declines more dramatically in the harder plus-maze task than in the Y-maze task and that systemic glucose (1.0 mL of 250 mg/kg i.p., 30 min before testing) reverses the drop in extracellular glucose observed during Y-maze training. (From McNay et al.[47] Reprinted with permission by the National Academy of Sciences, U.S.A.) (b) Mean extracellular glucose concentrations in young (3 mo) and old (24 mo) Fisher 344 rats. Note that the hippocampus glucose levels decline to a greater extent and recover much more slowly in old rats than they do in young rats. (From McNay and Gold.[46] Reprinted with permission.)

equate levels for optimal cognitive functioning. As task difficulty rises, demands on cerebral glucose may increase, even in healthy young brains.[48,49]

Changes in available glucose may alter local cerebral metabolism,[50] may modify neurophysiological properties of neurons via changes in ion channel activity,[51] and may interact with the output of neurochemical systems,[21] perhaps by providing substrates for the synthesis of various neurotransmitters.

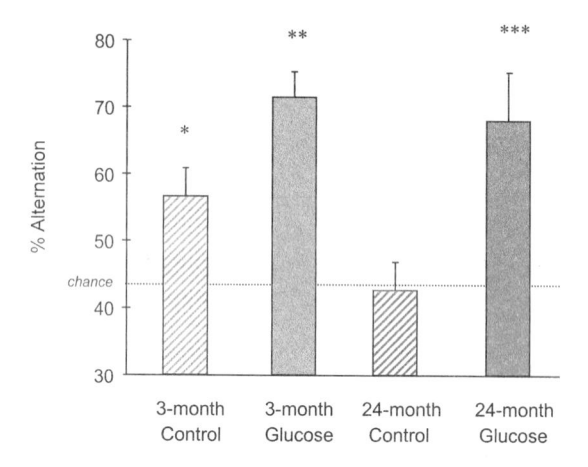

FIGURE 7. **Effects of systemic glucose on performance on spontaneous alternation in a plus-maze, a hippocampal-dependent task.** Glucose significantly enhances performance relative to saline-treated controls in both young (3 mo) and old (24 mo) rats. Note also that under control conditions old rats show deficits on this task relative to young rats and that glucose reverses age-related deficits. $*P < 0.05$ vs. 24-month control; $**P < 0.05$ vs. 3-month control; $***P < 0.05$ vs. 24-month control and not significantly different vs. 3-month glucose group. (From McNay and Gold.[46] Reprinted with permission.)

CONCLUSIONS AND DIRECTIONS

Many lines of research with laboratory animals and humans support the findings that glucose enhances cognition through modulation of memory formation. Perhaps systemic glucose acts at highly activated neural sites, (i.e., those brain areas involved in solving the task at hand), restoring depleted provisions of extracellular glucose, and maximizing information flow through these brain areas. Though the neural mechanisms underlying glucose's actions are not fully understood, several candidates have been elucidated, including production of precursors of neurotransmitters through byproducts of glucose metabolism and the inactivation of K-ATP channels through the production of ATP.[51]

Like physiological health, attention to the cognitive aspects of nutrition has become important for understanding the aging process and for developing treatments or diets to maintain cognitive health across the lifespan. Several key issues in the study of nutrition and cognition remain, including the specific dietary factors responsible for long-term neural health and for cognitive enhancement. It is seemingly paradoxical that acute glucose treatments enhance cognitive function, while chronic glucose consumption may lead to degeneration of neural and other tissue across the life span via metabolic stress following the production of oxygen free radicals.[52] However, as mentioned above, processes through which acute rises in blood glucose enhance cognition may act by providing precursors for neurotransmitter synthesis or other neurochemicals from glycolysis and may not solely rely on oxidative metabolic actions of glucose. Furthermore, the neural site of action of glucose is likely to be distant and distinct from absolute values of blood levels, such that the relationship between enhancement and blood glucose is not linear. Sorting out the neural mechanisms of glucose's actions will help to resolve these and other issues of nutrition and aging.

More broadly, for the field of healthy aging we need to fit glucose into a full spectrum of physiological responses to the environment. In one sense, glucose is a product of nutrition, but in another sense, changes in circulating glucose is a product of neuroendocrinologic sequelae of stress. Other hormones, including adrenal cortical[53,54] and gonadal steroids such as estrogen,[55,56] may play important roles in maintaining cognitive and brain health across the aging process.

ACKNOWLEDGMENTS

This work was supported by NSF Grants IBN-0081061, NS32914, AG07648 and by private donors. I wish to thank Lisa Savage for comments on this manuscript.

REFERENCES

1. WACHS, T.D. 1995. Relation of mild-to-moderate malnutrition to human development: correlational studies. J. Nutr. **125:** 2245S–2254S.
2. LA RUE, A., K.M. KOEHLER, S.J. WAYNE, et al. 1997. Nutritional status and cognitive functioning in a normally aging sample: a 6-y reassessment. Am. J. Clin. Nutr. **65:** 20–29.
3. FRANCHI, F., G. BAIO, A.G. BOLOGNESI, et al. 1998. A review on the relations between the vitamin status and cognitive performances. Arch. Gerontol. Geriatr. **6S:** 207–214.
4. POLLITT, E., S. CUETO & E.R. JACOBY. 1998. Fasting and cognition in well- and undernourished schoolchildren: a review of three experimental studies. Am. J. Clin. Nutr. **67:** 779S–784S.
5. DESCHAMPS, V., P. BARBERGER-GATEAU, E. PEUCHANT, et al. 2001. Nutritional factors in cerebral aging and dementia: epidemiological arguments for a role of oxidative stress. Neuroepidemiology **20:** 7–15.
6. KOROL, D.L. & P.E. GOLD. 1998. Glucose, memory and aging. Am. J. Clin. Nutr. **67:** 764S–771S.
7. GOLD, P.E. 2001. Cognitive enhancers in rodents and humans. In Animal Research and Human Health: Advancing Human Welfare Through Behavioral Science. M.E. Carroll & J.B. Overmeir, Eds.: 293–304. American Psychological Association. Washington, DC.
8. STONE, W.S., K. COTTRILL, D. WALKER, et al. 1988. Blood glucose and brain function: interactions with CNS cholinergic systems. Behav. Neural. Biol. **50:** 325–334.
9. PARSONS, M.W. & P.E. GOLD. 1992. Scopolamine-induced deficits in spontaneous alternation performance: attenuation with lateral ventricle injections of glucose. Behav. Neural Biol. **57:** 90–92.
10. RAGOZZINO, M.E., G. ARANKOWSKY-SANDOVAL & P.E. GOLD. 1994. Glucose attenuates the effect of combined muscarinic-nicotinic blockade on spontaneous alternation. Eur. J. Pharmacol. **256:** 31–36.
11. PARENT, M.B. & P.E. GOLD. 1997. Intra-septal infusions of glucose potentiate inhibitory avoidance deficits when co-infused with the GABA agonist muscimol. Brain Res. **748:** 317–320.
12. RAGOZZINO, M.E., M.E. PARKER & P.E. GOLD. 1992. Spontaneous alternation and inhibitory avoidance impairments with morphine injections into the medial septum: Attenuation by glucose administration. Brain Res. **597:** 241–249.
13. RAGOZZINO, M.E. & P.E. GOLD. 1994. Task-dependent effects of intra-amygdala morphine injections: Attenuation by intra-amygdala glucose injections. J. Neurosci. **14:** 7478–7485.

14. STONE, W.S. & P.E. GOLD. 1988. Sleep and memory relationships in intact old and amnestic young rats. Neurobiol. Aging **9:** 719–727.
15. WINOCUR, G. & S. GAGNON. 1998. Glucose treatment attenuates spatial learning and memory deficits of aged rats on tests of hippocampal function. Neurobiol. Aging **19:** 233–241.
16. GOLD, P.E., J. VOGT & J.L. HALL. 1986. Posttraining glucose effects on memory: Behavioral and pharmacological characteristics. Behav. Neural Biol. **46:** 145–155.
17. MESSIER, C. & N.M. WHITE. 1987. Memory improvement by glucose, fructose, and two glucose analogs: a possible effect on peripheral glucose transport. Behav. Neural Biol. **48:** 104–27.
18. LEE, M.K., S. GRAHAM & P.E. GOLD. 1988. Memory enhancement with posttraining intraventricular glucose injections in rats. Behav. Neurosci. **102:** 591–595.
19. WHITE, N.M. 1991. Peripheral and central memory-enhancing actions of glucose. *In* Peripheral Signaling of the Brain: Role in Neural-Immune Interactions, Learning and Memory. R.C.A. Frederickson, J.L. McGaugh & D.L. Felten, Eds.: 421–441. Hogrefe and Huber. Toronto, Ontario.
20. GREENWOOD, C.E., & G. WINOCUR. 2001. Glucose treatment reduces memory deficits in young adult rats fed high-fat-diets. Neurobiol. Learning Memory **75:** 179–189.
21. RAGOZZINO, M.E., K.E. UNICK & P.E. GOLD. 1996. Hippocampal acetylcholine release during memory testing in rats: Augmentation by glucose. Proc. Natl. Acad. Sci USA **93:** 4693–4698.
22. HALL, J.L. & P.E. GOLD. 1986. The effects of training, epinephrine, and glucose injections on plasma glucose levels in rats. Behav. Neural Biol. **46:** 156–176.
23. BARNES, C.A. 2001. Plasticity in the aging central nervous system. Int. Rev. Neurobiol. **45:** 339–354.
24. CRAIK, F.I.M. 1994. Memory changes in normal aging. Curr. Dir. Psychol. Sci. **3:** 155–158.
25. ZACKS, R.T., L. HASHER & K.Z.H. LI. 2000. Human memory. *In* The Handbook of Aging and Cognition, 2nd ed. F.I.M. Craik & T.A. Salthouse, Eds.: 293–357. Lawrence Erlbaum. Mahwah, NJ.
26. GOLD, P.E., J.L. MCGAUGH, L.L. HANKINS, *et al.* 1981. Age dependent changes in retention in rats. Exp. Aging Res. **8:** 53–58.
27. BENTON, D., P.Y PARKER & R.T. DONOHOE. 1996. The supply of glucose to the brain and cognitive functioning. J. Biosoc. Sci. **28:** 463–479.
28. BENTOURKIA, M., A. BOL, A. IVANOIU, *et al.* 2000. Comparison of regional cerebral blood flow and glucose metabolism in the normal brain: effect of aging. J. Neurol. Sci. **181:** 19–28.
29. MESSIER, C. & M. GAGNON. 2000. Glucose regulation and brain aging. J. Nutr. Hlth. Aging **4:** 208–213.
30. HALL, J.L., L.A. GONDER-FREDERICK, W.W. CHEWNING, *et al.* 1989. Glucose enhancement of performance on memory tests in young and aged humans. Neuropsychologia **27:** 1129–1138.
31. MANNING, C.A., J.L. HALL & P.E. GOLD. 1990. Glucose effects on memory and other neuropsychological tests in elderly humans. Psychol. Sci. **1:** 307–311.
32. CRAFT, S., G. ZALLEN & L.D. BAKER. 1992. Glucose and memory in mild senile dementia of the Alzheimer type. J. Clin. Exp. Neuropsychol. **14:** 253–267.
33. CRAFT, S., C.G. MURPHY & J. WEMSTROM. 1994. Glucose effects on complex memory and nonmemory tasks: the influence of age, sex, and glucoregulatory response. Psychobiology **22:** 95–105.
34. BENTON, D., D.S. OWENS & P.Y PARKER. 1994. Blood glucose influences memory and attention in young adults. Neuropsychologia **32:** 595–607.
35. MESSIER, C., M. GAGNON & V. KNOTT. 1997. Effect of glucose and peripheral glucose regulation on memory in the elderly. Neurobiol. Aging **18:** 297–304.
36. NEWCOMER, J.W., S. CRAFT, R. FUCETOLA, *et al.* 1999. Glucose-induced increase in memory performance in patients with schizophrenia. Schizophrenia Bull. **25:** 321–335.
37. PARSONS, M. & P.E. GOLD. 1992. Glucose enhancement of memory in elderly humans: an inverted-U dose-response curve. Neurobiol. Aging **13:** 401–404.

38. MANNING, C.A., M.W. PARSONS & P.E. GOLD. 1992. Anterograde and retrograde enhancement of 24-hour memory by glucose in elderly humans. Behav. Neural Biol. **58:** 125–130.
39. MANNING, C.A., W.S. STONE, D.L. KOROL, et al. 1998. Glucose enhancement of 24-hour memory retrieval in healthy elderly humans. Behav. Brain Res. **93:** 71–76.
40. MANNING, C.A., M. RAGOZZINO & P.E. GOLD. 1993. Glucose enhancement of memory in patients with Alzheimer's disease. Neurobiol. Aging **14:** 523–528.
41. DONOHOE, R. & D. BENTON. 1999. Cognitive functioning is susceptible to the level of blood glucose. Psychopharmacology **145:** 378–385.
42. MARTIN, P.Y & D. BENTON. 1999. The influence of a glucose drink on a demanding working memory task. Phsyiol. Behav. **67:** 69–74.
43. DONOHOE, R.T. & D. BENTON. 2000. Glucose tolerance predicts performance on tests of memory and cognition. Physiol. Behav. **71:** 395–401.
44. KAPLAN, R.J., C.E. GREENWOOD, G. WINOCUR, et al. 2000. Cognitive performance is associated with glucose regulation in healthy elderly persons and can be enhanced with glucose and dietary carbohydrates. Am. J. Clin. Nutr. **72:** 825–836.
45. MCNAY, E.C. & P.E. GOLD. 1999. Extracellular glucose concentrations in the brain. J. Neurochem. **73:** 2222–2223.
46. MCNAY, E.C. & P.E. GOLD. 2001. Age-related differences in hippocampal ECF glucose concentration during behavioral testing and following systemic glucose administration. J. Gerontol. Biol. Sci. **56A:** B66–B71.
47. MCNAY, E.C., T.M. FRIES & P.E. GOLD. 2000. Decreases in rat extracellular hippocampal glucose concentration associated with cognitive demand during a spatial task. Proc. Natl. Acad. Sci. USA **97:** 2881–2885.
48. DONOHOE, R. & D. BENTON. 1999. Declining blood glucose levels after a cognitively demanding task predict subsequent memory. Nutr. Neurosci. **2:** 413–424.
49. SCHOLEY, A.B., S. HARPER & D.O. KENNEDY. 2001. Cognitive demand and blood glucose. Physiol. Behav. **73:** 585–592.
50. RAGOZZINO, M.E., K. HELLEMS, R.C. LENNARTZ, et al. 1995. Pyruvate infusions into the septal area attenuate spontaneous alternation impairments induced by intraseptal morphine injections. Behav. Neurosci. **109:** 1074–1080.
51. STEFANI, M.R., G.M. NICHOLSON & P.E. GOLD. 1999. ATP-sensitive potassium channel blockade enhances spontaneous alternation performance in the rat: a potential mechanism for glucose-mediated memory enhancement. Neuroscience **93:** 557–563.
52. JOSEPH, J.A., N.A. DENISOVA, D. BIELINSKI, et al. 2000. Oxidative stress protection and vulnerability in aging: putative nutritional implications for intervention. Mech. Ageing Dev. **116:** 141–153.
53. LUPIEN, S.J., M. DELEON, S. DESANTI, et al. 1998. Cortisol levels during human aging predict hippocampal atrophy and memory deficits. Nat. Neurosci. **1:** 69–73.
54. MCEWEN, B.S. 2000. Effects of adverse experiences for brain structure and function. Biol. Psychiatry **48:** 713–714.
55. SHERWIN, B.B. 1997. Estrogen effects on cognition in menoapusal women. Neurology **48:** S21–S26.
56. KOROL, D.L. & C.A. MANNING. 2001. Effects of estrogen on cognition: implications for menopause. *In* Animal Research and Human Health: Advancing Human Welfare Through Behavioral Science. M.E. Carroll & J.B. Overmier, Eds.: 305–322. American Psychological Association. Washington DC.

Ascorbic Acid, Blood Pressure, and the American Diet

GLADYS BLOCK

University of California, Berkeley, California 94720, USA

> ABSTRACT: A large controlled study supported by the NIH, the DASH study (Dietary Approaches to Stop Hypertension), demonstrated that a diet rich in fruits and vegetables can reduce blood pressure in persons with moderate elevation in blood pressure (BP). Fruits and vegetables are important sources of antioxidants such as vitamin C and carotenoids. We conducted a study in which we fed people a diet deficient in vitamin C for 30 days, followed for another 30 days by a diet adequate in vitamin C. Their blood levels of vitamin C and blood pressure (BP) were tracked. Plasma vitamin C was inversely related to diastolic blood pressure one month later (correlation = −0.48, $P < 0.0001$). Persons whose blood levels of vitamin C went down the furthest on depletion had the highest blood pressure one month later. Persons in the lowest one-fourth of the plasma vitamin C distribution had diastolic BP 7 mm Hg higher than did those in the upper one-fourth of the plasma ascorbic acid distribution. Multivariate control for age, body mass index, other plasma antioxidants, and dietary energy, calcium, fiber, sodium, and potassium did not reduce the plasma vitamin C effect. We believe that this indicates that the tissue stores of vitamin C may be important in regulating blood pressure. It is often thought that Americans' intake of vitamin C is ample, since the average intake is about 100 mg/day. However, this average level obscures the fact that substantial numbers of people actually have habitually low intake levels and low blood levels. African Americans tend to have low blood levels of vitamin C as well as the highest risk of hypertension. Low intake of antioxidant-rich fruits and vegetables may be one of the causes of hypertension.
>
> KEYWORDS: hypertension; blood pressure; nutrition; vitamin C; ascorbic acid; antioxidants

The DASH study, "Dietary Approaches to Stop Hypertension,"[1] demonstrated that a diet rich in fruits and vegetables can significantly reduce blood pressure (BP) in persons with moderate BP elevation. Fruits and vegetables are major sources of antioxidants, as well as of fiber and potassium. While a varied diet composed of many nutrients probably confers greater benefits than any single nutrient, it is important to determine whether a particular nutrient played a major role. In this study we examined the role of vitamin C and several other antioxidants in influencing BP in a controlled-diet study.

Address for correspondence: Gladys Block, Ph.D., 426 Warren Hall, School of Public Health, University of California, Berkeley, California 94720. Voice: 510-643-7896; fax: 510-643-6981.
gblock@uclink4.berkeley.edu

Numerous cross-sectional studies found highly significant inverse relationships ($P < 0.001$) between BP and plasma vitamin C. However, cross-sectional studies do not provide strong evidence for a causal relationship, because of correlations among nutrients in both food and plasma. Intervention studies would be preferable, but most of those that have been conducted have had various methodologic problems that make them difficult to interpret.[2] Many were very small, some had no control group or permitted placebo subjects to take multivitamins, or they did not exclude smokers, did not control alcohol or other dietary intake, and did not control body weight changes or other factors that might affect blood pressure. A few intervention studies have been conducted since the review by Ness et al.[3–5]

Considerable laboratory research has shown redox status to be important in several blood pressure–relevant biological systems. Because of that research, and the research on vitamin C and blood pressure, we examined whether vitamin C status or other antioxidant status is associated with blood pressure in a 17-week feeding study in a normotensive sample of 68 men.

METHODS

The National Cancer Institute (NCI) conducted this study in collaboration with the U.S. Department of Agriculture (USDA). The study was approved by the Human Subjects Committees of NCI and USDA, and informed consent was obtained. The design and methods have been reported in detail elsewhere.[6–8]

Study Design

Sixty-eight healthy men aged 30–59 years were recruited from the Beltsville, Maryland area. Persons who had smoked within the prior six months were excluded so that the effects of dietary vitamin C intake could be examined unconfounded by smoking's effect on BP and plasma vitamin C. Mean age was 40.6 years (range 30–59), mean weight 80.9 kg (range 59.3–100.8), and mean BMI 25.7 (range 18.1–34.9).

All participants underwent one month of stabilization on 60 mg/day vitamin C, then one month of vitamin C depletion (weeks 1–5) followed by one month of repletion (weeks 6–9). This pattern was then repeated: depletion (weeks 10–13), repletion (weeks 14–17). Subjects did not smoke, drink alcohol, use aspirin, or consume any supplements or food other than that provided by the study during the entire 17-week controlled-diet period. Energy intake was adjusted weekly to prevent weight gain or loss. Physical activity, stress, sickness, and other factors were recorded daily.

Diets

Diets consisted of a 14-day rotating menu of typical American foods. During depletion, the diet contained 9 mg of vitamin C per day provided by fruits and vegetables containing little vitamin C: pear nectar, grape juice, apple juice, pears, fruit cocktail, applesauce, canned plums, raisins, pinto beans, iceberg lettuce, cucumber, celery, beets, corn, carrots, zucchini, mashed potatoes, mixed vegetables and mushrooms. For repletion, subjects were randomized to receive 117 mg vitamin C from one of three sources: oranges, broccoli, or vitamin C supplement. The vitamin C supplement group continued to eat the fruits and vegetables in the depletion diet, listed above. The oranges and broccoli were assayed twice weekly, and amounts adjusted to maintain identical dosages throughout the study.

Subjects were monitored during meals, and uneaten food was collected and weighed; uneaten food had no effect on average vitamin C intake. Daily reports of protocol violations were obtained, and were negligible; this was confirmed in a final, post-reimbursement anonymous questionnaire, which again indicated that reported dietary violations were minor, and had no effect on average energy, vitamin C, or other nutrient intake. These monitoring procedures are similar to those of the DASH study, and indicate excellent compliance with the dietary regimen.

Beginning in week 9, the end of the first repletion period, BP was measured using a Critikon Dinamap Model 8100 Portable Blood Pressure Monitor (Critikon, Inc., Tampa, FL).[9] Measurement was repeated three times, and the average of the last two measures was used in the analyses.

Fasting venous blood was obtained every two weeks during the depletion periods (weeks 3, 5, 11, and 13), and every week during the repletion periods (weeks 6, 7, 8, 9, 14, 15, 16, and 17). For vitamin C assays, plasma was stabilized with 10% metaphosphoric acid, and concentration was determined spectrophotometrically using 2,4-dinitrophenylhydrazine,[10] which correlates highly with HPLC methods.[11] Plasma was also assayed for carotenoids, retinol, selenium, and alpha- and gamma-tocopherol at the same weeks as plasma ascorbate, and for cholesterol at weeks 1, 5, 9, 13, and 17.

Statistical Analyses

As noted, blood pressure measurement did not begin until week 9, after one full depletion–repletion cycle. As we have shown elsewhere,[6] this resulted in incomplete stabilization of vitamin C status at the end of that period. One-third of subjects had not reached a plateau in plasma vitamin C at the end of the first repletion, and half had not reached a plasma plateau at the end of the second repletion. Consequently, *change* in blood pressure at the ends of depletion and repletion was not an appropriate study outcome since in either case it did not represent a steady-state vitamin C status. Consequently, the main outcome to be examined is the effect of baseline tissue stores (as reflected in plasma vitamin C retained after one month of depletion) on subsequent BP. Multiple regression, analysis of variance, t-tests and Pearson correlations were calculated using SAS version 6.12, with significance at $P < 0.05$.

RESULTS

Subjects had a mean diastolic blood pressure (DBP) at week 9 of 73 mm Hg (range 53–97 mm Hg) and mean systolic blood pressure (SBP) of 122 mm Hg (range 103–143 mm Hg.). Their ethnic distribution was 57 Caucasian, 8 African American and 3 Asian. Age, weight, and body mass index (BMI) were positively associated with BP; for age and DBP ($r = +0.33$, $P = 0.006$) (data not shown).

During the last two weeks of depletion 1 (weeks 4–5), mean plasma vitamin C was 26.9 mmol/L (0.47 mg/dL), and more than 80% of subjects had levels above 22.7 mmol/L (0.40 mg/dL), often considered the lower level of "normal."[12] At

TABLE 1. Correlation of week-9 diastolic BP with plasma vitamin C at two time points

	Correlation (r)	Significance (P)	Percent of DBP variance explained ($R^2 \times 100$)
Ascorbate at week 5 (end of depletion)	−0.48	<0.0001	23
Ascorbate at week 9 (end of repletion)	−0.31	<0.01	9

TABLE 2. Risk of having week-9 diastolic BP above 80 mm Hg or systolic BP above 120

Week-5 plasma vitamin C		Diastolic blood pressure		Systolic blood spressure	
		OR		OR	
Unadjusted odds ratio					
> = 22.7 µmol/L	(0.4 mg/dL)	1.00[a]		1.00[a]	
< = 22.7 µmol/L	(0.4 mg/dL)	6.00	P = 0.03	1.90	P = 0.02
Adjusted odds ratio[b]					
> = 22.7 µmol/L	(0.4 mg/dL)	1.00		1.00	
< = 22.7 µmol/L	(0.4 mg/dL)	7.3	P = 0.08	4.00	P = 0.02

[a]Reference category.
[b]In logistic regression analysis adjusting for age, BMI, energy, sodium, and fiber. None of the variables other than plasma vitamin C approached statistical significance.

week 9, after four weeks of repletion, subjects attained a mean plasma vitamin C of 71.6 mmol/L (1.26 mg/dL).

TABLE 1 shows the relationship of week 9 DBP to plasma vitamin C measured at week 5 and week 9. Plasma vitamin C at week 5 was significantly and inversely correlated with DBP ($r = -0.48$, $P < 0.0001$). Plasma carotenoids (alpha- and beta-carotene, lutein, lycopene), tocopherols (alpha- and gamma-tocopherol), retinol, and selenium were also examined. None of these other plasma nutrients approached statistical significance or exceeded a correlation of $r = 0.22$ (data not shown). The same pattern was true for systolic BP, although weaker in these bivariate analyses.

Multiple regression analyses were performed, controlling for numerous other risk factors. No other variable had a significant inverse association with DBP. Each quartile increase in plasma vitamin C at week 5 was associated with 2.4 mm Hg lower diastolic BP at week 9, $P = 0.003$, after control for age, BMI, energy, sodium, and fiber (data not shown). The source of vitamin C (oranges, broccoli, pills) was not itself significant in analysis of variance ($P = 0.89$) and did not alter the significance of the vitamin C effect. Plasma vitamin C was also inversely associated with systolic BP, but was not statistically significant.

TABLE 2 shows a multiple regression analysis of the risk of having week 9 diastolic BP above 80 mm Hg, or week 9 systolic BP above 120 mm Hg, by whether the subjects' week 5 plasma vitamin C was above or below a conventional definition of "normal."[12] Having a plasma vitamin C below "normal" at week 5 was associated with a statistically significant increased risk of elevated BP for both diastolic and

TABLE 3. Vitamin C intake and plasma levels among men in the U.S. population

	Mean	SD	5th	10th	25th	50th	75th	90th	95th
Dietary intake (mg/day)[a]	101.6	102.6	8.5	15.3	33.7	72.4	136.0	221.8	291.0
Plasma levels (mg/dL)[b]	0.67	0.47	0.07	0.13	0.32	0.67	0.95	1.16	1.37

[a]Based on 2-day data from the Continuing Survey of Food Intakes by Individuals (CSFII), 1996.
[b]Based on serum data from the Third National Health and Nutrition Examination Survey (NHANES III), 1989–94.

systolic BP. Only 4% of those whose plasma vitamin C remained at or above "normal" had diastolic BP above 80 mm Hg, compared with 25% of those with lower plasma vitamin C. The association remained at or near statistical significance, even after adjustment for age, BMI, and dietary variables.

Nationally representative data on vitamin C intake and plasma levels reveal that a substantial proportion of the adult male population in the United States has low levels of vitamin C (TABLE 3). The dietary intake data are derived from the two-day data from the Continuing Survey of Food Intakes by Individuals (CSFII). Intake averaged over two days represents a more stable estimate of the true distribution of intake than would intake for a single day. While the mean intake of 101.6 mg/day is slightly above the RDA of 90 mg/day for men, the median value of 72.4 mg/day indicates that more than 50 percent of men failed to consume the RDA amount. Even more troublesome, 25 percent of American men consumed one-third of the RDA or less per day, and 10 percent of the population consumed 15.3 mg/day or less.

The serum data in TABLE 3 are derived from the Third National Health and Nutrition Examination Survey (NHANES III). They reveal that the low dietary intake data described above are reflected in the distribution of serum values. A level of 0.4 mg/dL is considered the lower limit of "normal;"[12] more than 25% of American men have blood concentrations below that level. Seventy-five percent of men are below what can be considered an optimum level of approximately 1.0 mg/dL, a level easily attainable with a diet rich in fruits and vegetables.

DISCUSSION

This study indicates that plasma vitamin C is inversely associated with blood pressure, even in healthy persons with normal blood pressure. This was true both at blood and dietary vitamin C somewhat lower than those of most Americans, and at levels higher than most Americans. This result was consistent with extensive cross-sectional results in the literature, but this study design improves on cross-sectional as well as on other intervention designs. Habituation to a study and regression to the mean[13] cannot be the explanation of the results, because we did not select subjects on the basis of elevated blood pressure, and did not begin blood pressure measurement until week 9. Body weight changes and dietary intake, including fat, potassium and calcium, were controlled by the study. Subjects did not smoke or drink during the study, which could have caused alterations in vitamin C status or BP. Numerous plasma nutrients were examined, including carotenoids and vitamin E, and they were neither significant themselves nor did they affect the significance of the vitamin C variable. Numerous potential confounders were evaluated, and none was found to alter the plasma vitamin C effect.

The dietary intakes of vitamin C in this study are relevant to intakes in Western societies. During repletion, subjects received 117 mg/day, an amount easily obtained in a normal diet and approximately equal to the average American intake. The vitamin C that was fed during the depletion period, 9 mg/day, is lower than the intake of most Americans, but the *blood* vitamin C levels seen during depletion are found in a substantial proportion of the U.S. population. The average plasma vitamin C during the last two weeks of depletion was 26.9 mmol/L (0.47 mg/dL); in NHANES III, more than 20 percent of American men in this age range had blood vitamin C levels this low or lower. Among African American men, approximately 30 percent had blood vitamin C values in this range.[14] In this context it is notable that African Americans have higher rates of hypertension.[15] This study, as well as other research,[16] suggests that some of the hypertension among African Americans may be due to low plasma vitamin C levels.

Considerable research supports a number of biological mechanisms that could explain a relationship between plasma vitamin C and BP. Ascorbic acid has been shown to prevent free radical inhibition of prostacyclin synthetase; prevent nitric oxide inhibition of release of endothelium-derived relaxing factor (EDRF); promote endothelial prostacyclin production; and to have effects on smooth muscle contractility of peripheral blood vessels, on aortic collagen, and other mechanisms.[17–22] Our study suggests that *tissue levels* of vitamin C are relevant to maintenance of desirable blood pressure. Tissue levels are difficult to measure, but the week 5 blood levels, coming after a month of low intake, indirectly reflect long-term tissue stores. Persons who enter a depletion period without full tissue stores are less able to maintain plasma levels during depletion, and fall to a lower plasma level than persons with adequate tissue stores. Thus, the fact that plasma vitamin C was most strongly associated with BP at that time point provides an important clue, suggesting tissue levels as the key to normal BP maintenance.

Numerous human organs and tissues import vitamin C against a concentration gradient; adrenal and pituitary glands have approximately 100 times the plasma concentration, and liver, spleen, pancreas, brain, and eye lens have approximately 20–30-fold the plasma concentration in both rats and guinea pigs and in humans.[23] It is likely that when confronted with chronic marginal intake, certain key organs may have higher priority than vascular cells or other organs related to blood pressure, leading to chronic marginal insufficiency relative to their optimal requirements. Thus, we believe that the week 5 data suggest that *body stores* of vitamin C may be associated with BP.

It has been estimated[24] that a reduction of 2 mm Hg in average population DBP could be associated with 14% fewer strokes and 8% less coronary heart disease. The data in TABLE 3 suggest the possibility of important reductions in BP if adequate vitamin C tissue stores are achieved and maintained. Long-term, well-designed interventions are clearly needed, but this study provides substantial evidence for a possible role for vitamin C in preventing elevated blood pressure.

ACKNOWLEDGMENTS

We acknowledge the assistance of William Campbell, John Canary, Arlene Salbe, Joseph Vanderslice, Elaine Wolfe, Ida Tateo, and the staff of the Beltsville USDA Human Studies Facility.

REFERENCES

1. APPEL, L.J. et al.—DASH COLLABORATIVE RESEARCH GROUP. 1997. A clinical trial of the effects of dietary patterns on blood pressure. N. Engl. J. Med. **336:** 1117–1124.
2. NESS, A.R., D. CHEE & P. ELLIOTT. 1997. Vitamin C and blood pressure: an overview. J Hum. Hypertens. **11:** 343–350.
3. DUFFY, S.J. et al. 1999. Treatment of hypertension with ascorbic acid. Lancet **354:** 2048–2049.
4. MILLER, E.R. III et al. 1997. The effect of antioxidant vitamin supplementation on traditional cardiovascular risk factors. J. Cardiovasc. Risk **4:** 19–24.
5. GALLEY, H.F. et al. 1997. Combination oral antioxidant supplementation reduces blood pressure. Clin. Sci. **92:** 361–365.
6. BLOCK, G. et al. 1999. Body weight and prior depletion affect plasma ascorbate levels attained on identical vitamin C intake: a controlled-diet study. J. Am. Coll. Nutr. **18:** 628–637.
7. MANGELS, A.R. et al. 1993. The bioavailability to humans of ascorbic acid from oranges, orange juice and cooked broccoli is similar to that of synthetic ascorbic acid. J. Nutr. **123:** 1054–1061.
8. BLOCK, G. et al. 2001. Ascorbic acid status and subsequent diastolic and systolic blood pressure. Hypertension **37:** 261–267.
9. 1986. Survey of Studies Involving the Dinamap Vital Signs Monitor. Critikon, Inc. Tampa, FL.
10. U.S. DEPARTMENT OF HEALTH AND HUMAN SERVICES, PUBLIC HEALTH SERVICE. 1979. Laboratory Procedures Used by the Clinical Chemistry Division, for the Second National Health and Nutrition Examination Survey (NHANES II) 1976–1980. IV: Analytical Methods, Vitamin C. Centers for Disease Control, Clinical Chemistry Division. Atlanta, GA.
11. SAUBERLICH, H.E. et al. 1989. Ascorbic acid and erythorbic acid metabolism in non-pregnant women. Am. J. Clin. Nutr. **50:** 1039–1049.
12. 1992. Current Medical Diagnosis & Treatment.: 1278. Appleton & Lange. Norwalk, CT.
13. KNAPP, H.R. 1996. Nutritional aspects of hypertension. In Present Knowledge in Nutrition. E.E. Ziegler & L.J. Filer, Eds.: 438–444. ILSI Press. Washington, DC
14. FULWOOD, R., C.L. JOHNSON & J.D. BRYNER—NATIONAL CENTER FOR HEALTH STATISTICS. 1982. Hematological and Nutritional Biochemistry Reference Data for Persons 6 Months–74 Years of Age: United States, 1976–80. Vital and Health Statistics. Series 11–No.232. DHHS Pub. No. (PHS) 83–1682. Public Health Service. Washington, DC.
15. GILLUM, R. 1991. Cardiovascular diseases in the United States: an epidemiological overview. In Cardiovascular Diseases in Blacks. E. Saunders, Ed.: 3–14. F.A. Davis. Philadelphia, PA.
16. TOOHEY, L., M.A. HARRIS, K.G.D. ALLEN & C.L. MELBY. 1996. Plasma ascorbic acid concentrations are related to cardiovascular risk factors in African-Americans. J. Nutr. **126:** 121–128.
17. SOLZBACH, U., B. HORNIG, M. JESERICH & H. JUST. 1997. Vitamin C improves endothelial dysfunction of epicardial coronary arteries in hypertensive patients. Circulation **96:** 1513–1519.
18. KANANI, P.M. et al. 1999. Role of oxidant stress in endothelial dysfunction produced by experimental hyperhomocyst(e)inemia in humans. Circulation **100:** 1161–1168.
19. VALLANCE, P., A. CALVER & J. COLLIER 1992. The vascular endothelium in diabetes and hypertension. J. Hypertens. **10** (Suppl. 1): S25–S29.

20. TOIVANAN, J.L. 1987. Effects of selenium, vitamin E and vitamin C on human prostacyclin and thromboxane synthesis in vitro. Prostaglandins Leukotrienes Med. **26:** 265–280.
21. LEVINE, G.N. *et al.* 1996. Ascorbic acid reverses endothelial vasomotor dysfunction in patients with coronary artery disease. Circulation **93:** 1107–1113.
22. SIOW, R.C. *et al.* 1999. Vitamin C protects human vascular smooth muscle cells against apoptosis induced by moderately oxidized LDL containing high levels of lipid hydroperoxides. Arterioscler. Thromb. Vasc. Biol. **19:** 2387–2394.
23. HORNIG, D.H. 1975. Distribution of ascorbic acid, metabolites and analogues in man and animals. Ann. N.Y. Acad. Sci. **258:** 103–118.
24. MACMAHON, S. *et al.* 1990. Blood pressure, stroke, and coronary heart disease. Part 1: Prolonged differences in blood pressure: prospective observation studies corrected for the regression dilution bias. Lancet **335:** 765–774.

Toward Mechanism-based Antioxidant Interventions

Lessons from Natural Antioxidants

VALERIAN E. KAGAN,[a] ELENA R. KISIN,[b] KAZUAKI KAWAI,[a] BEHICE F. SERINKAN,[a] ANATOLY N. OSIPOV,[a] ELENA A. SERBINOVA,[c] IRA WOLINSKY,[d] AND ANNA A. SHVEDOVA[b]

[a]*Department of Environmental and Occupational Health, University of Pittsburgh, Pittsburgh, Pennsylvania 15260, USA*

[b]*Health Effects Laboratory Division, Pathology and Physiology Research Branch, NIOSH, Morgantown, West Virginia, USA*

[c]*Bertek Pharmaceuticals, Inc., Foster City, California, USA*

[d]*University of Houston, Houston, Texas, USA*

> ABSTRACT: It is generally accepted that one of the major and important contributions to skin aging, skin disorders, and skin diseases results from reactive oxygen species. More than other tissues, the skin is exposed to numerous environmental chemical and physical agents, such as ultraviolet light, causing oxidative stress. Accelerated cutaneous UV-induced aging, photo aging, is only one of the harmful effects of continual oxygen radical production in the skin. Interestingly, our ELISA assays of 8-oxo-2′–deoxyguanosine in skin of young and old Balb/c mice showed that cumene hydroperoxide–induced accumulation of the biomarker of oxidative DNA damage in skin of 32-week-old mice occurred independently of their vitamin E status, while no accumultaion of oxo^8-dG was detectable in the skin of young animals. This suggests that vitamin E is not the major protector of skin against cumene hydroperoxide–induced oxidative stress. Production and accumulation of apoptotic cells is one of the characteristic features of skin damage by oxidative stress that, in the absence of effective scavenging by macrophages, dramatically enhances oxidative damage and inflammatory response. In our model experiments, we demonstrated that Cu-OOH induces significant oxidative stress in phospholipids of normal human epidermal keratinocytes (NHEK) whose characteristic feature is an early and profound oxidation of phosphatidylserine (PS), likely related to PS externalization. Since externalized PS is a signal for recognition of apoptotic cells by macrophage scavenger receptors, PS oxidation may be translatable into elimination of thus damaged NHEKs. Experiments are now underway to determine whether inhibition of PS oxidation by antioxidants may interfere with improtant signaling functions of oxidative stress in eliminating apoptotic cells.
>
> KEYWORDS: vitamin E; natural antioxidants; prooxidant; signaling pathways

Address for correspondence: Valerian E. Kagan, 3343 Forbes Ave., Pittsburgh, PA 15260. Voice: 412-383-2136.
kagan@pitt.edu.

Many theories have been advanced to account for the aging process. For example, the aging process has been attributed to molecular cross-linking, changes in immunologic function, damage by free radical reactions, senescence genes, and most recently, to telomere shortening. No single theory is generally accepted: "This remarkable process remains a mystery," and "it is doubtful that a single theory will explain all the mechanisms of aging."[1] Among more than 300 theories to explain the aging phenomenon, the free radical theory of aging, postulated first by D. Harman, is the most popular and widely tested, and is based on the chemical nature and ubiquitous presence of free radicals. Numerous studies emphasized the role of free radicals in DNA damage—both nuclear as well as mitochondrial—the oxidative stress they impose on cells, the role of antioxidants, the presence of autoantibodies, and their overall impact on the aging process.[2]

In the United States, the average life expectancy at birth rose from 69.7 years in 1960 to 75.7 years in 1994. Interestingly, since the 1960s the percentage of the population of the United States taking antioxidant supplements has increased to a value of 40–50% today. These data are in accord with beneficial effects expected from the growing use of antioxidant supplements since the 1960s to decrease disease and enhance life span and the widespread publicity about the ability of fruits and vegetables to decrease disease by depressing free radical–reaction damage.[3] This suggests that development of new mechanism-based antioxidant approaches combined with monitoring of oxidative stress/antioxidant status may be central to understanding the mechanisms of aging and developing novel optimized strategies for increased life span.

OPTIMIZING ANTIOXIDANT PROTECTION AGAINST OXIDATIVE STRESS

Redox Requirements

The intra- and extracellular regulation of relatively low reactive one- or two-electron reduction intermediates of molecular oxygen, such as superoxide and hydrogen peroxide, is successfully achieved by several specialized enzymes: different types of superoxide dismutases, catalase, and peroxidases (for a current review see Thiele et al.[4]). Other radical intermediates—hydroxyl, alkoxyl, and peroxyl radicals—are so reactive that they cannot be effectively controlled by these enzymatic mechanisms and require additional specialized systems for their management. Indeed, Mother Nature has created a unique network of small antioxidants that includes both lipid-soluble and water-soluble molecules. Notably, these molecules located in different compartments of cells closely interact with each other such that the overall antioxidant protection is very efficient. It is tempting to believe that supplementation with additional amounts of natural antioxidants or use of synthetic low molecular weight antioxidant molecules may offer relatively simple and effective ways to control oxidative stress. These expectations, however, should be based on detailed knowledge of antioxidant mechanisms and pathways that are essential for uninterrupted and physiologically justified antioxidant protection in specific intracellular environments.

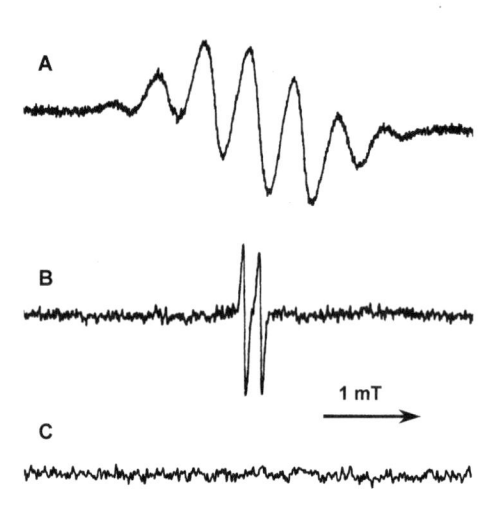

FIGURE 1. ESR spectra of α-tocopherol phenoxyl and ascorbate radicals produced upon UVB irradiation. α-Tocopherol suspension (0.1 mM) in SDS (100 mM) was irradiated with 290 nm light in the absence (**A**) or in the presence (**B**) of 0.5 mM ascorbate. Irradiation of ascorbate solution without α-tocopherol gave no ESR signal (**C**).

There are several critical requirements for a molecule that should be fulfilled in order to create a perfect and effective new antioxidant that include but are not limited to: (1) effective radical scavenging; (2) low reactivity of antioxidant radicals towards vital intracellular components; (3) low level of one-electron enzymatic metabolism of antioxidants; and (4) lack of interference with endogenous antioxidant networks, resulting in wasteful consumption of their resources. Vitamin E represents probably one of the best examples of a "perfect" lipid-soluble antioxidant in membranes and lipoproteins, where it can interact and be recycled by other lipid-soluble antioxidants (e.g., coenzyme Q)[5] and water-soluble antioxidants (e.g., vitamin C and thiols).[6] In addition, vitamin E can be regenerated from its radical by electron transport in mitochondria and endoplasmic reticulum.[7] Despite significant advantages that vitamin E's properties render to accomplish its role as interactive component of the antioxidant network, these same redox features of vitamin E may cause adverse effects under some circumstances. For example, it has been demonstrated that the vitamin E radical can directly attack lipids in lipoproteins and cause oxidative damage rather than antioxidant protection when the rate of oxidation-initiating radicals is high enough.[8] This prooxidant effect of vitamin E is only observable in the absence of other components of antioxidant network such as vitamin C or coenzyme Q, which can prevent unwanted direct interaction of the vitamin E radical with vital biomolecules.

Under some conditions, however, the recycling properties of vitamin E may cause adverse effects. Formation of the vitamin E radical, vitamin E phenoxyl radical, can be triggered by UVB light. We have demonstrated that UVB-induced vitamin E radicals can be reduced by vitamin C both in model systems and in skin.[9] As shown in FIGURE 1, UVB-induced vitamin E phenoxyl radical readily observable in the EPR

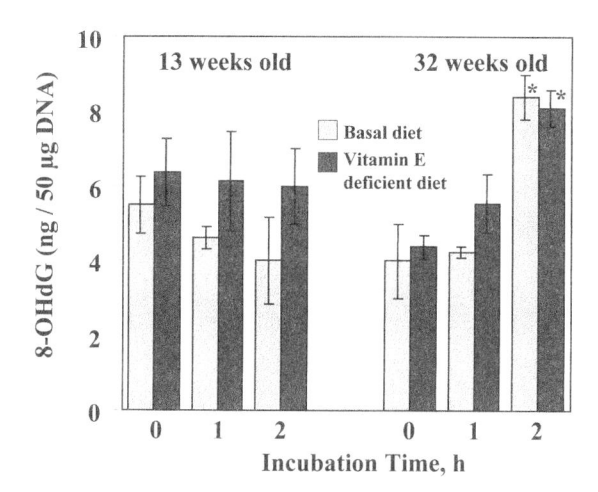

FIGURE 2. Levels of 8-oxo-2′-deoxyguanosine (oxo^8-dG) in skin of young and old Balb/c mice with different levels of vitamin E after exposure to cumene hydroperoxide. *Conditions:* Weaning Balb/c female mice were given vitamin E–deficient or –sufficient diets for 10 or 29 weeks. Levels of vitamin E in skin of mice given basal diet for 10 and 29 weeks were 98.5 ± 11.6 and 52.3 ± 7.9 pmol/mg, respectively. Levels of vitamin E in skin of mice given vitamin E–deficient diet for 10 and 29 weeks were 2.4 ± 0.7 and 0.62 ± 0.11 pmol/mg, respectively. *Treatment:* 100 µL cumene hydroperoxide (12 mmol/kg) were applied topically on the dorsal side. Mice were scarified after 1 or 2 hours postexposure. ELISA determination of oxo^8-dG was performed according to the manufacturer's instructions as described in the kit obtained from Genox Corporation (Baltimore, MD) after isolation of DNA using a chaotropic agent, NaI (obtained from Wako Chemical Co., Richmond, VA), as described by Helbock *et al.*[10] $P < 0.05$ vs. control.

spectra upon irradiation of vitamin E disappeared and was substituted by a typical doublet signal of vitamin C (ascorbate) radical. Given that UVB irradiation of vitamin C does not produce any signal in the EPR spectra in the absence of vitamin E, these data indicate that reduction of vitamin E phenoxyl radical was responsible for the spectral changes observed. This effect was also documented by UVB-induced generation of ascorbate radicals from endogenous vitamin C in mouse skin homogenates that was strictly dependent on the amount of vitamin E present in skin. Thus vitamin E that acts as a well-known protective skin antioxidant in the dark may also induce oxidative stress under UVB exposure. This suggests that under specific conditions, when skin is exposed to UVB irradiation, vitamin E may act as a photo-sensitizer catalytically consuming and destroying endogenous pools of vitamin C as a mechanism of wasteful vitamin E redox-recycling. Obviously, direct radical scavenging effects of vitamin E are also realized under the same conditions. As a result, the outcome of anti- versus prooxidant overall action of vitamin E will depend on specific conditions (i.e., intensity of UVB-irradiation and concentrations of vitamin E and vitamin C).

Interestingly, an accelerated cutaneous UV-induced aging (photoaging) is known as one of the harmful effects of continual oxidative stress in the skin. Interestingly, our ELISA assays of 8-oxo-2′-deoxyguanosine (oxo^8-dG) in skin of young and old

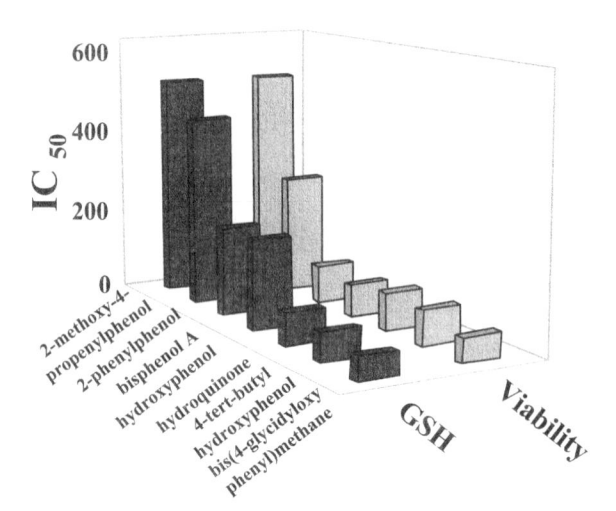

FIGURE 3. Comparison of cytotoxicity and GSH oxidation in normal human epidermal keratinocytes exposed to phenolic compounds. Normal human epidermal keratinocytes were incubated in phenol-free KGM-2 basal medium in the presence of seven phenolic compounds for 18 h at 37°C in 96-well plates. After the incubation, cells were washed twice with PBS, pH 7.4. GSH was measured using ThioGlo-1™ (10 µM) as described by Kagan et al.[13] Cell viability was determined using 10% Alamar Blue, as described by Keane et al.[14]

Balb/c mice showed that cumene hydroperoxide–induced accumulation of this biomaker of oxidative DNA damage in skin of 32-week old mice occurred independently of their vitamin E status (after keeping the animals on vitamin E–sufficient or vitamin E–deficient diets, respectively) while no accumulation of oxo^8-dG was detectable in the skin of young (13-week old) animals (FIG. 2).[10] This suggests that vitamin E is likely not the major protector of skin against cumene hydroperoxide–induced oxidative stress.

Vitamin E may exhibit its prooxidant activity only under some exquisite conditions. There are many examples of molecules that are good donors of electrons and hence extraordinary effective scavengers of oxidation-initiating radicals. In fact, many mono- and polyphenolic compounds have an appropriate electron-donating capacity to reduce peroxyl, alkoxyl, and hydroxyl radicals. Not all of them, however, may be good candidates for antioxidant protection. The major problem is that the products of their one-electron oxidation, the respective phenoxyl radicals, are sufficiently reactive to directly oxidize important targets in cells and biological fluids. Which intracellular constituents exactly are the targets that may suffer from oxidation by antioxidant phenoxyl radicals depends, to a large extent, on the redox potentials of phenoxyl radicals as well as on steric hindrance of the phenoxyl moiety by the surrounding groups. In the absence of vitamin C, intracellular thiols may be the most susceptible targets to attack by phenoxyl radicals. FIGURE 3 shows how different concentrations of environmentally and occupationally relevant phenolic compounds affect viability and levels of GSGH in cultures of normal human epidermal keratinocytes (NHEK). One can see that there is a strong correlation between the abil-

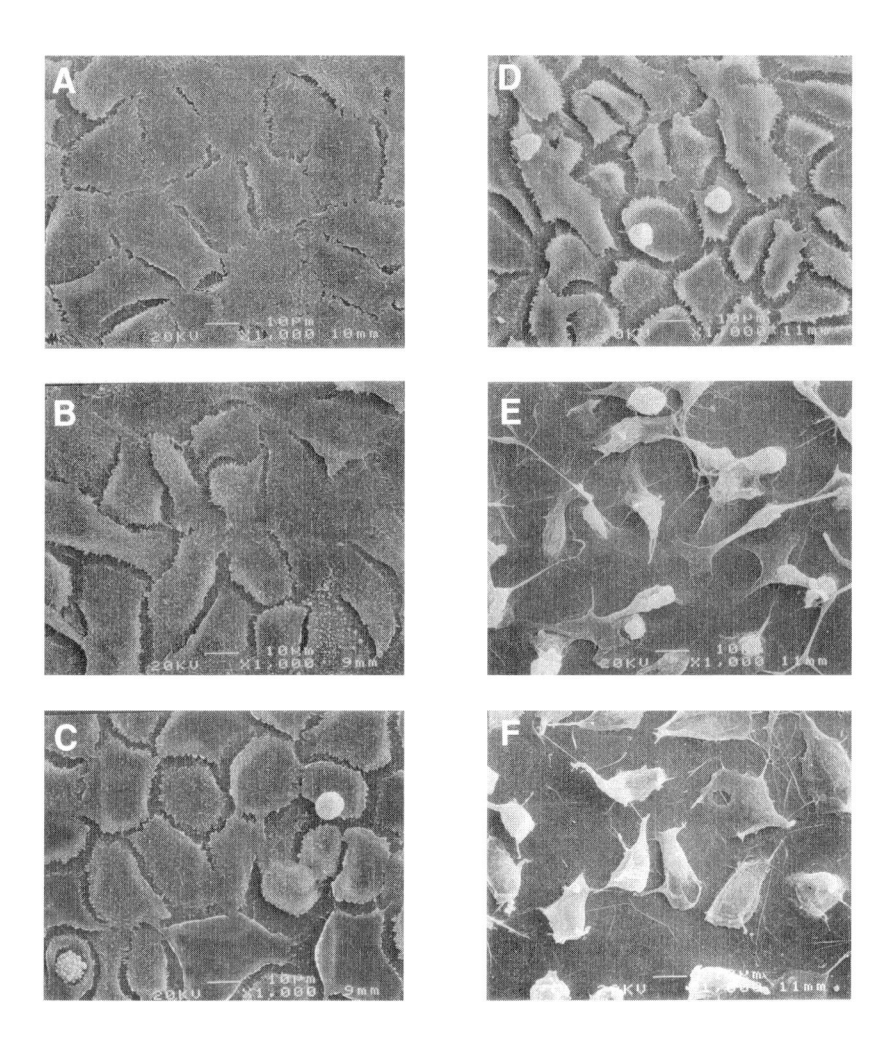

FIGURE 4. Scanning electron microphotographs of normal human epidermal keratinocytes exposed to bisphenol. Keratinocyte separation from monolayers in tissue cell culture, loss of keratinocytes, and altered cell surface homogeneity seem to be suitable for characterizing differences in keratinocyte morphology after bisphenol exposure. The signs of flattening keratinocyte cell surface, reduction of the size, and blurring of the cell borders were observed after exposure of keratinocyte cell cultures to bisphenol (**D–F**). Overall, confident signs of cell shrinking were evident after exposure to 200 μM bisphenol. Altered cell integrity was clearly visible 18 h after 300–500 μM bisphenol exposure (**E–F**). *Conditions:* Normal human epidermal keratinocytes were incubated in phenol-free KGM-2 basal medium in the absence and in the presence of 50–500 μM bisphenol for 18 h at 37°C in chamber slides. After the incubation, cells were washed twice with PBS, pH 7.4, and scanning microscopy was performed. (**A**) control cells; (**B**) after incubation with 50 μM of bisphenol; (**C**) after incubation with 100 μM of bisphenol; (**D**) after incubation with 200 μM of bisphenol; (**E**) after incubation with 300 μM of bisphenol; (**F**) after incubation with 500 μM of bisphenol.

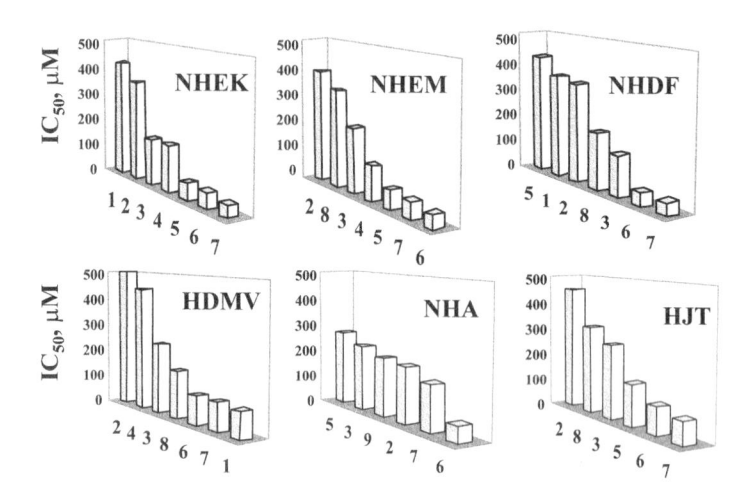

FIGURE 5. Effectiveness of glutathione (GSH) oxidation in different human cell lines exposed to phenolic compounds. Human cells (normal human keratinocytes, NHEK; normal human melanocytes, NHEM; normal human fibroblasts, NHDF; normal human astrocytes, NHA; normal human dermal microvascular cells, NHMV; and human Jurkat cells, HJT) were incubated in phenol-free KGM-2 basal medium in the presence of phenolic compounds for 18 h at 37°C in 96-well plates. After the incubation, cells were washed twice with Na-phosphate buffer, pH 7.4. GSH was measured using ThioGlo-1™ (10 μM) as described by Kagan et al.[13] *Columns:* (1) 2-methoxy-4-propenylphenol; (2) 2-phenylphenol; (3) bis(4-hydroxyphenyl)dimethylmethane (4) hydroxyphenol; (5) 1,4-benzenediol; (6) 4-*tert*-butylhydroxyphenol; (7) bis(4-glycidyloxyphenyl)methane; (8) 4-*tert*-butylphenol; (9) phenol.

ity of these phenolic compounds to deplete GSH and their cytotoxicity. Morphological features of cytotoxicity of phenolic compounds to keratinocytes exemplified by the effects of bisphenol on NHEK are shown on FIGURE 4. This reveals gradual keratinocyte separation from monolayers in tissue cell culture, altered cell surface homogeneity, and finally damage and loss of keratinocytes after exposure to bisphenol.

It should be noted that different types of peroxidase activity in NHEK (e.g., peroxidase activity of prostagladin synthase) can catalyze one-electron oxidation of phenolics and generate their phenoxyl radicals. Moreover, not only keratinocytes but also other types of cells in normal human skin, such as melanocytes, fibroblasts, astrocytes, dermal microvascular cells, as well as Jurkat cells, display a similar similarity between depletion of GSH and loss of viability upon exposure to different phenolic compounds (FIGS. 5 and 6). Since vitamin C is not usually present in culture growth media, it is not present at any significant levels in cultured cells. This implies that protection of cultured cells from toxic effects of phenoxyl radicals does not involve their reduction due to interaction with vitamin C. In the presence of vitamin C, one can envision that generation of phenoxyl radicals may be causative to depletion of vitamin C that will precede oxidation of GSH and protein thiols. In any case, formation of reactive phenoxyl radicals by oxidative stress or as a result of enzymatic one-electron metabolism may be associated with further enhancement of oxidative

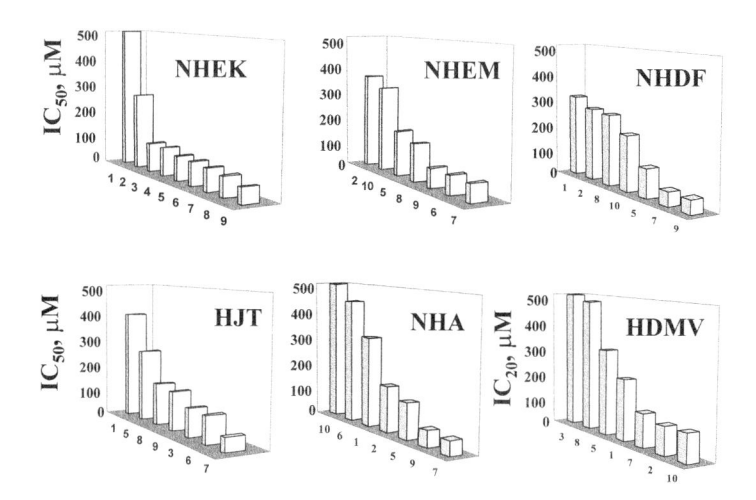

FIGURE 6. Cytotoxicity of phenolic compounds to different human cell lines. Human cells (normal human keratinocytes, NHEK; normal human melanocytes, NHEM; normal human fibroblasts, NHDF; normal human astrocytes, NHA; normal human dermal microvascular cells, NHMV; and human Jurkat cells, HJT) were incubated in phenol-free KGM-2 basal medium in the presence of phenolic compounds for 18 h at 37°C in 96-well plates. After incubation, cells were washed twice with Na-phosphate buffer, pH 7.4. Cell viability was determined using 10% Alamar Blue as described by Keane et al.[14] *Columns:* (1) 2-methoxy-4-propenylphenol; (2) 2-phenylphenol; (3) bis(4-hydroxyphenyl)dimethylmethane; (4) hydroxyphenol; (5) 1,4-benzenediol; (6) 4-*tert*-butylhydroxyphenol; (7) bis(4-glycidyloxyphenyl)methane; (8) 4-*tert*-butylphenol; (9) phenol; (10) 4-allyl-2-methoxyphenol.

stress rather than protective effects of phenolic compounds if their redox characteristics are compatible with direct oxidation of essential intracellular constituents.

Requirements Related to Essential Signaling Pathways

When cellular production of reactive radical intermediates overwhelms the capacity of its antioxidant network, damage to cellular macromolecules such as lipids, protein, and DNA may ensue. As a result "oxidative stress" may contribute to the pathogenesis of a number of human diseases. Recent studies, however, have also implicated alterations in cellular redox state, production of reactive oxygen species as well as organic radical intermediates, and resulting oxidative modifications of proteins in normal physiological signaling (e.g., by growth factors, cytokines) (for a review, see paper of Thannickal and Fanburg[11]). Moreover, phospholipid oxidation products can also serve as signaling molecules with potent physiologic effects.[12] It seems that blockade of these fundamental signaling pathways by antioxidants may interfere with the fulfillment of their physiologic functions. Therefore, design of new potent antioxidants should take into consideration these important consequences that potent antioxidants may exert via their interference into signaling pathways.

Production and accumulation of apoptotic cells is one of characteristic features of tissue damage by oxidative stress that in the absence of effective scavenging by macrophages dramatically enhances oxidative damage and inflammatory response.

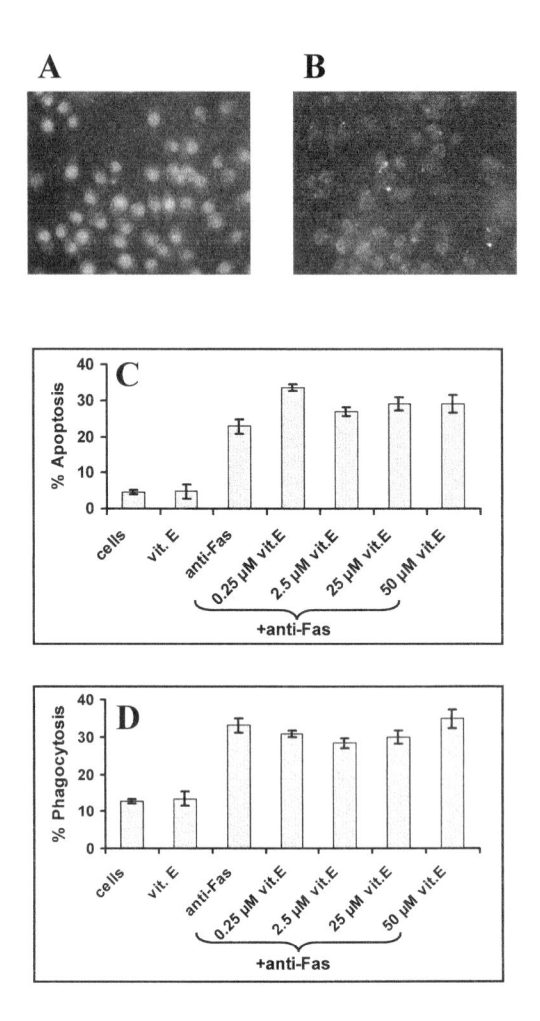

FIGURE 7. Vitamin E does not affect phagocytosis of apoptotic Jurkat cells. Typical fluorescence microphotographs showing phagocytosis of control Jurkat cells by J774A.1 macrophages (**A**) and Fas-triggered apoptotic Jurkat cells (**B**). Quantitative results on Fas-triggered apoptosis and phagocytosis of apoptotic cells are shown in panels **C** and **D**, respectively. Exposure to anti-Fas agonistic antibody induced apoptosis in 33 ± 2% of Jurkat cells in the absence of vitamin E. Pretreatment with vitamin E did not affect the yield of Fas-induced apoptosis (**C**). Phagocytosis of apoptotic Jurkat cells by J774A.1 macrophages (25 ± 3%) was not significantly affected by vitamin E in the concentration range 0.25–50 μM (**D**). Apoptosis was induced in Jurkat cells by anti-Fas agonistic antibody (250 ng/10^6 cells) after preincubation of the cells with different concentrations of vitamin E (0.25–50μM) for 48 h. J774A.1 macrophage cell line was used for phagocytosis assay. Target Jurkat cells (typically 30 × 10^6) were labeled with 0.5 mM Cell Tracker Green^{TM} (Molecular Probes, Eugene OR) in serum-free medium for 15 min at 37°C and cultured at 10^6 cells/mL in the presence of anti-Fas agonistic antibody. After labeling, cells were washed and resuspended in serum-containing RPMI medium. Fluorescently labeled cells were added to macrophages

While oxidative stress has been implicated as an initiator of apoptosis in at least some of these conditions, generation of reactive oxygen species and subsequent oxidative stress has also been demonstrated to be a component of a final common pathway of apoptotic execution via mitochondrial dysfunction. It is well established that mitochondrial permeability transition and departure of cytochrome c, the hallmarks of apoptosis, are associated with excessive generation of radical intermediates and oxidative stress. What is not known is whether there is any specialized mechanistic role(s) for ROS and oxidative stress in guiding or directing apoptotic pathways and outcomes.

Importantly, apoptotic cell death is not accompanied by inflammatory response due to safe engulfment and digestion of damaged cells by macrophages. This critical function of macrophages is mediated by the specific interactions of their cognate receptor(s) with an anionic phospholipid, phosphatidylserine (PS), appearing on the surface of cells undergoing apoptosis. Normally, most cells maintain asymmetric distribution of phospholipids across plasma membrane such that aminophospholipids—PS and phosphatidylethanolamine (PE)—are mainly confined to the inner leaflet of plasma membrane. This is accomplished by a specialized enzymatic system, aminophospholipid translocase (APT). Apoptotic cells lose the ability to sustain this vital asymmetry and allow for externalization of PS (and PE) from the inner leaflet of plasma membrane to its outer surface, due to inhibition of APT and activation of "scramblase," an enzymatic activity responsible for bidirectional nonspecific translocation of phospholipids.

We have recently established that apoptosis induced by various stimuli in a number of different cells is accompanied by selective oxidation of PS that was significantly more pronounced than oxidation of other more abundant phospholipids (PE, phosphatidylcholine). We further demonstrated that PS oxidation is involved in the mechanisms responsible for PS externalization in apoptotic cells and its subsequent recognition by macrophage receptors. Therefore, antioxidants may possess dramatic effects on PS externalization and hence macrophage recognition/phagocytosis of apoptotic cells. This is because inhibition of PS oxidation may result in failure of its externalization and interaction with macrophages, hence producing an exuberant inflammatory response. Therefore, it is critical to determine whether various antioxidants are capable of inhibiting PS oxidation during execution of apoptotic program in cells.

In a series of preliminary experiments, we studied the ability of vitamin E to affect phagocytosis of apoptotic Jurkat cells (in which apoptosis was induced by anti-Fas agonistic antibody) by a macrophage cell line, J.774A.1. We found that in the concentration range from 5 to 50 µM, vitamin E did not cause any changes in the effectiveness of phagocytosis (FIG. 7). This suggests that vitamin E is not likely to in-

---

pretreated with 1 mg/mL Hoechst 33342 fluorescent dye at a ratio of 10:1, and the mixture was incubated for 1 h at 37°C. Phagocytosis was evaluated by two-color fluorescence analysis (Hoechst 33342 and Cell Tracker Green™) using a Nikon ECLIPSE TE 200 fluorescence microscope (Tokyo, Japan) equipped with a digital Hamamatsu CCD camera (C4742-95-12NRB) and analyzed using MetaImaging Series™ software version 4.6 (Universal Imaging Corp., Downingtown, PA). At least 300 macrophages/experimental condition were counted. Phagocytosis data are reported as percent phagocytes positive for uptake.

terfere with the apoptotic signaling pathway dependent on PS externalization. In separate experiments with Jurkat cells, however, we established that a combination of catalase/SOD was able to inhibit both oxidation of PS and phagocytosis of Fas-triggered Jurkat cells. Therefore, it is imperative that antioxidants are tested as potential inhibitors of oxidation reactions of specific molecules that may be important for vital signaling pathways.

ACKNOWLEDGMENT

This work was supported by NIH 1RO1HL64145-01A1.

REFERENCES

1. HARMAN, D. 1998. Aging: phenomena and theories. Ann. N. Y. Acad. Sci. **854:** 1–7.
2. ASHOK, B. T. & R. ALI. 1999. The aging paradox: free radical theory of aging. Exp. Gerontol. **34:** 293–303
3. HARMAN, D. 1998. Extending functional life span. Exp. Gerontol. **33:** 95–112.
4. THIELE, J.J. et al. 2001. The antioxidant network of the stratum corneum. Curr. Probl. Dermatol. **29:** 26–42.
5. STOYANOVSKY, D.A. et al. 1995. Ubiquinone-dependent recycling of vitamin E radicals by superoxide. Arch. Biochem. Biophys. **323:** 343–351.
6. KAGAN, V.E. et al. 1992. Dihydrolipoic acid—a universal antioxidant both in the membrane and in the aqueous phase. reduction of peroxyl, ascorbyl and chromanoxyl radicals. Biochem. Pharmacol. **44:** 1637–1649.
7. PACKER, L. et al. 1989. Mitochondria and microsomal membranes have a free radical reductase activity that prevents chromanoxyl radical accumulation. Biochem. Biophys. Res. Commun. **159:** 229–235.
8. STOCKER, R. 1994. Lipoprotein oxidation: mechanistic aspects, methodological approaches and clinical relevance. Curr. Opin. Lipidol. **5:** 422–433.
9. GORBUNOV, N.V. et al. 1996. NO-redox paradox: direct oxidation of alpha-tocopherol and alpha-tocopherol-mediated oxidation of ascorbate. Biochem. Biophys. Res. Commun. **219:** 835–841.
10. HELBOCK, H.J., K.B. BECKMAN & B.N. AMES. 1999. 8-Hydroxydeoxyguanosine and 8-hydroxyguanine as biomarkers of oxidative DNA damage. Methods Enzymol. **300:** 156–166.
11. THANNICKAL, V.J. & B.L. FANBURG. 2000. Reactive oxygen species in cell signaling. Am. J. Physiol. Lung Cell. Mol. Physiol. **279:** L1005–L1028.
12. REDDY, S. et al. 2001. Mitogen-activated protein kinase phosphatase 1 activity is necessary for oxidized phospholipids to induce monocyte chemotactic activity in human aortic endothelial cells. J. Biol. Chem. **276:** 17030–17035.
13. KAGAN, V.E. et al. 1999. Mechanism-based chemopreventive strategies against etoposide-induced acute myeloid leukemia: free radical/antioxidant approach. Mol. Pharmacol. **56:** 494–506.
14. KEANE, R.W. et al. 1997. Activation of CPP32 during apoptosis of neurons and astrocytes. J. Neurosci. Res. **48:** 168–180.

Role of Mitochondria in Oxidative Stress and Aging

GIORGIO LENAZ, CARLA BOVINA, MARILENA D'AURELIO, ROMANA FATO, GABRIELLA FORMIGGINI, MARIA LUISA GENOVA, GIOVANNI GIULIANO, MILENA MERLO PICH, UGO PAOLUCCI, GIOVANNA PARENTI CASTELLI, AND BARBARA VENTURA

Dipartimento di Biochimica "G. Moruzzi," Università di Bologna, Via Irnerio 48, 40126 Bologna, Italy

ABSTRACT: The mitochondrial respiratory chain is a powerful source of reactive oxygen species (ROS), considered as the pathogenic agent of many diseases and of aging. We have investigated the role of Complex I in superoxide radical production and found by combined use of specific inhibitors of Complex I that the one-electron donor in the Complex to oxygen is a redox center located prior to the sites where three different types of coenzyme Q (CoQ) competitors bind, to be identified with an Fe-S cluster, most probably N2, or possibly an ubisemiquinone intermediate insensitive to all the above inhibitors. Short-chain coenzyme Q analogues enhance superoxide formation, presumably by mediating electron transfer from N2 to oxygen. The clinically used CoQ analogue idebenone is particularly effective, raising doubts about its safety as a drug. The mitochondrial theory of aging considers somatic mutations of mitochondrial DNA induced by ROS as the primary cause of energy decline; in rat liver mitochondria, Complex I appears to be most affected by aging and to become strongly rate limiting for electron transfer. Mitochondrial energetics is also deranged in human platelets upon aging, as demonstrated by the decreased Pasteur effect (enhancement of lactate production by respiratory inhibitors). Cells counteract oxidative stress by antioxidants: CoQ is the only lipophilic antioxidant to be biosynthesized. Exogenous CoQ, however, protects cells from oxidative stress by conversion into its reduced antioxidant form by cellular reductases. The plasma membrane oxidoreductase and DT-diaphorase are two such systems: likewise, they are overexpressed under oxidative stress conditions.

KEYWORDS: oxidative stress; bioenergetic defects; coenzyme Q; rotenone

INTRODUCTION

The occurrence of oxidative stress, caused by reactive oxygen species, is considered as a major etiological and/or pathogenic agent of most diseases;[1] moreover, it is believed that ROS are involved in the progressive deterioration of cell structures accompanying aging.[2–4] The free radical theory of aging[5,6] was based on the idea

---

Address for correspondence: Professor Giorgio Lenaz, Dipartimento di Biochimica "G. Moruzzi," Via Irnerio 48, 40126 Bologna, Italy. Voice: +39 051 2091229; fax: +39 051 2091217.
lenaz@biocfarm.unibo.it

that cells, continuously exposed to ROS, are progressively damaged in their most vital macromolecules. The implication of mitochondria both as producers and as targets of ROS[4,7,8] has been the basis for the mitochondrial theory of aging;[9,10] the theory postulates that random alterations of mitochondrial DNA (mtDNA) in somatic cells are responsible for the energetic decline accompanying senescence. It was proposed that accumulation of somatic mutations of mtDNA, induced by exposure to ROS, leads to errors in the mtDNA-encoded polypeptides; these errors are stochastic and randomly transmitted during mitochondrial division and cell division. The consequence of these alterations, which affect exclusively the four mitochondrial complexes involved in energy conservation, would be defective electron transfer and oxidative phosphorylation. Respiratory chain defects may become associated with increased ROS production, thus establishing a vicious circle.[11]

The primary role of ROS in the stochastic theories of aging elicits, on one hand, a better understanding of the cellular sources of these damaging species and of the factors modulating their production, and, on the other, a search for agents capable of controlling excessive ROS production and propagation of ROS-induced damages.

MITOCHONDRIAL COMPLEX I AS A SOURCE OF THE SUPEROXIDE RADICAL

The mitochondrial respiratory chain is a powerful source of ROS, primarily the superoxide radical and consequently hydrogen peroxide, either as a product of mitochondrial superoxide dismutase (SOD)[12] or by spontaneous disproportionation. It was calculated that 1–4% of oxygen reacting with the respiratory chain is incompletely reduced to ROS.[13] Their production may increase in state 4 with respect to state 3[14] because oxygen concentration increases and the level of reduced one-electron donors in the respiratory chain is concomitantly increased.[15]

There are two major respiratory chain regions where ROS are recognized to be produced, one being Complex I (NADH coenzyme Q reductase)[17–19] and the other Complex III (ubiquinol cytochrome c reductase) (cf. Ref. 4).

In Complex III, antimycin is known not to completely inhibit electron flow from ubiquinol to cytochrome c: the antimycin-insensitive reduction of cytochrome c is mediated by superoxide radicals; the source of superoxide in the enzyme may be either cytochrome b_{566},[16] or ubisemiquinone,[17] or Rieske's iron-sulfur center.[18] Ubisemiquinone is relatively stable only when protein-bound[19] and therefore the CoQ pool in the lipid bilayer is no source of ROS. The role of ubiquinone within ROS production deserves some comment, since it has been described both as a prooxidant[14,17,20] and as a powerful antioxidant[21,22] (cf. below).

Early experiments proved the involvement of Complex I in ROS production;[23] addition of either NADH at low concentration or of NADPH, which feeds the electrons at decreased rate into the Complex, led to copious ROS production detected by lipid peroxidation; on the other hand, addition of NADH at high concentration, but in presence of rotenone, also induced peroxidation. In another study,[24] water-soluble CoQ homologues used as electron acceptors from isolated Complex I stimulated H_2O_2 production in the order $CoQ_1 > CoQ_0 > CoQ_2$, whereas CoQ_6 and CoQ_{10} were inactive; the rate of H_2O_2 production was partly inhibited by rotenone, indicating that water-soluble quinones may react with oxygen when reduced at sites both prior and subsequent to the rotenone block. There is evidence that the one-electron donor to oxygen in Complex I is a nonphysiological quinone reduction site different from the physiological site(s);[25,26] the former, hydrophilic, site reduces several quinones to the corresponding semiquinone forms, which are unstable and can reduce oxygen to superoxide. This mechanism is shared by several quinones, including such drugs as anthracyclines[27] and the clinically employed CoQ analogue, idebenone.[28] However, auto-oxidation of fully reduced quinones,[29] such as those formed by NADH CoQ reductase past the rotenone inhibition site, is also a source of ROS, but this effect exclusively pertains to hydrophilic quinones, and not to the physiological hydrophobic ubiquinol. Finally, in view of the experiments of Takeshige et al.,[23] the hydrophilic, rotenone-insensitive site can apparently reduce oxygen to superoxide in the absence of intermediate acceptors. More recent studies confirmed that Complex I is a major source of superoxide production in several types of mitochondria[30] and localized the oxygen- reducing site between the ferricyanide and the quinone reduction sites.[31]

Structural changes in Complex I may also enhance ROS production. This has been ascertained in some Complex I defects induced by nuclear DNA mutations,[32,33] but there are reasons to believe that also mitochondrial DNA defects affecting Complex I, such as three mutations causing Leber's hereditary optic neuropathy (LHON),[34] are accompanied by increased ROS production. Recently, Barrientos and Moraes[35] developed a cellular model of partial Complex I defect that closely resembles LHON. In this model, besides the respiratory defect, they described increased ROS production and induction of apoptotic cell death. Moreover, a single study showed that viability of LHON cybrids, carrying the common 11778 mutation, had an increased sensitivity to oxidative stress compared to the wild-type parental cell line.[36]

We have investigated the role of Complex I in superoxide radical production in bovine heart submitochondrial particles (SMP). Complex I of the mitochondrial respiratory chain represents the first site of oxidative phosphorylation. The enzyme is still scarcely understood due to its utter complexity[37] (43 subunits in mammals, 7 of which are encoded by mitochondrial DNA, and several prosthetic groups including FMN, at least 7 iron-sulfur clusters, and a few molecules of protein-bound coenzyme Q). The natural acceptor is CoQ dissolved in the lipid bilayer (2,3-dimethoxy-5-methyl-6-polyprenyl-1,4-benzoquinone); however, the enzyme assay requires using artificial acceptors, including homologues and analogues of the natural CoQ (mostly CoQ_{10}), binding both the physiological site and additional nonphysiological site(s) upstream.[38]

Complex I is inhibited by several compounds, almost all binding the hydrophobic subunits, three classes of which have been distinguished on the basis of the interaction sites;[39] their use allows the enzyme to be functionally dissected in relation to its multiple sites of interaction. Among the inhibitors, there are some short-chain homologues of the natural CoQ, such as CoQ_2 and CoQ_3 (but not CoQ_1) acting both as (poor) acceptors and as inhibitors.[38] Present knowledge in fact indicates that the features of the side chain in position 6 are critical for CoQ function as electron acceptor.[40] The mechanism by which these homologues inhibit is not understood, although the active form appears to be the reduced one: it is puzzling that analogues having a side chain of the same length but saturated and linear, such as decylubiquinone (DB), are inactive as inhibitors but very active as acceptors.

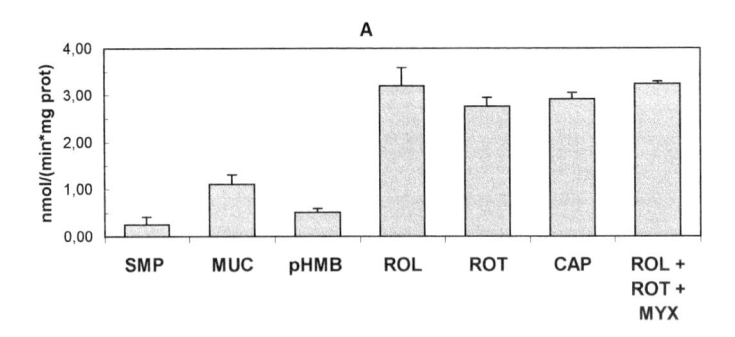

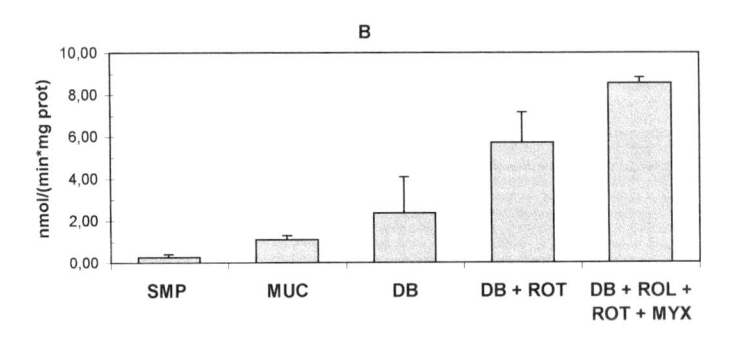

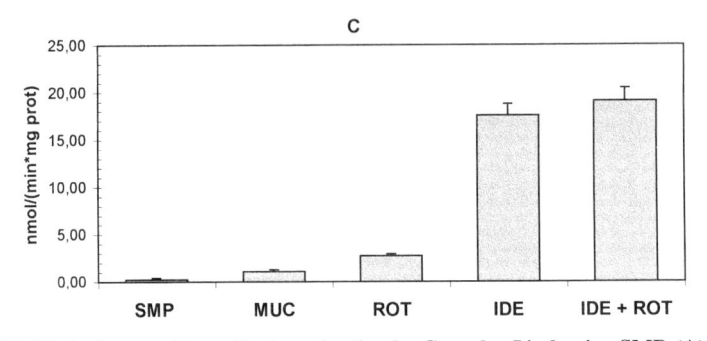

FIGURE 1. Superoxide radical production by Complex I in bovine SMP. (**A**) In presence of 125 μM NADH and no Complex I acceptor; mucidin (1.8 μM) was added to inhibit Complex III in all samples except where indicated (SMP). Inhibitor concentrations: *p*-hydroxymercuribenzoate (FeS-cluster inhibitor), 59 μM; rolliniastatin-2 (Center A inhibitor), 0.2 nmol/mg protein; rotenone (Center B inhibitor), 0.2 nmol/mg protein; capsaicin (Center C inhibitor), 4 μmol/mg protein. (**B**) In presence of 125 μM NADH, 1.8 μM mucidin and (when indicated) 60 μM decyl-ubiquinone (DB) as acceptor. Inhibitor concentrations: rotenone, 0.2 nmol/mg protein; rolliniastatin-2, 0.2 nmol/mg protein; myxothiazol (Center C inhibitor), 230 nmol/mg protein. Inhibitor classes are according to the nomenclature of Degli Esposti.[39] (**C**) In presence of 1.8 μM mucidin and idebenone, 2 μmol/mg protein. Abbreviations: MUC, mucidin; pHMB, *p*-hydroxymercuribenzoate; ROL, rolliniastatin-2; ROT, rotenone; CAP, capsaicin; MYX, myxothiazol; DB, decyl-ubiquinone; IDE, idebenone.

We have exploited the effects of different Complex I inhibitors and quinone acceptors to dissect the sites and mechanism of one-electron transfer to oxygen with superoxide formation, investigated by the method of SOD-sensitive epinephrine oxidation to adrenochrome.[41] In order to functionally isolate superoxide production by Complex I only, its formation by Complex III was prevented using mucidin, an inhibitor of center o (out). We avoided using antimycin A, since this center i (in) inhibitor is known to enhance superoxide formation,[4] and myxothiazol, another center o inhibitor that however also inhibits Complex I.[42]

Addition of NADH to mucidin-inhibited SMP promotes superoxide formation that is enhanced to similar extents by Complex I inhibitors belonging to all three classes and by combinations thereof (FIG. 1A). Contrary to the findings of Barja,[31] we observed very low superoxide production in noninhibited SMP. Addition of short-chain analogues and homologues of CoQ enhances superoxide formation of noninhibited Complex I, and this enhancement is further stimulated by Complex I inhibitors (FIG. 1B). Among the quinones tested, idebenone is particularly effective in inducing a dramatic increase of superoxide production (FIG. 1C). Since idebenone is clinically used in mitochondrial cytopathies and neurodegenerative diseases,[43] its strong prooxidant effect raises doubts on its safety as a drug. On the other hand, Complex I inhibitors acting at the level of iron-sulfur clusters, such as *p*-hydroxymercuribenzoate,[31] inhibited superoxide production. Similar results were ob-

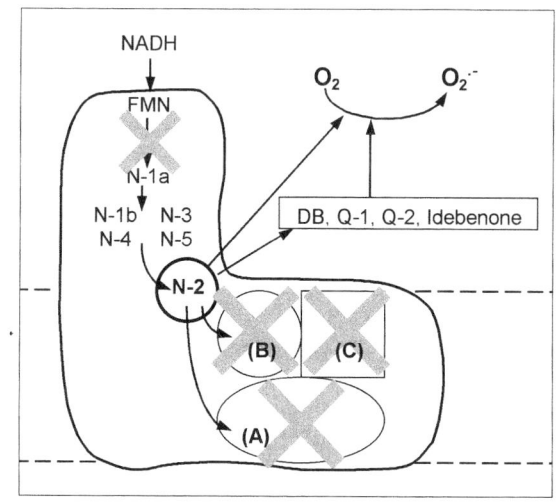

FIGURE 2. A model of electron transfer and the site of superoxide production by Complex I. The scheme follows the model of Degli Esposti[39] and depicts FeS-cluster N2 as the source of electrons to bound ubiquinone (Center B) and to the ubiquinone molecule deriving from the pool (Center A). The two deriving semiquinones dismutate so that Center B contains oxidized ubiquinone, while the reduced ubiquinone (ubiquinol) moves to Center C, from where it is released to the pool. The effect of different inhibitors and acceptors (see text) is compatible with FeS-cluster N2 as the source of one electron to oxygen or to exogenous quinones (in place of the endogenous bound CoQ), which, in turn, reduce oxygen monoelectronically. Idebenone behaves both as an acceptor and as a type A inhibitor.

tained with SMP obtained from rat heart and rat liver, although the latter were significantly less active in superoxide formation (not shown).

The fact that a combination of inhibitors acting on three quinone-binding sites of the Complex enhances superoxide formation suggests that the site of oxygen reduction lies upstream of the quinone-binding sites of the Complex. It is also known that the ubisemiquinone EPR signal in Complex I is rotenone sensitive.[44] The electron donor to the first molecule of bound ubiquinone in the Complex is most probably the FeS cluster N2.[44,45] It is likely that this center is also the electron donor to oxygen either directly or via one-electron reduction of several exogenous quinones (FIG. 2). In agreement with this interpretation, preliminary studies in CoQ-depleted and reconstituted mitochondria indicated that endogenous CoQ is not required for superoxide generation. Thus, exogenous quinones are preferentially reduced at the physiological site in place of the ubiquinone pool, but a low though significant percentage of the quinone molecules can directly react, in place of endogenous bound quinones, with N2 (or, anyway, a rotenone-insensitive species upstream of the block of all three classes inhibitors).

MITOCHONDRIAL BIOENERGETIC DEFECTS IN AGING

The subject of age-dependent changes in mitochondrial bioenergetics abounds in conflicting data, for example, reporting declines of respiratory enzymes or ATPase activity or being unable to find significant differences (cf. Ref. 4). However, energy-defective cells may undergo elimination by apoptosis;[46] the continuous cell elimination when mitochondria become deficient would prevent observing important energetic changes in the remaining population.

If the energetic impairment derives from a stochastic damage to the mitochondrial genes, then it is important to select the mitochondrial activity that is most likely to be affected. Since 7 of the 13 structural genes in mtDNA encode for polypeptides in Complex I, then it is Complex I that is most likely to undergo functional alterations.[47] Unfortunately the assay of Complex I activity suffers from serious problems due to the choice of the best quinone to be used as electron acceptor;[40] in our laboratory it was found useful, when possible, to assay this activity indirectly[48] by exploiting the *pool equation:*[49]

$$V_{obs} = (V_o \cdot V_r)/(V_o + V_r)$$

whereby the rate of CoQ reduction (V_r) is related to total rate of NADH oxidation by oxygen (V_{obs}) and to rate of ubiquinol oxidation (V_o). Using this method, significant decreases of NADH CoQ reductase activity, undetected by the direct assay, were revealed in liver and heart mitochondria from 24-month old rats,[48] presumably by providing more accurate values of NADH CoQ reductase activity.

A decrease of an individual enzyme activity in a metabolic pathway is meaningful only if it is able to affect the rate of the whole pathway, and this will depend on the degree of *flux control* exerted by the individual step:[50] in the respiratory chain, Complex I is present in lowest amounts,[51] and then it is presumably the rate-limiting step of aerobic NADH oxidation; however, this is not true for the oxidation of NAD-linked substrates in phosphorylating mitochondria.[52,53] In mitochondrial diseases,

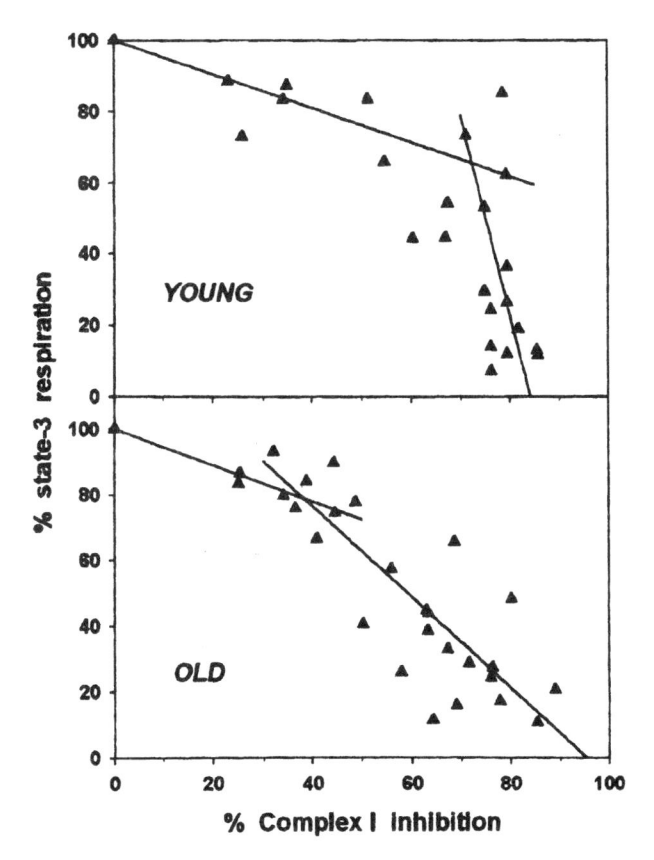

FIGURE 3. Threshold curves of glutamate-malate supported State 3 respiration in liver mitochondria from young (*upper plot*) and old rats (*lower plot*). Each point comes from the experimental titration curves with rotenone of State 3 respiration in intact coupled mitochondria and of NADH CoQ reductase activity studied using DB as acceptor in sonicated mitochondria, and represents the percent rate of State 3 respiration as a function of the percentage of Complex I inhibition for the same rotenone concentration.

the flux control coefficient at Site I in permeabilized cells was found to dramatically increase.[54] We have addressed this point in respiration of liver mitochondria from young and old rats, and found that the threshold for decrease of NAD-linked State 3 respiration by Complex I inhibition by rotenone was dramatically increased in the old animals (FIG. 3) (cf. Ref. 55), indicating that Complex I becomes strongly rate-limiting in the old.

Another approach employed in our laboratory for recognition of possible early changes not only in postmitotic cells, but also in short-living cells, such as blood platelets, has been looking for specific changes linked to subunits encoded for by mtDNA; by analogy with previous findings in LHON,[56] it was found that rotenone sensitivity of NADH CoQ reductase was significantly decreased in platelets from old individuals.[57] The same change was exhibited by nonsynaptic mitochondria from rat brain cortex[58] and in rat liver mitochondria.[55]

The search for a sensitive marker of aging in man, representing an individual index of biological age and predisposition to age-related diseases, must take into consideration mitochondrial function; since such a function may only be investigated in cells containing mitochondria, blood platelets may represent a unique system[59] in that they possess mitochondria and afford easy sampling without invasive procedures. Moreover, platelets were proposed as a possible marker of acquired neurological diseases, bearing some biological similarities with neurons.[60] The rational use of platelets as a biomarker of mitochondrial lesions rests on the assumption that alterations occurring in senescence and in age-related diseases are present in all cells, and that platelets may signal generalized bioenergetic deficiencies.[4,61]

It is known that platelets rely on glycolysis as well as mitochondrial oxidative phosphorylation for their energy supply:[59] the main function of platelets is their energy-dependent aggregation process,[62] a part of the mechanism of blood clotting, physiologically elicited via exocytosis of their secretory granules.

An alteration of Complex I activity in platelet mitochondria in aged individuals is indicated by the increase of I_{50} of rotenone inhibition,[57] similar to that detected in rat brain cortex mitochondria.[58] Since, as already mentioned, rotenone binds the hydrophobic sector of the enzyme that is involved in proton translocation, the altered inhibitor sensitivity may represent an indication of altered energy conservation. A quantitative determination of glycolytic and mitochondrial ATP can be provided by the Pasteur effect:[63] a decreased mitochondrial function stimulates glycolysis in order to maintain a constant ATP synthesis, and meanwhile pyruvate is reduced to lactate to regenerate oxidized pyridine nucleotides. Since, in the absence of mitochondrial function, the stoichiometric ratio for glucose breakdown in the glyc-

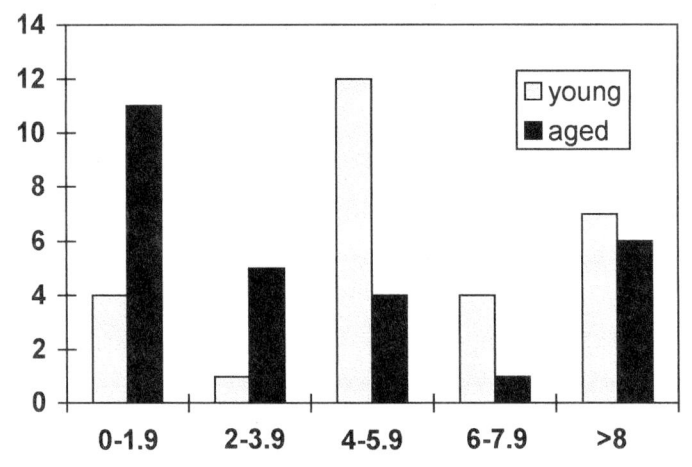

FIGURE 4. Class distribution of the ratio of mitochondrial ATP over glycolytic ATP in platelets from young (19–30 years) and old (65–87 years) individuals. The ratio corresponds to the ratio of Δ-lactate (lactate produced in presence of antimycin A minus basal lactate produced in absence of inhibitor) over basal lactate.[64] (Modified from FIG. 3 in D'Aurelio et al.[64])

olytic pathway is two ATP and two lactate molecules per glucose, it follows that the lactate production stimulated by inhibition of respiration is equivalent to the correspondingly inhibited production of ATP by mitochondria.

Lactate production by washed platelets is strongly enhanced by antimycin A inhibition of mitochondrial respiration; the Δ-lactate production in presence and absence of antimycin A represents the amount of ATP produced *via* oxidative phosphorylation in physiological conditions, whereas the basal lactate production represents glycolytic ATP.[59] Both the Δ-lactate and the ratio of oxidative ATP over glycolytic ATP are significantly decreased in aged individuals[55,64] (FIG. 4).

COENZYME Q AS AN ANTIOXIDANT

Cells contain enzymatic systems capable of converting ROS into less toxic or nontoxic species;[1] the coordinate action of superoxide dismutase and peroxidases (glutathione peroxidase being of particular importance) detoxifies superoxide to water; if the action of superoxide dismutase is, however, not accompanied by that of peroxidases, the accumulation of hydrogen peroxide would instead induce production of the damaging hydroxyl radical by means of the Fenton reaction.[65]

Other defense systems include metal-binding proteins, preventing the prooxidant action of heavy metals, metabolic intermediates acting as free radical scavengers, and *antioxidants* largely taken in the organism by nutrition, such as ascorbic acid, vitamin E, carotenes, polyphenols, and flavonoids.[1]

Among antioxidants a special position is held by coenzyme Q (CoQ_{10} in humans), the only lipid-soluble antioxidant that is normally synthesized by the organism.[66] Its strong hydrophobicity, due to the long isoprenoid chain at the 6-position, causes it to be inserted in the membrane phospholipid bilayer.

The biosynthesis of CoQ is particularly complex;[67] the benzoquinone ring is synthesized from the essential amino acid phenylalanine up to 4-hydroxy-benzoate, whereas the isoprenoid chain is formed by a pathway common to that of cholesterol and dolichol biosynthesis. CoQ biosynthesis requires the dietary intake of several vitamin cofactors: it is therefore conceivable that one or more such factors may become limiting under physiological or pathological conditions,[66] thus slowing down ubiquinone biosynthesis and inducing a ubiquinone deficiency state.

Besides its bioenergetic role, as a component of the mitochondrial respiratory chain, CoQ is also a component of extramitochondrial redox chains,[68] whose function, among others, would be to remove excess reducing power formed by glycolysis when mitochondrial respiration is decreased.[46,69,70]

As an antioxidant, the reduced form of CoQ is exploited either directly upon superoxide or indirectly on lipid radicals;[21,22] ubiquinol can also act together with vitamin E (α-tocopherol) by regenerating the active form from the tocopheroxyl radical.[71,72]

The antioxidant action of ubiquinol yields the ubisemiquinone radical; this species is converted back to its antioxidant form by re-reduction, which occurs through the electron transfer chain in mitochondria, and is operated by various quinone reductases present in different cell fractions.[73–75]

Studies in perfused rat liver[76] and in isolated rat hepatocytes[74] clearly showed the antioxidant effect of exogenous added CoQ_{10}. The anticancer quinone glycoside,

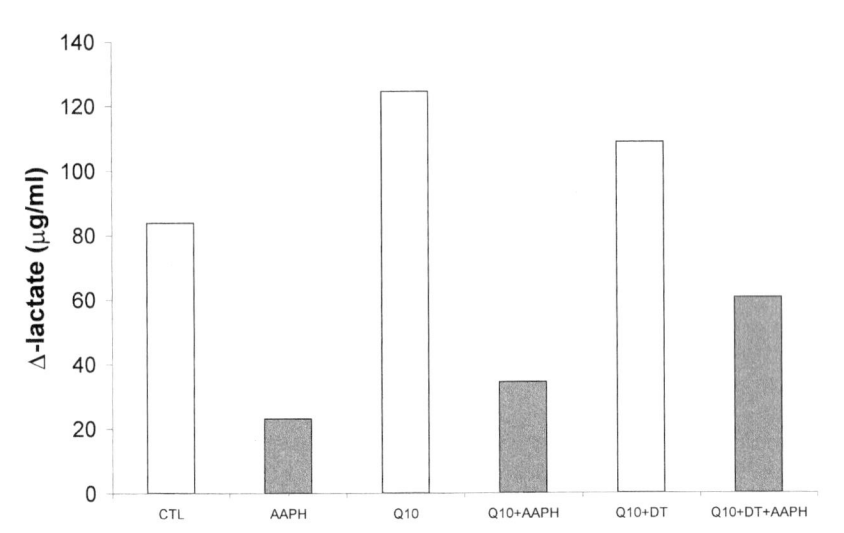

FIGURE 5. Δ-lactate values in platelets subjected to an oxidative stress and effect of oxidized CoQ in presence and absence of a reducing system. Oxidative stress was accomplished in washed platelets by incubation with 50 mM 2,2'-azobis-2-amidinopropane (AAPH) for 3 hours at 37°C during the incubation for Δ-lactate determination (cf. legend of FIG. 4 and Ref. 64). The samples had been preincubated for 1 hour with or without addition of different CoQ suspensions at room temperature with stirring. The CoQ sample (20 μM) was a soluble formulation, guttaQuinon™, kindly donated by Dr. F. Enzmann of MSE Pharmazeutika GmbH, Bad Homburg, Germany. The reducing system consisted of 150 μM β-NADPH and 1000 units of DT-diaphorase (a kind gift from Dr. J. Segura-Aguilar).

adriamycin, induces an oxidative stress by enhancing ROS production in mitochondria and endoplasmic reticulum. In hepatocytes, adriamycin enhances ROS production: concomitantly, endogenous CoQ is reoxidized and the mitochondrial membrane potential falls. Incubation of the cells with exogenous CoQ_{10} prevents ROS formation and protects both reduced CoQ and the $\Delta\Psi_{mit}$. The cytosolic enzyme DT-diaphorase seems to be responsible for reduction of both endogenous and exogenous CoQ, as shown by the effect of dicoumarol, an inhibitor of DT-diaphorase, preventing the protective action of exogenous CoQ addition.[74] Studies in platelets from transfusional buffy coats also showed protection by added CoQ of the mitochondrial function, investigated by way of the Pasteur effect (see above); the protection was enhanced by addition of an exogenous source of CoQ reduction, such as purified DT-diaphorase in presence of NADPH (unpublished results) (FIG. 5).

We have found an increase of plasma membrane oxidoreductase, including an increase of DT-diaphorase (its dicoumarol-sensitive portion) in insulin-dependent diabetic patients (TABLE 1), whose mitochondrial function was also found to be affected (unpublished data); such an increase may be related (in addition to the necessity of releasing the excess of cytosolic reducing power[69]) to a higher requirement for the reduced antioxidant form of CoQ, due to the oxidative stress occurring in diabetes.[77]

TABLE 1. Plasma membrane oxidoreductase (PMOR) activity of lymphocytes from 32 controls and 33 insulin-dependent diabetic patients

	No dicoumarol	10 µM dicoumarol
Controls	0.93 ± 0.21	0.91 ± 0.1
Patients	1.72 ± 0.53^a	1.25 ± 0.3^a

NOTE: Activity was expressed in nmol dichlorophenol indophenol (DCIP) reduced by intracellular NADH per minute per 10^7 cells. The dicoumarol-sensitive activity is equated to DT-diaphorase.
[a]Significantly different from controls, $P < 0.001$

If aging is the result of prolonged oxidative stress, an adequate antioxidant supply might counter the process. The content of vitamin antioxidants depends on dietary intake, and it may be subjected to decreases due to deficient intestinal absorption and bad dietary habits of the aged. CoQ, being synthesized, is a special case. Some studies have shown a decrease in CoQ with age;[48,78,79] however, this is not true for brain, where high levels are maintained throughout aging,[80,81] in accordance with the steady level of nonaprenyl-4-hydroxybenzoate transferase.[82] Nevertheless, even if the levels of CoQ and other antioxidants do not dramatically fall with aging, we must consider that the antioxidant defenses should actually strongly *increase* to cope with the enhanced oxidative stress.

In some instances of acute or subacute stress this is actually the case: the CoQ plasma level in the rat doubles by simple sham operation,[83] indicating that surgical stress can induce increased ubiquinone release from tissues and/or increased biosynthesis. On the other hand, a stronger metabolic stress, such as liver resection, followed by regeneration,[83] can exhaust the CoQ biosynthesis capability, yielding lowered plasma CoQ levels.

Senescence is associated with increased incidence of degenerative diseases, such as Parkinson's and Alzheimer's diseases, and age-linked macular degeneration; these diseases often have a strong genetic component, which is, however, associated with exogenous factors, among which oxidative stress and mitochondrial involvement may be major triggering factors.[4,61,84–86] A decrease of CoQ_{10} and of antioxidant defenses in plasma was found in our laboratory in patients affected by age-related macular degeneration of the retina.[87]

The proposal of an antioxidant therapy, as an attempt to reduce or retard the damaging effect of ROS in aging and age-related degenerative diseases, is strongly supported by the excellent results obtained in Alzheimer's disease and Huntington's disease.[84,88] The use of CoQ as a dietary supplement requires its distribution to deficient tissues. Dietary CoQ is quickly taken into blood, where it is mainly transported by LDL[89] and rapidly incorporated in liver and reticuloendothelial cells. The uptake of CoQ_{10} by other tissues has not been shown in nutritional experiments in the rat,[90] although there are indirect observations suggesting its incorporation in tissues when the endogenous levels are lowered.[88] In spite of the lack of uptake of dietary CoQ_{10} by rat heart mitochondria, the exogenous quinone was found to strongly protect mitochondria from oxidative changes.[91]

ACKNOWLEDGMENTS

This work was supported in part by PRIN "Longevity Determinants in Humans," MURST, Rome.

REFERENCES

1. DIPLOCK, A.T. 1994. Antioxidants and disease prevention. Molec. Aspects Med. **15**: 293–376.
2. HARMAN, D. 1981. The aging process. Proc. Natl. Acad. Sci. USA **78**: 7124–7128.
3. SHIGENAGA, M.K., T.M. HAGEN & B.N. AMES. 1994. Oxidative damage and mitochondrial decay in aging. Proc. Natl. Acad. Sci. USA **91**: 10771–10778.
4. LENAZ, G. 1998. Role of mitochondria in oxidative stress and aging. Biochim. Biophys. Acta **1366**: 53–67.
5. HARMAN, D. 1956. Aging: a theory based on free radical and radiation chemistry. J. Gerontol. **11**: 298–300.
6. HARMAN, D. 1988. Free radicals in aging. Mol. Cell. Biochem. **84**: 55–61.
7. CHANCE, B., H. SIES & A. BOVERIS. 1979. Hydroperoxide metabolism in mammalian organs. Physiol. Rev. **59**: 527–605.
8. ERNSTER, L. 1993. Lipid peroxidation in biological membranes: mechanisms and implications. *In* Active Oxygen, Lipid Peroxides and Antioxidants. K. Yagi, Ed.: 1–38. CRC Press. Boca Raton, FL.
9. MIQUEL, J. *et al.* 1980. Mitochondrial role in cell aging. Exp. Gerontol. **15**: 575–591.
10. LINNANE, A.W. *et al.* 1989. Mitochondrial DNA mutations as an important contributor to ageing and degenerative diseases. Lancet **i**: 642–645.
11. OZAWA, T. 1997. Genetic and functional changes in mitochondria associated with aging. Physiol. Rev. **77**: 425–464.
12. FRIDOVICH, I. 1986. Superoxide dismutases. Adv. Enzymol. **58**: 61–97.
13. RICHTER, C. 1988. Do mitochondrial DNA fragments promote cancer and aging? FEBS Lett. **241**: 1–5.
14. BOVERIS, A. & B. CHANCE. 1973. The mitochondrial generation of hydrogen peroxide: general properties and effect of hyperbaric oxygen. Biochem. J. **134**: 707–716.
15. SKULACHEV, V.P. 1996. Role of uncoupled and non-coupled oxidations in maintenance of safely low levels of oxygen and its one-electron reductants. Q. Rev. Biophys. **29**: 169–202.
16. NOHL H. & W. JORDAN 1986. The mitochondrial site of superoxide formation. Biochem. Biophys. Res. Commun. **138**: 533–539.
17. TURRENS, J.F., A. ALEXANDRE & A.L. LEHNINGER. 1985. Ubisemiquinone is the electron donor for superoxide formation by complex III of heart mitochondria. Arch. Biochem. Biophys. **237**: 408–414.
18. DEGLI ESPOSTI, M. *et al.* 1990. The oxidation of ubiquinol by the isolated "Rieske" iron–suplhur protein in solution. Arch. Biochem. Biophys. **283**: 258–265.
19. TRUMPOWER, B.L. 1981. New concepts on the role of ubiquinone in the mitochondrial respiratory chain. J. Bioenerg. Biomembr. **13**: 1–24.
20. NOHL, H. *et al.* 1996. Conditions allowing redox-cycling ubisemiquinone in mitochondria to establish a direct redox couple with molecular oxygen. Free Radic. Biol. Med. **20**: 207–213.
21. BEYER, R.E. & L. ERNSTER. 1990. The antioxidant role of Coenzyme Q. *In* Highlights of Ubiquinone Research. G. Lenaz *et al.*, Eds.: 191–213. Taylor & Francis. London.
22. ERNSTER, L. & G. DALLNER. 1995. Biochemical, physiological and medical aspects of ubiquinone function. Biochim. Biophys. Acta **1271**: 195–204.
23. TAKESHIGE, K., K. TAKAYANAGI & S. MINAKAMI. 1980. Biochemical, physiological and medical aspects of ubiquinone function. *In* Biomedical and Clinical Aspects of Coenzyme Q. Vol. 2: 15–26. Y. Yamamura *et al.*, Eds. Elsevier. Amsterdam.
24. CADENAS, E. *et al.* 1977. Production of superoxide radicals and hydrogen peroxide by NADH-ubiquinone reductase and ubiquinol-cytochrome c reductase from beef-heart mitochondria. Arch. Biochem. Biophys. **180**: 248–257.

25. DEGLI ESPOSTI, M. *et al.* 1996. The specificity of mitochondrial complex I for ubiquinones. Biochem. J. **313:** 327–334.
26. GLINN, M.A., C.P. LEE & L. ERNSTER. 1997. Pro- and anti-oxidant activities of the mitochondrial respiratory chain factors influencing NAD(P)H-induced lipid peroxidation. Biochim. Biophys. Acta **1318:** 246–254.
27. DAVIES, K.J.A. & J.H. DOROSHOW. 1986. Redox cycling of anthracyclines by cardiac mitochondria. I. Anthracycline radical formation by NADH dehydrogenase. J. Biol. Chem. **261:** 3060–3067.
28. DEGLI ESPOSTI, M. *et al.* 1996. The interaction of Q analogs, particularly hydroxydecyl benzoquinone (idebenone), with the respiratory complexes of heart mitochondria. Arch. Biochem. Biophys. **330:** 395–400.
29. CADENAS, E., P. HOCHSTEIN & L. ERNSTER. 1992. Pro- and antioxidant functions of quinones and quinone reductases in mammalian cells. Adv. Enzymol. **65:** 97–146.
30. BARJA, G. 1999. Mitochondrial oxygen radical generation and leak: sites of production in states 4 and 3, organ specificity, and relation to aging and longevity. J. Bioenerg. Biomembr. **31:** 347–366.
31. HERRERO, A. & G. BARJA. 2000. Localization of the site of oxygen radical generation inside the complex I of heart and nonsynaptic brain mammalian mitochondria. J. Bioenerg. Biomembr. **32:** 609–616.
32. ROBINSON, B.H. 1998. Human complex I deficiency: clinical spectrum and involvement of oxygen free radicals in the pathogenicity of the defect. Biochim. Biophys. Acta **1364:** 271–286.
33. RAHA, S. & B.H. ROBINSON. 2000. Mitochondria, oxygen free radical, disease and ageing. Trends Biochem. Sci. **25:** 502–508.
34. HOWELL, N. 1997. Leber hereditary optic neuropathy: how do mitochondrial DNA mutations cause degeneration of the optic nerve? J. Bioenerg. Biomembr. **29:** 165–173.
35. BARRIENTOS, A. & C.T. MORAES. 1999. Titrating the effects of mitochondrial complex I impairment in the cell physiology. J. Biol. Chem. **274:** 16188–16197.
36. WONG, A. & G. CORTOPASSI. 1997. MtDNA mutations confer cellular sensitivity to oxidant stress that is partially rescued by calcium depletion and cyclosporin A. Biochem. Biophys. Res. Commun. **239**: 139–145.
37. BRANDT, U. 1997. Proton-translocation by membrane-bound NADH:ubiquinone-oxidoreductase (complex I) through redox-gated ligand conduction. Biochim. Biophys. Acta **1318:** 79–91.
38. LENAZ, G. 1998. Quinone specificity of complex I. Biochim. Biophys. Acta **1364**: 207–221.
39. DEGLI ESPOSTI, M. 1998. Inhibitors of NADH-ubiquinone reductase: an overview. Biochim. Biophys. Acta **1364:** 222–235.
40. FATO, R. *et al.* 1996. Steady-state kinetics of the reduction of Coenzyme Q analogs by Complex I in bovine heart mitochondria and submitochondrial particles. Biochemistry **35:** 2705–2716.
41. BOVERIS, A. 1984. Determination of the production of superoxide radicals and hydrogen peroxide in mitochondria. Methods Enzymol. **105:** 429–435.
42. DEGLI ESPOSTI, M. *et al.* 1993. Complex I and Complex III of mitochondria have common inhibitors acting as ubiquinone antagonists. Biochem. Biophys. Res. Commun. **190:** 1090–1096.
43. GILLIS, J.C., P. BENFIELD & D. MCTAVISH 1994. Idebenone. A review of its pharmacodynamic and pharmacokinetic properties, and therapeutic use in age-related cognitive disorders. Drugs Aging **5:** 133–152.
44. YAGI, T. *et al.* 1998. Procaryotic complex I (NDH-1), an overview. Biochim. Biophys. Acta **1364:** 125–133.
45. OHNISHI, T. 1998. Iron-sulfur clusters/semiquinones in complex I. Biochim. Biophys. Acta **1364:** 186–206.
46. LAWEN, A. *et al.* 1994. The universality of bioenergetic disease: the role of mitochondrial mutation and the putative interrelationship between mitochondria and plasma membrane NADH oxidoreductase. Molec. Aspects Med. **15:** s13–s27.
47. LENAZ, G. *et al.* 1997. Mitochondrial complex I defects in aging. Mol. Cell Biochem. **174:** 329–333.

48. GENOVA, M.L. et al. 1995. Major changes in Complex I activity in mitochondria from aged rats may not be detected by direct assay of NADH-coenzyme Q reductase. Biochem. J. **311:** 105–109.
49. KRÖGER, A. & M. KLINGENBERG. 1973. The kinetics of redox reactions of ubiquinone related to the electron transport activity of the respiratory chain. Eur. J. Biochem. **34:** 358–368.
50. KACSER, A. & J.A. BURNS. 1979. Molecular democracy: who shares the controls? Biochem. Soc. Trans. **7:** 1149–1160.
51. CAPALDI, R.A. 1982. Arrangement of proteins in the mitochondrial inner membrane. Biochim. Biophys. Acta **694:** 291–306.
52. DAVEY, G.P. & J.B. CLARK. 1996. Threshold effects and control of oxidative phosphorylation in nonsynaptic rat brain mitochondria. J. Neurochem. **66:** 1617–1624.
53. MORENO-SANCHEZ, R. et al. 1991. Distribution of control of oxidative phosphorylation in mitochondria oxidizing NAD-linked substrates. Biochim. Biophys. Acta **1060:** 284–292.
54. KUZNETSOV, A.V. et al. 1997. Application of inhibitor titrations for the detection of oxidative phosphorylation defects in saponin-skinned muscle fibers of patients with mitochondrial diseases. Biochim. Biophys. Acta **1360:** 142–150.
55. LENAZ, G. et al. 2000. Mitochondrial bioenergetics in aging. Biochim. Biophys. Acta **1459:** 397–404.
56. DEGLI ESPOSTI, M. et al. 1994. Functional alterations of mitochondrially encoded ND-4 subunit associated with Leber's hereditary optic neuropathy. FEBS Lett. **352:** 375–379.
57. MERLO PICH, M. et al. 1996. Inhibitor sensitivity of respiratory complex I in human platelets: a possible biomarker of ageing. FEBS Lett. **380:** 176–178.
58. GENOVA, M.L. et al. 1997. Decrease of rotenone inhibition as a sensitive parameter of Complex I damage in brain non-synaptic mitochondria of aged rats. FEBS Lett. **410:** 467–469.
59. HOLMSEN, H. 1987. Biochemistry of the platelet: energy metabolism. In Hemostasis and Thrombosis. R.W. Colman, Ed.: 631–643. Lippincott. Philadelphia.
60. DA PRADA, M. et al. 1988. Platelets as a model for neurones? Experientia **44:** 115–126.
61. SCHAPIRA, A.H.V. 1998. Human Complex I defects in neurodegenerative diseases. Biochim. Biophys. Acta **1364:** 261–270.
62. DE GAETANO, G. 1981. Platelets, prostaglandins and thrombotic disorders. Clin. Haematol. **10:** 297–326.
63. HOLMSEN, H. & L. ROBKIN. 1980. Effects of antimycin A and 2-deoxyglucose on energy metabolism in washed human platelets. Thromb. Haemost. **42:** 1460–1472.
64. D'AURELIO, M. et al. 2001. Decreased Pasteur effect in platelets of aged individuals. Mech. Ageing Dev. **122:** 823–833.
65. CROFT, S. et al. 1992. An ESR investigation of the reactive intermediate generated in the reaction between Fe^{2+} and H_2O_2 in aqueous solution: direct evidence for the formation of the hydroxyl radical. Free Radical Res. Commun. **17:** 21–39.
66. APPELKVIST, E.L. et al. 1994. Regulation of coenzyme Q biosynthesis. Molec. Aspects Med. **15S:** 37–46.
67. ANDERSSON, M. et al. 1994. Modulations in hepatic branch-point enzymes involved in isoprenoid biosynthesis upon dietary and drug treatments of rats. Biochim. Biophys. Acta **1214:** 79–87.
68. CRANE, F.L. & P. NAVAS. 1997. The diversity of coenzyme Q function. Molec. Aspects Med. **18:** s1–s6.
69. LARM, J.A. et al. 1994. Up-regulation of the plasma membrane oxidoreductase as a prerequisite for the viability of human Namalwa rho 0 cells. J. Biol. Chem. **269:** 30097–30100.
70. MORRE, D.M., G. LENAZ & D.J. MORRE. 2000. Surface oxidase and oxidative stress propagation in aging. J. Exp. Biol. **203:** 1513–1521.
71. KAGAN, V., E. SERBINOVA & L. PACKER. 1990. Antioxidant effects of ubiquinones in microsomes and mitochondria are mediated by tocopherol recycling. Biochem. Biophys. Res. Commun. **169:** 851–857.
72. ERNSTER, L., P. FORSMARK & K. NORDENBRAND. 1992. The mode of action of lipid-soluble antioxidants in biological membranes: relationship between the effects of

ubiquinol and vitamin E as inhibitors of lipid peroxidation in submitochondrial particles. BioFactors **3**: 241–248.
73. VILLALBA, J.M. *et al.* 1995. Coenzyme Q reductase from liver plasma membrane: purification and role in trans-plasma-membrane electron transport. Proc. Natl. Acad. Sci. USA **92:** 4887–4891.
74. BEYER, R.E. *et al.* 1996. The role of DT-diaphorase in the maintenance of the reduced antioxidant form of Coenzyme Q in membrane systems. Proc. Natl. Acad. Sci. USA **93:** 2528–2532.
75. TAKAHASHI, T. *et al.* 1995. The role of DT-diaphorase in the maintenance of the reduced antioxidant form of Coenzyme Q in membrane systems. Biochem. J. **309:** 883–890.
76. VALLS, V. *et al.* 1994. Protective effect of exogenous Coenzyme Q against damage by adriamycin in perfused rat liver. Biochem. Mol. Biol. Int. **33:** 633–642.
77. LOW, P.A., K.K. NICKANDER & H.J. TRITSCHLER. 1997. The roles of oxidative stress and antioxidant treatment in experimental diabetic neuropathy. Diabetes **46:** S38–42.
78. KALÈN, A. *et al.* 1990. Uptake and metabolism of dolichol and cholesterol in perfused rat liver. Lipids **25**: 93–99.
79. BEYER, R.E. *et al.* 1985. Tissue Coenzyme Q (ubiquinone) and protein concentrations over the life span of the laboratory rat. Mech. Ageing Dev. **32**: 267–281.
80. BATTINO, M. *et al.* 1995. Coenzyme Q content in synaptic and nonsynaptic mitochondria from different brain regions of the ageing rat. Mech. Ageing Dev. **78**: 173–187.
81. SÖDERBERG, M. *et al.* 1990. Lipid composition of different regions of the human brain during aging. J. Neurochem. **54:** 415–423.
82. ANDERSSON, M. *et al.* 1995. Age-dependent modifications in the metabolism of mevalonate pathway lipids in rat brain Mech. Ageing Dev. **85:** 1–14.
83. FORMIGGINI, G. *et al.* 1996. Coenzyme Q depletion in rat plasma after partial hepatectomy. Biochem. Mol. Biol. Int. **39:** 1135–1140.
84. BEAL, M.F. 1998. Mitochondrial dysfunction in neurodegenerative diseases. Biochim. Biophys. Acta **1366:** 211–223.
85. GÖTZ, M.E. *et al.* 1994. Oxidative stress: free radical production in neural degeneration. Pharm. Ther. **63:** 37–122.
86. ZARBIN, M.A. 1998. Age-related macular degeneration: review of pathogenesis. Eur. J. Ophthalmol. **8:** 199–206.
87. BLASI, M.A. *et al.* 2001. Does coenzyme Q10 play a role in opposing oxidative stress in patients with age-related macular degneration? Ophthalmologica **215:** 51–54.
88. BEAL, M.F. 1999. Coenzyme Q10 administration and its potential for treatment of neurodegenerative diseases. BioFactors **9:** 261–266.
89. KARLSSON, J. *et al.* 1993. Ubiquinone and alpha-tocopherol in plasma; means of translocation or depot. Clin Invest. **71S:** 84–91.
90. ZHANG, Y., M. TURUNEN & E.L. APPELKVIST 1996. Restricted uptake of dietary coenzyme Q is in contrast to the unrestricted uptake of alpha-tocopherol into rat organs and cells. J. Nutr. **126:** 2089–2097.
91. HUERTAS, J.R. *et al.* 1999. Virgin olive oil and coenzyme Q10 protect heart mitochondria from peroxidative damage during aging. Biofactors **9:** 337–344.

Programmed Death Phenomena: From Organelle to Organism

VLADIMIR P. SKULACHEV

Department of Bioenergetics, A. N. Belozersky Institute of Physico-Chemical Biology, Moscow State University, Moscow 119899, Russia

ABSTRACT: Programmed death phenomena appear to be inherent not only in living cells (apoptosis), but also in subcellular organelles (e.g., self-elimination of mitochondria, called mitoptosis), organs (organoptosis), and even whole organisms (phenoptosis). In all these cases, the "Samurai law of biology"—it is better to die than to be wrong—seems to be operative. The operation of this law helps complicated living systems avoid the risk of ruin when a system of lower hierarchic position makes a significant mistake. Thus, mitoptosis purifies a cell from damaged and hence unwanted mitochondria; apoptosis purifies a tissue from unwanted cells; and phenoptosis purifies a community from unwanted individuals. Defense against reactive oxygen species (ROS) is probably one of the primary evolutionary functions of programmed death mechanisms. So far, it seems that ROS play a key role in the mito-, apo-, organo-, and phenoptoses, which is consistent with Harman's theory of aging. Here a concept is described that tries to unite Weismann's hypothesis of aging as an adaptive programmed death mechanism and the generally accepted alternative point of view that considers aging as an inevitable result of accumulation in an organism of occasional injuries. It is suggested that injury accumulation is monitored by a system(s) actuating a phenoptotic death program when the number of injuries reaches some critical level. The system(s) in question are organized in such a way that the lethal case appears to be a result of phenoptosis long before the occasional injuries make impossible the functioning of the organism. It is stressed that for humans these cruel regulations look like an atavism that, if overcome, might dramatically prolong the human life span.

KEYWORDS: apoptosis; aging; mitochondria; mitoptosis; programmed death of an organism; phenoptosis; reactive oxygen species

INTRODUCTION

More than 18 centuries ago, the Roman physician and naturalist Galen introduced the term *apoptosis*, which in Greek means defoliation. He paid attention to the fact that the autumnal defoliation, preventing the plant from being broken by snow in the winter, occurs only if a plant is alive. Now it is clear that the mechanism of this phenomenon means that in the autumn some cells in the leaf stem commit suicide. Dur-

Address for correspondence: Vladimir P. Skulachev, Department of Bioenergetics, A. N. Belozersky Institute of Physico-Chemical Biology, 4 Khokhlova str., Bldg. A, Moscow State University, Moscow 119899, Russia. Fax: +7-095-939-0338.
skulach@genebee.msu.su

ing the last 20 years, it has been shown that suicide programs are inherent in many (apparently in *all*) types of cells in multicellular organisms. Phenomena of programmed cell death are called, after Galen, apoptosis.

Apoptosis is the fate of (1) many embryonic cells that transiently appear during ontogenesis, (2) cells of the immune system that produce antibodies to their own proteins, (3) cells with damaged DNA, proteins, or lipids, and (4) "homeless" cells that, for example, have accidentally left their place in a corresponding tissue. The latter case is especially demonstrative. The extracellular space contains so-called growth factors, that is, tissue-specific proteins that bind with receptors on the cell surface. This binding switches off a cell suicide program that in the absence of the growth factor sends the cell to apoptosis. If a cell escapes from its tissue, it immediately finds itself in a medium lacking the necessary grow factor, an event initiating apoptosis. In fact, cells of multicellular organism resemble serious hypochondriacs who require a constant stimulus to stay alive.[1]

This situation is most probably a particular case of a general principle that I have dubbed the "Samurai law of biology."[2] It can be formulated briefly as follows: it is better to die than to be wrong; or, in more detail, any biological system from organelle to organism possesses a program of self-elimination. This suicide program is actuated when the system appears to be dangerous for any other system of higher position in the biological hierarchy.

MITOPTOSIS, APOPTOSIS, AND ORGANOPTOSIS

Mitoptosis, Programmed Elimination of Mitochondria

In 1992, my coworker Dmitry Zorov and his colleagues suggested that mitochondria possess a mechanism of self-elimination.[3] This function was ascribed to the so-called permeability transition pore (PTP). The PTP is a rather large nonspecific channel located in the inner-mitochondrial membrane. The PTP is permeable for compounds of molecular mass < 1.5 kDa. The PTP is usually closed. A current point of view is that PTP opening results from some modification and conformation change of the ATP/ADP antiporter, the protein normally responsible for exchange of extramitochondrial ADP for intramitochondrial ATP. Oxidation of Cys56 in the antiporter seems to convert it to the PTP in a way that is catalyzed by another mitochondrial protein, cyclophilin.[4–6] When opened, the PTP makes impossible the performance of the main mitochondrial function, that is, coupling of respiration with ATP synthesis. This is due to the collapse of the membrane potential and pH gradient across the inner-mitochondrial membrane that mediate respiratory phosphorylation. Membrane potential is also a driving force for import of cytoplasmic precursors of mitochondrial proteins. Moreover, it is strictly required for the proper arrangement of mitochondrially synthesized proteins in the inner membrane of the mitochondrion. Thus, repair of the PTP-bearing mitochondrion ceases, and the organelle perishes.[7–10]

It is noteworthy that the above scheme of elimination of a mitochondrion does not require any extramitochondrial proteins. It can be initiated by a signal originating from a particular mitochondrion, such as reactive oxygen species (ROS) produced by the mitochondrial respiratory chain. ROS seem to oxidize the crucial SH-group in the ATP/ADP antiporter, thereby actuating the elimination process. This is why one can consider this effect as the programmed death of the mitochondrion (mitochondrial suicide). For this event, I coined the word *mitoptosis*, by analogy with apoptosis, the programmed death of the cell.[7] I also suggested that the biological function of mitoptosis is the purification of the intracellular population of mitochondria from those that became dangerous for the cell because their ROS production exceeded their ROS scavenging capacity.[7–10] This situation may well be a particular case of the above-mentioned Samurai law.

It seems very probable that antioxidant defense is not the only function of mitoptosis. However, at least some alternative mitoptotic functions require ROS to be formed as mediators of mitoptosis. For example, disappearance of mitochondria during the maturation of the mammalian erythrocytes starts with initiation (in some yet unknown way) of 15-lipoxygenase, producing fatty acyl hydroperoxides of mitochondrial phospholipids. These hydroperoxides seem to react with $CoQH^•$ in an Fe^{2+}-dependent way so that $OH^•$ is generated.[11] The latter apparently causes the opening of the PTP, an event actuating mitoptosis, followed by autophagia of perishing mitochondria by lysosomes[12,2] (just as apoptosis of cells is followed by consumption of these cells by macrophages). Thus, the entire process can be described by equation (1):

$$\text{signal} \to [ROS]\uparrow \to \text{mitoptosis}. \qquad (1)$$

as if the evolutionary primary antioxidant system were later used for quite other purposes.[1]

Massive Mitoptosis Results in Apoptosis

Opening of the PTP leads to an osmotic imbalance between the mitochondrial matrix and cytosol, swelling of the matrix and, consequently, the loss of integrity of the outer-mitochondrial membrane, thus releasing the intermembrane proteins into the cytosol. Among them, four proteins are of interest in this context: cytochrome *c*, apoptosis-inducing factor (AIF), the *s*econd *m*itochondrial apoptosis-*a*ctivating protein (Smac; also abbreviated DIABLO), and procaspase 9.[13–22] All these proteins are somehow involved in apoptosis.

AIF was the first mitochondrial component for which the ability to activate apoptosis was revealed.[13] AIF is a flavoprotein of sequence resembling that of dehydroascorbate reductase, an enzyme found in the intermembrane space of plant mitochondria.[14] The reductase regenerates ascorbate, the main water-soluble antioxidant, from dehydroascorbate, using NADH as the reductant. One might speculate that AIF was originally used by mitochondria as an antioxidant enzyme and later was employed by the cell as an apoptosis-activating factor.[2] When released from mitochondria, AIF goes to the nucleus and activates a nuclease that decomposes nuclear DNA.[14]

The route of cytochrome *c*–mediated cell death was shown to be more complicated.[15–18] In cytosol, cytochrome *c* combines with very high affinity with a cytosolic protein called *a*poptosis *p*rotease–*a*ctivating *f*actor 1 (Apaf-1) and dATP. The complex, in turn, combines with an inactive protease precursor, procaspase 9, to form the *apoptosome*. As a result, several procaspase 9 molecules are placed near each other, and they cleave each other to form active caspase 9. When formed, caspase 9 attacks procaspase 3 and cleaves it to form active caspase 3, a protease that hydrolyses certain enzymes occupying key positions on the metabolic map. This causes cell death. At least in some tissues, procaspase 3 and some other procaspases are also localized mainly in the intermembrane space.[20]

Smac, the fourth proapoptotic protein of the intermembrane space, was recently shown to bind cytoplasmic *i*nhibitors of *a*poptosis-activating *p*roteins (IAPs), which suppress the activities of caspases 9, 3, and others. Smac•IAP complexes lack the antiapoptotic activity inherent in the free IAPs.[21,22]

Considering these data, the following scenario of the final steps of the defense of a tissue from mitochondrion-produced ROS seems to be most likely. ROS induce PTP opening and, consequently, release of cytochrome *c* and other proapoptotic proteins from mitochondria to the cytosol. If this occurs in a small fraction of ROS-overproducing mitochondria, these mitochondria die. The cytosol concentrations of proapoptotic proteins released from the dying mitochondria appear to be too low to induce apoptosis. If, however, more and more mitochondria become ROS overproducers, the concentrations in question reach a level sufficient for the induction of apoptosis. This results in purification of the tissue from the cells whose mitochondria produce too many ROS.[1]

It should be stressed that dysfunction of mitochondria per se can be a reason for cell death in tissues where phosphorylating respiration is the major source of ATP. However, apoptosis caused by cytochrome *c* and other intermembrane "death proteins" occurs much earlier than the mitochondrial dysfunction results in exhaustion of ATP. On the contrary, dATP and/or ATP are required for apoptosis (e.g., to actuate the apoptosome formation; see above). It looks as if cytochrome *c* and other mitochondrial "death proteins," when they appear in large amounts in the cytosol, represent a signal for the cell that something is dramatically wrong with its mitochondrial population.[23] Such a cell commits suicide, following the Samurai law.

In 1994, I postulated a scheme that mitoptosis is an event preceding apoptosis.[8] In the same year, Newmeyer and coauthors published the first indication of a requirement of mitochondria for apoptosis.[24] Quite recently, Tolkovsky and her coworkers presented direct proof of the mitoptosis concept.[25,26] In the first set of experiments, axotomized sympathetic neurons deprived of neuron growth factor were studied. It was found that such neurons died within a few days, showing cytochrome *c* release and other typical features of apoptosis. However, the cells survive if a pan-caspase inhibitor Boc-Asp (O-methyl)-CH$_2$F (BAF) was added a day after the growth factor deprivation. The cell survival was due to the fact that the mitochondrion-linked apoptotic cascade was interrupted downstream of the mitochondria. Electron microscopy showed that in the majority of such cells *all the mitochondria disappear within three days* after the BAF addition (FIG. 1A).[25] Later, the same group reported[26] that a similar effect could be shown using such classical experimental models of apoptosis as HeLa cells treated with staurosporin. Again, addition of BAF to the staurosporin-treated cells resulted in (1) the cells living longer and (2) mitochondria disappearing within several days. This was shown to be accompanied by disappearance of mitochondrial DNA as well as the cytochrome oxidase subunit IV encoded by nuclear DNA. On the other hand, nuclear DNA, Golgi apparatus, endoplasmic reticulum, centrioles, microtubules, and plasma membrane remained undamaged. Mitoptosis was prevented by overexpression of antiapoptotic protein Bcl-2, which is known to affect mitochondria upstream from the cytochrome *c* release.

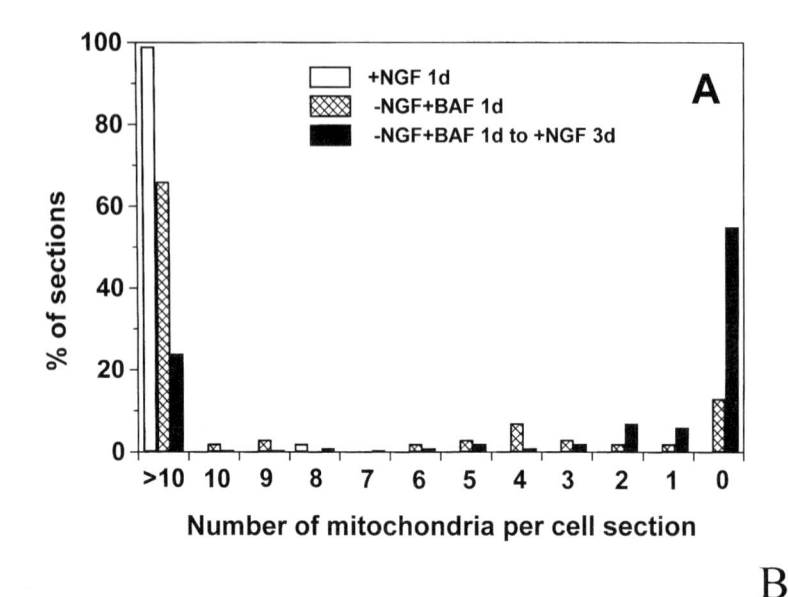

FIGURE 1. Mitoptosis in sympathetic neurons after nerve grow factor (NGF) deprivation and inhibition of apoptosis by pan-caspase inhibitor Boc-Asp(o-methyl)-CH2F (BAF). (**A**) Up to 202 individual cell sections from each of the three treatments, namely (1) 1 day with NGF, (2) 1 day without NGF and with BAF, and (3) 1 day without NGF and with BAF to subsequent 3 days with NGF, were sorted into 12 groups (section containing 0–10 or >10 mitochondria per cell section). Cells with NGF contained 59±10 mitochondria per section (From Fletcher et al.[25]). (**B**) A scheme explaining results of the above experiment. Apoptotic signal (NGF deprivation) reaches mitochondria (1), which multiply the signal via BAF-sensitive caspase activation and induce fast apoptosis (2). Moreover, slow apoptoses can be induced in BAF-resistant fashions. They can be mitochondrion independent (3) or mitochondrion dependent. In the latter case, mitoptosis takes place (4), an event entailed by a cell death (5). It should be stressed that the three types of apoptosis may differ not only in mechanisms but also final manifestations of the death program. *Solid* and *dashed lines*, fast and slow processes, respectively.

Apparently, disappearance of mitochondria in the apoptotic cells without BAF could not be seen since the cells die too quickly to reveal mitoptosis and subsequent autophagia of dead mitochondria. On the other hand, inhibition of apoptosis at a postmitochondrial step prevented fast death of the cells so that there was time for mitoptosis to be completed (FIG. 1B).

It should be mentioned that the cells without mitochondria could not grow and died within a week. Tolkovsky and coworkers described this as "energy starvation" and called this type of cell death *limokonia*, which is the Greek term for starvation.[25] However, the situation might be more complicated. Perhaps a cell recognizing disappearance of the entire mitochondrial population commits suicide, following the Samurai law. Another possibility is that the cell monitors the ATP level, rather than the presence of mitochondria per se, and goes to apoptosis just because of a decrease in this crucial parameter when mitochondria disappear. In any case, the death program for cells lacking mitochondrion must be caspase independent. It is noteworthy in this context that such types of apoptosis have already been described. For instance, AIF, when released from mitochondria, can send a cell to apoptosis with no caspases involved.[14]

Similarly, the PTP is probably not the sole mechanism of mitoptosis. Possible involvement of the PTP can be recognized by adding cyclosporin A, a specific PTP inhibitor. Unfortunately, cyclosporin A was not tried in Tolkovsky's experiments.

On the other hand, in our group it was found that cytochrome *c* release and apoptosis induced by staurosporin are cyclosporin A resistant, in contrast to those induced by tumor necrosis factor (TNF) (B.V. Chernyak and coauthors, in preparation). Such release does not require the PTP. Instead, protein-permeable channels seem to be formed by a complex of the proapoptotic protein Bax and porin in the outer-mitochondrial membrane (for review, see Ref. 1).

Organoptosis, Programmed Elimination of Organs

In the preceding section, programmed death at the subcellular and cellular levels was considered. Now we shall deal with similar phenomena in supercellular systems. It is clear that massive apoptosis of cells composing an organ should eliminate the organ. This process we call *organoptosis*. For example, consider the disappearance of the tail of a tadpole when it converts to a frog. It was recently reported by Kashiwagi *et al.*[27] that addition of thyroxine (a hormone known to cause regression of the tail in tadpoles) to severed tails surviving in a special medium caused shortening of the tails that occurred within hours. The following chain of events was elucidated:

thyroxine $\to$ NO synthase induction $\to [NO]\uparrow \to$ inactivation of catalase

(2)

and glutathione peroxidase by NO $\to [H_2O_2]\uparrow \to$ apoptosis.

Generally, H_2O_2 and NO seem to operate as intercellular mediators of apoptosis, a function that must be especially important for any case of programmed death at levels higher than cellular. Using these small penetrating molecules, an organism can organize elimination of, for example, tissue regions infected by a virus. At least in some cases, infected cells have been shown to produce H_2O_2 not only to commit suicide but also to organize apoptosis in nearby cells that are probable targets for the virus during the expansion of the infection. As a result, a "dead area" is organized around the infected cell (for details, see Refs. 1 and 28).

PHENOPTOSIS, PROGRAMMED DEATH OF AN ORGANISM

Obviously, massive apoptosis in an organ of vital importance, resulting in organoptosis, must entail death of the entire organism. On the face of it, such an event should be regarded as a lethal pathology of no biological sense. However, this may not be the case if the organism in question is a member of a community of other individuals. Here, altruistic death of individuals may appear to be useful for a superorganismal unit, a mechanism for adaptation of the group to a changing environment. Thus, the chain of events: "mitoptosis $\rightarrow$ apoptosis $\rightarrow$ organoptosis" can, in principle, be supplemented with one more step, that is, the programmed death of an organism. I call such an event *phenoptosis*. Phenoptosis can be defined as *a mechanism purifying kin or community from individuals that are not longer wanted.*[1,29–31]

Phenoptosis among Unicellular Organisms

For unicellular organisms, programmed death of a cell is phenoptosis. It is already clear that the bacterial cell has suicide programs that are actuated when there is something wrong with the cell.

For instance, bacteria have a protein that monitors DNA damage. It is called RecA. DNA damage activates RecA, which hydrolyses the LexA repressor.[32] This results in derepression of genes encoding (1) proteins of SOS DNA repair and (2) the short-lived protein SulA. The latter binds FtsZ, a protein that forms a division ring so that cell division appears to be blocked. Surprisingly, the $sulA^-$ mutant is many-fold less sensitive to the same DNA damage (caused by quinolone antibiotics) than the wild-type bacterium.[33] Lewis[34] suggested that SulA, besides binding FtsZ, sends a signal for cell suicide. He hypothesized that such a phenoptotic signal is realized by an autolysin, a peptidoglycan hydrolase causing decomposition of the cell wall and, in turn, phenoptosis of bacteria reaching the stationary growth phase or treated with some antibiotics (see below). Another possibility is that a long-term arrest of the cell division per se is a suicide signal, as illustrated in FIGURE 2. Lewis concluded that "$sulA^-$ mutants have an enormous survival advantage over the wild type, yet the immediate benefit of greater survival of $sulA^-$ cells is apparently outweighed by the longer-term disadvantage due to the loss of the ability to eliminate defective cells." [34]

The SulA story is very instructive in that a unicellular organism commits suicide due to DNA damage long before this damage per se becomes incompatible with the life of the organism. This means that a cell usually dies when DNA is damaged because of a suicide signal rather than because of a dysfunction of DNA. Such a strategy is consistent with the principle formulated above: it is better to die than to be wrong. This insures the genetic program against dangerously modified DNA that can result from its accidental damage.

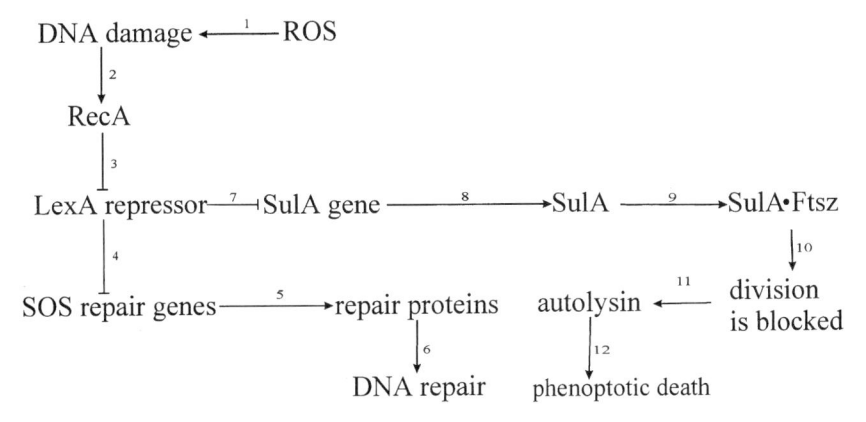

```
DNA damage ←—1—— ROS
    │ 2
    ↓
  RecA
    │ 3
    ↓
LexA repressor ——7—→ SulA gene ————8————→ SulA ———9———→ SulA·Ftsz
    │ 4                                                      │ 10
    ↓                                          11            ↓
SOS repair genes ——5—→ repair proteins   autolysin ←——— division
                         │ 6                  │ 12         is blocked
                         ↓                    ↓
                      DNA repair       phenoptotic death
```

FIGURE 2. Regulation of DNA repair, cell division, and phenoptosis in bacteria. 1, DNA damage caused by ROS (or by any other agents) activates RecA protein (2), which hydrolyses the LexA repressor (3), a protein that previously arrested the SOS repair genes (4), and the SulA gene (7); 5, formation of the DNA repair proteins; 6, DNA repair; 8, formation of SulA protein, which binds the FtsZ protein required for cell division (9); 10, the division ceases, an event actuating the autolysin-mediated phenoptosis (11, 12). (Modified from Lewis[34]).

Lewis[34] listed in his excellent review some other examples of phenoptosis in bacteria. Among these are (1) active lysis of the mother cell of *Bac. subtilis* during sporulation, which is required to release spores; (2) lysis of some cells of *S. pneumoniae* to release DNA, which is picked up by other cells that did not lyse; and (3) lysis of *S. pneumoniae* caused by penicillin. In the latter case, a mutant was selected that was resistant not only to lysis by penicillin but also by several other antibiotics acting on quite different targets. In spite of the absence of the *lysis* response, all the antibiotics tested were shown to inhibit *growth* of the mutant bacteria just as that of the wild type, a fact showing that the antibiotics were able to act normally against their targets in the mutant cells.

Quite recently, the mechanism of this phenomenon was elucidated by Tuomanen and coworkers.[35] It proved to be related to the peptide involved in the so-called "quorum-sensing" effect. It was found that bacteria (in this study, *S. pneumoniae*) always excrete a peptide composed of 27 amino acid residues (Pep-27). When the number of growing bacteria in a medium increases, this entails elevation of Pep-27, which appears to be an agent inducing the autolysin-mediated lysis of the *S. pneumoniae* cells. In this way, phenoptosis regulates the level of bacteria in the environment, apparently optimizing their number under given ambient conditions. Pep-27 production was shown to strongly increase when something was wrong with the bacterium. This is why a wide range of antibiotics affecting various targets in the bacterial cell induce lysis—one more example of the operation of Samurai law–linked phenoptosis.

In *E. coli*, three suicide mechanisms that are activated by the appearance of a phage in the cell interior have been described. One of them is the formation of ion-permeable channels in the bacterial membrane, whereas the two others are the activation of a protease or ribonuclease specifically cleaving a protein (EF-T$_u$) or RNA

($tRNA^{Lys}$) respectively, that is, components required for protein synthesis. Since corresponding death programs are encoded by plasmid or a prophage integrated into the bacterial genome, Lewis suggested that the cell suicide "is a result of competition of parasitic DNAs, with the host as a battlefield."[34] In any case, it is obvious that the phage-induced suicide is favorable for the bacterial community, purifying it from the phage-infected cells. This is why this kind of mechanism was conserved by evolution (reviewed in Refs. 36 and 30).

In all of the above cases, the mechanisms of programmed death of bacteria are carried out by proteins that are quite different from those involved in apoptosis of animal cells. On the other hand, some domains inherent in animal pro- and antiapoptotic factors have already been found in bacteria. Perhaps, they are involved in other phenoptotic programs (for reviews, see Refs. 34 and 37).

Phenoptosis has already been documented in unicellular eukaryotes. Fröhlich and coworkers[38] reported that in the yeast *Saccharomyces cerevisiae* small amounts of H_2O_2 caused cell shrinkage, appearance of phosphatidyl serine in the outer-membrane leaflet, chromatin condensation and margination, and cleavage of DNA, all these events resembling the H_2O_2-induced apoptosis in multicellular organisms. A protein synthesis inhibitor suppressed the death program initiated by H_2O_2.

A programmed death apparently took place in experiments of Longo *et al.*,[39] when the yeast *S. cerevisiae* was kept in expired minimal medium. Expression of the animal antiapoptotic protein Bcl-2 prolonged the life of the yeast cells under these conditions. Death did not occur within the measured period of time (12 days) if pure water was used in place of the expired minimal medium. Similar relationships (except for the Bcl-2 effect) were revealed with some bacteria. It was suggested that such strategy represents an altruistic suicide of the majority of cells to allow a small number of cells to survive in the minimal media. This cannot help when nutrition is completely absent (water instead of a minimal medium), so the cells use a strategy another than phenoptosis.[34]

A programmed death mechanism seems to be operative in protozoa. In *Tetrahymena*, staurosporin was reported to induce morphological changes resembling those in apoptotic animal cells. The transcription inhibitor actinomycin D prevented the killing by staurosporin.[40]

Age-independent Phenoptosis among Multicellular Organisms: Possible Role of Bacterial Toxins

A higher organism seriously infected by a dangerous pathogen is an unwanted guest for the community, just as a phage-infected *E. coli* cell is for a population of these bacteria. From a superorganismal point of view, quick death of such an individual might be a cruel but radical solution to the problem, being the last line of the antiepidemic defense. This means that a population of organisms possessing a mechanism to purify the community from badly infected individuals will have reproductive advantage compared with that lacking such a mechanism.

Perhaps the above reasoning might explain the diphtheria toxin paradox. Diphtheria is induced by *Corynebacterium*, which excretes a protein toxin composed of larger and smaller domains. The larger domain is recognized by a special receptor in the plasma membrane of a cell of a macroorganism. After binding with the receptor, the toxin translocates its smaller domain through the plasma membrane. When it appears on the inner surface of the plasma membrane, the smaller domain is cleaved and released into the cytosol. Here it operates as an enzyme that catalyzes ADP-ribosylation of diphthamide, a histidine derivative inherent in the elongation factor 2 (EF-2). This modification of EF-2 is inhibitory, so protein synthesis in the target cell ceases.

Diphthamide, the toxin target, is found only in a single protein (EF-2), where it is present in a single copy. It is formed by posttranslational modification of a histidine residue of EF-2, the modification being catalyzed by a system composed of five individual enzymes that are not involved in other metabolic processes (for review, see Refs. 41–43 & 86).

On the face of it, diphtheria toxin is a typical biochemical weapon invented by a bacterium to fight a macroorganism. However, such an explanation is difficult to reconcile with the fact that all attempts to find diphthamide function(s) other than to be attacked by bacterial toxins have failed. Animal cells with mutant EF-2 that cannot be ADP ribosylated by diphtheria toxin show normal protein synthesis and differ from the wild-type cells in only one property—they are diphtheria-toxin resistant. The impression arises that the sole function of diphthamide is to kill a cell and, under heavy infection, an organism. Certainly, it is impossible to exclude that someday a useful function of diphthamide will be discovered. However, even if that occurred and one could say that diphtheria toxin is a weapon used by corynebacteria to kill their enemy, the situation would still be paradoxical. For corynebacteria, an animal is a growth medium rather than an enemy. The death of the macroorganism is an undesirable event from the "corynebacterial point of view." Even more, epidemic growing to pandemic is in fact catastrophic for pathogenic bacteria that will disappear when all the macroorganisms that can be infected die.

Perhaps, *Corynebacterium*–macroorganism relationships represent a type of quorum-sensing effect mediated by the toxin. Let us assume that originally diphtheria toxin was invented by the bacteria as a weapon against other microorganisms (diphthamide has been found in some archea[44] and yeast[42]). However, further evolution resulted in a situation in which the toxin, besides its primary function (weapon), is used to induce phenoptosis of a macroorganism, thereby preventing an epidemic that is equally dangerous for both macroorganisms and bacteria. If this were the case, the situation with diphtheria would be symmetric to that with infection of *E. coli* by a phage (see above), when appearance of a phage inside the cell initiates a phenoptotic mechanism, killing the infected bacterium (in some cases, by means of inhibition of its protein synthesis, see above) to prevent massive reproduction of phage in this bacterium. It might be important for understanding of evolution of the diphtheria toxin mechanism that this toxin be encoded by the bacteriophage β genome integrated into the corynebacterial genome, just as $EF-T_u$–attacking protease is encoded by a prophage in the *E. coli* genome. Following this logic, we can suppose that killing of a badly infected individual by the toxin would prevent expansion of the epidemic and save the population. If a population lost such a mechanism, it would fail to purify itself from infected individuals and disappear, since it could not survive the epidemic. Certainly, such a suggestion presumes that corynebacteria lacking toxin are still unwanted guests for the macroorganism.

It should be noted that the principle of action of diphtheria toxin is not unique. The action mechanism of toxin A excreted by *Pseudomonas aurogenosa* is almost identical to that of the diphtheria toxin (only the toxin receptors are different).[43] One may think, therefore, that the diphthamide system defends populations not only from diphtheria, but from a group of dangerous infections.

On the other hand, there are some other potentially phenoptotic systems that might perform a similar defense function. For instance, the dysentery pathogen produces a toxin that stops the host protein synthesis with no diphthamide involved.[43] Cholera and pertussis toxins, like diphtheria toxin and toxin A, have their own receptors in the plasma membrane of the host cell and catalyze ADP-ribosylation of an intracellular protein, but the targets are different. For cholera, it is the α-subunit of G_s protein activating adenylate cyclase, whereas for pertussis toxin it is the α-subunit of G_i that inhibits the same enzyme. In both cases, normal regulation of [cAMP] is damaged, so β- and $α_2$-adrenergic receptions become impossible.[45,46]

The murine plague toxin seems to block the β-adrenergic receptor, causing circulatory collapse. In contrast to the above-mentioned toxins, which are actively excreted by bacteria, the plague toxin is associated primarily with the bacterial cell wall until cell death and lysis. Thus, it should be attributed to so-called "endotoxins."[47] Such a feature is rather surprising if one regards the plague toxin as a weapon used by the bacterium in its struggle with the macroorganism. Even more surprising is the final result of the toxin action, circulatory collapse, killing the macroorganism and hence the pathogenic bacteria living in this organism.

Again, the paradox is explained if we assume that plague toxin is used by the animals to purify their population from badly infected individuals. It is remarkable that the toxin in question is especially effective in killing rats and mice, whose populations form natural reservoirs of the plague infection.

Similar relationships seem to be inherent in septic shock. All the features of septic shock indicate that the death of an ill individual is well organized by the macroorganism itself, the role of the pathogen being rather passive. "Endotoxin," causing sepsis, is a lipopolysaccharide (LPS) forming the outer layer of the wall of Gram-negative bacteria. The toxicity of endotoxin is absolutely dependent on the presence of an endotoxin-binding protein in blood and some receptors in the plasma membrane of the patient's cells. Sepsis is accompanied by massive formation of TNF and other cytokines that induce apoptosis of these cells. Knockout of genes coding for these proteins as well as inhibition of the receptors (for review, see Refs. 48 and 49) or of caspases[50] decreases the toxicity of LPS. In fact, LPS looks like a signal of the appearance (in blood and tissues) of Gram-negative bacteria, which may be especially dangerous because their LPS-containing wall protects them from attack by the antibacterial systems of the macroorganism. This effect apparently represents a generalized response of an organism to *any* Gram-negative bacteria, including noninfectious ones. This explains why sepsis can be noncontagious.[1,30]

Certainly, phenoptosis is the last line of defense for a community of organisms against infection. If the amount of pathogen in an individual is not too high, the same LPS signal is used by the organism to attract leukocytes to the infected region of a tissue. The formation of cytokines by leukocytes is LPS dependent. Moreover, LPS induces synthesis of mitochondrial uncoupling proteins that are apparently responsible for hyperthermia, bringing the body temperature to a value that is nonpermissive for the bacteria.[51] If the extent of infection is not too high, these measures are useful for the organism. This is why the common opinion concerning sepsis is that it represents an overuse by the macroorganism of its defensive antimicrobial tools. However, such a point of view fails to explain why a control mechanism to prevent this potentially very dangerous system from killing the organisms has not been invented during the evolution of these organisms.[1,2,30]

Within the framework of this concept, the patient–pathogen relationships can be described as the interaction of the three types of mechanisms: (1) attack of the patient's cells by pathogen toxins, (2) activation of antibacterial defense of the macroorganism, and (3) generation of a phenoptotic signal when the level of infection exceeds some critical value. The situation may be complicated by the fact that sometimes the same compound is involved in two of these mechanisms. For instance, diphtheria toxin seems to be not only the pathogen weapon, but also the phenoptosis-inducing agent. On the other hand, bacterial LPS apparently participates in both the bactericidal system and the initiation of phenoptosis.

PHENOPTOSIS AND AGING

Weismann's Hypothesis Revisited

More than a century ago, August Weismann hypothesized that death of old individuals had been invented by biological evolution as a kind of adaptation. He wrote: "Worn-out individuals are not only valueless to the species, but they are even harmful, for they take the place of those which are sound…I consider that death is not a primary necessity but that it has been secondarily acquired as an adaptation. I believe that life is endowed with a fixed duration, not because it is contrary to its nature to be unlimited, but because the unlimited existence of individuals would be a luxury without any corresponding advantage."[52]

Weismann's hypothesis on aging as an adaptive mechanism was strongly criticized by Medawar,[53] who assumed that aging could not have developed during the course of biological evolution. Medawar in fact assumed that, under natural conditions, the majority of organisms die before they become old. This assumption, however, cannot be applied to some periods of evolution of many species.[54]

Moreover, Medawar did not take into account a possibility that individuals with changes in their genomes can dramatically affect the fate of a population even if they amount to only a very small part of the population. Muir and Howard[55] recently published an excellent example illustrating this statement. A fish with an inserted human growth factor gene was studied. This transgenic animal had increased growth rate. In a mixed population of modified and unmodified animals, the larger modified males attracted four times as many mates as their smaller rivals. However, only two-thirds of the modified animals survived to reproductive age. Thus, the modification decreased the reproductive potential of the fish. Calculations showed that the whole population would become extinct within just 40 generations if 60 transgenic fish joined a population of 60,000 fish. Even a single transgenic individual could have such an effect, although extinction would take a longer time. This study gave a quantitative description to practices applied for many years as a defense against some insects. To the insect population, some sterilized males were added, which resulted in extinction of the population, since the balance between reproduction and death of insects appears to be shifted toward death.

In the already cited review of Lewis, the author wrote: "It is quite possible that the main danger unicellular organisms face are not competitions, pathogens or lack of nutrients, but their own kin turning into "unhopeful monsters" causing death of the population."[34] Muir and Howard's work clearly shows that this statement should be extended to multicellular animals for which an "antimonster" defense is perhaps even more important than for a bacterium because of the much higher complexity of their organization. The very fact that a simple change in activity of a single gene in a small minority of organisms composing a population can be sufficient to kill this population points to existence of a very well-organized system preventing changes in the genome. It is this system that allows a species to exist for millions of years in changing environmental conditions.

The system must include special measures (1) to prevent oxidative and any other kind of damage to the genome, (2) to repair damage to the genome, and (3) to purify the population from genetically impaired individuals. Damage accumulates with age. Therefore, death because of aging can be regarded as a type-3 mechanism.[1] However, biological evolution would be impossible if all changes in genomes were completely blocked. Fortunately, such a risk is practically excluded since defense of the genome cannot be absolute.

Adverse Conditions Increase the Mutation Rate

An attractive suggestion is that organisms can regulate their mutation rate, suppressing this rate under optimal conditions and stimulating it when the conditions change in an unfavorable direction. Mao et al.[56] described an example of this kind for *E. coli*. They reported that growth of an *E. coli* strain lacking lactose permease on lactose-containing medium resulted in a 500-fold increase in mutagenesis.

For aerobic organisms, an increase in mutagenesis due to adverse environmental conditions might be a direct consequence of higher respiration rate, when more energy is required to survive in a more hostile environment. A higher respiration rate requires a larger number of respiratory chain enzymes per cell. This increases the probability for electron carriers of the initial and middle spans of respiratory chain to be attacked by O_2, resulting in the generation of $O_2^{\bullet-}$. This, in turn, increases the probability of oxidative damage to DNA. More mutations lead to higher probability of the appearance of new traits. If a useful trait appears, it can be conserved by means of natural selection. This facilitates survival under new conditions and, hence, decreases respiration and mutagenesis.[57]

During the course of evolution, this simple scheme could be modified, such that special mechanism(s) were developed that stimulate ROS-dependent mutagenesis under unfavorable changes in the environment. The same goal might also be achieved independently of ROS, for example, by suppression of DNA repair.[58] Such regulations may well be a molecular basis for a "mutator," a system responsible for maintenance of the mutation rate at a level higher than zero.[56,59]

Finding of a novel useful trait and, hence, adaptation to new conditions can be accelerated if the generations of the evolving organism change more frequently. This means a short life span and high reproduction rate. Again, short life span under adverse conditions may be a direct consequence of the influence of a hostile environment. A more sophisticated mechanism could include regulated phenoptosis, when aggravation of conditions switches on a death program (FIG. 3).

In this context, an observation by Reznick[60] may be mentioned. The author reported that when guppies that had not previously encountered predation were sub-

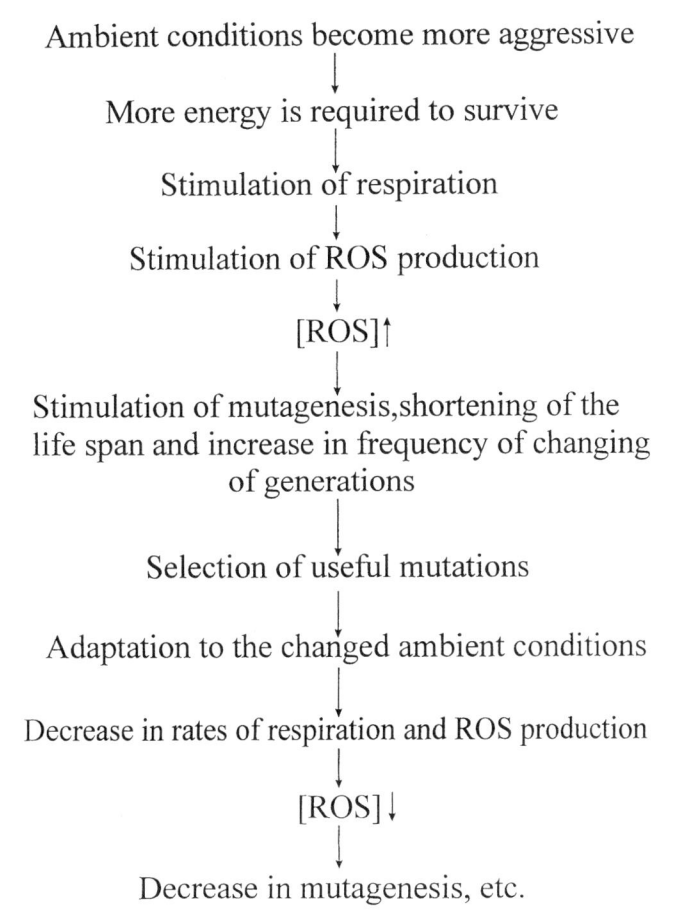

Ambient conditions become more aggressive
↓
More energy is required to survive
↓
Stimulation of respiration
↓
Stimulation of ROS production
↓
[ROS]↑
↓
Stimulation of mutagenesis, shortening of the life span and increase in frequency of changing of generations
↓
Selection of useful mutations
↓
Adaptation to the changed ambient conditions
↓
Decrease in rates of respiration and ROS production
↓
[ROS]↓
↓
Decrease in mutagenesis, etc.

FIGURE 3. ROS-mediated control of mutagenesis and life span under changing conditions. For explanations, see the text. (From Skulachev[1]).

jected to predation for five years, they reached fertility at an earlier age and had a shortened life span even if predators were again excluded from the medium (for discussion, see Ref. 54).

Thus, age-dependent phenoptosis might be involved in the purification of a population from unwanted (useless or dangerous) individuals as well as in regulation of the frequency of change of generations.[1]

Phenoptosis of Multicellular Organisms That Reproduce Only Once

In some of such species, the organism is constructed in a way predetermining death shortly after reproduction. Remember mayflies. Their imagoes die in a few days since they cannot eat, due to lack of a functional mouth, and their intestines are filled with air.[52] In the mite *Adactylidium*, the young hatch inside the mother's body and eat their way out,[61] just as spores formed inside a *Bac. subtilis* cell are released to the outer medium by lysis of the cell (see above). However, much more often a special phenoptotic program is switched on immediately after the act of reproduction. The male of some squids dies just after transferring his spermatophore to a female.[62] The female of some spiders eats the male after copulation. Bamboo can live for 15–20 years reproducing vegetatively but then, in the year of florescence, dies immediately after the ripening of the seeds. The pacific salmon dies soon after spawning, and this happens due to actuation of a specific corticosteroid-mediated program (rather than to exhaustion of the forces required for life), since dysfunction of the adrenal cortex prevents this kind of sudden death (for discussion, see Refs. 1, 29, 52, 61).

Aging of Repeatedly Reproducing Organisms: Why Is It Slow?

On the face of it, also in these organisms, age-dependent phenoptosis might be organized as sudden death. Bowles[63] mentioned that a marine bird species was found that suddenly dies at about age 50, without any indications of aging. However, this is certainly an exception rather than a rule.

For evolution of repeatedly reproducing organisms, slow aging should be expected to have a considerable advantage over acute phenoptosis. The function of an age-dependent phenoptosis is to reduce the pollution of the population by long-lived ancestors, thereby stimulating progressive evolution. Slow phenoptosis facilitates performance of this function. In fact, the appearance of a useful trait may compensate for unfavorable effects of aging within certain time limits, thereby giving some reproductive advantage to an individual acquiring such a trait. A strong, large-bodied deer, even after reaching a rather old age, still has a better chance than his younger but weaker rival to win a spring battle for a female or to escape from wolves.[29]

POSSIBLE MECHANISMS OF THE AGE-DEPENDENT PHENOPTOSIS

End Under-replication of Linear DNA: Role of the Telomere

Bowles[63] suggested that, historically, the living cell invented the first specialized mechanism of aging when linear DNA was used instead of the circular DNA inherent in the majority of bacteria and *Archae*. This event immediately resulted in a specific kind of DNA aging, a process consisting of replication-linked shortening of DNA. Such shortening inevitably accompanies replication of linear DNA, since even now the replication complex operates with linear DNA in the same way as it does with circular DNA. To produce an exact copy of a template, this complex should have some nucleotide residues to the left and to the right from the place where it combines with DNA. This is always the case if it deals with a circular DNA. However, with a linear DNA, the operation of this mechanism results in under-replication of the ends of the DNA molecule, as was first indicated by Olovnikov.[64] The question arises why eukaryotes, during many millions of years of their evolution, failed to improve such an important enzyme as that carrying out DNA replication, to adapt it to linear DNA, while at the same time they solved many much more difficult problems. According to Bowles,[63] it happened first of all because under-replication is a mechanism applied by unicellular eukaryotes to accelerate the change of generations by shortening of the life span.

Apparently, this mechanism was eventually perfected such that special noncoding sequences (telomeres) were added to the ends of linear DNA. The shortening of the telomere could be used by the cell to count cell divisions without damaging those DNA sequences that encode RNA. Thus, the old (genetic) DNA function was separated from the new one, that is, the cell division counting.

It is not yet clear whether telomere shortening determines the life span of multicellular organisms or only of some cells composing these organisms. It has been suggested that the limited number of divisions determined by telomere shortening is a line of anticancer defense of higher organisms, since knockout of a gene required for telomere formation inhibits some kinds of cancerogenesis.[34,65] On the other hand, there are some indications that the intact telomere is unfavorable for the development of other kinds of cancer[66] (for discussion, see Ref. 67). In any case, it is obvious that under-replication of DNA had already appeared in unicellular eukaryotes, that is, long before carcinogenesis, so their application in anticancer defense must represent the modification of another, much older function.[1]

Quite recently, Sasajima and coworkers[68] reported that the average length of telomeres in hepatocytes of people older than 80 is almost twofold shorter than those of children below the age of 8. Similar dynamics were revealed in cells of digestive tract mucosa, in spite of the fact that the renewal times for hepatocytes and mucosal cells are quite different, that is, 480–620 and 3–7 days, respectively. Thus, such a parameter of DNA aging as the telomere shortening seems to be constant for various types of somatic cells of the same organism. This certainly means that the shortening cannot be a simple function of the number of the DNA replications but is controlled by some regulatory system of the entire organism. Remarkably, this type of organismal control does not work in cancer cells. It was found that in hepatocarcinoma cells the telomere shortening occurs faster than in hepatocytes (as well as in mucosal cells),[69] although in hepatocarcinoma cells telomerase is operative, whereas in hepatocytes it is not.[70]

These observations are consistent with the hypothesis that coordinated telomere shortening is a mechanism of age-dependent phenoptosis. For a better understanding of this intriguing phenomenon, it would be desirable to correlate the telomere shortening rates in different somatic cells of one and the same individual since the deviation of data for different individuals is rather large.[68] Another important goal is to compare the telomere-shortening rate in various species of the same class of organisms strongly differing in life span (e.g., in two nematodes with maximal life spans varying by more than a 1000-fold range[71]). By the way, the very fact that two organisms of the same systematic group and, hence, of similar structure differ so strongly in life span may be additional evidence for the conclusion that the life span is not a simple function of complexity of the organism, but rather a regulated parameter.[52]

Another unclear problem is how the telomere shortening is related to ischemic diseases, the most common of age-dependent lethal pathologies.

Ischemic Diseases and Cancer

Heart attack and stroke resemble to some degree the already described septic shock (see above). In all these cases, death is usually a result of massive apoptosis of a great number of cells in an organ of vital importance. However, in contrast to septic shock, when apoptosis is a reaction to the appearance in the organism of bacterial LPS, apoptosis in heart attack and stroke is most probably a result of reoxygenation of these organs after anoxia, which is a consequence of ischemia. It was suggested that anoxia is accompanied by the reduction of intracellular Fe^{3+} to Fe^{2+}, which is an excellent reducing agent for H_2O_2 in the Fenton reaction, forming $OH^{\bullet}$, the most aggressive ROS. This actuates ROS-linked apoptosis not only in cells really damaged during ischemia, but also in a large number of bystanders. Thus, a rather small necrotic region that, as a rule, cannot cause dysfunction of the organ appears to be surrounded by a much larger region of cells that died because of apoptosis.[2,30] This explains why inhibitors of apoptosis have favorable effects on animals when these agents are immediately applied after experimental heart or brain ischemia and traumatic brain injury (for review, see Ref. 1).

It is noteworthy in this context that ischemia of isolated mouse hearts has a much stronger damaging effect on DNA of the cardiomyocytes if the hearts are obtained from 22- to 24-month-old mice rather than from 6- to 7-month-old ones.[72]

Again, as in the case of septic shock, the question arises why the organism allows overuse of the apoptotic machinery, resulting in death of an individual. The answer may be found if we take into account that (1) ischemic diseases are clearly age dependent, (2) they represent the major reason for death of old individuals, and (3) if death because of aging is a result of the operation of some suicide program, ischemic diseases might be regarded as mechanisms of death signal execution (K. Lewis, personal communication).

Following this logic, we might speculate that cancer, the third (after heart attack and stroke) reason for death of old people, might also be a phenoptotic mechanism that is operative in those individuals whose antiapoptotic system is still dominating over the proapoptotic one even in old age. It is suggested that apoptosis is a line of anticancer defense (see the preceding section). If this is the case, decreased apoptosis *lowers* the risk of death because of ischemic diseases but *increases* this risk because of cancer.[1,30] It is well established that cancer, like heart attack and stroke, is a disease of old, rather than young, people (for review, see Ref. 73). At least partially, the increase in the frequency of cancer in old age is due to mutations in the p53 gene. The protein encoded by this gene performs functions similar to those of RecA in bacteria. One of these is the generation of a cell suicide signal in response to DNA damage. Mutations in the p53 gene are inherent in about 50% of all cases of malignant transformation (for review, see Ref. 1). In some other cases, malignization was shown to correlate with superproduction of the antiapoptotic protein Bcl-2.[74]

It is worth noting that the three above-listed diseases, if not urgently treated in a proper way, are fast and lethal (fast terminal stage of age-dependent phenoptosis), differing in this respect from numerous chronic diseases slowly developing because of accumulation of metabolic and structural defects in old organisms (slow preliminary stage of this phenoptosis). The defects in question per se might entail death of an individual, since some vital function may become impossible due to the mentioned defects. However, at least in some cases, the death seems to come long before the function really ceases, just as occurs at suborganismal levels. Here the Samurai principle means switching on the phenoptotic program when some essential deviation from normal functioning of the organism is no longer compensated for by stabilization systems and is recognized by a mechanism that generates a suicide signal.

For instance, oxidative damage of DNA due to the age-dependent decline in antioxidant defense[75] is recognized by a p53-mediated system. This apparently occurs first of all in the telomere part of the DNA, which is more sensitive to ROS than the main part of the chromosome.[76] p53 sends an apoptotic signal, and a cell with damaged telomere DNA dies. This may result in death of the organism if in some organ so many cells were sent to apoptosis that functioning of the organ ceased.[1]

Oxidative stress can be a result of (1) occasional imbalance of the antioxidant and prooxidant systems, or (2) deliberate actuation of the death program according to equation (3)

$$\text{suicide signal} \to \text{ROS}\uparrow \to \text{mitoptosis} \to \text{apoptosis} \to \text{phenoptosis} \qquad (3)$$

The above reasoning may be regarded as a modern version of the classical Harman theory of the ROS-induced mechanism of aging.[77]

Quite recently, Pfeuty and Gueride[78] reported that, at least for senescence of some cells in culture, the scheme shown by equation 3 seems to take place. Under the conditions used, rabbit articular chondrocytes showed up to 23 doublings. Then growth arrest occurred, which was followed by cell death. It was found that at two-thirds of the cell life span, H_2O_2 production suddenly increased by a factor of more than 10. The effect disappeared in time. p21, a protein overproduced in senescent cells, was induced with the peak of H_2O_2 formation.

One more piece of evidence for the above concept was furnished in 1999 by Pelicci and coworkers.[79] They reported that (1) mice lacking a particular 66-kDa protein (p66[shc]) lived 30% longer than control animals, and (2) fibroblasts derived from these mice did not respond to an H_2O_2 addition by initiating apoptosis.

It is clear from these data that p66[shc] is involved in ROS-induced apoptosis. Apparently in young mice it helps to purify the organism from ROS-overproducing cells. This is good for the organism and might, in principle, prolong its life. However, the same function of p66[shc] appears to be involved in a phenoptotic cascade (see above, equation 3), and this effect becomes dominating in old mice. As a result, p66[shc] shortens the life span (for discussion, see Refs. 1 and 80).

The same reasoning can be used to explain the recent observation of Kirkwood and coworkers[81] who found a positive correlation of the life span of various mammals and the *in vitro* resistance of their fibroblasts to oxidative stress.

Some Specific Features of Human Aging

In many animal species, including higher monkeys, the females die soon after their reproductive period is over, a fact that can be regarded as one more example of phenoptosis. Humans are unique in that they have a life span that is twice as long as other primates. This is partially due to the fact that the postreproductive period of the female is strongly extended. Lewis proposed that "the transmission of knowledge from grandparents to progeny serves as a driving force for extending human longevity…It is further suggested that in early human societies, older individuals who are no longer useful could increase their reproductive success by activating a programmed aging mechanism, which would result in channeling of resources to progeny."[82] Actually, there is a correlation between mortality and such psychological factors as a lack of emotional support and low mastery, that is, the belief that one is able to control his or her own life.[83]

In terms of the phenoptosis concept, this means that the processing of a death signal actuated in old monkeys is not realized in old humans while sufficient emotional support is present. This inhibition disappears and the death signal becomes operative when this support is lowered.

The biochemical mechanisms involved in such regulation of life span are obscure. Nevertheless, the fact is that psychological factors can really cause "biochemical suicide." "Voodoo death" is the most demonstrative illustration for this statement. Voodoo death is the term for a situation where a victim dies after hearing that he or she is subjected to sorcery. Instances and descriptions of voodoo death occur in the anthropology of many native peoples. Eastwall[84] discussed two cases of this kind among Australian aborigines, mentioning that dehydration of the victim's body was the most probable reason for the lethal pathology taking no more than a few days.

The age-dependent phenoptosis occurring in civilized societies is apparently carried out by other mechanisms, usually resulting in heart and brain ischemia diseases or cancer. Here the disappearance of adequate reaction to oxidative stress (see the preceding section) may well be involved. However, a lot of work should be done to elucidate the whole chain of events between external or internal death signals and lethal pathology as well as the very nature of these signals. When this work is completed, a chance may appear to dramatically increase the human life span.

It should be emphasized that, for humans, phenoptosis, if it exists, should be regarded as an animal atavism. Metchnikoff[85] stated in 1907: "Traits of animal origin are inherent in human, who appeared as a result of a long cycle of development. Achieving a level of mental development, which is unknown among animals, he retains many traits that are not only unnecessary for him, but even obviously harmful." Phenoptosis must be attributed to the most harmful among such traits. In wild nature, phenoptosis is useful first of all for survival and evolution of communities of organisms in aggressive environments. Humans organize their lives to minimize dependence on environmental conditions. Even a phenoptotic function such as defense against asocial monsters (that can appear in the progeny of old parents due to mutations accumulating with age) may be replaced by, say, social regulations forbidding the bearing of children beyond some critical age.[1]

CONCLUSIONS

In this paper, we started with programmed death of intracellular organelles and then considered similar phenomena at the levels of cells and organs; then, moving along this line, we came to phenoptosis, programmed death of an organism. The latter idea, suggested by Weismann[52] in the end of nineteenth century, is now revisited with the proverb: "we can see something only if we already saw it before." Identification of programmed death mechanisms at the suborganismal levels makes acceptance of a similar concept much easier at the level of an entire organism. For sure, phenoptosis takes place in wild nature, being inherent in quite different species from bacteria to higher animals. The possibility has been discussed that phenoptosis also occurs among humans. Here fast death of badly infected individuals was regarded as an example of programmed death of an organism, preventing expansion of an epidemic. As to aging, it was assumed to include two phenoptotic stages, namely, slow (age-dependent accumulation of injuries) and fast (biochemical suicide of the organism by means of stroke, heart attack, or cancer), occurring when the degree of injuries reached some critical level required to initiate the death program.

Some facts supporting the above concept were summarized. However, it is quite obvious that these observations do not yet allow discrimination between the two concepts of aging that have been discussed since Weismann,[52] that is, death because of accumulation of occasional injuries, or operation of a suicide program.

Remarkably, these two hypotheses, always regarded as alternative, may, in fact, be complementary if we assume that accumulation of injuries actuates a suicide program long before the damage due to these injuries per se becomes sufficient to kill the organism. In this case, the Samurai law forces an organism, recognizing some defects in functioning of the most important systems, to commit biochemical suicide.

For practical medicine the phenoptosis hypothesis has an obvious advantage over the alternative point of view accepted by the majority of gerontologists, since it promises significant prolongation of active life by decelerating (or even eliminating) aging. To do this, we should exclude the death signals or block mechanisms of their processing. These goals will be realistic when we reveal the nature of the signals and the biochemistry of the processing mechanisms.

[NOTE ADDED IN PROOF]: Quite recently, two pieces of evidence concerning the above concept were published. Severin and Hyman[87] reported that a yeast pheromone, namely α-factor (a peptide produced by haploid cells of the α mating type), induces programmed death of cells of the opposite (*a*) type. The program was found to include a protein kinase of the pheromone cascade and, like apoptosis in higher organisms, production of reactive oxygen species, a cyclosporin A–sensitive event, and cytochrome *c*. It requires mitochondrial DNA and protein synthesis. The death-inducing pheromone concentrations were higher than those required for mating. However, even without the added pheromone, programmed death of the above features could be observed if α cells were mixed with *a* cells. These relationships can be accounted for assuming that the pheromone is a compound that not only is favorable for mating but also kills cells failing to mate. This should (1) force the population to switch from the vegetative to sexual reproduction and (2) accelerate changes of generations, stimulating thereby adaptation, that is, a search for new traits when conditions change for the worse. Thus, yeast seems to be a form of life that oscillates between short-lived and long-lived modes, the oscillation being a mechanism of adaptation to changing conditions. In fact, Severin and Hyman's data are in line with Weismann's paradoxical hypothesis that death can be a kind of adaptation. The next (and the most important!) problem is to determine to what degree such a principle can be applied to higher organisms.

Donehower and coworkers[88] generated mice with a deletion in the *p53* gene that expresses a truncated RNA capable of encoding a carboxyl-terminal 24 kDa fragment of p53. Mutant ($p53^{+/m}$) mice exhibited enhanced p53 activity and resistance to spontaneous tumors. In fact, none of the thirty-five $p53^{+/m}$ mice developed overt, life-threatening tumors, whereas over 45% $p53^{+/+}$ and over 80% $p53^{+/-}$ mice, respectively, developed such tumors. Surprisingly to the authors, the mutant mice lived *shorter* by about 25%. Shortening of the life span proved to be a result of an increase in the aging rate. Aging included such traits as reduction of body weight; loss of mass of liver, kidney, and spleen; lymphoid and muscle atrophy; osteoporosis; and hunchbacked spine.

These data may be explained assuming that p53, performing its "guard of genome" function, (1) assures longevity by causing cells that have damaged DNA and that would become malignant to commit apoptotic suicide, but (2) decreases life span by causing the apoptosis of cells with shortened telomeres that are still quite functional. As a result, p53 may be involved in optimization of the life span of organisms. Mechanistically, the two p53-linked effects seem to be different, the latter specifically including p66^{shc}. Thus one may hope to prolong life span by a concerted activating of p53 and inhibiting p66^{shc}.

ACKNOWLEDGMENTS

The author is very grateful to Dr. K. Lewis for useful advice and discussion. This work was supported by the Ludwig Institute for Cancer Research (Grant RBO 863) and the Russian Foundation for Basic Research (Grant 00-15-97799).

REFERENCES

1. SKULACHEV, V.P. 2001. The programmed death phenomena, aging and the Samurai law of biology. Exp. Gerontol. **36:** 995–1024.
2. SKULACHEV, V.P. 2000. Mitochondria in the programmed death phenomena; a principle of biology: "It is better to die than to be wrong." IUBMB Life **49:** 365–372.
3. ZOROV, D.B., K.W.KINNALLY & H. TEDESCI. 1992. Voltage activation of heart inner mitochondrial membrane channels. J. Bioenerg. Biomembr. **24:** 119–124.
4. ZORATTI, M. & I. SZABO. 1995. The mitochondrial permeability transition. Biochim. Biophys. Acta **1241:** 139–176.
5. HALESTRAP, A.P., K.-Y.WOODFIELD & C.P.CONNERN. 1997. Oxidative stress, thiol reagents, and membrane potential modulate the mitochondrial permeability transition by affecting nucleotide binding to the adenine nucleotide translocase. J. Biol. Chem. **272:** 3346–3354.
6. COSTANTINI, P., A.-S. BELZACQ, H.L. VIEIRA, et al. 2000. Oxidation of a critical thiol residue of the adenine nucleotide translocator enforces Bcl-2-independent permeability transition pore opening and apoptosis. Oncogene **19:** 307–314.
7. SKULACHEV, V.P. 1998. Uncoupling: new approaches to an old problem of bioenergetics. Biochim. Biophys. Acta **1363:** 100–124.
8. SKULACHEV, V.P. 1994. Lowering of intracellular O_2 concentration as a special function of respiratory systems of cells. Biochemistry (Moscow) **59:** 1433–1434.
9. SKULACHEV, V.P. 1996. Role of uncoupled and non-coupled oxidations in maintenance of safely low levels of oxygen and its one-electron reductants. Q. Rev. Biophys. **29:** 169–202.
10. SKULACHEV, V.P. 1996. Why are mitochondria involved in apoptosis? Permeability transition pores and apoptosis as selective mechanisms to eliminate superoxide-producing mitochondria and cell. FEBS Lett. **397:** 7–10.
11. SCHNURR, K., M. HELLWING, B. SEIDEMANN, et al. 1996. Oxygenation of biomembranes by mammalian lipoxygenases: the role of ubiquinone. Free Radic. Biol. Med. **20:** 11–21.
12. LEMASTERS, J.J., A.-L. NIEMINEN, T. QIAN, et al. 1998. The mitochondrial permeability transition in cell death: a common mechanism in necrosis, apoptosis and autophagy. Biochim. Biophys. Acta **1366:** 177–196.
13. SUSIN, S.A., N. ZAMZAMI, M. CASTEDO, et al. 1996. Bcl-2 inhibits the mitochondrial release of an apoptogenic protease. J. Exp. Med. **184:** 1331–1341.

14. SUSIN, S.A., H.K. LORENZO, N. ZAMZAMI, et al. 1999. Molecular characterization of mitochondrial apoptosis-inducing factor. Nature **397:** 441–446.
15. LIU, X., C. NAEKYUNG, J.YANG, et al. 1996. Induction of apoptotic program in cell-free extracts: requirement for dATP and cytochrome c. Cell **86:** 147–157.
16. YANG, J., X. LIU, K. BHALLA, et al. 1997. Prevention of apoptosis by Bcl-2: release of cytochrome c from mitochondria blocked. Science **275:** 1129–1132.
17. KLUCK, R.M., E. BOSSY-WETZEL, D.R. GREEN & D.D. NEWMEYER. 1997. The release of cytochrome c from mitochondria: a primary site for Bcl-2 regulation of apoptosis. Science **275:** 1132–1136.
18. KLUCK, R.M., S.J. MARTIN, B.M. HOFFMAN, et al. 1997. Cytochrome c activation of CPP32-like proteolysis plays a critical role in Xenopus cell-free apoptosis system. EMBO J. **16:** 4639–4649.
19. SUSIN, S.A., H.K. LORENZO, N. ZAMZAMI, et al. 1999. Mitochondrial release of caspase-2 and -9 during the apoptotic process. J. Exp. Med. **189:** 381–393.
20. SAMALI,A., J. CAI, B. ZHIVOTOVSKY, D.P. JONES & S. ORRENIUS. 1999. Presence of a pre- apoptotic complex of pro-caspase-3, Hsp60 and Hsp10 in the mitochondrial fraction of Jurkat cells. EMBO J. **18:** 2040–2048.
21. DU, C., M. FANG, Y. LI, et al. 2000. Smac, a mitochondrial protein that promotes cytochrome c-dependent caspase activation by eliminating IAP inhibition. Cell **102:** 33–42.
22. VERHAGEN, A.M., P.G. EKERT, M. PAKUSCH, et al. 2000. Identification of DIABLO, a mammalian protein that promotes apoptosis by binding to and antagonizing IAP proteins. Cell **102:** 43–53.
23. LI, K., Y. LI, J.M. SHELTON, et al. 2000. Cytochrome c deficiency causes embryonic lethality and attenuates stress-induced apoptosis. Cell **101:** 389–399.
24. NEWMEYER, D.D., D.M. FARSCHON & J.C. REED. 1994. Cell-free apoptosis in Xenopus egg extracts: inhibition by Bcl-2 and requirement for an organelle fraction enriched in mitochodria. Cell **79:** 353–364.
25. FLETCHER, G.C., L. XUE, S.K. PASSINGHAM & A.M. TOLKOVSKY. 2000. Death commitment point is advanced by axonomy in sympathetic neurons. J. Cell Biol. **150:** 741–754.
26. XUE, L., G.C. FLETCHER & A.M. TOLKOVSKY. 2001. Mitochondria are selectively eliminated from eukaryotic cells after blockade of caspases during apoptosis. Curr. Biol. **11:** 361–365.
27. KASHIWAGI, A., H. HANADA, M. YABUKI, et al. 1999. Thyroxine enhancement and the role of reactive oxygen species in tadpole tail apoptosis. Free Radic. Biol. Med. **26:** 1001–1009.
28. SKULACHEV, V.P. 1998. Possible role of reactive oxygen species in antiviral defense. Biochemistry (Moscow) **63:** 1438–1440.
29. SKULACHEV, V.P. 1997. Aging is a specific biological function rather than the result of a disorder in complex living systems: biochemical evidence in support of Weismann's hypothesis. Biochemistry (Moscow) **62:** 1191–1195.
30. SKULACHEV, V.P. 1999. Mitochondrial physiology and pathology; concept of programmed death of organelles, cells and organisms. Mol. Aspects Med. **20:** 139–184.
31. SKULACHEV, V.P. 1999. Phenoptosis: programmed death of an organism. Biochemistry (Moscow) **64:** 1418–1426.
32. WALKER, G.C. 1996. The SOS response of Escherichia coli. In Escherichia coli and Salmonella. Cellular and Molecular Biology. F.C. Neidhard, R.I. Curtiss, J.L. Ingraham, C.C.L. Lin, K.B. Low, B. Magasanik, W.S. Reznikoff, M. Riley, M. Schaechter & H.E. Umbarger, Eds. ASM Press. Washington.
33. PIDDOCK, L.J. & R.N. WALTERS. 1992. Bactericidal activities of five quinolones for Escherichia coli strains with mutations in genes encoding the SOS response or cell decision. Antimicrob. Agents Chemother. **36:** 819–825.
34. LEWIS, K. 2000. Programmed death in bacteria. Microbiol. Mol. Biol. Rev. **64:** 503–514.
35. NOVAK, R., E. CHARPENTIER, J.S. BRAUN & E. TUOMANEN. 2000. Signal transduction by a death signal peptide: uncovering the mechanism of bacterial killing by penicillin. Mol. Cell **5:** 49–57.
36. RAFF, M.C. 1998. Cell suicide for beginners. Nature **396:** 119–122.

37. BAKAL, C.J. & J.E. DAVIES. 2000. No longer an exclusive club: eukaryotic signalling domains in bacteria. Trends Cell Biol. **10:** 32–38.
38. MADEO, F., E. FRÖHLICH, M. LIGR, et al. 1999. Oxygen stress: a regulator of apoptosis in yeast. J. Cell Biol. **145:** 757–767.
39. LONGO, V.D., L.M. ELLERBY, D.E. BREDESEN, et al. 1997. Human Bcl-2 reverses survival defects in yeast lacking superoxide dismutase and delays death of wild- type yeast. J. Cell Biol. **137:** 1581–1588.
40. CHRISTENSEN, S.T., J. CHEMNITZ, E.M. STRAARUP, et al. 1998. Staurosporine-induced cell death in *Tetrahymena thermophila* has mixed characteristics of both apoptotic and autophagic degeneration. Cell Biol. Int. **22:** 591–598.
41. LONDON, E. 1992. Diphtheria toxin: membrane interaction and membrane translocation. Biochim. Biophys. Acta **1113:** 25–51.
42. KIMATA, Y. & K. KOHNO. 1994. Elongation factor 2 mutants deficient in diphthamide formation show temperature-sensitive cell growth. J. Biol. Chem. **269:** 13497–13501.
43. SPIRIN, A.S. 1983. Molecular Biology. Ribosome structure and protein biosynthesis. Vysshaya Shkola. Moscow.
44. RAIMO, G., M. MASULLO, A. PARENTE, et al. 1992. Molecular, functional and structural properties of an archaebacterial elongation factor 2. Biochim. Biophys. Acta **1132:** 127–132.
45. MEKALANOS, J.J., R.J.COLLIER & W.R. ROMING. 1979. Enzymatic activity of cholera toxin. II. Relationships to proteolytic processing, disulfide bond reduction, and subunit composition. J.Biol. Chem. **254:** 5855–5861.
46. LENCER, W.I., T.R. HIRST & R.K. HOLMES. 1999. Membrane traffic and the cellular uptake of cholera toxin. Biochim. Biophys. Acta **1450:** 177–190.
47. PERRY, R.D. & J.D. FETHERSTON. 1997. *Yersinia pestis*—etiologic agent of plague. Clin. Microbiol. Rev. **10:** 35–66.
48. KLOSTERHALFEN, B. & R.S. BHARDAJ. 1998. Septic shock. Gen. Pharmac. **31:** 25–32.
49. FENTON, M.J. & D.T. GELONBOCK. 1998. LPS-binding proteins and receptors. J. Leukocyte Biol. **64:** 25–32.
50. HOTCHKISS, R.S., K.W. TINSLEY, P.E. SWANSON, et al. 1999. Prevention of lymphocyte cell death in sepsis improves survival in mice. Proc. Natl. Acad. Sci. USA **96:** 14541–14546.
51. CORTEZ-PINTO, H., S.Q. YANG, H.Z. LIN, et al. 1998. Bacterial lipopolysaccharide induces uncoupling protein-2 expression in hepatocytes by a tumor necrosis factor-α-dependent mechanism. Biochem. Biophys. Res. Commun. **251:** 313–319.
52. WEISMANN, A. 1889. Essays upon heredity and kindred biological problems. Claderon Press. Oxford.
53. MEDAWAR, P.B. 1952. An unsolved problem of biology. H.K. Lewis. London.
54. BOWLES, J.T. 2000. Shattered: Medawar's test tubes and their enduring legacy of chaos. Med. Hypotheses **54:** 326–339.
55. MUIR, W.M. & R.D. HOWARD. 1999. Possible ecological risks of transgenic organism release when transgenes affect mating success: sexual selection and the Trojan gene hypothesis. Proc. Natl. Acad. Sci. USA **96:** 13853–13866.
56. MAO, E.F., L. LANE, J. LEE & J.H. MILLER. 1997. Proliferation of mutators in a cell population. J. Bacteriol. **179:** 417–422.
57. SKULACHEV, V.P. 1999. The dual role of oxygen in aerobic cells. *In* Biosciences 2000. Current Aspects and Prospects for the Next Millenium. Ch. A. Pasternak, Ed.: Vol. 1: 173–193. Imperial College Press. London.
58. SNIEGOWSKI, P.D., P.J. GERRISH & R.E. LENSKI. 1997. Evolution of high mutation rates in experimental populations of *E. coli*. Nature **387:** 703–705.
59. PENNISI, F. 1998. How the genome readies itself for evolution. Science **281:** 1131–1134.
60. REZNICK, D. 1997. Life history evolution in guppies (*Poecilia reticulata*): guppies as a model for studying the evolutionary biology of aging. Exp. Gerontol. **32:** 245–258.
61. KIRKWOOD, T.B.L. & T. CREMER. 1982. Cytogerontology since 1881: a reappraisal of August Weismann and a review of modern progress. Hum. Genet. **60:** 101–121.
62. NESIS, K.N. 1997. Cruel love among the squids. *In* Russian Science; Withstand and Revive. A.V. Byalko, Ed. Nauka-Physmatlit. Moscow. (Russian).

63. BOWLES, J.T. 1998. The evolution of aging: a new approach to an old problem of biology. Med. Hypotheses **51:** 179–221.
64. OLOVNIKOV, A.M. 1971. Principles of marginotomy in template synthesis of polynucleotides Dokl. Akad. Nauk SSSR **201:** 1496–1498 (Russian).
65. CHIN, L., S.E. ARTANDI, Q. SHEN, et al. 1999. p53 deficiency rescues the adverse effects of telomere loss and cooperates with telomere dysfunction to accelerate carcinogenesis. Cell **97:** 527–538.
66. RUDOLPH, K.L., S. CHANG, H.W. LEE, et al. 1999. Longevity, stress response, and cancer in aging telomerase-deficient mice. Cell **96:** 701–712.
67. DE LANGE, T. & T. JACKS. 1999. For better or worse? Telomerase inhibition and cancer. Cell **98:** 273–275.
68. TAKUBO, K., K.-I. NAKAMURA, N. IZUMIYAMA, et al. 2000. Telomere shortening with aging in human liver. J. Gerontol. **55A:** B533–B536.
69. MIURA, N., I. HORIKAWA, A. NISHIMOTO, et al. 1997. Progressive telomere shortening and telomerase reactivation during hepatocellular carcinogenesis. Cancer Genet. Cytogenet. **93:** 56–62.
70. KOJIMA, H., O. YOKOSUKA, F. IMAZEKI, et al. 1997. Telomerase activity and telomere length in hepatocellular carcinoma and chronic liver disease. Gastroenterology **112:** 493–500.
71. GEMS, D. 2000. Longevity and ageing in parasitic and free-living nematodes. Biogerontology **1:** 289–307.
72. AZHAR, G., W. GAO, L. LIU & J.Y. WEI. 1999. Ischemia-reperfusion in the adult mouse heart. Influence of age. Exp. Gerontol. **34:** 699–714.
73. ANISIMOV, V.N. 1983. Carcinogenesis and aging. Adv. Cancer Res. **40:** 265–324.
74. CHIPUK, J.E., M. BHAT, A.Y. HSING, et al. 2001. Bcl-xL blocks TGF-b1-induced apoptosis by inhibiting cytochrome *c* release and not by directly antagonizing Apaf-1-dependent caspase activation in prostate epithelial cells. J. Biol. Chem. **276:** 26614–26621.
75. FRENKEL-DENKBERG, G., D. GERSHON & A.P. LEVY. 1999. The function of hypoxia-inducible factor 1 (HIF-1) is impaired in senescent mice. FEBS Lett. **462:** 341–344.
76. VON ZGLINICKI, T., G. SARETZKI, W. DOCKE & C. LOTZE. 1995. Mild hyperoxia shortens telomeres and inhibits proliferation of fibroblasts: a model for senescence? Exp. Cell Res. **220:** 186–193.
77. HARMAN, D. 1956. Aging: a theory based on free radical and radiation chemistry. J. Gerontol. **11:** 298–300.
78. PFEUTY, A. & M. GUERIDE. 2000. Peroxide accumulation without major mitochondrial alteration in replicative senescence. FEBS Lett. **468:** 43–47.
79. MIGLIACCIO, E., M. GIORGIO, S. MELE, et al. 1999. The p66^{shc} adaptor protein controls oxidative stress response and life span in mammals. Nature **402:** 309–313.
80. SKULACHEV, V.P. 2000. The p66^{shc} protein: a mediator of the programmed death of an organism? IUBMB-Life **49:** 177–180.
81. KAPAHI, P., M.E. BOULTON & T.B.L. KIRKWOOD. 1999. Positive correlation between mammalian life span and cellular resistance to stress. Free Radic. Biol. Med. **26:** 495–500.
82. LEWIS, K. 1999. Human longevity: an evolutionary approach. Mech. Ageing Dev. **109:** 43–51.
83. PENNINX, B.W., T. VAN TILBURG, D.M. KRIEGSMAN, et al. 1997. Effects of social support and personal coping resources on mortality in older age. Am. J. Epidemiol. **146:** 510–519.
84. EASTWELL, H.D. 1987. Voodoo death in Australian aborigines. Psychiatr. Med. **5:** 71–73.
85. METCHNIKOFF, I. 1907. The prolongation of life: optimistic studies. Heinemann. London.
86. MOSS, J. & M. VAUGHAN, Eds. 1990. ADP-ribosylating toxins and G proteins. Insights into signal transduction. American Society for Microbiology, Washington.
87. SEVERIN, F.F. & A.A. HYMAN. 2002. Pheromone induces programmed cell death in *S. cerevisiae*. Curr. Biol. Accepted.
88. TYNER, S.D., S. VENKATACHALAM, J. CHOL, et al. 2002. p53 mutant mice that display early ageing-associated phenotypes. Nature **415:** 45–53.

Melatonin Reduces Oxidant Damage and Promotes Mitochondrial Respiration

Implications for Aging

RUSSEL J. REITER, DUN XIAN TAN, LUCIEN C. MANCHESTER, AND MAMDOUH R. EL-SAWI

*Department of Cellular and Structural Biology,
The University of Texas Health Science Center, San Antonio, Texas 78229-3900, USA*

ABSTRACT: Melatonin has a number of properties as a consequence of which it could be beneficial to animals as they age. Of particular interest are its ubiquitous actions as a direct and indirect antioxidant and free radical scavenger. Besides directly detoxifying a variety of reactive oxygen and reactive nitrogen species, at least one product that is formed as a result of these interactions is also a potent free radical scavenger. Thus, the product that is formed when melatonin detoxifies hydrogen peroxide, that is, N^1-acetyl-N^2-formyl-5-methoxykynuramine is an efficient scavenger, at least equivalent to melatonin itself. This antioxidant cascade increases the ability of melatonin to resist oxidative damage. Other actions of melatonin, such as stimulation of antioxidative enzymes also improves its status as an antioxidant. Finally, recent observations documenting melatonin's ability to stimulate electron transport and ATP production in the inner-mitochondrial membrane also has relevance for melatonin as an agent that could alter processes of aging. These findings, coupled with diminished melatonin production in advanced age, has prompted scientists to consider melatonin in the context of aging. As of this writing there is no definitive evidence to prove that melatonin alters the rate of aging, although data relating to melatonin deferring some age-related degenerative conditions is accumulating rapidly.

KEYWORDS: melatonin; oxygen-based radicals; nitrogen-based radicals; oxidative phosphorylation; mitochondria; aging

INTRODUCTION

The recent impetus for studies related to the role of oxygen-based and nitrogen-based free radicals and reactants with aging[1,2] has its origin with speculations and findings generated almost 50 years ago.[3,4] Certainly no individual has had a more enduring influence in the field than D. Harman,[5,6] who over the last 40 years has persisted in providing the enthusiasm and support for this now burgeoning field.[7,8] A tremendous amount of scientific effort has been directed at identifying the actual

---

Address for correspondence: Russel J. Reiter, Department of Cellular and Structural Biology, The University of Texas Health Science Center, 7703 Floyd Curl Drive, Mail Code 7762, San Antonio, TX 78229-3900. Voice: 210/567-3859; fax: 210/567-6948.
  Reiter@uthscsa.edu

Ann. N.Y. Acad. Sci. 959: 238–250 (2002). © 2002 New York Academy of Sciences.

role of radicals and related reactants in the processes of aging and the progression of a variety of age-related diseases.[9,10] This brief review summarizes what is known about the role of melatonin as a direct and indirect antioxidant and its potential relationship to aging and diseases of the aged. For additional details, more extensive reviews can be consulted.[11,12]

MELATONIN AS AN ANTIOXIDANT

Roughly 10 years ago melatonin was discovered to be a direct scavenger of the highly toxic hydroxyl radical ($^{\bullet}$OH).[13] This finding was unexpected, inasmuch as prior to that discovery melatonin had been exclusively known as a hormone of the pineal gland that mediated fluctuations in reproductive physiology in seasonal breeding animals and for its role in circadian functions.[14] In the study of Tan et al.,[13] the $^{\bullet}$OH-scavenging activity of melatonin was confirmed by means of electron spin resonance (ESR) spectroscopy of an adduct formed by the spin trap 5,5-dimethylpyrroline-N-oxide and the $^{\bullet}$OH. Melatonin, like a number of other antioxidants, detoxifies radicals via electron donation. The ability of melatonin to donate one electron has been verified using cyclic voltametry (FIG. 1). The finding that melatonin is a

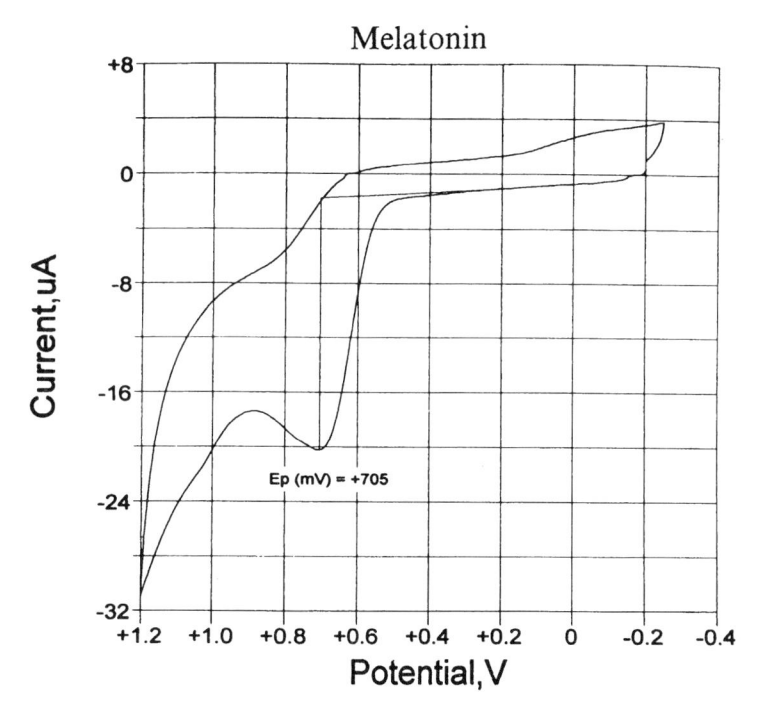

FIGURE 1. Cyclic voltametry of melatonin. This FIGURE illustrates that melatonin donates a single electron, as indicated by the anodic wave at Ep(a) of +705 mV. FIGURE was provided by Dr. R. Kohen, Hadassah University, Jerusalem, Israel.

TABLE 1. Summary of the reactants, both free radicals and free radical-related agents, which have been shown to be scavenged by melatonin. Also shown are the products that are formed as a consequence of the reported interactions.

Reactant scavenged	Product generated	References
Singlet oxygen ($^1O_2$)	N^1-Acetyl-N^2-formyl-5-methoxytryptamine	25–27
Hydrogen peroxide (H_2O_2)	N^1-Acetyl-N^2-formyl-5-methoxytryptamine	27–29
Hydroxyl radical (•OH)	Cyclic 3-hydroxymelatonin	13, 15–24
Hypochlorous acid (HOCl)	2-Hydroxymelatonin	30
Nitric oxide (NO•)	N-Nitrosomelatonin	31–33
Peroxynitrite/peroxynitrous acid (ONOO⁻)/ONOOH)	Cyclic 2-hydroxymelatonin; cyclic 3-hydroxymelatonin; 1-hydroxymelatonin; 6-hydroxymelatonin; 1-nitrosomelatonin	34, 35
Peroxyl radical (LOO•)[a]	—	36–38

[a]Despite some early reports claiming melatonin is a highly effective LOO• scavenger, more recent studies have not supported this conclusion. Despite this, melatonin strongly inhibits *in vivo* lipid peroxidation.

highly effective •OH scavenger is important because this particular radical is considered to be highly reactive and readily damages lipids, proteins, and DNA. It may account for up to 50% of the free radical damage organisms sustain.

Confirmation of the interaction of melatonin with the •OH has been confirmed in many publications using a variety of techniques, including additional ESR studies,[15,16] reduction in melatonin fluorescence,[17] monitoring the absorption of the indolyl radical,[18] production of 2,3-dihydrobenzoate,[19] formation of cyclic 3-hydroxymelatonin (cyclic 3-OHM),[20] and kinetic studies with terephthelic acid[21] and methane sulfonic acid.[22] Melatonin scavenges the •OH both *in vitro*[15–19,21,22] and *in vivo*.[20,23] The rate constant for the scavenging of the •OH by melatonin is 2.7–4.0 × 10^{10} m⁻¹s⁻¹.[17,24]

Melatonin's ability to detoxify toxic reactants, however, is not confined to its ability to scavenge the •OH. TABLE 1 summaries other reactants that are scavenged by melatonin as well as the products that are believed to be generated as a result of these interactions. This combination of detoxifying processes undoubtedly contributes to the efficiency of melatonin in protecting against free radical damage.

The toxicity of the individual oxygen and nitrogen-based reactants that are produced in organisms varies widely. It is generally conceded that the most devastatingly reactive agents are the •OH and the peroxynitrite anion (ONOO⁻) (FIG. 2). Besides being capable of directly damaging macromolecules, the ONOO⁻ is also believed to degrade into the •OH.[39] Specifically, what percentage of the total oxidative damage that an organism sustains is due to the •OH and ONOO⁻ is difficult to determine. Nevertheless, melatonin's ability to neutralize these reactants before they damage macromolecules in the vicinity of where they are produced is presumably an important aspect of the indole's antioxidative actions. Certainly, melatonin has been shown to effectively reduce free radical–mediated oxidative damage to polyunsatu-

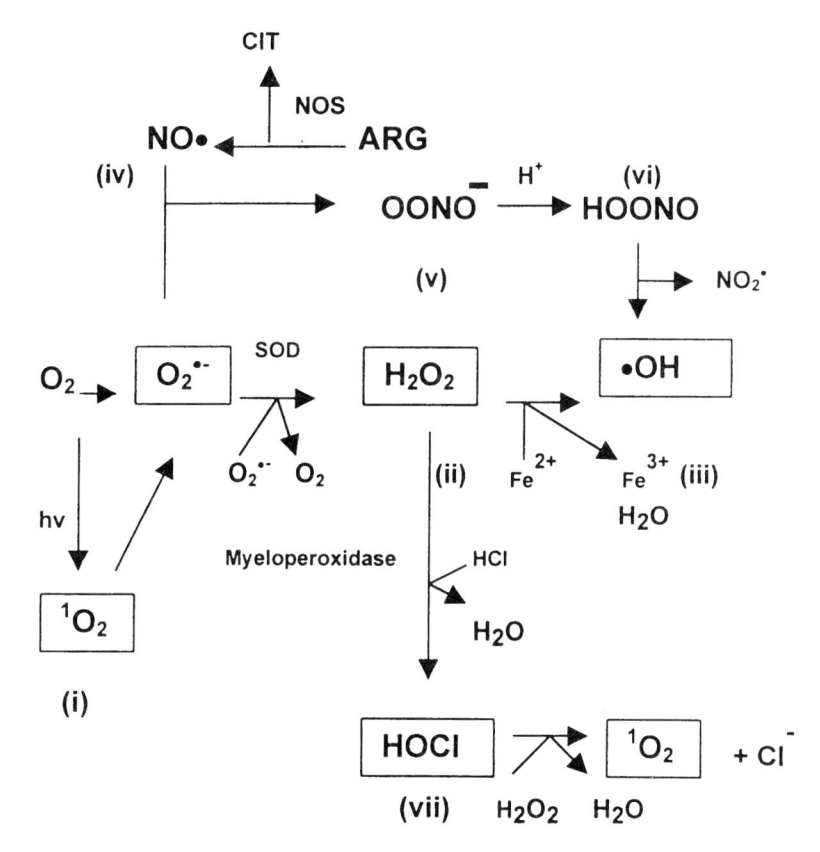

FIGURE 2. Oxygen metabolism and the production of reactive oxygen and nitrogen species. The most reactive of these, namely, the hydroxyl radical ($^\bullet$OH) and the peroxynitrite anion (ONOO$^-$) indiscriminately mangle all molecules, including lipids, proteins, and DNA. The resulting damage, often referred to as oxidative stress, is commonly estimated by measuring the levels of oxidatively damaged macromolecules. Among others, as summarized in the text, melatonin directly detoxifies the $^\bullet$OH and ONOO$^-$, thereby reducing the level of oxidative stress. The symbols i–vii identify the reactants that melatonin directly detoxifies.

rated fatty acids (PUFA) within cellular membranes,[40–42] proteins throughout the cell,[43,44] and both nuclear[45,46] and mitochondrial DNA.[47,48] Each of these macromolecules is capable of being damaged by $^\bullet$OH and ONOO$^-$.

If in fact melatonin prevents the destruction of PUFA, proteins, and DNA by direct free radical–scavenging processes, then it must be in the neighborhood of these molecules when the damaging radicals are generated, that is, melatonin must be in membranes, cytosol, nucleus, and in mitochondria. The close proximity of melatonin to the site of toxic reactant generation is a necessity for providing protection, because these highly reactive agents have a very short half-life and migrate extremely short distances before they mutilate a molecule, that is, the damage they create is always within the immediate vicinity of where they are produced. It is estimated, for example, that the •OH travels no more than a couple of molecular diameters and has an estimated half-life of 1×10^{-9} s[49] before it ravages a macromolecule. Likewise, it is indiscriminate in terms of the molecule it mutilates. What this means is that any free radical scavenger, including melatonin, must be at the site of free radical generation to provide what is referred to as on-site protection.[50]

The implications of the findings summarized above in terms of melatonin's protective actions suggests it is widely distributed within cells. Melatonin's high lipophilicity is well documented,[51] and it is somewhat hydrophilic as well.[52] Measurements of its intracellular distribution and differential concentrations, however, have only been sparingly investigated. The studies to date suggest higher concentrations of melatonin in the nucleus[53,54] and mitochondria[55] than in other portions of the cell. These data must be considered preliminary, however, and the need for more extensive research regarding the subcellular distribution of melatonin is obvious. Of interest is that the mRNAs for the key enzymes required for melatonin synthesis have been found in a large number of cells, suggesting that, besides its uptake from the blood, melatonin may actually be produced in many cells[56] where it could function as an antioxidant. Although these findings are suggestive, the widespread intracellular production of melatonin requires documentation.

Direct scavenging of toxic species is only one means by which melatonin protects against oxidative stress. It also promotes other intracellular activities that help cells rid themselves of toxic reactants. There is now evidence from a variety of publications that shows that melatonin causes the metabolism of reactive species to innocuous products via the stimulation of antioxidative enzymes (FIG. 3). Some of the most important antioxidative enzymes are the superoxide dismutases (SOD), glutathione peroxidases (GPx) and glutathione reductase (GRd). Both physiological and pharmacological doses of melatonin have been shown to increase either gene expression[57] for these enzymes or actually increase enzyme activities.[58,59] Furthermore, increased oxidative stress diminishes the activities of the toxic reactant–metabolizing enzymes, responses that are reversed by melatonin.

SOD is an enzyme that causes the dismutation of $O_2^{-•}$ to H_2O_2. This reduces any damage $O_2^{-•}$ may induce as well as lowers the likelihood of its coupling with NO• to generate the $ONOO^-$ (Fs 2). This latter consequence is especially important in light of the high reactivity of $ONOO^-$.[60]

GPx metabolizes H_2O_2 and lipid hydroperoxides to nonreactive products. Thus, the stimulation of this enzyme by melatonin[58] is important in reducing steady state levels of the •OH, inasmuch as H_2O_2 is its precursor (FIG. 2). In the process of metabolizing H_2O_2 to nonreactive products, glutathione (GSH) is used as a substrate and is oxidized to its disulfide (GSSG). Normally, in excess of 97% of the total glutathione in cells is maintained in the reduced state, that is, as GSH. To ensure this occurs, GSSG is quickly metabolized back to GSH by GRd. Since melatonin stimulates GRd,[58] it benefits the recycling of glutathione and helps to maintain the GSH:GSSG ratio highly in favor of the former.[61] Besides influencing the recycling of glutathione, melatonin also promotes its *de novo* synthesis by stimulating the activity of its rate-limiting enzyme, γ-glutamyl-cysteine synthetase.[62] These actions of melatonin on glutathione synthesis and recycling are considered important given glutathione's central role in reducing intracellular oxidative stress.[63]

As mentioned above, NO• besides being an important gaseous neurotransmitter, can have negative consequences when it is produced in excess. The bulk of its tox-

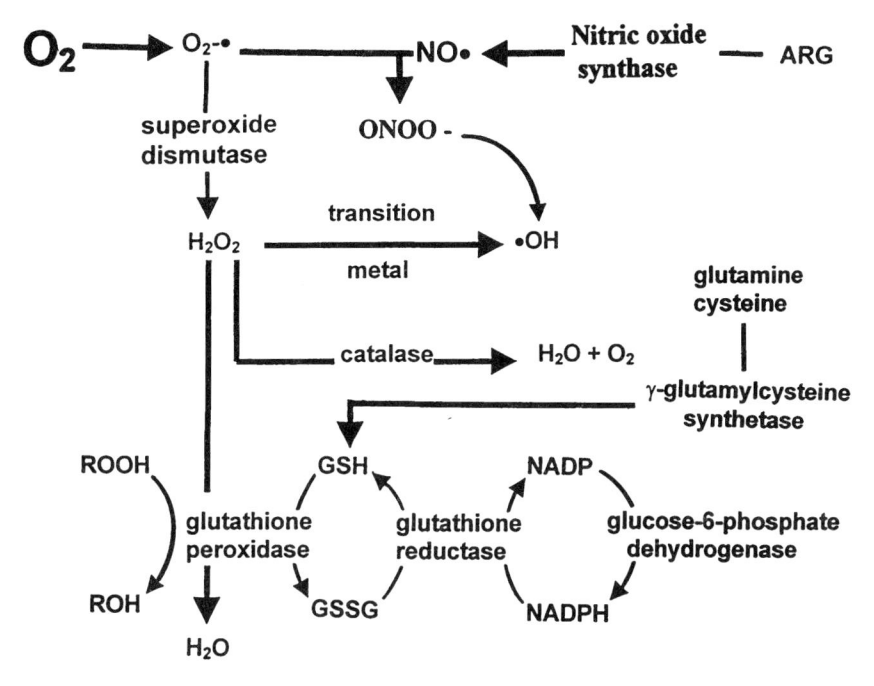

FIGURE 3. Some of the major antioxidative enzymes are depicted in this FIGURE. The superoxide anion radical ($O_2^{-\bullet}$) is dismutated by superoxide dismutase, of which there are several isoforms, to hydrogen peroxide (H_2O_2), the precursor of the devastatingly reactive hydroxy radical ($^{\bullet}OH$). Melatonin aids in the reduction of $^{\bullet}OH$ generation by stimulating H_2O_2-metabolizing enzymes, the glutathione peroxidases. Melatonin also enhances the activity of glutathione reductase, helping to keep most of the glutathione within cells in the reduced state. Additionally, melatonin stimulates γ-glutamylcysteine synthetase, the rate limiting enzyme in glutathione (GSH) production, thereby helping to keep this intracellular antioxidant in high concentrations.

icity is secondary to its coupling with $O_2^{-\bullet}$ and the generation of $ONOO^-$ (FIG. 2).[60] Melatonin lowers steady state concentrations of $NO^{\bullet}$ in two ways. As noted above, it directly scavenges this nitrogen-based reactant,[31–33] but it also limits its production while inhibiting its synthesis by lowering the activity of nitric oxide synthase (NOS).[64] Under conditions of high $NO^{\bullet}$ production, NOS functions as a proxidative enzyme that melatonin holds in check.

Given melatonin's many direct and indirect actions as an antioxidant, its ready uptake, its ability to cross all morphophysiological barriers, and its distribution to presumably all cells in the organism, it is not surprising that it has been shown to be so widely protective against oxidative damage in virtually every organ.[65–67] How these individual actions of melatonin contribute to its overall protection against free radical injury is undetermined. Also, still to be investigated is melatonin's interactions with other well-known antioxidants, such as vitamin C, vitamin E, and β-carotene. Not uncommonly, combinations of antioxidants may have additive and/or synergistic actions given their ability to recycle one another.

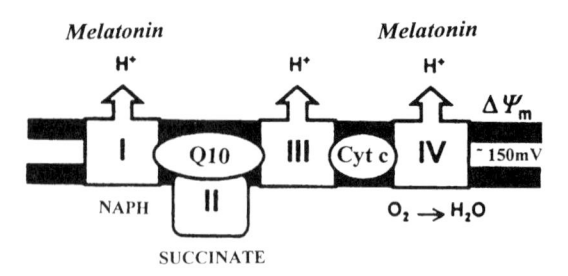

FIGURE 4. Schematic representation of electron flow through the ETC of the inner-mitochondrial membrane. Also shown are the proposed sites at which melatonin acts to increase the efficiency of electron transport and OXPHOS. By doing so, it is presumed that melatonin limits electron leak and the generation of free radicals and enhances ATP production.

MELATONIN AND MITOCHONDRIAL PHYSIOLOGY

In the last two decades much has been written about the potential central role of the mitochondrial dysfunction in the processes of aging.[8,68,69] Since the mitochondria are the site of utilization of the bulk of the inspired oxygen (O_2), they are also the site of abundant free radical generation. This is reflected in the high rate of mitochondrial DNA damage relative to the damaged products measured in nuclear DNA. In mitochondria, 90% of the organism's O_2 is used by a single enzyme, cytochrome oxidase (C-IV).[70] Aerobic organisms generate energy in the form of ATP via the process of oxidative phosphorylation (OXPHOS), which involves a multienzymatic process that permits the transfer of electrons through the electron transport chain (ETC). The ETC consists of four complexes with the transfer of electrons between them being driven by the reduced forms of ubiquinone (UQ) and cytochrome c.

Most O_2 taken into cells is reduced to water, a process that requires the addition of four electrons. The intermediate steps result in the formation of $O_2^{-\bullet}$, H_2O_2, and $^\bullet OH$, corresponding to the reduction of O_2 by one, two, or three electrons, respectively. The production of these reactants accounts for the widespread molecular abuse that mitochondria especially, but other parts of the cell as well, sustain. Damage at the mitochondrial level can seriously jeopardize ATP production and lead to death of cells via apoptosis or necrosis.

There are at least three observations that make the potential presence of melatonin in mitochondria likely and suggest a role for this molecule in mitochondrial physiology. Thus, the mitochondrion as an organelle is believed to derive from bacteria that have been shown to produce melatonin.[71] Second, mitochondria do not produce GSH but rather they take it up from the cytoplasm. Since melatonin stimulates cytoplasmic GSH synthesis, there are significant implications for mitochondria, inasmuch as they use and recycle this thiol in large amounts. Third, melatonin interferes with the ability of cyanide to block C-IV of the mitochondrial ETC.[72]

Against this backdrop, several groups have examined the effect of melatonin at the mitochondrial level. A metabolic effect of melatonin on mitochondria was initially described by De Atenor et al.,[73] while Gilad and coworkers[74] found that melatonin added to cultured 5774 macrophages reversed the inhibition of mitochondrial respiration caused by $ONOO^-$. Additionally, melatonin was shown to reduce the NADPH-dependent peroxidation of lipids in mitochondria derived from human placenta.[75] Finally, the inhibition of C-I of the ETC by MPTP is prevented by melatonin.[76]

When given *in vivo*, melatonin was found to increase liver and brain (the only two organs investigated) mitochondrial C-I and C-IV activities in a time-dependent manner; by 120–180 min following melatonin administration, the activities of these complexes had returned to preinjection levels.[55] When rats were given ruthenium red, a toxin that impairs mitochondrial metabolism, including a reduction in ETC and ATP synthesis, a significant reduction in mitochondrial C-I and C-IV was measured; these changes were counteracted in those rats also treated with melatonin.[77] In a related study, melatonin was also found to restore mitochondrial GPx activity that was inhibited by ruthenium red.

The protective effects of melatonin were also documented in isolated mitochondria prepared from rat neural and hepatic tissues.[55] In this study, oxidative stress was induced using *tert*-butyl-hydroperoxide (*t*-BHP); this molecule reduced GPx and GRd activities in the mitochondria and significantly increased oxidized GSH levels, that is, GSSG. Each of these changes was reversed when mitochondria were treated with melatonin, but vitamins C and E were incapable of doing so. Likewise, *N*-acetylcysteine, a precursor of glutathione, was unable to prevent the changes induced by *t*-BHP.

Additional investigations of the interactions of melatonin with mitochondrial ETC showed that the indole increased the activities of C-I and C-IV in a dose-dependent manner (FIG. 4); the effect became significant when melatonin levels reached 1 nM, the estimated intracellular concentration of melatonin.[55] Also, melatonin counteracted cyanide-induced inhibition of C-IV. The changes induced by melatonin were also found to be associated with a rise in ATP production; this was true for untreated mitochondria and in mitochondria depleted of ATP with cyanide.

Collectively, these findings suggest that melatonin may have a significant role in maintaining mitochondrial homeostasis and increasing the efficiency of electron transport.[78] Although this has not been measured to date, melatonin would also be expected to reduce electron leak and thereby lower reactive oxygen species generation. These actions, coupled with melatonin's ability to maintain the stability of the inner-mitochondrial membrane,[79] indicate that the indole may be important for optimal electron transport and energy production, processes that are known to be diminished during aging when melatonin levels wane.

POTENTIAL LINKS BETWEEN MELATONIN AND AGING

A number of theories have proposed that melatonin modifies some processes of aging.[12] Some of these ideas evolved because endogenous melatonin production diminishes in advanced age in all species in which it has been investigated, including humans.[80] While the deterioration of function during aging correlates with the loss of melatonin, there is no proof that the two are related. There are data, however, suggesting that they may be.[81,82]

The impetus for a proposed relationship between melatonin and senescence derives, in part, from melatonin's ability to function as an antioxidant and free radical scavenger. There are certainly a variety of age-associated diseases, particularly of the brain, where free radicals are believed to be involved in the pathological process. This being the case, antioxidants would be of potential benefit to these degenerative conditions. In this regard, melatonin has been examined for its ability to forestall some of the signs of brain aging.[9,83] Diseases of particular interest have been Alzheimer's disease, Parkinsonism and Huntington's disease.[83–85] In the bulk of the studies where melatonin has been tested in experimental models of these diseases, its efficacy in reducing neuronal degradation and loss has been attributed to its ability to function as a ubiquitous and multifaceted free radical scavenger and antioxidant.

Tests of melatonin's ability to alter longevity per se have not been totally conclusive.[86] According to Pierpaoli and Regelson,[87] melatonin given to mice in the drinking water at night prolonged maximal like span. When melatonin was given during the day, however, it was ineffective. Similar studies, of which there have been only a few, have had similarly ambiguous outcomes when survival was the major endpoint.[83,86]

Pinealectomy, which deprives the animal of its endogenous melatonin rhythm, has been shown to hasten oxidative damage in a variety of organs throughout a lifetime, although in this study no evidence was provided that loss of the pineal gland actually shortened like span; that is, the animals were killed before they died.[88] What the study did show is that earlier pinealectomy (at two months of age) caused substantial accumulations of products of lipid peroxidation, oxidized DNA, and damaged protein in many organs when the animals reached 25 months of age, relative to those rats in which the pineal gland was left intact. Furthermore, the animals lacking their pineal gland had relatively less fluid cellular membranes (usually associated with increased products of lipid peroxidation) than did the intact rats. Because of the large number of endpoints that were measured, the report is suggestive of the ability of endogenously produced melatonin to slow the accumulation of oxidatively damaged molecules, which are usually taken as evidence of age-related deterioration. No definitive proof, however, was provided for melatonin being the deficient factor that resulted in what appeared to be accelerated aging.

CONCLUDING REMARKS

Knowledge concerning the ability of physiological, and especially pharmacological, doses of melatonin to prevent and/or defer what is referred to as oxidative stress has advanced rapidly in the last half decade.[9,40,66,89] Many of the mechanisms by which melatonin detoxifies oxygen and nitrogen-based reactants have been defined.[25,65,78,90] Additionally, melatonin's protective actions against an uncommonly wide variety of processes and toxins that generate oxidizing agents have been documented.[49,91] A major unanswered question, however, relates to the precise relationship of melatonin to senescent decline, a process widely believed to be, in part, a result of the persistent bludgeoning of macromolecules by free radicals.

REFERENCES

1. HALLIWELL, B. & J.M.C. GUTTERIDGE. 1989. Free Radicals in Biology and Medicine. Clarendon Press. Oxford, UK.
2. GRISHAM, M.B. 1992. Reactive Metabolites of Oxygen and Nitrogen in Biology and Medicine, R.G. Landes Co. Austin, TX.
3. HARMAN, D. 1956. Aging: a theory based on free radical and radiation chemistry. J. Gerontol. **11:** 298–300.
4. GERSHMAN, R., D.L. GILBERT, S.W. NYE, et al. 1954. Oxygen poisoning and x-irradiation: a mechanism in common. Science **119:** 623–626.
5. HARMAN, D. 1972. The biologic clock: the mitochondria? J. Am Geriatr. Soc. **20:** 145–147.
6. HARMAN, D. 1993. Free radicals and age-related degenerative diseases. *In* Free Radicals in Aging. B.P. Yu, Ed.: 205–222. CRC Press. Boca Raton, FL.
7. POLI, G., E. CADENAS & L. PACKER, Eds. 2000. Free Radials in Brain Pathophysiology. Marcel Dekker. New York.
8. DE GREY, D.N.J. 1999. The Mitochondrial Free Radial Theory of Aging. R.G. Landes Co. Austin, TX.
9. REITER, R.J. 1995. Oxidative processes and antioxidative defense mechanisms in the aging brain. FASEB J. **9:** 526–533.
10. TAYLOR, A. & T. NOVELL. 1997. Oxidative stress and antioxidant function in relation to risk of cataract. *In* Antioxidants in Disease Mechanisms and Therapy, H. Sies, Ed.: 516–536. Academic Press. San Diego, CA.
11. POEGGELER, B., R.J. REITER, D.X. TAN, et al. 1993. Melatonin, hydroxyl radical-mediated oxidative damage and aging: a hypothesis. J. Pineal Res. **14:** 151–158.
12. REITER, R.J. 1995. The pineal gland and melatonin in relation to aging: a summary of the theories and of the data. Exp. Gerontol. **30:** 199–212.
13. TAN, D.X., L.D. CHEN, B. POEGGELER, et al. 1993. Melatonin: a potent, endogenous hydroxyl radical scavenger. Endocrine J. **1:** 57–60.
14. REITER, R.J. 1991. Pineal melatonin: cell biology of its synthesis and of its biological interactions. Endocrine Rev. **12:** 151–180.
15. SUSA, N., S. UENO, Y. FURUKUSA, et al. 1997. Potent protective effect of melatonin on chromium (VI)-induced DNA single strand breaks, cytotoxicity and lipid proxidation in primary cultures of rat hepatocytes. Toxicol. Appl. Pharmacol. **144:** 377–384.
16. BRÖMME, H.J., W. MÖRKE, E. PESCHKE, et al. 2000. Scavenging effect of melatonin on hydroxyl radials generated by alloxan. J. Pineal Res. **29:** 201–208.
17. POEGGELER, G., R.J. REITER, R. HARDELAND, et al. 1996. Melatonin and structurally related, endogenous indoles act as potent electron donors and radical scavengers in vitro. Redox Rept. **2:** 179–184.
18. STASICA, P., P. ULANSKI & J.M. ROSIAK. 1998. Melatonin as a hydroxyl radical scavenger. J. Pineal Res. **25:** 65–66.
19. KHALDY, H. G. ESCAMES, J. LEON, et al. 2000. Comparative effects of melatonin, L-deprenyl, Trolox and ascorbate in the suppression of hydroxyl radical formation during dopamine autoxidation in vitro. J. Pineal Res. **29:** 100–107.
20. TAN, D.X., L.C. MANCHESTER, R.J. REITER, et al. 1998. A novel melatonin metabolite, cyclic 3-hydroxymelatonin: a biomarker of in vivo hydroxyl radical generation. Biochem. Biophys. Res. Commun. **253:** 614–620.
21. PÄHKLA, R., M. ZILMER, T. KULLISAR & L. RÄGO. 1998. Comparison of the antioxidant activity of melatonin and pinoline in vivo. J. Pineal Res. **24:** 96–101.
22. BANDYOPADHYAY, D., K. BISWAS, V. BANDYOPADHYAY, et al. 2000. Melatonin protects against stress-induced gastric lesions by scavenging hydroxyl radicals. J. Pineal Res. **29:** 143–151.
23. LI, X.J., J. GU, A.Z. ZHANG & R.Y. SUN. 1997. Melatonin decreases production of hydroxyl radicals during cerebral ischemia-reperfusion. Acta Pharm. Sin. **18:** 394–396.
24. MATUSZEK, Z., K. RESZKA & C.F. CHIGNELL. 1997. Reaction of melatonin and related indoles with hydroxyl radical: ESR and spin trapping investigators. Free Radic. Biol. Med. **23:** 367–372.

25. HARDELAND, R., R.J. REITER, B. POEGGELER & D.X. TAN. 1993. The significance of the metabolism of the neurohormone melatonin: antioxidant protection and formation of bioactive substances. Neurosci. Biobehav. Rev. **17:** 347–357.
26. MARSHALL, K.A., R.J. REITER, B. POEGGELER, *et al.* 1996. Evaluation of the antioxidant activity of melatonin in vitro. Free Radic. Biol. Med. **21:** 307–315.
27. ZANG L.Y., G. COSMA, H. GARDNER & V. VALLYNATHAN. 1998. Scavenging of reactive oxygen species by melatonin. Biochem. Biophys. Acta **1425:** 467–477.
28. ADRISANO, V., C. BERTUCCI, A. BATTAGLIA & V. CAVRINI. 2000. Photostability of drugs: photodegradation of melatonin and its determination in commercial formulations. J. Pharmaceut. Biomed. Anal. **23:** 15–23.
29. TAN, D.X., L.C. MANCHESTER, R.J. REITER, *et al.* 2001. Melatonin directly scavenges hydrogen peroxide: a potentially new metabolic pathway of melatonin biotransformation. Free Radic. Biol. Med. **29:** 1177–1185.
30. DELLEGAR, S.M., S.A. MURPHY, A.E. BOUNE, *et al.* 1999. Identification of factors affecting the rate of deactivation of hypochlorous acid by melatonin. Biophys. Biochem. Res. Commun. **257:** 431–439.
31. NODA, Y., A. MORI, R. LIBURTY & L. PACKER. 1999. Melatonin and its precursors scavenger nitric oxide. J. Pineal Res. **27:** 159–163.
32. TURJANSKI, A.G., F. LEONIK, R.E. ROSENSTEIN, *et al.* 2000. Scavenging of NO by melatonin. J. Am. Chem. Soc. **122:** 10468–10469.
33. TURJANSKI, A.G., D.A. SAINZ, F. DOCTOROVICH, *et al.* 2001. Nitrosation of melatonin by nitric oxide: a computational study. J. Pineal Res. **31:** 97–101.
34. ZHANG, H., G.L. SQUADRITO, R. UPPU & W.A. PRYOR. 1999. Reaction of peroxynitrite with melatonin: a mechanistic study. Chem. Res. Toxicol. **12:** 526–534.
35. BLANCHARD, B., D. POMPON & C. DUCROQ. 2000. Nitrosation of melatonin by nitric oxide and peroxynitrite. J. Pineal Res. **29:** 184–192.
36. PIERI, C., M. MORONI, F. MARCHESELLI & R. RECCHIONI. 1995. Melatonin is an efficient antioxidant. Arch. Gerontol. Geriatr. **20:** 159–165.
37. LIVREA, M., L. TESORIERE, D. D'ARPA & M. MORREALE. 1997. Reaction of melatonin with lipoperoxyl radicals in phospholipid bilayers. Free Radic. Biol. Med. **23:** 706–711.
38. ANTUNES, F., L.R.C. BARCLAY, K.O. INGOLD, *et al.* 1999. On the antioxidant activity of melatonin. Free Radic. Biol. Med. **26:** 117–128.
39. PRYOR, W. & G. SQUADRITO. 1995. The chemistry of peroxynitrite: a product from the reaction of nitric oxide with superoxide anion. Am. J. Physiol. **268:** L699–L722.
40. REITER, R.J., L. TANG, J.J. GARCIA & A. MUÑOZ-HOYOS. 1997. Pharmacological actions of melatonin in free radical pathophysiology. Life Sci. **60:** 2255–2271.
41. CUZZOCREA, S., G. COSTANTINO, E. GITTO, *et al.* 2000. Protective effects of melatonin in ischemic brain injury. J. Pineal Res. **29:** 217–227.
42. KARBOWNIK, M., D.X. TAN, L.C. MANCHESTER & R. J. REITER. 2000. Renal toxicity of the carcinogen δ-aminolevulinic acid: antioxidant effects of melatonin. Cancer Lett. **161:** 1–7.
43. KIM, S.J., R.J. REITER, W. QI, *et al.* 2000. Melatonin prevents oxidative damage to protein and lipid induced by ascorbate –Fe3+-EDTA: comparison with glutathione and α-tocopherol. Neuroendocrinol. Lett. **21:** 269–276.
44. CUZZOCREA, S., E. MAZZON, I. SERRIANO, *et al.* 2001. Melatonin reduces dinitrobenzene sulfonic acid-induced colitis. J. Pineal Res. **30:** 1–12.
45. TAN D.X., R.J. REITER, L.D. CHEN, *et al.* 1994. Both physiological and pharmacological levels of melatonin reduce DNA adduct formation induced by the carcinogen safrole. Carcinogenesis **15:** 315–318.
46. QI, W., R.J. REITER, D.X. TAN, *et al.* 2000. Increased levels of oxidatively damaged DNA induced by chromium (III) and H_2O_2: protection by melatonin and related molecules. J. Pineal Res. **29:** 54–61.
47. PAPPOLLA, M.A., Y.J. CHYAN, B. POEGGELER, *et al.* 1999. Alzheimer's b protein mediated oxidative damage of mitochondrial DNA: protection by melatonin. J. Pineal Res. **27:** 226–229.
48. WAKATSUKI, A., Y. OKATANI, K. SHINOHARA, *et al.* 2001. Melatonin protects fetal rat brain against oxidative mitochondria damage. J. Pineal Res. **30:** 22–28.

49. REITER, R.J., D.X. TAN, C. OSUNA & E. GITTO. 2000. Actions of melatonin in the reduction of oxidative stress. J. Biomed. Sci. **7:** 444–458.
50. FRAGA, C.G., M.K. SHIGENAGA, J.W. PARK, et al. 1990. Oxidative damage to DNA during aging: 8-hydroxy-2′-deoxyguanosine in rat organ DNA and urine. Proc. Nat. Acad. Sci. USA **87:** 4533–4537.
51. COSTA, E.J., R.H. LOPES & M.T. LAMY-FREUND. 1995. Permeability of pure lipid bilayers to melatonin. J. Pineal Res. **19:** 123–126.
52. SHIDA, C.S., A.M.L. CASTRUCCI & M.T. LAMY-FREUND. 1994. High melatonin solubility in aqueous medium. J. Pineal Res. **16:** 198–201.
53. MENENDEZ-PELAEZ, A. & R.J. REITER. 1993. Distribution of melatonin in mammalian tissues: relative importance of nuclear verses cytosolic localization. J. Pineal Res. **15:** 59–69.
54. MENENDEZ-PELAEZ, A., B. POEGGELER, R.J. REITER, et al. 1993. Nuclear localization of melatonin in different mammalian tissues: immunocytochemical and radioimmunoassay evidence. J. Cell. Biochem. **53:** 373–382.
55. MARTIN, M., M. MACIAS, G. ESCAMES, et al. 2000. Melatonin but not vitamins C and E maintain glutathione homeostasis in t-butyl hydroperoxide-induced mitochondrial oxidative stress. FASEB J. **14:** 1677–1679.
56. STEFULJ, J., M. HÖRTNER, M. GHOSH, et al. 2001. Gene expression of the key enzymes of melatonin synthesis in extrapineal tissues of the rat. J. Pineal Res. **30:** 243–247.
57. ANTOLIN, I., C. RODRIQUEZ, R.M. SAINZ, et al. 1996. Neurohormone melatonin prevents cell damage: effect on gene expression for antioxidative enzymes. FASEB J. **10:** 882–890.
58. PABLOS, M.I., R.J. REITER, G.G. ORTIZ, et al. 1998. Rhythms of glutathione peroxidase and glutathione reductase in brain of chick: their inhibition by light. Neurochem. Int. **32:** 69–75.
59. ALBARRAN, M.T., S. LOPEZ-BURILLO, M.I. PABLOS, et al. 2001. Endogenous rhythms of melatonin, total antioxidant status and superoxide dismutase activity in several tissues of chick and their inhibition by light. J. Pineal Res. **30:** 227–233.
60. BECKMAN, J.S. & W.H. KOPPENOL. 1996. Nitric oxide, superoxide, and peroxynitrite: the good, the bad and the ugly. Am. J. Physiol. **271:** 427–437.
61. HARA, M., M. YOSHIDA, H. NISHIJIMA, et al. 2001. Melatonin, a pineal secretory product with antioxidant properties, protects against cisplatin-induced nephrotoxicity in rats. J. Pineal Res. **30:** 129–138.
62. URATA, Y., S. HONMA, S. GOTO, et al. 1999. Melatonin induces γ-glutamylcysteine synthetase mediated by activator protein-1 in human vascular endothelial cells. Free Radic. Biol. Med. **27:** 838–847.
63. MEISTER, A. 1980. Glutathione metabolism and its selective modification. J. Biol. Chem. **263:** 17205–17208.
64. POZO, D., R.J. REITER, J.M. CALVO & J.M. GUERRERO. 1997. Inhibition of nitric oxide synthase and cyclic GMP production by melatonin via complex formation with calmodulin. J. Cell. Biochem. **45:** 430–442.
65. TAN, D.X., L.C. MANCHESTER, R.J. REITER, et al. 2000. Significance of melatonin in antioxidative defense system: reactions and products. Biol. Signals Recept. **9:** 137–159.
66. REITER, R.J. 2000. Melatonin: lowering the high price of free radicals. News Physiol. Sci. **15:** 246–250.
67. KARBOWNIK, M. & R.J. REITER. 2000. Antioxidative effects of melatonin in protection against cellular damage caused by ionizing radiation. Proc. Soc. Exp. Biol. Med. **225:** 9–22.
68. SOHAL, R.S. 1997. Role of mitochondria and oxidative stress in the aging process. *In* Mitochondria, Free Radicals and Neurodegenerative Disease. M.F. Beal, N. Howell, & I. Bodis-Wallmer, Eds.: 99–107. Wiley-Liss. New York.
69. BARJA, G. 1999. Mitochondrial oxygen radical generation and leak: sites of production in states 4 and 3, organ specificity, and relation to aging and longevity. J. Bioenerg. Biomembr. **31:** 347–366.
70. NATHAN, A.T. & M. SINGER. 1999. Mitochondria and neuronal survival. Br. Med. Bull. **55:** 96–108.

71. MANCHESTER, L.C., B. POEGGELER, F.L. ALVARES, et al. 1995. Melatonin immunoreactivity in the photosynthetic prokaryote *Rhodospirillum rubrum*: implications for an ancient antioxidant system. Cell. Mol. Biol. Res. **41:** 321–325.
72. YAMAMOTO, H.A. & H.W. TANG. 1996. Preventive effect of melatonin against cyanide-induced seizures and lipid peroxidation in mice. Neurosci. Lett. **207:** 89–92.
73. DE ANTENOR, M.S., I.R. DE ROMERO, E. BRAUCKMANN, et al. 1994. Effects of the pineal gland and melatonin on the metabolism of oocytes in vitro and in ovulation in *Bufo arenarum*. J. Exp. Zool. **268:** 436–441.
74. GILAD, E., S. CUZZOCREA, B. ZINGARELLI, et al. 1997. Melatonin is a scavenger of peroxynitrite. Life Sci. **60:** PL169–PL174.
75. MILCZAREK, R., J. KLIMEK & L. ZELEWSKI. 2000. Melatonin inhibits NADPH-dependent lipid peroxidation in human placental mitochondria. Horm. Metab. Res. **32:** 84–85.
76. ABSI, E., A. AYALA, A. MACHADO & J. PARRADO. 2000. Protective effect of melatonin against the 1-methyl-4-phenylpyridinium-induced inhibition of Complex I of the mitochondrial respiratory chain. J. Pineal Res. **29:** 40–47.
77. MARTIN, M., M. MACIAS, G. ESCAMES, et al. 2000. Melatonin-induced increased activity of the respiratory chain complexes I and IV can prevent mitochondrial damage induced by ruthenium red in vivo. J. Pineal Res. **28:** 242–248.
78. ACUÑA-CASTROVIEJO, D., M. MARTIN, M. MACIAS, et al. 2001. Melatonin, mitochondria, and cellular bioenergetics. J. Pineal Res. **30:** 65–74.
79. GARCIA, J.J., R.J. REITER, J. PIE, et al. 1999. Role of pinoline and melatonin in stabilizing hepatic microsomal membranes against oxidative damage. J. Bioenerg. Biomembr. **31:** 609–616.
80. REITER, R.J. 1992. The aging pineal gland and its physiological consequences. Bio Essays **14:** 169–175.
81. REITER, R.J. 1997. Aging and oxygen toxicity: relation to changes in melatonin. Age **20:** 201–213.
82. REITER, R.J., M.I. PABLOS, M.T. AGAPITO & J. M. GUERRERO. 1996. Melatonin in the context of the free radical theory of aging. Ann. N.Y. Acad. Sci. **786:** 362–378.
83. REITER, R.J. 1998. Oxidative damage in the central nervous system: protection by melatonin. Prog. Neurobiol. **56:** 359–384.
84. REITER, R.J., J. CABRERA, R.M. SAINZ, et al. 1999. Melatonin as a pharmacological agent against neuronal loss in experimental models of Huntington's disease, Alzheimer's disease and Parkinsonism. Ann. N.Y. Acad. Sci. **890:** 471–484.
85. PAPPOLLA, M.A., Y.J. CHYAN, B. POEGGELER, et al. 2000. An assessment of the antioxidant and the antiamyloidogenic properties of melatonin: implications for Alzheimer's disease. J. Neural Transm. **107:** 203–231.
86. REITER, R.J. 2000. Melatonin and aging. *In* The Science of Geriatrics. J.E. Mosley, H.J. Armbrecht, R.M. Coe & B. Vellas, Eds.: Vol. I: 323–333. Springer. New York.
87. PIERPAOLI, W. & W. REGELSON. 1991. Pineal control of aging: effect of melatonin and pineal grafting on aging mice. Proc. Natl. Acad. Sci. USA **91:** 787–791.
88. REITER, R.J., D.X. TAN, S.J. KIM, et al. 1999. Augmentation of indices of oxidative damage in life-long melatonin-deficient rats. Mech. Aging Develop. **110:** 157–173.
89. REITER, R.J., D.X. TAN, D. ACUÑA-CASTROVIEJO, et al. 2000. Melatonin: mechanisms and actions as an antioxidant. Curr. Top. Biophys. **24:** 171–183.
90. REITER, R.J., D.X. TAN, L.C. MANCHESTER & W. QI. 2001. Biochemical reactivity of melatonin with reactive oxygen and nitrogen species: a review of the literature. Cell Biochem. Biophys. **34:** 237–256.
91. REITER, R.J., D.X. TAN, L.C. MANCHESTER & J.R. CALVO. 2002. Antioxidative capacity of melatonin. *In* Handbook of Antioxidants. E. Cadenas & L. Packer, Eds.: 565–613. Marcel Dekker. New York.

Metabolic Alterations and Shifts in Energy Allocations Are Corequisites for the Expression of Extended Longevity Genes in *Drosophila*

ROBERT ARKING,[a] STEVEN BUCK,[a] DAE-SUNG HWANGBO,[a] AND MARK LANE[b]

[a]*Department of Biological Sciences, Wayne State University, Detroit, Michigan 48202, USA*

[b]*Laboratory of Neurosciences, National Institute on Aging, National Institutes of Health, Baltimore, Maryland 21224, USA*

ABSTRACT: Evolutionary theories suggest that the expression of extended longevity depends on the organism's ability to shift energy from reproduction to somatic maintenance. New data led us to reexamine our older data and integrate the two into a larger picture of the genetic and metabolic alterations required if the animal is to live long. Our Ra normal-lived control strain can express any one of three different extended longevity phenotypes, only one of which involves significant and proportional increases in both mean and maximum longevity and thus a delayed onset of senescence. This phenotype is dependent on the up-regulation of the antioxidant defense system (ADS) genes and enzymes. Animals that express this phenotype typically have a pattern of altered specific activities in metabolically important enzymes, suggesting they are necessary to support the $NAD^+/NADP^+$ reducing system required for the continued high ADS enzyme activities. Fecundity data suggests that the energy required for this higher level of somatic maintenance initially came from a reduced egg production. This was only transient, however, for the females significantly increased their fecundity in later generations while still maintaining their longevity. The energy required for this enhanced fecundity was probably obtained from an increased metabolic efficiency, for the mitochondria of the La long-lived strain are metabolically more efficient and have a lower leakage of reactive oxygen species (ROS) to the cytosol. Selection pressures that do not lead to these shifts in energy allocations result in extended longevity phenotypes characterized by increased early survival or increased late survival but not by a delayed onset of senescence.

KEYWORDS: extended longevity phenotypes; metabolic alterations; energy allocations; genes; aging; *Drosophila*; free radicals; ROS; antioxidant defense systems; somatic maintenance; fecundity; mathematical modeling

Address for correspondence: Robert Arking, Department of Biological Sciences, Wayne State University, Detroit, Michigan 48202. Voice: 313-577-2891; fax: 313-577-6891.
rarking@biology.biosci.wayne.edu

INTRODUCTION

We used artificial selection to generate long-lived strains of *Drosophila* and over the years have done a series of comparative experiments in order to deduce what processes had been significantly altered and therefore might play an important role in the expression of the extended longevity phenotype. A review of all the work done on these strains, including mutational analysis, has been recently presented.[1] The essential characteristic of the long-lived La strain, resulting from this treatment, is that it lives long due to a delayed onset of senescence brought about by an early and specific up-regulation of the antioxidant defense system (ADS) genes.[2–4] New information allows us to integrate that finding into a larger picture of the genetic and metabolic alterations required if the animal is to express the extended longevity phenotype.

THE THREE PHENOTYPES OF EXTENDED LONGEVITY

One particularly striking point that emerged from our experiments was the fact that our normal-lived Ra control strain was capable of giving rise to three different types of extended longevity phenotypes when subjected to three different stimuli.[5] Only one of these phenotypes (type 1, in our terminology) involved significant and proportional increases in both the mean and maximum life span values. These are, of course, the characteristics that denote what is usually meant when we talk about a significant increase in longevity. The other two phenotypes involve increases in early (type 2) or late (type 3) adult survival but not both, and these lead to increases in mean longevity but not to significant and proportional increases in maximum longevity.

In our hands, the type 1 extended longevity phenotype is only expressed in organisms who are significantly more resistant to oxidative stress.[6,7] The type 2 phenotype seems to be associated with organisms who have a decreased resistance to oxidative stress and an enhanced P450 activity.[8] The type 3 phenotype is likely associated with increased expression of hsp genes and gene products.

Thus, the Ra strain can give rise to three different phenotypes, all of which increase the mean longevity and therefore technically bring about an "extended longevity" phenotype. However, only the type 1 ADS-dependent phenotype brings about a delayed onset of senescence, which is really the important aspect of current aging studies. The data presented below suggests that a metabolic reorganization involving both the ADS genes and the mitochondria are involved in the expression of this phenotype. Changing the expression of key genes seems to bring about a supporting metabolic reorganization of the organism.

METABOLIC ENZYMES AND LONGEVITY

Our biomarker data[2] suggested that the earliest determining event in the expression of the extended longevity phenotype took place early in adult life at about 5–7 days of age. Other data[3–4,7] documented the specific up-regulation of the ADS genes and enzymes beginning at this age. We also determined whether any metabolic changes occurred, and if they were general or specific in nature,[9] by assaying the

TABLE 1. Enzymes that show repeatable significant differences in the various selected strains relative to their progenitor strains[a]

Selected Strains	L	2L	RevL
Phenotype:	Long-lived	Long-lived	Normal-lived
Progenitor Strain:	R	R	L
Increase	AK		NADPHdia
	HK	HK	
		NADHdia	
	PGM	PGM	
		XDH	
	G6PDH		
Decrease	NADPHdia	NADPHdia	
		GAPDH	GPI
			G6PDH
			G3PDH
			HK
			ICD
			MDH
			ME

[a]Data taken from Buck and Arking.[9] The enzymes listed show significant concordant changes in replicate strains of each strain type. Each assay was based on the values of three dependent samples in each replicate strain. See original reference for experimental details and data on other strains.

specific activity of 17 metabolically important enzymes in 5- to 7-day-old flies of 13 strains variously selected for different longevities. The relevant data, summarized in TABLE 1, suggests that there are specific metabolic changes associated with the up-regulated ADS enzyme activities characteristic of the long-lived strains.

Those data[9] strongly suggest that the Lab strains are likely to have a higher flux through the pentose shunt. This generates increased levels of NADPH, which is used for the detoxification of peroxides formed after the dismutation of superoxide by CuZnSOD.[10] The elevated ADS activities known to occur in these strains require correspondingly elevated NADPH levels if the enzymes are to function effectively. These can be produced by the pentose shunt. Classic insect biochemistry studies have shown that insects usually have a deficient NADPH reoxidizing system;[11] thus the activity of the pentose shunt depends on the rate of reoxidation of NADPH. The down-regulation of NADPHdia would release the $NADP^+$-dependent inhibition of G6PDH, thereby increasing the metabolic flux through the pentose shunt, and increasing the reduction of the $NADP^+$ produced by the ADS enzymes. This scenario would require a higher G6PDH activity, which is observed. Isocitrate dehydrogenase (ICD) not only regulates the flux through the TCA cycle but also generates NADPH. The enzymes glucose-6-phosphate dehydrogenase (G6PDH) and ICD both generate NADPH, and both have been implicated in influencing life span in *Drosophila* by

TABLE 2. Pleiotropic effects of selection for delayed fecundity on fecundity are transient

Generation of selection	Percent of La life span in which the mean daily fecundity of the La female < Ra female	Total eggs/female/lifetime Ra	Total eggs/female/lifetime La	La/Ra Life Span Ratio
F1	100%	1726	620	0.81
F5	76%	1752	1288	1.13
F9	16%	766	906	1.37
F13	15%	562	1170	1.22
F21	2%	1195	1516	1.64

other investigations.[12,13] We conclude that the Lab strains have extended their longevity by using a metabolic strategy based on the significant up-regulation of the ADS system (particularly CuZnSOD and MnSOD in the case of the La strains[4] or catalase in the case of the Lb strains[7]), coupled with the significant up-regulation of the pentose shunt in both cases. Reverse selecting the Lab strains for a normal life span yields the RevL$_{ab}$ strains. These strains show a mirror-image pattern of ADS[4,7] and metabolic enzyme increases and decreases relative to their Lab progenitor strains (TABLE 1), thus showing that the two sets of enzymes are coupled and essential to the expression of the extended longevity phenotype.

By contrast, the 2Lab strains appear to have a significantly reduced flux through the pentose shunt and apparently depend on an increased flux through the glycolytic and TCA cycle. They also have a significant increase in their XDH activity, the product of which is a nonenzymatic ROS scavenger. Presumably these may function as a NADP$^+$-reducing system for the elevated ADS genes presumably involved in these strains, in much the same manner as ascorbic acid is known to function in the reduction of oxidized glutathione or vitamin E.[14] We conclude that the 2Lab strains have extended their longevity by using a metabolic strategy based on the significant up-regulation of the ADS system (as evidenced by their significant resistance to oxidative stress[14]) coupled with a significant increase in uric acid to function as the required NADP$^+$-reducing system.

Both the Lab and 2Lab strategies can be interpreted as an increased energy expenditure on somatic maintenance. We conclude that theories based on differential energy allocations, such as the disposable soma theory of Kirkwood[16] or the optimality theory of Partridge and Barton,[17] might be able to empirically explain, at least in part, the mechanisms underlying the transformation of a normal longevity phenotype to an extended longevity phenotype. There are some conceptual problems, however, with this conclusion that we will address in the next two sections.

LONGEVITY AND FECUNDITY: ANOTHER LOOK AT ANTAGONISTIC PLEIOTROPY

In TABLE 2, we present a summary of previously unpublished fecundity data for the Ra and La strains during the course of the original selection experiment.[18,19] It may be seen that the initial results of selection for delayed female fecundity showed that fecundity really was significantly decreased in the (presumptive) La strain relative to the Ra control strain. In the F1 generation, this is demonstrated not only by the fact that the total lifetime fecundity of the Ra females was 2.8-fold greater than that of the F1 La females, but also by the fact that the mean fecundity (eggs/female/day/lifetime) of the Ra females was greater than the La females on every day of their life. By the F5 generation, the La females had about doubled their mean fecundity, and in fact the older La females outperformed the older Ra females during the last 12% of their life span. By the time of the next measurement, the F9 Ra females had a higher mean daily fecundity than the La females only over the initial 22% (12 days) of their mean life span. After day 13, the La females outperformed them, thus accounting for the higher total number of eggs per lifetime for the La females relative to the Ra females. By F13 onwards, the Ra animals not only continued to lay fewer total eggs per female per lifetime than did the La animals, but their once higher mean daily fecundity now became progressively compressed to the first 10 (F13) or 4 (F21) days of their life. The Lb data (not shown) suggests that the same phenomenon happened in the sister strain as well.

When we reported some of these fecundity results at the time, we focused only on the F21 data and suggested that the higher mean daily fecundity of the young Ra females relative to the young La females "…implies that the effects of the early eggs on inclusive fitness are probably greater than are the effects of the later eggs" (Ref. 20, p. 13) and that "…the early reproductive superiority of control strains relative to the NDC-L strain has been previously noted and reported as evidence supporting the pleiotropic gene theory of life span evolution…." (Ref. 19, p. 214).

Those conclusions were true enough so far as they went, but since they did not address the transient nature of this pleiotropic response, they implicitly assumed that the evolutionary tradeoff of reduced fecundity for long life was a permanent feature of the extended longevity phenotype. It is not, and since it was a transient feature only, then this implies that the La females used the time of the first five to nine generations of selection to somehow reorganize themselves so that by the end of selection they had the ability to both be more fecund and live longer than the nonselected Ra control animals. This outcome was not explicitly predicted by theory. We need to understand what processes might have been reorganized during this interval and how this relates to the selection process.

MATHEMATICAL MODELING OF THE Ra STRAIN

Since the La animal is known to have the same mean daily metabolic rate as does the Ra animal,[21,22] then the extra energy needed for this improved somatic maintenance must be obtained at the expense of some other variable. Mathematical modeling of the Ra strain's metabolic energy expenditures on reproduction and somatic maintenance suggests that the typical Ra female is exercising an optimal allocation of energy to these two compartments.[23] Indeed, the fecundity data and longevity data (not shown) for the short-lived Ea female suggests that she suffers from a lack of somatic maintenance relative to the Ra female. Mathematical modeling also suggests that decreasing the energy spent on egg production would significantly increase life span.[23] In the case of the La female, increasing the flux through the pentose shunt and using the reduced NADPH generated therein to oxidize the ADS enzymes instead of being used to generate more ATP, represents an increase in the amount of energy being used for somatic maintenance.

If this is actually the operative strategy being used by the La female, then it must follow that there should be a deleterious effect on reproduction, but the above reexamination of the fecundity data showed that the deleterious reproductive effects on the La animal were transient and have all but disappeared by the F21 generation. The outcome of this contradiction is that the evolutionary tradeoff implicit in the antagonistic pleiotropy theory is not a one-time event but is rather a dynamic and transient process. Thus, although the shift of energy from reproduction might be sufficient to start the processes necessary to longevity, it is not required to maintain these processes over the long term. How then does the La female obtain sufficient energy to be both fecund and long-lived?

LA AND RA MITOCHONDRIA ARE DIFFERENT FROM ONE ANOTHER

What other processes were altered during the first five to nine generations of selection that eventually enabled the La animal to be both fecund and long-lived? We believe that the energy not expended on reproduction was used by these animals to reorganize their mitochondria and their metabolism. Let us examine the available data.

We showed that the mean daily metabolic rates of the Ra and La animals were statistically identical.[21] Ross[22] confirmed these findings, using animals from sister strains to our own and extended them by showing that the La mitochondria have significantly lower age-specific rates of mitochondrial H_2O_2 production TABLE 3). Young La mitochondria are around 20% less leaky than are comparably aged Ra mitochondria. In addition to this difference in absolute values, the La mitochondria show a much slower rate of increase in H_2O_2 production.

The simplest interpretation of these data is that the mitochondrial membrane of the La animal suffers less oxidative damage due to the generation of ROS than do the Ra mitochondria.[22] Barja and his colleagues[25] have shown that the mitochondria of long-lived vertebrates have significantly lower levels of fatty acid unsaturation than do the mitochondria of short-lived vertebrates. This low double bond content in their mitochondrial lipids results from a redistribution of the types of fatty acids being synthesized and incorporated into the mitochondrial membrane and make the mitochondrial membrane significantly less sensitive to lipid peroxidation damage. Barja and his colleagues conclude that the capacity of longevous vertebrates to produce less mitochondrially derived H_2O_2 is thought to be due to their lower leakage of ROS from the mitochondria, which in turn might be due both to the altered membrane composition and their ability to maintain a lower degree of reduction of the complex I oxygen radical generator in the steady state condition. They also conclude that there is a robust correlation between the flux of free radical attack to mtDNA and the aging rate of vertebrates.

The above findings show that the La and Ra mitochondria differ in significant ways from one another and that these observed differences are consistent with those observed to be significantly related to life span differences in vertebrates. If these suggestions are correct, then the La mitochondria should be responsible for much of

TABLE 3. La mitochondria are less leaky than Ra mitochondria[a]

Age	nmol/min of H_2O_2/mg protein (mean value only) Ra	La	Percent difference of La relative to Ra at each age	Percent increase in H_2O_2 Ra	La
15	1.9	1.5	−21%		
29	2.1	1.7	−20%	11%	13%
42	3.1	2.0	−36%	48%	18%
58	4.1	2.5	−40%	32%	25%
70	—	2.8	—	—	12%

[a] Data taken from FIG. 3 of Ross.[22] See original reference for experimental details and variance estimates.

the life span differences noted in our strains. Driver and Tawadros[26] have critically tested this assumption by performing standard genetic crosses to produce a strain with a (mostly) Ra nuclear genome and (mostly) La mitochondria (designated as the La-mt strain). When the life span of this strain was compared to that of the control Ra-mt strain, the La-mt strain showed about a 25% increase in longevity that was nutrient dependent. This result demonstrates mitochondrial autonomy and suggests that the altered La mitochondria are largely, but not entirely, responsible for the increased longevity of our La strain. This finding is consistent with the data of Ross[22] and lends further weight to our assumption that the findings of Barja and colleagues may apply to flies as well.

A REVISED HYPOTHESIS

Given the new information presented here, what can we say about the nature of the events that probably took place during the selection process? And what is the impact of these new data on the evolutionary interpretation of our selection experiments? We now formulate a revised and dynamic view of the effects of selection on the flies.

The initial selection for delayed female fecundity gave rise to F1 animals whose fecundity was significantly reduced and delayed relative to the nonselected Ra controls (TABLE 3). This then represents an upsetting of the optimal energy allocations to somatic maintenance and reproduction characteristic of the Ra animal, which in the case of the Ra female are approximately 64 µL/O_2/day for reproduction and about 81 µL/O_2/day for somatic maintenance.[23] As much as 42.5% of the total energy available, or about 31% if averaged over the entire life span, is devoted to egg production.[23] This is a large number. Reducing the mean lifetime egg output by approximately 64% in the F1 generation reduces this cost to about 10% of total lifetime energy and frees up a great deal of energy that must therefore be allocated to somatic maintenance. The animals used this newly available energy in three ways:

- One was the up-regulation of the ADS genes. We have no data on the changes in this variable over the course of the first 21 generations of selection, but we assume that this happened in an incremental fashion. Part of the reason for this involved the necessity to divert NADPH from being used for ATP production and use it instead for the detoxification of peroxides formed after the dismutation of superoxide by CuZnSOD. Without this diversion of an energy-rich compound, it would have proven difficult to substantially increase ADS enzyme activities. Without such an increase, there would have been no selective pressure to up-regulate ADS gene transcription.

- Second was the shift to the pentose shunt (TABLE 1), presumably done in order to more easily supply the quantities of NADPH required to maintain the up-regulated ADS enzymes at their heightened activity.[4]

- Third was the alteration of the mitochondrial membrane fatty acid composition and other possible changes necessary to reduce the leakage of H_2O_2 from the mitochondria into the cytosol. This alteration was most likely driven by the conditions of our selection protocol, which required that all the animals used to found the next selection generation were taken from the first 300 adults to hatch following a 48-hour egg-laying period.[19] This not only selected for fast development of the larvae but also selected for maximal early fecundity of the females. Only those La females who rapidly increased their mean daily fecundity would contribute to the next generation. The concurrent selection for long life inherent in our selection protocol meant that they could not simply shift energy from maintenance back to reproduction. They were forced to adopt a new strategy. Presumably the energy freed up by the initial reduction in egg production was more or less captured by the ADS up-regulation/pentose shunt alterations discussed above. The only way to capture more energy was to increase the metabolic efficiency by reducing the ROS leakage across the mitochondrial membrane. The ~20% initial decrease in this leakage (TABLE 3) made available to the animal the ATPs eventually produced by those now-recaptured electrons. By reducing the ROS load in the cytosol, it also allowed for some reduction in the amount of ADS defenses and/or repair systems previously required to maintain the "youthful" state of the cell. This recaptured energy could now be diverted from somatic maintenance back to egg production, beginning with the F9 generation (TABLE 2).

The net result of these changes is an animal that can live long while still being very fecund. Why then is the world not overrun with long-lived *Drosophila*? It cannot be the reduced fecundity, for we have shown that it is transient and gives rise to a significantly increased fecundity. We have previously shown that all of our long-lived strains exhibit a significant reduction in developmental viability relative to the normal-lived strains, ranging from 3 to 18% reduction in the number of eggs giving rise to viable adults.[27] These numbers are evolutionarily significant and might arise from metabolic complications stemming from coordinating the three different metabolic alterations described above. The Ra animal may well be at an optimal level of energy expenditures for the developmental stages as well as for the adult stages.

GENES, ENERGY METABOLISM, AND EXTENDED LONGEVITY

The type 1 phenotype is also found in calorically restricted rodents.[28] Although the molecular mechanism(s) underlying the effects of caloric restriction is not yet definitively known, the physiological and molecular similarities between caloric restriction effects and the operation of the insulin-like signaling system (ISS) genes in *C. elegans* are such as to make it very plausible that caloric restriction works through the ISS genes in mammals as well, and this has been formally suggested by Lane.[29] The involvement of the ISS genes are certainly capable of conceptually explaining the altered fecundity, metabolism, and stress resistance of the calorically restricted mammal. We presented preliminary data[6] showing that down-regulation of the ISS genes in our Ra strain led to a type 1 extended longevity phenotype, in which these long-lived animals had a significantly higher resistance to oxidative stress. Our findings are consistent with the more detailed analyses put forth by Clancy *et al.*[30] and Tatar *et al.*,[31] which also demonstrate that mutational down-regulation of the ISS genes in *Drosophila* yields a type 1 phenotype. It seems as if all the type 1 mechanisms are united at a deep biological level by their effects on metabolism and oxidative stress resistance. Furthermore, similar sorts of metabolic reorganization have been reported in caloric-restriction experiments,[28] as is a report that energy restriction decreases proton leaks.[32] The phenomena are not limited to *Drosophila*. It is reasonable to conclude that all these ADS-dependent type 1 mechanisms must be affecting the same or overlapping pathways. We present in FIGURE 1 a model of just how the ADS, caloric restriction, and mitochondrial alteration interventions may be plausibly connected with one another and with extended longevity. The net result of these changes is to shift the cells, and therefore the organism, form a growth and reproduction strategy to one of survival and life maintenance. At the cellular level, this would likely be evidenced by a shift in the corresponding cell-signaling pathways, for instance, for P13K, and toward, for example, MAPK and ERK. Molecular mechanisms that impart stress resistance without the requisite metabolic alterations needed to shift energy from reproduction to somatic maintenance are most likely not capable of inducing the expression of a type 1 phenotype.[33]

A particular kind of metabolic reorganization is a necessary prerequisite for the expression of the type 1 extended longevity phenotype in our long-lived strains. This reorganization is a dynamic process involving both the mitochondrial and nuclear compartments and that eventually results in the increased metabolic efficiency of the La female adult. This reorganization frees up sufficient energy in a two-step process to support high levels of fecundity and somatic maintenance. This process is characterized by an initial drop in fecundity and corresponding increase in somatic maintenance followed by a reduction in mitochondrial ROS generation and corresponding increase in fecundity. Stress responses that do not induce such a metabolic reorganization can only induce a type 2 or type 3 extended longevity phenotype. We note that this hypothesis does not fully explain the longevity of the La male adult, but it is known that males and females likely use different genes and mechanisms to express their longevity.[34]

This conclusion marks a significant modification of the stress theories of longevity,[35,36] for it both imposes limits on the types of competent mechanisms and offers insight into their nature. While compatible with the antagonistic pleiotropy theory,[37]

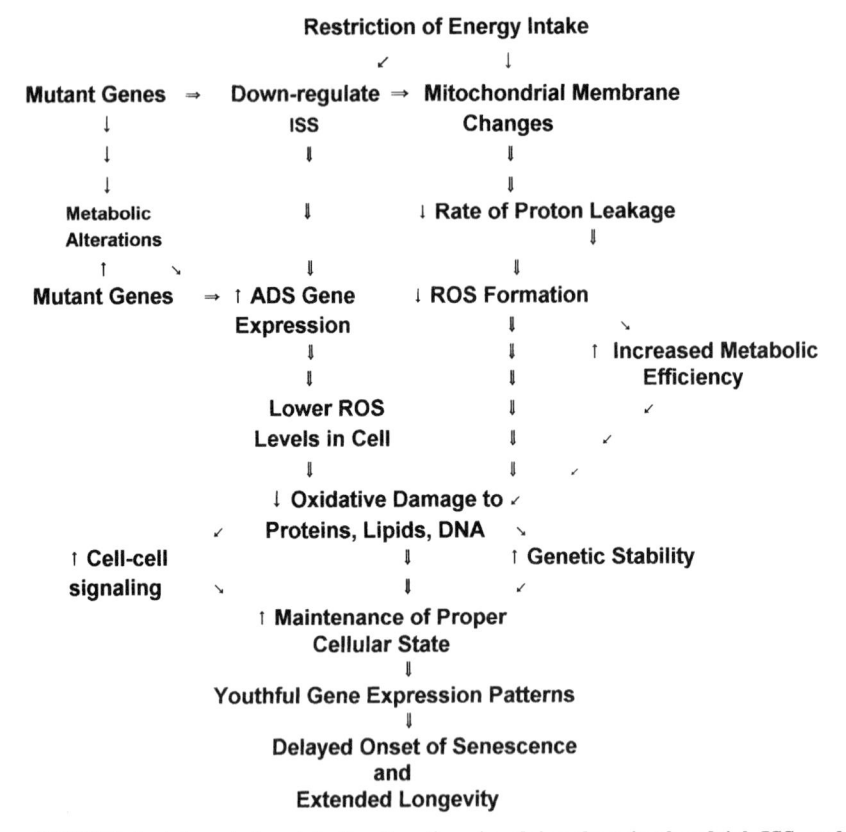

```
                          Restriction of Energy Intake
                                ↙        ↓
   Mutant Genes  →   Down-regulate  →  Mitochondrial Membrane
         ↓                 ISS                 Changes
         ↓                  ⇓                    ⇓
         ↓                  ⇓                    ⇓
      Metabolic             ⇓            ↓ Rate of Proton Leakage
     Alterations                                 ⇓
         ↑        ↘         ⇓                    ⇓
   Mutant Genes  →  ↑ ADS Gene            ↓ ROS Formation
                     Expression                  ⇓             ↘
                         ⇓                       ⇓        ↑ Increased Metabolic
                         ⇓                       ⇓              Efficiency
                      Lower ROS                  ⇓             ↙
                     Levels in Cell              ⇓          ↙
                         ⇓                       ⇓       ↙
                     ↓ Oxidative Damage to  ↙
                ↙     Proteins, Lipids, DNA   ↘
    ↑ Cell-cell              ⇓             ↑ Genetic Stability
     signaling   ↘           ⇓             ↙
                     ↑ Maintenance of Proper
                        Cellular State
                              ⇓
                  Youthful Gene Expression Patterns
                              ⇓
                     Delayed Onset of Senescence
                              and
                       Extended Longevity
```

FIGURE 1. Integrated metabolic alterations involving the mitochondrial, ISS, and ADS genes increase metabolic efficiency and alter optimal energy allocations to somatic maintenance versus reproduction. A synthesis of the interventions and mechanisms known to yield a type 1 extended longevity phenotype in the Ra strain of *Drosophila* and in other model organisms. There is a convergence of data on these interrelated mechanisms that can yield large decreases in oxidative stress and a concomitant enhancement of somatic maintenance. The mitochondrial reorganization can free up additional energy via an increased metabolic efficiency.

it suggests that the processes involved may be more complex than were initially envisioned. All of these questions deserve further consideration. A more detailed analysis of these processes and their applicability to other long-lived *Drosophila* was presented elsewhere.[24]

ACKNOWLEDGMENTS

RA was a Korean Science and Engineering Foundation "Expert Brain Pool" Visiting Research Professor at Pusan National University during the writing of this manuscript and appreciates the congenial and profitable interactions with Professors M.A. Yoo and H.Y. Chung during that time.

REFERENCES

1. ARKING, R. 2001. Gene expression and regulation in the extended longevity phenotypes of *Drosophila*. Ann. N.Y. Acad. Sci. **928:** 157–167.
2. ARKING, R. & R.A. WELLS. 1990. Genetic alteration of normal aging processes is responsible for extended longevity in *Drosophila*. Dev. Genetics **11:** 141–148.
3. DUDAS, S.P. & R. ARKING. 1995. A coordinate upregulation of antioxidant gene activities is associated with the delayed onset of senescence in a long-lived strain of *Drosophila*. J. Gerontol.: Biol. Sci. **50A:** B117–B127.
4. ARKING, R., V. BURDE, K. GRAVES, *et al.* 2000. Forward and reverse selection for longevity in *Drosophila* is characterized by alteration of antioxidant gene expression and oxidative damage patterns. Exp. Gerontol. **35:** 167–185.
5. ARKING, R., J. NOVOSELTSEVA, D-S. HWANGBO, V. NOVOSELTSEV & M. LANE. 2002. Genomic and phenotypic plasticity: multiple molecular mechanisms give rise to different types of extended longevity phenotypes in *Drosophila*. Submitted.
6. LANE, M., S. FELDMAN, D-S. HWANGBO & R. ARKING. 2000. Down-regulation of insulin signaling increases longevity in *Drosophila*. Poster presented at Gerontol. Soc. America Annual Meeting. Washington, D.C.
7. ARKING, R., V. BURDE, K. GRAVES, *et al.* 2000. Identical longevity phenotypes are characerized by different patterns of gene expression and oxidative damage. Exp. Gerontol. **35:** 353–373.
8. VETTRAINO, J., S. BUCK & R. ARKING. 2001. Direct selection for paraquat resistance in *Drosophila* results in a different extended longevity phenotype. J. Gerontol. A Biol. Sci. Med. Sci. **56:** B415–425.
9. BUCK, S.A. & R. ARKING. 2001. Metabolic alterations in genetically selected *Drosophila* strains with different longevities. J. Am. Aging Assoc. In press.
10. FEUERS, R.J., P.H. DUFFY, F. CHEN, *et al.* 1995. Intermediary metabolism and antioxidant systems. *In* Dietary Restriction: Implications for the Design and Interpretation of Toxicity and Carcinogenicity Studies. R.W. Hart, D.A. Neumann & R.T. Robertson, Eds.: 181–196. ILSI Press. Washington, D.C.
11. CHEFURKA, W. 1965. Intermediary metabolism of carbohydrates in insects. *In* The Physiology of Insecta. Chap. 11, Vol II. M. Rockstein, Ed. Academic Press. New York.
12. RIHA, V.F. & L.S. LUCKINBILL. 1996. Selection for longevity favors stringent metabolic control in *Drosophila melanogaster*. J. Gerontol. A Biol. Sci. Med. Sci. **51:** B284-294.
13. DA CUNHA, G.L. & A.K. DE OLIVEIRA. 1996. Citric acid cycle: a mainstream metabolic pathway influencing life span in *Drosophila melanogaster*? Exp. Gerontol. **31:** 705-715.
14. PACKER, L., S.U. WEBER & G. RIMBACH. 2001. Molecular aspects of α-tocotrienol antioxidant action and cell signalling. J. Nutr. (Suppl.) 369s–373s.
15. FORCE, A.G., T. STAPLES, S. SOLIMAN & R. ARKING. 1995. Comparative biochemical and stress analysis of genetically selected *Drosophila* strains with different longevities. Dev. Genet. **17:** 340–351.
16. KIRKWOOD, T.B.L. 1987. Immortality of the germ-live versus disposability of the soma. *In* Evolution of Longevity in Animals: A Comparative Approach. A.D. Woodhead & K.H. Thompson, Eds.: 209–218. Plenum. New York.
17. PARTRIDGE, L. & N.H. BARTON. 1993. Optimality, mutation and the evolution of ageing. Nature **362:** 305–311.
18. LUCKINBILL, L.S., R. ARKING, M.J. CLARE, *et al.* 1984. Selection for delayed senescence in *Drosophila melanogaster*. Evolution **38:** 996–1004.
19. ARKING, R. 1987. Successful selection for increased longevity in *Drosophila*: analysis of the survival data and presentation of a hypothesis on the genetic regulation of longevity. Exp. Gerontol. **22:** 199–220.

20. ARKING, R. 1987. Genetic and environmental determinants of longevity in *Drosophila*. *In* Evolution of Longevity in Animals: A Comparative Approach. A.D. Woodhead & K.H. Thompson, Eds.: 1–22. Plenum. New York.
21. ARKING, R., S. BUCK, R.A. WELLS & R. PRETZLAFF. 1988. Metabolic rates in genetically based long lived strains of *Drosophila*. Exp. Gerontol. **23:** 59–76.
22. ROSS, R.E. 2000. Age specific decreases in aerobic efficiency associated with increase in oxygen free radical production in *Drosophila melanogaster*. J. Insect Physiol. **46:** 1477–1480.
23. NOVOSELTSEV, V.N., R. ARKING, J.A. NOVOSELTSEVA & A.I. YASHIN. 2001. Evolutionary optimality applied to *Drosophila* experiments: hypothesis of constrained reproductive efficiency. Evolution. In press.
24. ARKING, R., S. BUCK, V.N. NOVOSELTSEV, D-S. HWANGBO & M. LANE. 2001. Genomic plasticity, energy allocations, and the extended longevity phenotypes of *Drosophila*. Aging Res. Rev. In press.
25. BARJA, G. 2000. The flux of free radical attack through mitochondrial DNA is related to aging rate. Clin. Ger. Res. **12:** 342–355.
26. DRIVER, C. & N. TAWADROS. 2000. Cytoplasmic genomes that confer additional longevity in *Drosophila melanogaster*. Biogerontology **1:** 255–260.
27. BUCK, S., J. VETTRAINO, A.G. FORCE & R. ARKING. 2000. Extended longevity in *Drosophila* is consistently associated with a decrease in developmental viability. J. Gerontol.: Biol. Sci. **55A:** B292–B301.
28. YU, B.P., D.Y. LEE, E.H. HWANG & B.O. LIM. 1999. Calorie restriction: a potent mechanistic solution to the oxygen paradox. *In* Research and Perspectives in Longevity: The Paradoxes of Longevity. J-M. Robine *et al.*, Eds.: 93–102. Springer-Verlag. Berlin.
29. LANE, M. 2000. Metabolic mechanisms of longevity: caloric restriction in mammals and longevity mutations in Caenorhabiditis elegans; A common pathway? AGE: J. Am. Aging Assoc. **23:** 1–7.
30. CLANCY, D.J., D. GEMS, L.G. HARSHMAN, *et al.* 2001. Extension of life-span by loss of CHICO, a *Drosophila* insulin receptor substrate protein. Science **292:** 104–106.
31. TATAR, M., A. KOPELMAN, D. EPSTEIN, *et al.* 2001. A mutant *Drosophila* insulin homolog that extends life-span and impairs neuroendocrine function. Science **292:** 107–110.
32. RAMSEY, J.J., M.E. HARPER & R. WEINDRUCK. 2000. Free Radic. Biol. Med. **29:** 946–968.
33. KIRK, K.L. 2001. Dietary restriction and aging: comparative tests of evolutionary hypotheses. J. Gerontol.: Biol. Sci. **56:** B123–129.
34. NUZHDIN, S.V., E.G. PASYUKOVA, C.L. DILDA, *et al.* 1997. Sex-specific quantitative trait loci affecting longevity in *Drosophila melanogaster*. Proc. Natl. Acad. Sci. USA **94:** 9734-9739.
35. PARSONS, P.A. 1995. Inherited stress resistance and longevity: a stress theory of ageing. Heredity **75:** 216–221.
36. JOHNSON, T.E., G.J. LITHGOW & S. MURAKIMI. 1996. Hypothesis: interventions that increase the response to stress affect the potential for effective life prolongation and increased health. J. Gerontol. Biol. Sci. **51A:** B392–B395.
37. WILLIAMS, G.C. 1957. Pleiotropy, natural selection and the evolution of senescence. Evolution **11:** 398–411.

Prevention of Mitochondrial Oxidative Damage Using Targeted Antioxidants

GEOFFREY F. KELSO,[a] CAROLYN M. PORTEOUS,[b] GILLIAN HUGHES,[b] ELIZABETH C. LEDGERWOOD,[b] ALISON M. GANE,[b] ROBIN A. J. SMITH,[a] AND MICHAEL P. MURPHY[c]

Departments of [a]Chemistry and [b]Biochemistry, University of Otago, Box 56, Dunedin, New Zealand

[c]MRC-Dunn Human Nutrition Unit, Wellcome Trust-MRC Building, Hills Road, Cambridge CB2 2XY, UK

ABSTRACT: Mitochondrial-targeted antioxidants that selectively block mitochondrial oxidative damage and prevent some types of cell death have been developed. These antioxidants are ubiquinone and tocopherol derivatives and are targeted to mitochondria by covalent attachment to a lipophilic triphenylphosphonium cation. Because of the large mitochondrial membrane potential, these cations accumulated within mitochondria inside cells, where the antioxidant moiety prevents lipid peroxidation and protects mitochondria from oxidative damage. The mitochondrially localized ubiquinone also protected mammalian cells from hydrogen peroxide–induced apoptosis while an untargeted ubiquinone analogue was ineffective against apoptosis. When fed to mice these compounds accumulated within the brain, heart, and liver; therefore, using these mitochondrial-targeted antioxidants may help investigations of the role of mitochondrial oxidative damage in animal models of aging.

KEYWORDS: mitochondria; antioxidants; ubiquinone; oxidative damage

INTRODUCTION

The mitochondrial respiratory chain is a major source of superoxide, and therefore mitochondria accumulate oxidative damage more rapidly than the rest of the cell, contributing to mitochondrial dysfunction and cell death in degenerative diseases and in aging.[1–5] One approach to preventing oxidative damage is to selectively target antioxidants to mitochondria.[6–8] The large membrane potential of 150–180 mV (negative inside) across the mitochondrial inner membrane can be used to deliver molecules to mitochondria.[6,7,9] Lipophilic cations pass easily through lipid bilayers because their charge is dispersed over a large surface area, and the potential gradient drives their accumulation into the mitochondrial matrix.[10,11] The uptake of lipophilic cations into mitochondria increases 10-fold for every 61.5 mV of mem-

---

Address for correspondence: Dr. Michael P. Murphy, MRC-Dunn Human Nutrition Unit, Wellcome Trust-MRC Building, Hills Road, Cambridge CB2 2XY, UK. Voice: +44-1223-252-900; fax +44-1223-252-905.

mpm@MRC-Dunn.cam.ac.uk

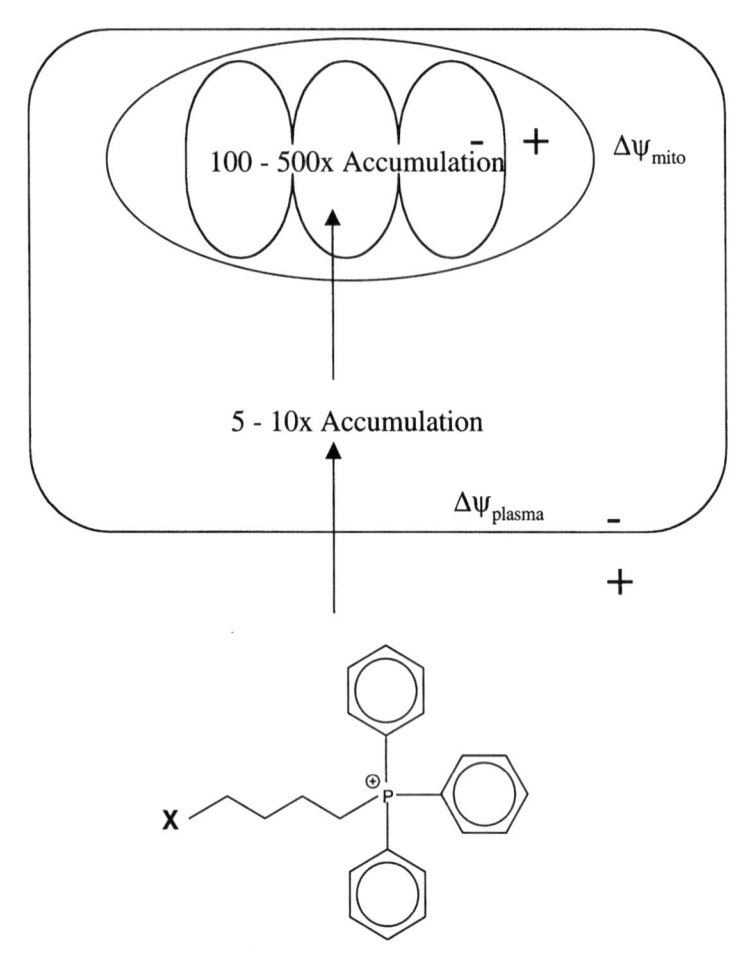

FIGURE 1. Uptake of lipophilic cations by cells and mitochondria. This schematic shows the uptake of a triphenylphosphonium moiety attached to a cargo molecule (X) into the cytoplasm from the extracellular environment driven by the plasma membrane potential. From the cytoplasm the compound is further accumulated into mitochondria, driven by the mitochondrial membrane potential. The mitochondrial and plasma membrane potentials ($\Delta\psi$) are indicated.

brane potential, leading to 100- to 500-fold accumulation, and uptake into cells is also driven by the plasma membrane potential (30–60 mV, negative inside) (FIG. 1).

Derivatives of ubiquinol and tocopherol are promising antioxidants to target to mitochondria by this procedure.[8,12] Mitochondrial ubiquinone is a respiratory chain component buried within the lipid core of the inner membrane where it accepts two electrons from complexes I or II, becoming reduced to ubiquinol which then donates electrons to complex III.[13] The ubiquinone pool *in vivo* is largely reduced, and ubiquinol is an effective antioxidant.[14–17] Ubiquinol acts as an antioxidant by donating a hydrogen atom from one of its hydroxyl groups to a lipid peroxyl radical, there-

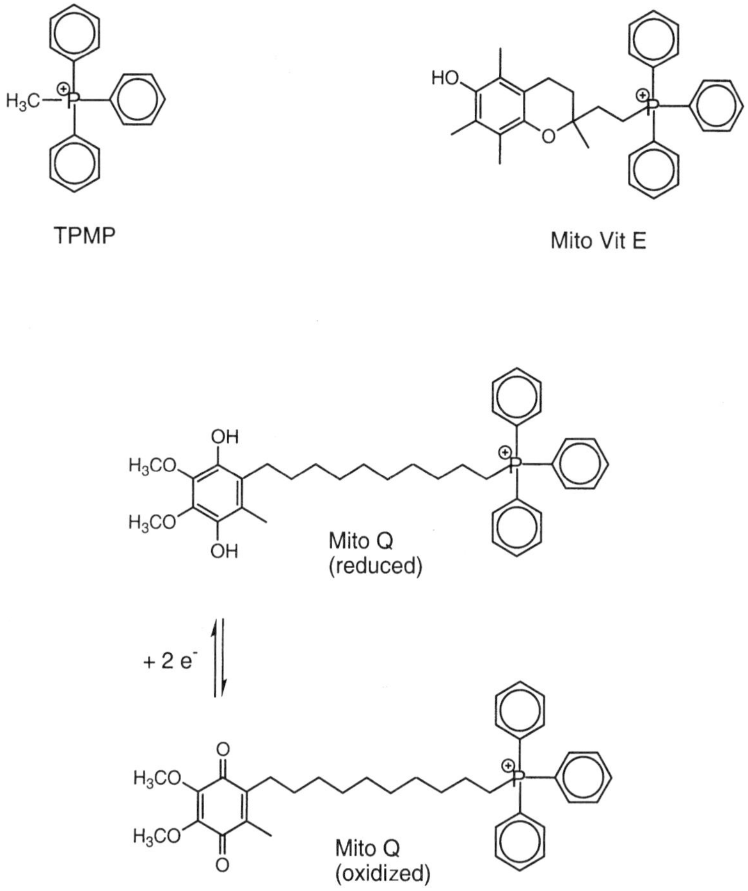

FIGURE 2. Compound structures. For mitoQ both the reduced (mitoquinol) and oxidized (mitoquinone) forms are shown.

by decreasing lipid peroxidation within the mitochondrial inner membrane.[17–19] The ubisemiquinone radicals thus formed disproportionate to ubiquinone and ubiquinol.[16,19,20] The respiratory chain then recycles ubiquinone back to ubiquinol to restore its antioxidant function. Vitamin E is another important antioxidant within the mitochondrial inner membrane and the tocopheroxyl radical thus formed is regenerated to active vitamin E by reaction with ubiquinol or ubisemiquinone.[14,16,19,21,22] Therefore ubiquinol and vitamin E cooperate to decrease mitochondrial oxidative damage.[15,16,19] To manipulate mitochondrial ubiquinone and tocopherol content *in vitro* and *in vivo,* we synthesized ubiquinone and tocopherol analogues selectively targeted to mitochondria by addition of a lipophilic triphenylphosphonium cation[23,24] (FIG. 2). Here we report on the antioxidant and antiapoptotic properties of these compounds and on their uptake into the brain, heart, and liver following feeding to mice.

MATERIAL AND METHODS

Mitochondrial Preparations and Incubations

Rat liver mitochondria were prepared by homogenization followed by differential centrifugation.[25] Beef heart mitochondria were isolated by standard procedures and membrane fragments prepared by sonication followed by centrifugation.[26] Protein concentrations were determined by the biuret assay using bovine serum albumin as a standard.[27] To measure membrane potential, rat liver mitochondria (2 mg protein/mL) were incubated for 3 min in 0.5 mL KCl medium supplemented with nigericin (1 µg/mL), 5 mM each of glutamate and malate, 1 µM TPMP (methyltriphenylphosphonium cation), and 100 nCi/mL [^{3}H]TPMP. After incubation the mitochondria were pelleted by centrifugation and the radioactivity in the pellet and supernatant measured by scintillation counting; the membrane potential was calculated from the Nernst equation, assuming a mitochondrial volume of 0.5 µL/mg protein and that 60% of the intramitochondrial TPMP was membrane bound.[28,29] The uptake of [^{3}H]mitoQ (mixture of mitoquinol and mitoquinone) by rat liver mitochondria was measured under the same conditions. Scanning spectra and kinetic measurements were made with an Aminco DW-2000 dual beam spectrophotometer using matched 1-mL quartz cuvettes at 20°C. Beef heart mitochondrial membranes were incubated in 50 mM potassium phosphate, pH 7.2. Rat liver mitochondria were incubated in KCl medium.

Oxidative Damage Assays

To measure thiobarbituric acid reactive species (TBARS), rat liver mitochondria (2 mg protein/mL) were incubated at 37°C with shaking for 45 min in 100 mM KCl, 10 mM Tris-HCl, pH 7.6. Then 0.8 mL aliquots were mixed with 400 µL 0.5% thiobarbituric acid in 35% HClO$_4$, heated at 100°C for 15 min, diluted with 3 mL water and extracted into 3 mL *n*-butanol. TBARS were determined fluorometrically (λ_{excite} = 515 nm; $\lambda_{emission}$ = 553 nm) and expressed as nmol malondialdehyde (MDA) by comparison with standard solutions of 1,1,3,3-tetraethoxypropane processed as above. Prior to analysing samples their mitoQ contents were brought to the same concentration to eliminate differences in MDA formation during heating and processing. To measure the membrane potential after exposure to oxidative damage, mitochondria were pelleted by centrifugation and resuspended in KCl medium; then their membrane potential was determined as described above.

Mammalian Cell Culture

The Jurkat human T lymphocyte line was grown at 37°C under humidified 95% air/5% CO$_2$ in RPMI 1640 supplemented with penicillin (100 U/mL), streptomycin (100 mg/mL), and 10% fetal calf serum. Apoptosis was induced by addition of hydrogen peroxide.[30] Caspase activation in lysed cell pellets was measured fluorometrically by the cleavage of DEVD-aminomethylcoumarin (AMC) and calibrated using an AMC standard curve.[31]

Animals

Female Swiss Webster mice (8–10 weeks, ~25–35 g) were used, supplied by the Department of Laboratory Animal Sciences, University of Otago. Mice were maintained at 22–23°C on a 12-hour light/dark cycle and had free access to drinking water and to standard solid chow, or to a complete liquid diet. All experiments were approved by the University of Otago animal ethics committee. The more water soluble compounds (TPMP and MitoVit E) were fed in the drinking water, while the less water soluble MitoQ was fed in a complete liquid diet,[32] which entirely replaced solid food. The dose was determined by monitoring water or liquid food consumption. Mouse weight, appearance, and behavior were monitored continually to gauge health. To determine compound distribution in mice, the mice were killed by cervical dislocation and bled. A blood sample was collected in an EDTA tube and precipitated with 1 vol 20% TCA on ice; then the supernatant was collected. The liver, brain (cerebrum, cerebellum, and brain stem), kidneys, heart, adipose tissue (intraperitoneal), and skeletal muscle (gastrocnemius and quadriceps) were collected and weighed. All tissues were homogenized in 4 mL STE (250 mM sucrose, 10 mM Tris-HCl, pH 7.4, 1 mM EGTA) using a 1 Ultraturrax homogenizer for 1–2 × 30 s, and the radioactive content of the homogenate was determined by scintillation counting in Optiphase Hi Safe II using an LKB Rack Beta scintillation counter with appropriate quench corrections. The content of the compound was expressed in nmol/g wet weight tissue, calculated from the specific activity of administered compound.

Compounds

TPMP was from Sigma; MitoVit E and MitoQ were synthesized as described.[23,24,33] Tritiated TPMP (50–60 Ci/mmol) was from American Radiolabelled Chemicals Inc. [^{3}H]-enriched MitoVit E and Mito Q were synthesized, as described previously,[23,24] and gave solutions of specific activities 200–800 mCi/mol for MitoVit E and 30 mCi/mL for MitoQ.

RESULTS AND DISCUSSION

MitoQ Reduction by the Respiratory Chain and Uptake by Isolated Mitochondria

The mitochondrially targeted quinol, 10-(6′-ubiquinolyl)decyltriphenylphosphonium, and quinone, 10-(6′-ubiquinonyl)decyltriphenylphosphonium, are shown in FIG. 2. Here they are called mitoquinol (10-(6′-ubiquinolyl)decyltriphenylphosphonium) (reduced) and mitoquinone (10-(6′-ubiquinonyl)decyltriphenylphosphonium) (oxidized), respectively, and mitoQ refers to a mixture of redox forms. To determine whether the respiratory chain could reduce mitoquinone, we incubated it with beef heart mitochondrial membranes and recorded its spectrum (FIG. 3A, $t = 0$). Addition of the respiratory substrate succinate reduced mitoquinone to mitoquinol (FIG. 3A). Mitoquinone–mitoquinol interconversion was then measured continuously by monitoring mitoquinone at 275 nm (FIG. 3B). Mitoquinone was reduced by beef heart mitochondrial membranes and succinate, and this reduction was blocked by the complex II inhibitor malonate (FIG. 3B). In other experiments chemically reduced mitoquinol was oxidized by mitochondrial membranes, and this oxidation was blocked

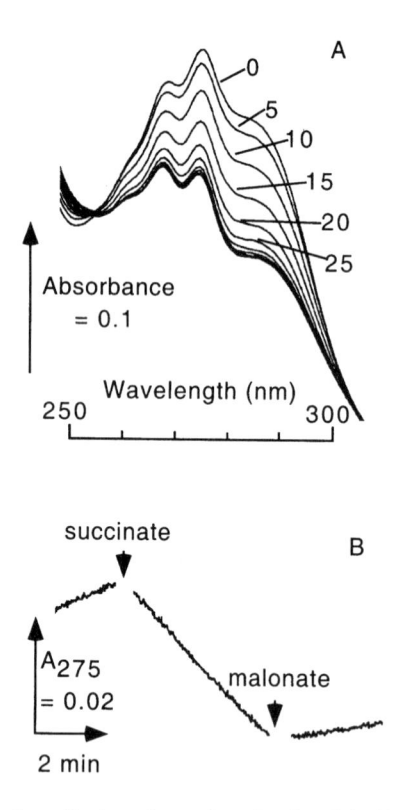

FIGURE 3. Reduction of mitoquinone by mitochondria. Panel A: 50 μM mitoQ was incubated with beef heart mitochondrial membranes and the spectrum of mitoquinone recorded ($t = 0$). Then antimycin (5 μM) and succinate (5 mM) were added and further spectra acquired at 5-minute intervals ($t = 5$–25). **Panel B:** Beef heart mitochondrial membranes (20 μg protein/mL) were incubated with rotenone (8 μg/mL) and mitoQ (50 μM). A_{275} was monitored continuously, and succinate (5 mM) and malonate (20 mM) were added where indicated.

by the complex III inhibitor myxothiazol.[23] Tritiated mitoQ was taken up rapidly by energized mitochondria and addition of the uncoupler carbonyl cyanide p-trifluoromethoxyphenylhydrazone (FCCP) caused its immediate efflux (FIG. 4), as was also the case for MitoVit E.[24] In other experiments we showed that these compounds were also taken up by mitochondria in cells.[23,24]

Antioxidant Properties of MitoQ

To quantitate the antioxidant efficacy of mitoQ, mitochondria were incubated with ferrous iron, and the accumulation of MDA was measured as a marker of lipid peroxidation (FIG. 5A). This oxidative damage also disrupted mitochondrial function as indicated by a decrease in the membrane potential (data not shown). Incubation with mitoQ prevented both the accumulation of MDA (FIG. 5A) and the disruption to mitochondrial function caused by oxidative stress (data not shown). To

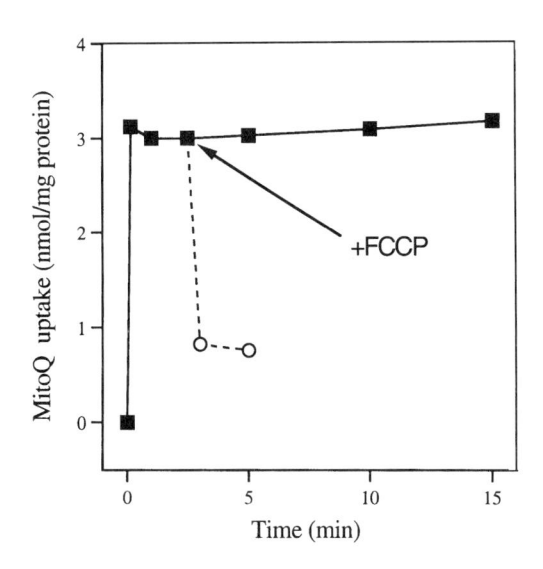

FIGURE 4. Uptake of mitoQ by energized mitochondria. Rat liver mitochondria were incubated in KCl medium supplemented with 10 mM succinate, rotenone (8 μg/mL), nigericin (1 μg/mL), 10 μM mitoQ, and 2.5 nCi [^{3}H]mitoQ/mL. Mitochondrial mitoQ uptake was determined at various times (*filled squares*). Where indicated 300 nM FCCP was added after 2.5 min mitoQ accumulation (*open circles*). This gave the same final mitoQ accumulation as when FCCP was present from the start of the incubation (data not shown). Data are means of duplicate determinations. In all cases the range is smaller than the symbols. This shows a typical experiment that was repeated on two separate mitochondrial preparations.

determine whether mitoquinone or mitoquinol was the effective antioxidant we oxidized mitoQ to mitoquinone and prevented its reduction by the respiratory chain by including malonate and rotenone in the incubation. Under these conditions mitoquinone did not block lipid peroxidation (FIG 5A). By contrast, when mitoQ was reduced to mitoquinol by the respiratory chain, oxidative damage was prevented (FIG. 5A). The simple lipophilic cation TPMP did not prevent lipid peroxidation (FIG. 5A). Therefore the antioxidant activity of mitoQ is due to its reduced ubiquinol moiety. Similar protection against mitochondrial oxidative damage was found for Mito-Vit E.[24] Importantly after mitoQ was oxidized by a reactive oxygen species, it was rapidly recycled to its active form by the respiratory chain. Therefore these compounds are taken up into mitochondria within cells and protect mitochondrial function from oxidative damage. MitoQ is recycled back to its active antioxidant form by the respiratory chain after having detoxified a reactive oxygen species.

Prevention of Apoptosis by MitoQ

The oxidant hydrogen peroxide induces apoptosis by releasing cytochrome *c* from mitochondria into the cytoplasm where it activates caspases.[30] Of particular interest is whether cytochrome *c* release induced by hydrogen peroxide is caused directly by mitochondrial oxidative damage or is a secondary consequence of cytoplasmic redox changes.[30] In addition it is of interest to see if mitochondrially

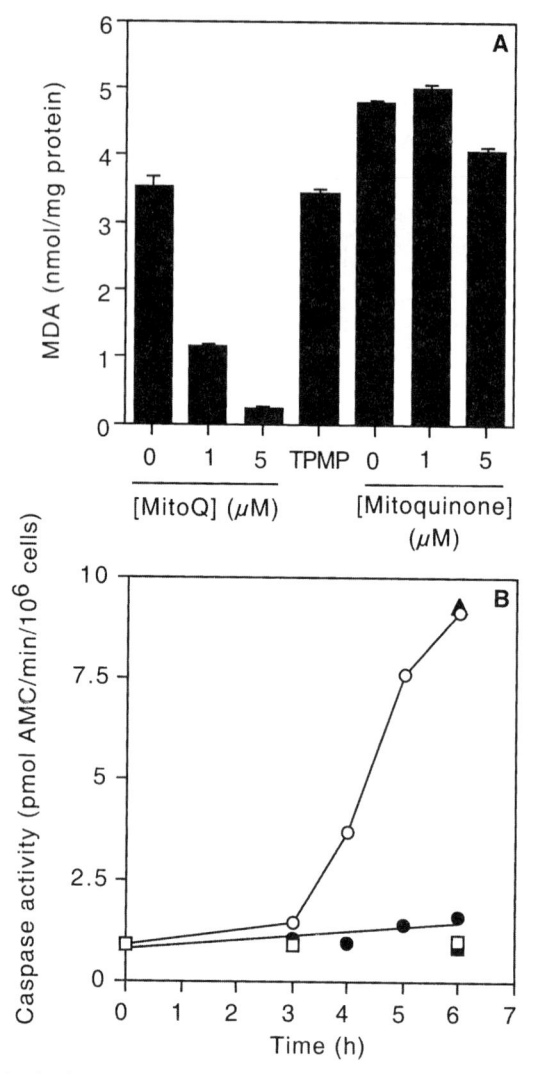

FIGURE 5. Antioxidant efficacy of mitoQ. Panel A: Mitochondria were incubated with 10 mM succinate, 8 μg/mL rotenone, in the presence or absence of mitoQ or TPMP (5 μM). For some incubations malonate (20 mM) was present, and mitoQ was oxidized completely to mitoquinone before addition by incubation at basic pH. After preincubation for 5 min, ferrous sulfate (50 μM) was added, and 40 mins later MDA formation was quantitated. Data are means ± range of duplicate determinations. **Panel B:** Jurkat cells (5×10^6) in 5 mL medium were preincubated for 30 min with no additions (*open circles*) or with 1 μM mitoQ (*filled circles*), and then 150 μM hydrogen peroxide was added and cells were harvested at various times and their caspase activity measured as the rate of DEVD-AMC cleavage. Without hydrogen peroxide there was no caspase activation either in the absence (*open squares*) or presence of 1 μM mitoQ (*filled squares*). Preincubation with 1 μM TPMP did not decrease caspase activation by hydrogen peroxide (*filled triangle*). The FIGURE shows a typical experiment repeated on five separate cell preparations.

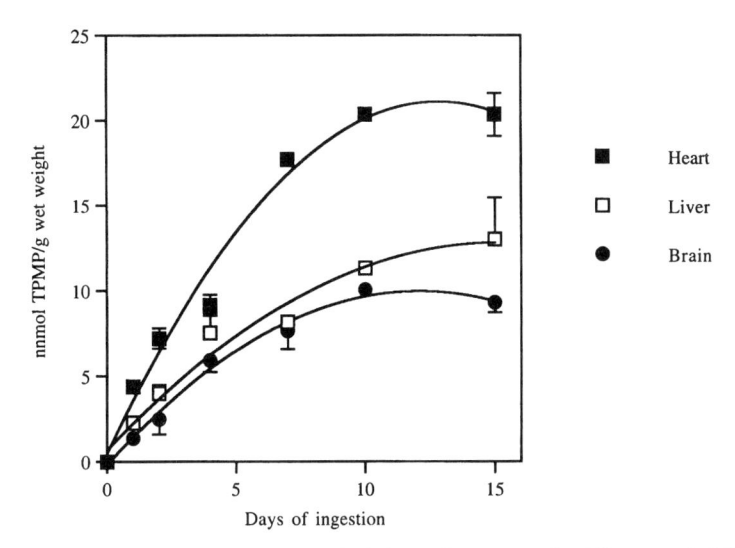

FIGURE 6. Distribution of orally administered compounds. Mice were fed 500 μM [^{3}H]TPMP (0.25 Ci/mol) in their drinking water. Pairs of mice were fed for the indicated times, and the content of TPMP was then determined. Data are means ± range.

targeted antioxidants can block oxidative damage-induced apoptosis. Therefore we investigated the effect of mitoQ on hydrogen peroxide–induced apoptosis. Addition of hydrogen peroxide to Jurkat cells led to caspase activation and induction of apoptotic cell death 4 to 6 hours later (FIG. 5B). Preincubation with 1 μM mitoQ completely blocked caspase activation (FIG. 5B). To determine whether the mitochondrial localization of mitoQ was required for this protective effect, we compared mitoQ with Q_1 (ubiquinone-1), a quinol antioxidant that distributes evenly throughout the cell, and found that Q_1 did not block caspase activation (data not shown). We conclude that the mitochondrial localization of mitoQ increases its ability to block apoptosis induced by hydrogen peroxide.

Distribution of Lipophilic Cations within Animals

Lipophilic cations should disperse throughout the body and be taken up from the extracellular space into cells and then into mitochondria (FIG. 1). Furthermore they should pass across the blood–brain barrier and accumulate in brain mitochondria as well as in other tissues affected by mitochondrial dysfunction. To investigate the delivery and distribution of lipophilic cations within the body, we measured the uptake and distribution of the simple lipophilic cation TPMP (FIG. 6). We fed this compound to mice in their drinking water and found that mice could be maintained indefinitely on drinking water containing 500 μM TPMP, corresponding to a safe dose of 30–40 mg/kg/day. To determine how TPMP distributed between organs we fed mice 500 μM [^{3}H]TPMP in their drinking water and measured its uptake into various organs over time (FIG. 6). The lipophilic cation was taken up rapidly into the liver, brain, and heart, coming to a steady state after 7–10 days (FIG. 6). The toxicity and organ distribution of antioxidants linked to a triphenylphosphonium moiety should be similar to that of TPMP. This was confirmed by feeding mice mitoVit E in their drinking water. MitoVit E could be fed to mice safely for long periods at the same concentration as used for TPMP, and [^{3}H]MitoVit E gave a similar tissue distribution as for TPMP (data not shown). The more hydrophobic compound mitoQ was fed to mice in a complete liquid diet and could be fed at similar concentrations as for TPMP without toxic effects; the tissue distribution of [^{3}H]mitoQ was similar to that of TPMP. Therefore orally administered lipophilic cations became located predominantly in mitochondria.

CONCLUSION

To provide new approaches to investigate the role of mitochondrial oxidative damage in cell death, we synthesized the mitochondrially targeted antioxidants mitoQ and mitoVit E. These comprised a ubiquinone or tocopherol moiety attached to a triphenylphosphonium lipophilic cation. For mitoQ the ubiquinone moiety was found to cycle between its oxidized (mitoquinone) and reduced (mitoquinol) forms by exchanging electrons with the respiratory chain. Mitoquinol was an effective antioxidant protecting mitochondria from oxidative damage and was rapidly regenerated by the respiratory chain after detoxifying a reactive oxygen species. As anticipated, the triphenylphosphonium cation led to the rapid and reversible accumulation of mitoQ by isolated mitochondria and by mitochondria within cells. Therefore mitoQ is a mitochondrial-specific antioxidant. We investigated the effects of mitoQ on apoptotic cell death and showed that mitoQ prevented apoptosis caused by hydrogen peroxide. These findings demonstrate that mitochondrially targeted antioxidants such as mitoQ can be used to investigate the role of mitochondrial oxidative stress in cell death. As these compounds are taken up by mitochondria in mice they may also be of use in investigating the role of mitochondrial oxidative damage in animal models of aging.

ACKNOWLEDGMENTS

This work was supported by grants to M.P.M. and R.A.J.S. from the Health Research Council of New Zealand, and from the Marsden Fund, administered by the Royal Society of New Zealand. G.F.K. is a Foundation for Research, Science and Technology Bright Futures Scholar, and E.C.L. is an HRC repatriation fellow.

REFERENCES

1. WALLACE, D.C. 1999. Mitochondrial diseases in man and mouse. Science **283:** 1482–1488.
2. AMES, B.N., M.K. SHIGENAGA & T.M. HAGEN. 1993. Oxidants, antioxidants, and the degenerative diseases of aging. Proc. Natl. Acad. Sci. USA **90:** 7915–7922.
3. AMES, B.N., M.K. SHIGENAGA & T.M. HAGEN. 1995. Mitochondrial decay in aging. Biochem. Biophys. Acta **1271:** 165–170.
4. BECKMAN, K.B. & B.N. AMES. 1998. The free radical theory of aging matures. Physiol. Rev. **78:** 547–581.

5. MICHIKAWA, Y., F. MAZZUCCHELLI, N. BRESOLIN, et al. 1999. Aging-dependent large accumulation of point mutations in the human mtDNA control region for replication. Science **286:** 774–779.
6. MURPHY, M.P. 1997. Targeting bioactive compounds to mitochondria. Trends Biotechnol. **15:** 326–330.
7. MURPHY, M.P. & R.A.J. SMITH. 2000. Drug delivery to mitochondria: the key to mitochondrial medicine. Adv. Drug Deliv. Rev. **41:** 235–250.
8. MATTHEWS, R.T., L. YANG, S. BROWNE, et al. 1998. Coenzyme Q10 administration increases brain mitochondrial concentrations and exerts neuroprotective effects. Proc. Natl. Acad. Sci. USA **95:** 8892–8897.
9. CHEN, L.B. 1988. Mitochondrial membrane potential in living cells. Annu. Rev. Cell Biol. **4:** 155–181.
10. LIBERMAN, E.A., V.P. TOPALI, L.M. TSOFINA, et al. 1969. Nature **222:** 1076–1078.
11. AZZONE, G.F., D. PIETROBON & M. ZORATTI. 1984. Determination of the proton electrochemical gradient across biological membranes. Curr. Top. Bioenerget. **13:** 1–77.
12. LASS, A., M.J. FORSTER & R.S. SOHAL. 1999. Effects of coenzyme Q10 and alpha-tocopherol administration on their tissue levels in the mouse. Free Radic. Biol. Med. **26:** 1357–1382.
13. CRANE, F.L. 1977. Hydroquinone dehydrogenases. Annu. Rev. Biochem. **46:** 439–469.
14. LASS, A. & R.S. SOHAL. 1998. Electron transport-linked ubiquinone-dependent recycling of α–tocopherol inhibits autooxidation of mitochondiral membranes. Arch. Biochem. Biophys. **352:** 229–236.
15. KAGAN, V.E., E.A. SERBINOVA, D.A. STOYANOVSKY, et al. 1994. Assay of ubiquinones and ubiquinols as antioxidants. Methods Enzymol. **234:** 343–354.
16. MAGUIRE, J.J., D.S. WILSON & L. PACKER. 1989. Mitochondrial electron transport-linked tocoperoxyl radical reduction. J. Biol. Chem. **264:** 21462–21465.
17. ERNSTER, L., P. FORSMARK & K. NORDENBRAND. 1992. Biofactors **3:** 241–248.
18. TAKADA, M., S. IKENOYA, T. YUZURIHA & K. KATAYAMA. 1984. Simultaneous determination of reduced and oxidised ubiquinones. Methods Enzymol. **105:** 147–155.
19. INGOLD, K.U., V.W. BOWRY, R. STOCKER & C. WALLING. 1993. Autoxidation of lipids and antioxidation by α-tocopherol and ubiquinol in homogeneous solution and in aqueous dispersions of lipids. Proc. Natl. Acad. Sci. USA **90:** 45–49.
20. LAND, E.J. & A.J. SWALLOW. 1970. One-electron reactions in biochemical systems as studied by pulse radiolysis. 3. Ubiquinone. J. Biol. Chem. **245:** 1890–1894.
21. STOYANOVSKY, D.A., A.N. OSIPOV, P.J. QUINN & V.E. KAGAN. 1995. Ubiquinone-dependent recycling of vitamin E radicals by superoxide. Arch. Biochem. Biophys. **323:** 343–351.
22. MUKAI, K., S. KIKUCHI & S. URANO. 1990. Stopped-flow kinetic study of the regeneration reaction of tocopheroxyl radical by reduced ubiquinone-10 in solution. Biochim. Biophys. Acta **1035:** 77–82.
23. KELSO, G.F., C.M. PORTEOUS, C.V. COULTER, et al. 2001. Selective targeting of a redox-active ubiquinone to mitochondria within cells. J. Biol. Chem. **276:** 4588–4596.
24. SMITH, R.A.J., C.M. PORTEOUS, C.V. COULTER & M.P. MURPHY. 1999. Targeting an antioxidant to mitochondria. Eur. J. Biochem. **263:** 709–716.
25. CHAPPELL, J.B. & R.G. HANSFORD. 1972. Preparation of mitochondria from animal tissues and yeasts. In Subcellular components: preparation and fractionation. G.D. Birnie, Ed.: 77–91. Butterworths. London.
26. SMITH, A.L. 1967. Preparation, properties, and condition for assay of mitochondria: slaughterhouse material, small-scale. Methods Enzymol. **10:** 81–86.
27. GORNALL, A.G., C.J. BARDAWILL & M.M. DAVID. 1949. Determination of serum protein by means of the biuret reaction. J. Biol. Chem. **177:** 751–766.
28. SCOTT, I.D. & D.G. NICHOLLS. 1980. Energy transduction in intact synaptosomes. Biochem. J. **186:** 21–33.
29. BROWN, G.C. & M.D. BRAND. 1985. Thermodynamic control of electron flux though mitochondria cytochrome bc_1 complex. Biochem. J. **225:** 399–405.
30. HAMPTON, M.B. & S. ORENIUS. 1997. Dual regulation of caspase activity by hydrogen peroxide: implications for apoptosis. FEBS Lett. **414:** 552–556.

31. SCARLETT, J.L., P.W. SHEARD, G. HUGHES, *et al.* 2000. Changes in mitochondrial membrane potential during staurosporine-induced apoptosis in Jurkat cells. FEBS Lett. **475:** 267–272.
32. LIEBER, C.S. & L.M. DECARLI. 1986. The feeding of alcohol in liquid diets. Alcohol. Clin. Exp. Res. **10:** 550–553.
33. COULTER, C.V., G.F. KELSO, T-K. LIN, *et al.* 2000. Mitochondrially targeted antioxidants and thiol reagents. Free Radic. Biol. Med. **28:** 1547–1554.

Cognitive Impairment of Rats Caused by Oxidative Stress and Aging, and Its Prevention by Vitamin E

KOJI FUKUI,[a] NAO-OMI OMOI,[a] TAKAHIRO HAYASAKA,[a] TADASHI SHINNKAI,[b] SHOZO SUZUKI,[b] KOUICHI ABE,[c] AND SHIRO URANO[a]

[a]*Division of Biological Chemistry, Shibaura Institute of Technology, 3-9-14 Shibaura, Minato-ku, Tokyo 108-8548, Japan*

[b]*Tokyo Metropolitan Institute of Gerontology, Tokyo, Japan*

[c]*Vitamin E Information and Technology Section, Eisai Co., Ltd., Tokyo, Japan*

ABSTRACT: In order to verify whether brain damage caused by chronic oxidative stress induces the impairment of cognitive function, the ability of learning and memory was assessed using the water maze and the eight-arm radial maze tasks. Young rats showed significantly greater learning ability before the stress than the old and vitamin E–deficient rats. At five days after subjection to oxidative stress, the memory function of the young declined toward the level of that in the aged rats maintained under normal condition. This phenomenon is supported by the findings that the delayed-type apoptosis appeared in the CA1 region of the hippocampus of the young at five to seven days after the stress. Vitamin E supplementation to the young accelerated significantly their learning functions before the stress and prevented the deficit of memory caused by the stress. When rats were subjected to stress, thiobarbituric acid–reactive substance (TBARS), lipid hydroperoxides, and protein carbonyls were significantly increased in synaptic plasma membranes. It was found that ζ-potential of the synaptic membrane surface was remarkably decreased. These phenomena were also observed in the aged and vitamin E–deficient rats maintained under normal condition. These results suggest that oxidative damage to the rat synapse in the cerebral cortex and hippocampus during aging may contribute to the deficit of cognitive functions.

KEYWORDS: cognitive impairment; oxidative stress; brain damage; vitamin E

INTRODUCTION

Enhanced oxidative stress is known to produce reactive oxygen species (ROS) in biological systems. It has been recognized that ROS are generated as a consequence of the leakage of electrons from specific segments of the electron transport system

Address for correspondence: Shiro Urano, Division of Biological Chemistry, Shibaura Institute of Technology, 3-9-14 Shibaura, Minato-ku, Tokyo 108-8548, Japan. Voice: +81-3-5476-2429; fax: +81-3-5476-3162.
urano@sic.shibaura-it.ac.jp

in mitochondria and that ROS may attack several organs to induce various disorders.[1–3] Numerous evidence has indicated that ROS are crucial in the aging process and age-related pathophysiological degeneration.[4]

The brain and nervous system are highly susceptible to oxidative stress due to high concentrations of oxidizable substrates, a high rate of oxidative metabolic activity, and endogenous ROS production caused by dopamine oxidation. In addition, it is known that certain regions of the brain are enriched in iron, a metal that is catalytically involved in the production of ROS in living tissues.[5,6] One possible explanation of the etiopathogenesis for Alzheimer's disease (AD) and senile dementia of the Alzheimer's type (SDAT) suggests that ROS are mainly responsible for progressive and specific neuronal degeneration.[7] According to this hypothesis, it implies that ROS produced by oxidative stress may impair cognitive function, such as learning and memory.

Recently, we observed that when rats were subjected to hyperoxia as an oxidative stress, their nerve terminals were oxidatively damaged, that is, swelling of mitochondria; we also observed a quite abnormal accumulation of synaptic vesicles in the synapse, which includes the neurotransmitters. It was also found that acetylcholine release by the KCl stimulation was decreased by the stress.[8,9] These abnormalities were also found in aged rats maintained under normal conditions. These findings suggest that oxidative stress may induce the impairment of neurotransmission, resulting in a deficit of cognitive function during brain aging. However, although the degeneration of hippocampal cholinergic neurons is recognized as a key to AD and SDAT, it is still unclear whether the oxidative neurodegeneration during aging may involve a deficit of cognitive function. The purpose of the present study is to verify whether brain damage caused by chronic oxidative stress during aging induces the impairment of cognitive function and how the impairment is associated with oxidative damage to the nerve terminals in the brain.

MATERIAL AND METHODS

Animals

All experiments with animals were performed with permission by the Animal Protection and Ethics Committee of Shibaura Institute of Technology. Male Wistar rats, aged 3 and 25 months old, fed an ad libitum standard diet, were used. In order to assess the susceptibility against oxidative stress, vitamin E–deficient rats, fed a vitamin E–deficient diet for 9 weeks were also used. After evaluation of the learning ability in all groups, young animals were maintained under 100% oxygen at 20°C for 48 hours in oxygen chambers. The old rats and vitamin E–deficient rats were maintained without oxidative stress for 48 hours.

Behavioral Testing

All animals were tested for learning and memory using the Morris water maze task and the eight-arm radial maze task. In the water maze test, the bottom of the pool (140 cm in diameter and 45 cm in height) was divided quarterly by white colored lines, and the submerged transparent platform was placed in the center of one quadrant, which was maintained at 20°C. For pretraining, rats were allowed to swim freely in the pool for 60 s without the platform. Daily training consisted of one trial in which rats started for the fixed goal from three different start points; this was conducted for 20 consecutive days. Goal time and length of distance swum were measured, and the rate of decrease in swimming time and distance from their values at the first (unlearned) start was expressed as the learning rate. After all groups had completely learned the task, the rats were subjected to hyperoxia for 48 hours (except for the old rats and the vitamin E–deficient rats). The platform was removed, and the animals were placed on the site opposite the quadrant where the platform had been. The percentage of time spent in the quadrant where the platform had been was used as an assessment of memory retention. Under an eight-arm radial maze test, rats were placed into the central chamber of the apparatus and then allowed to explore the maze. The number of consecutive correct choices prior to reentry into a previously entered arm was considered an index of performance. Errors were also evaluated as the number of reentries into a previously visited arm. After evaluation of the learning ability in all groups, their memory functions were assessed using the same procedure described above.

Apoptosis Assay

After decapitation of the rat, the whole brain was immediately soaked in a fixation solution (3% paraformaldehyde, 0.1 M sodium cacodylate, 0.1 M tannic acid). The brain was cut using a microtome (50 mm/section), and the sections obtained were stained using an Apoptosis *in situ* Detection Kit (Wako Pure Chemical Industries, Ltd, Tokyo).

Isolation of Synaptosomes from Rat Brain Cerebral Cortex and Hippocampus

According to the discontinuous Ficoll density gradient centrifugation method, as previously reported,[8,9] nerve terminals were isolated as synaptosomes from cerebral cortex and hippocampus. The synaptosomes obtained were used immediately for all studies.

Analyses of Thiobarbituric Acid–reactive Substance (TBARS), Lipid Hydroperoxides, and Protein Carbonyls

According to the previous reports,[8] TBARS, lipid hydroperoxides, and oxidized protein formation were used as the indices of the oxidative damage of synapses in cerebral cortex and hippocampus.

Measurement of the Membrane Surface Potential of Rat Nerve Terminals

The ζ-potentials of rat synaptosomal plasma membranes in phosphate-buffered saline (pH 7.4) were measured electrophoretically using the LAZER ZEE model 501 apparatus (PEN KEN Co., New York).

Statistical Analysis

The results were presented as mean ± SE. All data were assessed using the two-way analysis of variance (ANOVA).

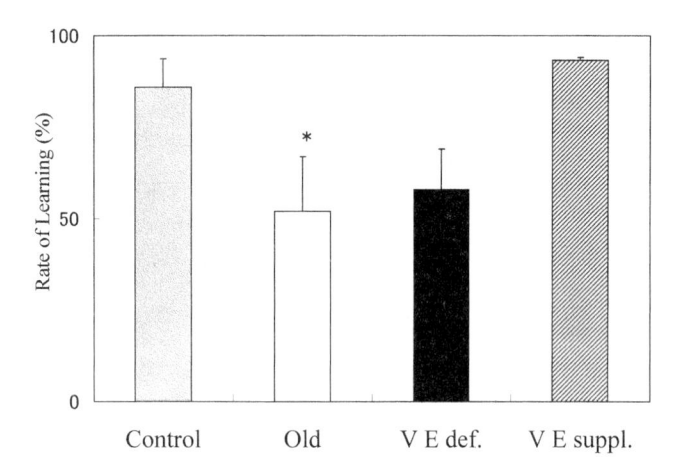

FIGURE 1. Influence of aging and vitamin E deficiency on the learning rate at the tenth trial using a Morris water maze task. *$P < 0.05$, versus the control rats; $n = 6$ each.

RESULTS AND DISCUSSION

Deficit of Learning and Memory in Rats Caused by Oxidative Stress and Aging

For the first trial in the water maze task, the learning rate of each group was expressed as 0% learning ability. Although the young control reached the platform within 20 s after only six trials, the old rats learned very slowly, and their abilities did not reach to 100% latency within 20 trials. Vitamin E–deficient rats also showed similar performances as the old ones (data not shown). When the learning ability is compared at the 10th trial, as shown in FIGURE 1, young rats have a significant higher ability when compared to that of the old rats and vitamin E–deficient rats. The maximum in the learning abilities of the old and vitamin E–deficient rats was remarkably low, about 50% of the rate of the young controls. In an assessment of the ability using the eight-arm radial task, young controls showed also a significant higher performance than the old and vitamin E–deficient rats (data not shown). When young rats were supplemented by vitamin E, their learning function was accelerated significantly before the stress. On the basis of these findings, it seems likely that the learning ability of rats may decline gradually during aging due to chronic oxidative stress, resulting from oxidative damage to the region for cognition, the cerebral cortex and hippocampus.

After rats learned the place of the platform in the water maze task, and any reward baits in the radial maze task, young rats and vitamin E–supplemented rats were subjected to hyperoxia as an oxidative stress for 48 hours. On the other hand, the old and vitamin E–deficient rats were maintained under air for 48 hours. Young rats showed impairment of memory retention in both tasks. As shown in FIGURE 2, in a water maze task, at five days after subjection to the oxidative stress, the memory function

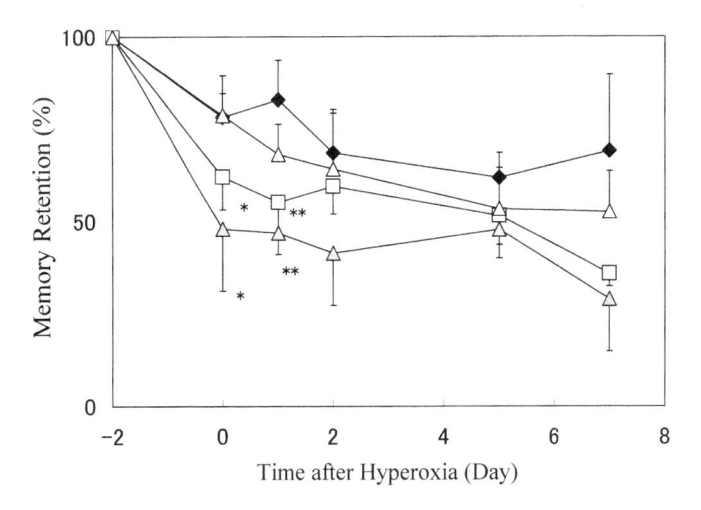

FIGURE 2. Effect of hyperoxia and aging on the memory retention using a Morris water maze task. $^*P<0.01$, $^{**}P<0.05$, versus the control rats. ◆, control; □, vitamin E–deficient; ▲, 24 month old; △, vitamin E–supplemented ($n = 6$ each).

of the young declined toward the level of that in the aged rats maintained under air for 48 hours. Interestingly, two days after the stress, the young controls maintained memory, but 5 to 7 days later after the stress, memory retention in the young was decreased. These phenomena are considered to be implicated in the induction of a delayed-type apoptosis of nerve cells caused by oxidative stress, resulting in a deterioration of space cognition. In order to confirm this hypothesis, we assessed the probability of an appearance of apoptosis in the hippocampus due to oxidative stress. Although just after the stress, the CA1 region of the hippocampus still maintained the normal feature (FIG. 3A), the delayed-type apoptosis appeared in the CA1 region of the young at seven days after the stress (FIG. 3B). The old rats maintained under air for 48 h also had apoptosis in the CA1 region (FIG. 3C). This cell damage caused by oxidative stress and during aging supports the findings that impairment in memory retention of young rats appeared at 5 to 7 days after the stress. In a radial maze task, the number of consecutive correct choices for the young control prior to reentry into a previously entered arm was significantly decreased after hyperoxia. Its ability declined toward the level of that in the aged rats maintained under air for 48 h, as shown in FIGURE 4A. The vitamin E supplementation for the young prevented the deficit of memory caused by the stress to some extent. The number of errors in the old rats and vitamin E–deficient rats increased significantly after the stress, and the vitamin E supplementation to the young prevented an increase in the number of errors (FIG. 4B). These results obtained here suggest that chronic oxidative stress may contribute to the deficit of the learning and memory function during aging, due to the neuronal apoptosis of the cerebral cortex and hippocampus, which are thought to control the learning and memory functions.

280   ANNALS NEW YORK ACADEMY OF SCIENCES

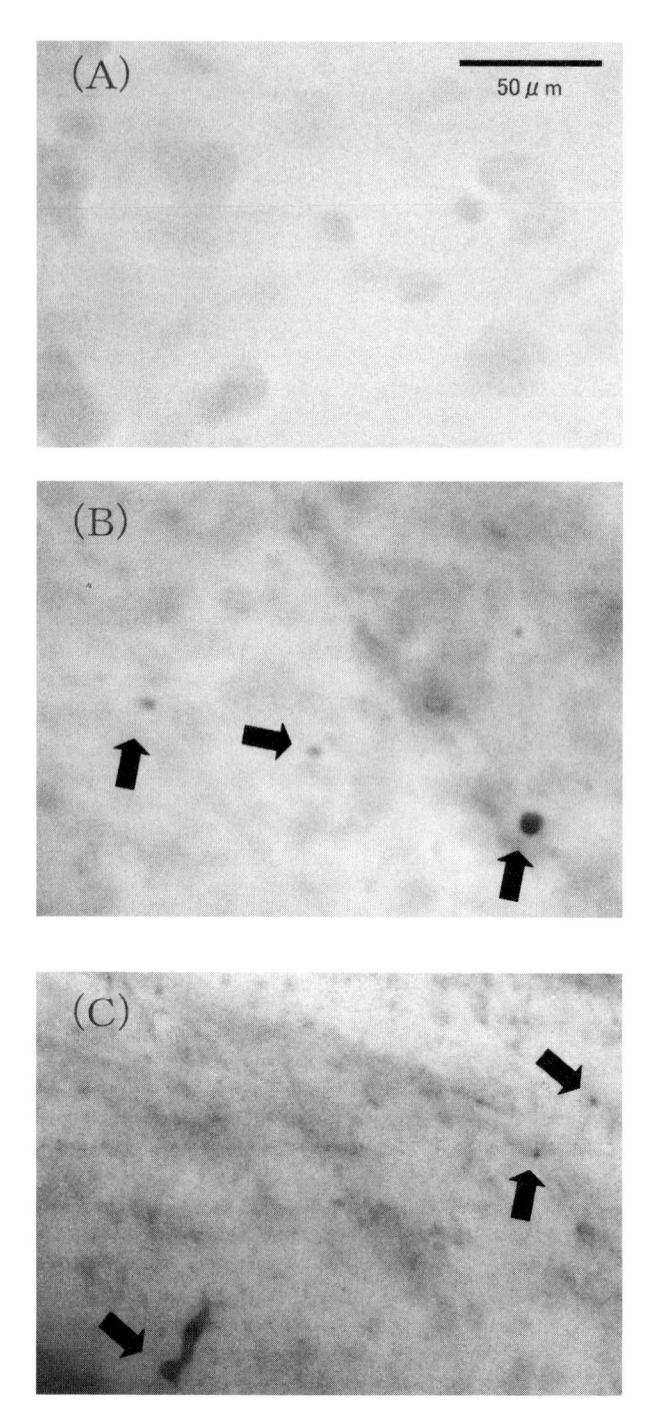

FIGURE 3. *See following page for legend.*

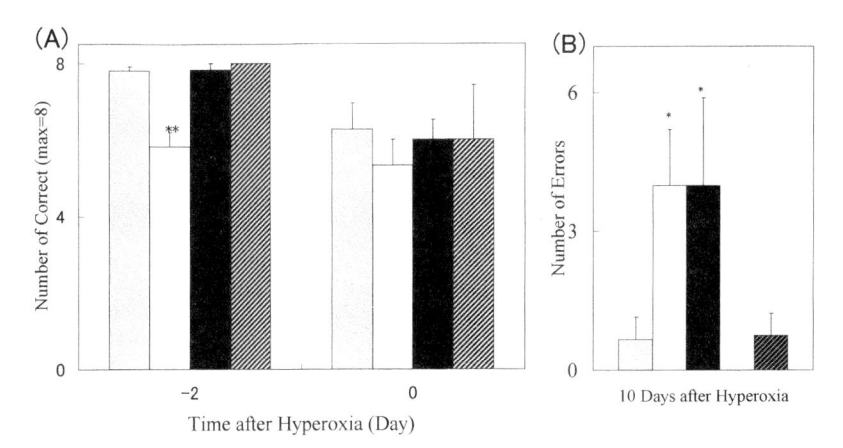

FIGURE 4. Memory retention before (A) and after (B) oxidative stress in an eight-arm radial performance. *Closed bars,* young control; *dotted bars,* 24 month old; *open bars,* vitamin E deficient; *slashed bars,* vitamin E supplement *$P < 0.01$, **$P < 0.05$, versus control. Vitamin E–deficient rats and 24-month-old rats were maintained under air, respectively.

The Damage to Brain Caused by Oxidative Stress

In order to verify whether deficit of cognitive performance of rats caused by oxidative stress involves oxidative injury to the rat brain, TBARS and lipid hydroperoxide levels were analyzed in synaptic membranes of rat cerebral cortex and hippocampus. As shown in TABLE 1, it was found that TBARS values in synaptic membranes of cerebral cortex and hippocampus of rats subjected to hyperoxia were significantly higher than those in the normal control. When vitamin E–deficient rats were maintained under air, the TBARS were also increased remarkably in both regions. Lipid hydroperoxides are another indicator of lipid peroxidation. The levels of lipid hydroperoxides in synaptic membranes of both regions were increased significantly by oxidative stress, aging, and vitamin E deficiency in a way similar to the changes in TBARS.

Protein carbonyls in the synaptic plasma membrane of whole brain were also increased remarkably by oxidative stress. These results suggest that nerve cells are extremely susceptible to oxidative stress and that the oxidative damage in nerve terminals caused by reactive oxygen species may induce declines in neurotransmission.

It has been considered that depolarization of the synaptic membrane surface is necessarily needed for neurotransmission. It is reasonable to consider that the nerve terminal damage caused by oxidative stress and aging may induce a deficit of depolarization of the membrane surface, resulting in a deterioration of the neurotransmission systems. As shown in FIGURE 5, the ζ-potential of synaptic membranes was significantly decreased by oxidative stress, aging, and vitamin E deficiency; on the

---

FIGURE 3. Appearance of delayed-type apoptosis caused by oxidative stress and aging in CA1 region of the hippocampus of rats. (**A**) Just after the stress; (**B**) at 7 days after the stress; (**C**) in the CA1 region of 24-month-old rats maintained under air. Magnification for each photograph is shown by the bar in **A**. Arrowhead shows apoptosis in CA1 region.

TABLE 1. Changes in the contents of TBARS, lipid peroxides, and protein carbonyls in synaptic membranes caused by hyperoxia and aging

Parameter	Control	Hyperoxia	Old[c]	Vit. E deficient[c]	Vit. E supplement[d]
TBARS (nmol/mg protein) cerebral cortex	2.38 ± 0.01	4.39 ± 1.30[a]	3.78 ± 0.89[b]	4.87 ± 2.02[a]	2.89 ± 0.15
Hippocampus	2.56 ± 0.06	4.23 ± 0.12[b]	3.18 ± 1.02[b]	3.84 ± 0.06[a]	2.38 ± 0.21
Lipid peroxides (pmol/mg protein) cerebral cortex	60.01 ± 10.23	111.14 ± 20.18[a]	80.15 ± 8.35[b]	92.38 ± 15.29[b]	61.83 ± 6.53
Hippocampus	67.83 ± 13.41	118.26 ± 18.79[a]	84.27 ± 5.83[b]	89.98 ± 16.86[b]	69.78 ± 5.88
Protein carbonyls (nmol/mg protein) cerebral cortex	1.62 ± 0.51	2.58 ± 0.48[b]	2.25 ± 0.26	2.24 ± 0.12[b]	1.41 ± 0.56
Hippocampus	1.25 ± 0.49	1.50 ± 0.58	1.48 ± 0.23	1.51 ± 0.36	1.27 ± 0.25

NOTE: Values are means ± SE, $n = 8$.
[a]$P < 0.01$.
[b]$P < 0.05$ versus control.
[c]Animals were maintained in air.
[d]Animals wer subjected to hyperoxia.

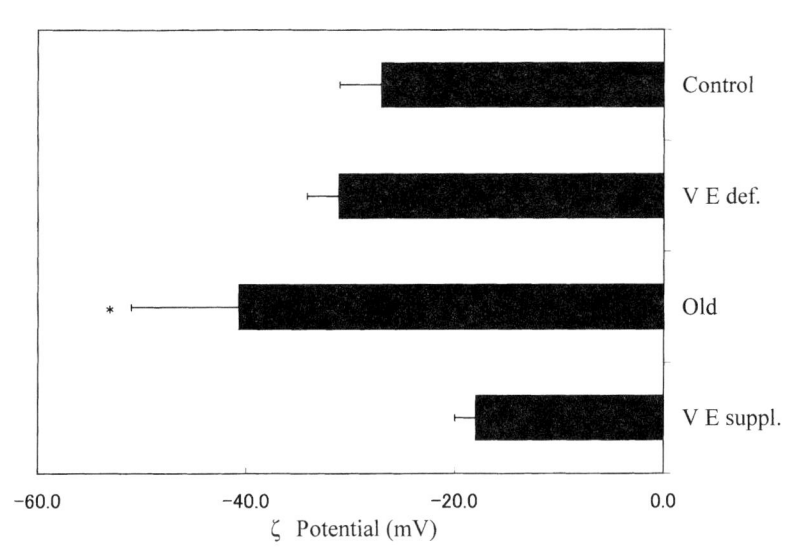

FIGURE 5. Changes in ζ-potential on synaptic membrane surface in rat brain caused by hyperoxia and aging, and its prevention by vitamin E. $^*P < 0.05$, versus control ($n = 6$ each).

contrary, vitamin E–supplemented rats showed the normal values even if they were subjected to hyperoxia.

In conclusion, results obtained in this study suggest that an oxidative degeneration of lipids and proteins in nerve terminal membranes may change the membrane surface potential, resulting in a deterioration of the neurotransmission systems due to a decline in the membrane fusion between nerve terminal membranes and synaptic vesicles, including the neurotransmitter. This consideration is consistent with our previous reports that synaptic vesicles accumulate abnormally in nerve terminals from oxidative stress and aging.[8,9] These reports imply that this damage in the cerebral cortex and hippocampus may induce a decline of cognitive function, such as learning and memory. Vitamin E protects the nervous system in the brain against oxidative stress during aging and, hence, prevents the decline of cognitive functions.

REFERENCES

1. RILEY, P.A. 1994. Free radical in biology: oxidative stress and the effect of ionizing radiation. Int. J. Radiat. Biol. **65:** 27–33.
2. BENZI, G. *et al.* 1992. The mitochondrial electron transfer alteration as a factor involved in the brain aging. Neurobiol. Aging **16:** 361–368.
3. SIGENAGA, M.K. *et al.* 1994. Oxidative damage and mitochondrial decay in aging. Proc. Natl. Acad. Sci. USA **91:** 10771–10778.
4. BEAL, M.F. 1995. Aging, energy, and oxidative stress in neurodegenerative diseases. Ann. Neurol. **38:** 357–366.
5. HALLIWELL, B. 1984. Oxidants and the central nervous system: some fundamental questions. Acta Neurol. Scand. **126:** 23–33.

6. FRANÇOIS, C. *et al.* 1981. Topographical and cytological localization of iron in rat and monkey brains. Brain Res. **215:** 317–322.
7. VOLICER, L. & P.B. CRINO. 1990. Involvment of free radicals in dementia of the Alzheimer's type: a hypothesis. Neurobiol. Aging **11:** 567–571.
8. URANO, S., Y. ASAI, S. MAKABE, *et al.* 1997. Oxidative injury of synapse and alteration of antioxidative defense systems in rats, and its prevention by vitamin E. Eur. J. Biochem. **245:** 64–70.
9. URANO, S., Y. SATO, T. OTONARI, *et al.* 1998. Aging and oxidative stress in neurodegeneration. BioFactors **7:** 103–112.

Reaction of Carnosine with Aged Proteins

Another Protective Process?

ALAN R. HIPKISS, CAROL BROWNSON, MARIANA F. BERTANI, EMILIO RUIZ, AND ALBERT FERRO

GKT School of Biomedical Sciences, King's College London,
Guy's Campus, London Bridge, London SE1 1UL, United Kingdom

ABSTRACT: Cellular aging is often associated with an increase in protein carbonyl groups arising from oxidation- and glycation-related phenomena and suppressed proteasome activity. These "aged" polypeptides may either be degraded by 20S proteasomes or cross-link to form structures intractable to proteolysis and inhibitory to proteasome activity. Carnosine (β-alanyl-L-histidine) is present at surprisingly high levels (up to 20 mM) in muscle and nervous tissues in many animals, especially long-lived species. Carnosine can delay senescence in cultured human fibroblasts and reverse the senescent phenotype, restoring a more juvenile appearance. As better antioxidants/free-radical scavengers than carnosine do not demonstrate these antisenescent effects, additional properties of carnosine must contribute to its antisenescent activity. Having shown that carnosine can react with protein carbonyls, thereby generating "carnosinylated" polypeptides using model systems, we propose that similar adducts are generated in senescent cells exposed to carnosine. Polypeptide-carnosine adducts have been recently detected in beef products that are relatively rich in carnosine, and carnosine's reaction with carbonyl functions generated during amino acid deamidation has also been described. Growth of cultured human fibroblasts with carnosine stimulated proteolysis of long-labeled proteins as the cells approached their "Hayflick limit," consistent with the idea that carnosine ameliorates the senescence-associated proteolytic decline. We also find that carnosine suppresses induction of heme-oxygenase-1 activity following exposure of human endothelial cells to a glycated protein. The antisenescent activity of the spin-trap agent α-phenyl-*N*-*t*-butylnitrone (PBN) towards cultured human fibroblasts resides in *N*-*t*-butyl-hydroxylamine, its hydrolysis product. As hydroxylamines are reactive towards aldehydes and ketones, the antisenescent activity of *N*-*t*-butyl-hydroxylamine and other hydroxylamines may be mediated, at least in part, by reactivity towards macromolecular carbonyls, analogous to that proposed for carnosine.

KEYWORDS: fibroblasts; endothelial; heme-oxygenase-1; proteasome; carbonyl; cross-links; oxidation; glycation; deamidation; adducts; PBN; hydroxylamines

Address for correspondence: Alan Hipkiss, Henriette-Raphael House, GKT School of Biomedical Sciences, King's College London, Guy's Campus, London Bridge, London SE1 1UL, U.K. Voice: +44-(0)207-848-6071; +fax: 44-(0)207-848-6399.
alan.hipkiss@kcl.ac.uk

CARNOSINE AND CELL SENESCENCE

Carnosine (β-alanyl-L-histidine) is a possible antioxidant[1–3] that has antisenescence activity; the dipeptide reverses the senescent phenotype within 1–2 weeks when added to cultured human fibroblasts.[4–6] It is suggested that properties additional to its antioxidant role are responsible for carnosine's rejuvenating effects.[7,8] First, it is difficult to understand how passive ROS-scavenging activity of typical antioxidant/free-radical scavengers could induce an active reversal of the senescent phenotype, and, second, better antioxidants and free-radical scavengers than carnosine do not provoke the rejuvenating effects.

Studies showed that carnosine could be a naturally occurring antiglycating agent,[9–12] as it protected proteins and peptides against modifications induced by a variety of deleterious aldehydes and ketones, including the lipid peroxidation product malondialdehyde. Indeed carnosine inhibited malondialdehyde-induced generation of polypeptide carbonyls and protein cross-linking,[12] modifications typical of aging. Carnosine's structure resembles preferred glycation sites in proteins, and it probably behaves as a sacrificial sink for deleterious sugars and aldehydes, such as malondialdehyde and 4-hydroxynonenal. Carnosine's antiglycating activity and aldehyde-scavenging potential have been confirmed by others.[13–17] That carnosine's concentration is highest in nonoxidative, glycolytic muscle[18] is consistent with its proposed aldehyde-scavenging activity, although this does not preclude its possible rapid consumption in other tissues.

The ability of carnosine to react with deleterious low-molecular-weight aldehydes is, however, yet another passive prophylactic activity and still does not explain its rejuvenating actions on cultured fibroblasts. It is therefore proposed that carnosine could activate the disposal of aberrant proteins that normally accumulate in se-

TABLE 1. The effect of carnosine on proteolysis in cultured human fibroblasts[a]

Percent Proteolysis Measured at	Grown with 30 mM carnosine Number of cell divisions			Grown without carnosine Number of cell divisions		
	39	44	63	39	44	63
At 1 hour	5.2	5.4	12.3	5.7	4.6	6.3
Plus 30 mM carnosine	6.2	8.0	13.3	6.2	6.0	6.1
At 4 hours	10.6	13.1	21.5	11.2	12.3	13.4
Plus 30 mM carnosine	11.8	15.7	20.0	12.6	13.2	14.6

[a]MRC-5 fibroblasts were grown as described by McFarland and Holliday.[4] Confluent cultures were radiolabeled with [^{14}C]leucine for 3 days. The medium and radiolabel were then removed; the cells were washed three times with PBS and then reincubated in growth medium supplemented with excess unlabeled leucine (20 mM), with or without 30 mM carnosine. Samples of medium (1 mL) were removed, trichloroacetic acid (TCA) added to 5%, and the radioactivity in the TCA-soluble fraction determined using a liquid scintillation spectrometer (Beckman). Proteolysis, indicated by the increase in TCA-soluble radioactivity over time, is expressed as a percentage of the total radioactivity incorporated into cell protein.

TABLE 2. Stimulation of loss of protein carbonyl groups by carnosine[a]

Incubation time	Carbonyl groups/mole protein
0 days	7.0
7 days	
No additions	5.2
Plus carnosine (50 mM)	3.0
Plus lysine (50 mM)	3.8

[a]Ovalbumin (10 mg/mL) was incubated with 100 mM methylglyoxal (MG) for 14 days and then dialyzed exhaustively to remove unreacted MG. The MG-treated ovalbumin was then reincubated at 37°C in 0.1 M phosphate buffer with/without either 50 mM carnosine or 50 mM lysine. Carbonyl groups present in the MG-treated protein were assayed by reactivity towards 2,4-dinitrophenylhydrazine as described.[22]

nescent cells. Indeed some preliminary studies showed that when cultured with carnosine, proteolysis of predominantly long-lived polypeptides was stimulated in fibroblasts as they approached their "Hayflick limit" (Ref. 19 and TABLE 1). This observation may be explained by either a stimulatory effect on the cells' proteolytic machinery and/or some action on the polypeptide substrates that facilitated their elimination. Ikeda et al.[20] found that carnosine induces expression of a number of genes in cultured fibroblasts, including the gene coding form vimentin, a protein that may play a role in endocytosis.[21] This observation is consistent with the idea that carnosine induces an up-regulation of a proteolytic activity. Much more work is required to confirm this likely possibility, however.

CARNOSINE AND AGED PROTEINS

Accumulation of protein carbonyl groups is often taken to be a biomarker of aging and an indicator of oxidative damage. Protein aging is the result of a number of predominantly postsynthetic modifications, including oxidation, glycation, and asparagine/glutamine deamidation. There is evidence that carnosine could be involved with all three of the above; its reactivity towards carbonyl functions could be a common factor that could theoretically facilitate the destruction or elimination of aged proteins from the cell.

CARNOSINE AND PROTEIN OXIDATION

Not only can carnosine prevent generation of carbonyl groups on proteins induced by malondialdehyde, hypochlorite, and methylglyoxal,[12] but it may also react directly with protein carbonyl groups (Ref. 22 and TABLES 2 and 3), producing protein-carbonyl-carnosine adducts or "carnosinylated" proteins,[23] thereby preventing cross-linking to other, unmodified protein.[22] Indeed γ-glutamyl-carnosine adducts have recently been detected by Karuda et al.[26] in beef products; conceivably the adducts derive from reaction of carnosine with glutamyl-semialdehyde in proteins

TABLE 3. The reaction of radiolabeled carnosine with methylglyoxal-treated ovalbumin[a]

Contents of incubation mixture	Radioactivity detected (cpm)
Untreated ovalbumin plus [^{14}C]carnosine	47
MG-treated ovalbumin plus [^{14}C]carnosine	833
MG-treated ovalbumin plus [^{14}C]carnosine plus 50 mM lysine	142

[a]Ovalbumin (10 mg/mL) was treated with 100 mM methyglyoxal (MG) for 2 weeks and then dialyzed exhaustively to remove unreacted MG. The MG-treated protein and control untreated ovalbumin were then incubated with [^{14}C]carnosine (5.8 nCi/mL) at 37°C in 10 mM phosphate buffer. After 3 weeks 400 µL were removed and protein precipitated with TCA (5%). The precipitate was washed three times in 5% TCA and redissolved in 0.5% NaOH (500 µL), and the radioactivity was determined in a liquid scintillation spectrometer.

formed from oxidation of arginine and proline residues. Alternatively/additionally carnosine may be involved in deamidation of asparagine and glutamine residues (see below).

Oxidized proteins are normally degraded by 20S proteasomes, but highly oxidized/cross-linked polypeptides can inhibit proteasome function.[24,25] Therefore it is at least conceivable that in cultured cells, carnosine, by reacting with protein carbonyls on oxidized proteins, could suppress inhibitory effects on proteasome activity and perhaps facilitate their proteolytic elimination. Our results (Ref. 19 and TABLE 1) are at least consistent with this proposal, but more studies are required. For example, does addition of carnosine stimulate proteolysis of oxidized protein in peroxide-treated cells, and are carnosinylated proteins proteolytic substrates or do they form inert lipofuscin-like structures? Very preliminary studies indicate that carnosine may be beneficial to the survival of peroxide-treated fibroblasts when added following removal of the oxidant (Kourousi, Rodriguez & Hipkiss, unpublished observations). If substantiated, these observations are consistent with our proposal, but much more work is required; for example, it is necessary to search for carnosinylated proteins in peroxide-treated cells and test their susceptibility to degradation by the proteasomes.

CARNOSINE AND PROTEIN GLYCATION

Another source of age-related aberrant protein is glycation,[26] the products of which are called advanced glycosylation end products (AGEs) and frequently possess carbonyl groups. Carnosine has been shown to protect cells[28] and proteins[29] against the deleterious effects of low-molecular-weight AGEs. Recent studies show that carnosine can protect cultured human endothelial cells (HUVEC) against glycated albumin, as judged by the dipeptide's ability to inhibit the up-regulation of heme-oxygenase-1 (HO-1) activity[29,30] following the cells' exposure to a protein-AGE (FIG. 1C). A similar result was obtained using fibroblasts obtained from a diabetic patient (FIG. 1A); however, the AGE did not induce HO-1 activity in cells from a nondiabetic control (FIG. 1B). The mechanism(s) whereby these protective effects are mediated remain to be elucidated, however, although direct reaction of the dipeptide with the AGE is one of a number of possibilities. It is also possible that carnos-

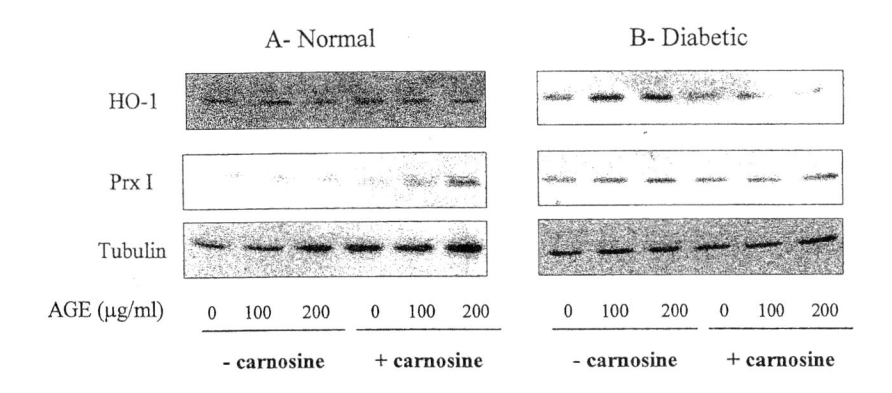

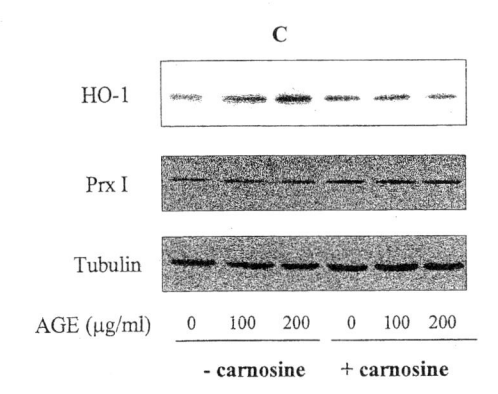

FIGURE 1. The effects of carnosine on AGE-induced heme-oxygenase-1 and peroxiredoxin-1 expression in (**A**) fibroblasts from a nondiabetic patient; (**B**) fibroblasts from a diabetic nephropathy patient; and (**C**) human umbilical vein endothelial cells (HUVEC). Confluent cell monolayers were pretreated with 20 mM carnosine for 24 hours and then challenged for 24 hours with 100 or 200 mg/mL protein-AGE (bovine serum albumin exposed to 100 mM glucose for 6 weeks at 37°C). Heme oxygenase-1 (HO-1) and peroxiredoxin-1 (Prx1) were detected by Western blotting of cell lysates with appropriate antibodies following SDS-PAGE.

ine's antioxidant activity could have a role here, as AGEs are reported to induce a hyperoxic effect following binding to RAGEs, the AGE receptors.[31]

CARNOSINE AND AMINO ACID DEAMIDATION

Deamidation of asparagine and glutamine residues in proteins is another source of age-related aberrant protein. Deamidation results in production of L or D forms of aspartic and glutamic acids, as well as isopeptide conformations where the side-chain carboxyl group (β or γ, respectively) becomes incorporated into the polypeptide backbone.[32] That a partial repair mechanism for this process[33] is widely distributed in nature indicates the biological importance of this type of postsynthetic change. Mice defective in the gene coding for the enzyme that initiates the repair, protein isoaspartate methyl transferase (PIMT or PCMT), accumulate large amounts of aberrant protein in their brains and usually die prematurely.[33]

It appears that carnosine may intervene during deamidation. Recent observations from food science show that covalent adducts between carnosine and polypeptide are found in beef soup preparations.[26,34] Further studies showed that if present during heat-induced deamidation of asparagine and glutamine, carnosine can react with the carbonyl species produced following loss of the amino group from the amide side chain of the amino acids generating β-aspartyl-carnosine and γ-glutamyl-carnosine adducts, respectively.[26] It appears that carnosine's amino group can form β- or γ-peptide bonds to the side chain carbonyls of the amino acids.[26] Interestingly, formation of the carnosine adducts proceeded about fourfold faster with asparagine deamidation than with glutamine.[26] A number of other products were also detected that contained either β-alanine or histidine, suggesting that cleavage of the peptide bond between β-alanine and histidine can occur. In the case of asparagine, 14 adducts were detected, whereas only 10 were detected when glutamine was incubated with carnosine.[26] It may be significant that three of the extra peptide adducts detected following asparagine's reaction with carnosine were particularly enriched with β-alanine, which could indicate that the peptide bond between β-alanine and histidine becomes particularly labile during/following the dipeptide's reaction with the asparginyl carbonyl derivative. This observation might explain the absence of β-aspartyl-carnosine adducts in the beef preparation, whereas γ-glutamyl-carnosine adducts were readily observed[26] as well as adducts containing β-alanine and histidine. Indeed is has been suggested that the presence of carnosinase, an enzyme that cleaves the bond between β-alanine and histidine, could influence carnosine's reactivity *in vivo*.[23]

COULD OTHER AGENTS THAT SUPPRESS SENESCENCE ALSO REACT WITH PROTEIN CARBONYL GROUPS?

The spin trap agent α-phenyl-*N*-*t*-butylnitrone (PBN) has been reported to delay senescence in cultured human fibroblasts.[35] It has apparently been assumed that PBN's antisenescent activity resides in its antioxidant/free-radical scavenging activities. However, Atamna *et el.*[36] recently showed that in fibroblasts PBN's hydrolysis product *N*-*t*-butylhydroxylamine was the active agent that delayed appearance of the senescent phenotype. Furthermore other hydroxylamines were also shown to possess similar antisenescent activity. It is suggested[37] that because hydroxylamines are generally reactive towards aldehydes and ketones, this property could better explain their antiaging activity toward cultured cells than exclusive antioxidant function, and that their antisenescent actions are similar to those proposed for carnosine.[23] Therefore it is speculated that protein-carbonyl-hydroxylamine adducts could be generated in PBN- and hydroxylamine-treated fibroblasts. Again a search for such adducts and an investigation of their proteolytic susceptibility could be fruitful.

Aminoguanidine is another agent that has been shown to suppress senescence in cultured cells.[38] This agent can also react with glycated polypeptides and AGEs,[39] perhaps similarly to that proposed for carnosine.[23] Hence aminguanidine's antisenescent activity might also be explained, at least partially, by reaction with oxidized/glycated polypeptides, thereby suppressing any deleterious interactions with other proteins and possibly facilitating their destruction.

ACTION OF ANTISENESCENT AGENTS *IN VIVO*

Carnosine and PBN have all been reported to delay senescence in senescence-accelerated mice (SAMP),[40,41] although better antioxidants than carnosine and PBN do not seem to possess antiaging activity *in vivo*. Assuming that the active agent of PBN *in vivo* is *N-t*-butylhydroxylamine,[36] the possibility arises that the antiaging mechanism of PBN and carnosine could reside at least partly in an ability to react with protein carbonyls, in addition to any antioxidant function. Such activity could explain the PBN-induced disappearance of protein carbonyls from gerbil brains and their rapid reappearance following its withdrawal.[42]

Kinetin also suppresses senescence in cultured cells and appears to possess both anti-oxidant and antiglycating activities.[43] As aging is multifactorial, pluripotency may therefore be a necessary quality for antiaging activity,[8,27] which PBN, kinetin and carnosine appear to possess.

Caloric restriction is the only reproducible method by which the average and maximal life span of many species can be extended.[44] Although many mechanisms have been proposed as explanations, few have been totally convincing, although the inhibitory effects of persistent hyperinsulinemia on proteasome activity in ad libitum fed animals[45–47] is attractive. Moreover maintenance of proteasome activity is important for DNA repair[48] and cell division,[49] and both show an age-related decline. The possible effects of carnosine, kinetin, aminoguanidine, and PBN in suppressing proteasome inhibition outlined above are consistent with such an explanation.

INTERRELATIONSHIP BETWEEN VARIOUS FORMS OF ABERRANT PROTEINS

It appears that many features of the aberrant proteins that accumulate with age are interrelated. For example, transcriptional frame-shift errors may increase with age,[50] erroneously synthesized proteins show an increased susceptibility to oxidative damage,[51] oxidative conditions increase asparagine/aspartate instability in proteins,[52] and asparagine/aspartate residue instability in DNA glycosylases and caspases could conceivably affect both DNA repair and apoptosis.[54] Coupled with the inhibitory effects of aberrant forms of ubiquitin and cross-linked proteins on 26S[53] and 20S[25] proteasome activity respectively, these observations demonstrate the not entirely unexpected synergy between various mechanistic explanations of aging and why pluripotent agents might be particularly successful for antiaging intervention.

CONCLUSIONS

Carnosine is one of a very few naturally occurring agents that can suppress the senescent phenotype in both cultured cells and possibly *in vivo*. Other antisenescent agents (PBN, aminoguanidine, and kinetin) appear to be pluripotent in their actions, like carnosine. In searching for possible mechanisms to explain the loss of the senescent phenotype, it is suggested that reaction with carbonyl groups present on proteins and other aged macromolecules is one property that carnosine, PBN, aminoguanidine, and kinetin could have in common. Carbonyls/aldehydes may also be generated at amino groups in some lipids and in DNA following spontaneous depurination/depyrimidation and base excision during repair. These proposals suggest novel routes for therapeutic intervention.

REFERENCES

1. BOLDYREV, A.A., V.E. FORMAZYUK & V.I. SERGIENKO. 1994. Biological significance of histidine-containing dipeptides with special reference to carnosine: chemistry, distribution, metabolism and medical applications. Sov. Sci. Rev. D. Physicochem. Biol. **13:** 1–60.
2. QUINN, P.R., A.A. BOLDYREV & V.E. FORMAZUYK. 1992. Carnosine: its properties, functions and potential therapeutic applications. Mol. Aspects Med. **13:** 379–444.
3. KOHEN, R., Y. YAMAMOTO, K.C. CUNDY & B.N. AMES. 1988. Antioxidant activity of carnosine, homocarnosine and anserine present in muscle and brain. Proc. Natl. Acad. Sci. USA **95:** 2175–2179.
4. MCFARLAND, G.A. & R. HOLLIDAY. 1994. Retardation of the senescence of cultured human diploid fibroblasts by carnosine. Exp. Cell Res. **212:** 167–175.
5. MCFARLAND, G.A. & R. HOLLIDAY. 1999. Further evidence for the rejuvenating effects of the dipeptide L-carnosine on cultured human diploid fibroblasts. Exp. Gerontol. **34:** 35–45.
6. HOLLIDAY, R. & G.A. MCFARLAND. 2000. A role for carnosine in cellular maintenance. Biochemistry (Moscow) **65:** 991–997.
7. HIPKISS, A.R., R. HOLLIDAY, G.A. MCFARLAND & J. MICHAELIS. 1993. Carnosine and senescence. Lifespan **4:** 1–3.
8. HIPKISS, A.R. 1998. Carnosine, a protective anti-ageing peptide? Int. J. Biochem. Cell Biol. **30:** 863–868.
9. HIPKISS, A.R., J. MICHAELIS & P. SYRRIS. 1995. Non-enzymic glycosylation of the dipeptide L-carnosine, a potential anti-protein-cross-linking agent. FEBS Letts. **371:** 81–85.
10. HIPKISS, A.R., J.E. PRESTON, D.T.M. HIMSWORTH, *et al.* 1997. Protective effects of carnosine against malondialdehyde induced toxicity towards cultured rat brain endothelial cells. Neurosci. Letts. **238:** 135–138.
11. HIPKISS, A.R., J. MICHAELIS, P. SYRRIS, *et al.* 1994. Carnosine protects proteins against in vitro glycation and cross-linking. Biochem. Soc. Trans. **22:** 399S.
12. HIPKISS, A.R., V.C. WORTHINGTON, D.T.J. HIMSWORTH & W. HERWIG. 1997. Protective effects of carnosine against protein modification mediated by malondialdehyde and hypochlorite. Biochim. Biophys. Acta **1380:** 46–54.
13. LEE, B.J., K.S. KANG, S.Y. NAM, *et al.* 1999. Effects of carnosine and related compounds on monosaccharide autoxidation and H_2O_2 formation. Korean J. Physiol. Pharmacol. **3:** 251–261.
14. SWEARENGIN, T.A., C. FITZGERALD & N.W. SEIDLER. 1999. Carnosine prevents glyceraldehyde 3-phosphate-mediated inhibition of aspartate aminotransferase. Mol. Toxicol. **73:** 307–309.
15. VINSON, J.A. & T.B. HOWARD. 1996. Inhibition of protein glycation and advanced glycation end products by ascorbic acid and other vitamins and nutrients. Nutr. Biochem. **7:** 659–663.

16. KULEVA, N.V. & Z.S. KOVALENKO. 1997. Change in the functional properties of actin by its glycation *in vitro*. Biochemistry (Moscow) **62:** 1119–1123.
17. DECKER, E.A., S.A. LIVISAY & S. ZHOU. 2000. A re-evaluation of the antioxidant activity of purified carnosine. Biochemistry (Moscow) **65:** 766–770.
18. ABE, H. 2000. Role of histidine-related compounds as intracellular proton buffering constituents in vertebrate muscle. Biochemistry (Moscow) **65:** 757–765.
19. HIPKISS, A.R., J. MICHAELIS, P. SYRRIS & M. DREMANIS. 1995. Strategies for extension of human lifespan. Perspect. Hum. Biol. **1:** 59–70.
20. IKEDA, D., S. WADA, C. YONEDA, *et al.* 1999. Carnosine stimulates vimentin expression in cultured rat fibroblasts. Cell Struct. Function **24:** 79–87.
21. SUN, W.B., B.L. HAN, Z.M. PENG, *et al.* 1998. Effect of aging on cytoskeletal system of Kupfer cell and its phagocytic capacity. World J. Gastroenterol. **4:** 70–77.
22. BROWNSON, C. & A.R. HIPKISS. 2000. Carnosine reacts with a glycated protein. Free Radic. Biol. Med. **28:** 1564–1570.
23. HIPKISS, A.R. & C. BROWNSON. 2000. Carnosine reacts with protein carbonyl groups: another possible role for the anti-ageing peptide? Biogerontology **1:** 217–223.
24. SITTE, N., M. HUBER, T. GRUNE, *et al.* 2000. Proteasome inhibition by lipofuscin/ceroid during postmitotic aging of fibroblasts. FASEB J. **14:** 1490–1498.
25. FRIGUET, B. & L.I. SZWEDA. 1997. Inhibition of the multicatalytic proteinase (proteasome) by 4-hydroxynonenal cross-linked protein. FEBS Lett. **405:** 21–25.
26. KURODA, M., R. OHTAKE, E. SUZUKI, *et al.* 2000. Investigation on the formation and the determination of γ-glutamyl-β-alanylhistidine and related isopeptide in the macromolecular fraction of beef soup stock. J. Agric. Food. Chem. **48:** 6317–6324.
27. BAYNES, J.W. & V.M. MONNIER. 1989. The Maillard reaction in aging, diabetes and medicine. Alan R. Liss. New York.
28. HIPKISS, A.R., J.E. PRESTON, D.T.M. HIMSWORTH, *et al.* 1998. Pluripotent protective effects of carnosine, a naturally occurring dipeptide. Ann. N. Y. Acad. Sci. **854:** 37–53.
29. HIPKISS, A.R. & H. CHANA. 1998. Carnosine protects proteins against methylglyoxal-mediated modifications. Biochem. Biophys. Res. Commun. **248:** 28–32.
30. HAMMES, H.P., A. BARTMAN, L. ENGEL & P. WULFROTH. 1997. Antioxidant treatment of experimental diabetic retinopathy with nicanartine. Diabetologia **40:** 629–634.
31. SCHMIDT, A.M., O. HORI, R. CAO, *et al.* 1996. RAGE—a novel cellular receptor for advanced glycation end products. Diabetes **45:** S77–S80.
32. GEIGER, T. & S. CLARKE. 1987. Deamidation, isomerization, and racemization at asparaginyl and aspartyl residues in peptides—succinimide-linked reactions that contribute to protein-degradation. J. Biol. Chem. **262:** 785–794.
33. LOWENSON, J.D., E. KIM, S.G. YOUNG & S. CLARKE. 2001. Limited accumulation of damaged proteins in L-isoaspartyl (D-aspartyl) *O*-methyltransfersase-deficient mice. J. Biol. Chem. **276:** 20695–20702.
34. KURODA, M. & T. HARADA. 2000. Incorporation of histidine and β-alanine into the macromolecular fraction of beef stock solution. J. Food Sci. **65:** 596–603.
35. CHEN, Q., A. FISCHER, J.D. REAGEN, *et al.* 1995. Oxidative DNA damage and senescence of human diploid fibroblast cells. Proc. Natl. Acad. Sci. USA **92:** 4337–4341.
36. ATAMNA, H., A. PALERMARTINEZ & B.N. AMES. 2000. *N-t*-butylhydroxylamine, a hydrolysis product of α-phenyl-*N-t*-butylnitrone, is more potent in delaying senescence in human lung fibroblasts. J. Biol. Chem. **275:** 6741–6748.
37. HIPKISS, A.R. 2001. On the anti-aging activities of aminoguanidine and *N-t*-butylhydroxylamine. Mech. Ageing Dev. **122:** 169–171.
38. FUJISAWA, H., T. NISHIKAWA, B.N. ZHU, *et al.* 1999. Aminoguanidine supplementation delays the onset of senescence in vitro in dermal fibroblasts-like cells from senescence-accelerated mice. J. Gerontol. **54:** 276–282.
39. LIGGINS, J. & A.J. FURTH. 1997. Role of protein-bound carbonyls in the formation of advanced glycosylation end-products. Biochim. Biophys. Acta **1361:** 123–130.
40. YUNEVA, M.O., E.R. BULYGINA, S.C. GALLANT, *et al.* 1999. Effect of carnosine on age-induced changes in senescence-accelerated mice. J. Anti-Aging Med. **2:** 337–342.
41. EDAMATSU, R., A. MORI & L. PACKER. 1995. The spin trap agent *N-tert*-α-phenyl-butylnitrone prolongs the life span of the senescence accelerated mouse. Biochem. Biophys. Res. Commun. **211:** 847–849.

42. BUTTERFIELD, D.A., B.J. HOWARD & S. YATIM. 1997. Free radical oxidation of brain proteins in accelerated senescence and its modulation by N-*tert*-butyl-α-phenylnitrone. Proc. Natl. Acad. Sci. USA **94:** 674–678.
43. RATTAN, S.I.S. & B.F.C. CLARK. 1994. Kinetin delays the onset of aging characteristics in human fibroblasts. Biochem. Biophys. Res. Commun. **201:** 665–672.
44. FORSTER, M.J., B.H. SOHAL & R.S. SOHAL. 2000. Reversible effects of long-term caloric restriction on protein oxidative damage. J. Gerontol. **55:** B522–B529.
45. HAMEL, F.G., R.G. BENNETT, K.S. MARMON, *et al.* 1997. Insulin inhibition of proteasome activity in intact cells. Biochem. Biophys. Res. Commun. **234:** 671–674.
46. FACCHINI, F.S., N.W. HUA, G.M. REAVEN, *et al.* 2000. Hyperinsulinemia: the missing link among oxidative stress and age-related disease? Free Radic. Biol. Med. **29:** 1302–1306.
47. KELLER, J.N., K.B. HANNI & W.R. MARKSBURY. 2000. Possible involvement of proteasome inhibition in aging: implications for oxidative stress. Mech. Ageing Dev. **113:** 61–70.
48. WEISSMAN, A.M. 2001. Themes and variations on ubiquitylation. Nat. Rev. Mol. Cell Biol. **2:** 169–178.
49. RAO, H., F. UHLMANN & A. VARSHAVSKY. 2001. Degradation of a cohesin subunit by the N-end rule pathway is essential for chromosome stability. Nature **410:** 955–959.
50. VAN DEN HURK, W.H., H.J.J. WILLEMS, M. BLOEMEN & G.J.M. MARTENS. 2001. Novel frameshift mutations near short simple repeats. J. Biol. Chem. **276:** 11496–11498.
51. DUKAN, S., A. FAREWELL, M. BALLESTEROS, *et al.* 2000. Protein oxidation in response to increased transcriptional and translational errors. Proc. Natl. Acad. Sci. USA **97:** 5746–5749.
52. INGROSSO, D., S. D'ANGELO, E. DI CARLO, *et al.* 2000. Increased methyl esterification of altered aspartyl residues in erythrocyte membranes in response to oxidative stress. Eur. J. Biochem. **267:** 4397–4405.
53. LAM, Y.A., C.M. PICKART, A. ALBAN, *et al.* 2000. Inhibition of the ubiquitin-proteasome system in Alzheimer's disease. Proc. Natl. Acad. Sci. USA **97:** 9902–9906.
54. HIPKISS, A.R. 2001. On the "struggle between chemistry and biology during aging"—implications for DNA repair, apoptosis and proteolysis, and a novel route of intervention. Biogerontology **2:** 173–178.

Pharmacological Interventions in Aging and Age-associated Disorders

Potentials of Propargylamines for Human Use

KENICHI KITANI,[a] CHIYOKO MINAMI,[a] TAKAKO YAMAMOTO,[a] SETSUKO KANAI,[b] GWEN O. IVY,[c] AND MARIA-CRISTINA CARRILLO[d]

[a]*National Institute for Longevity Sciences, Aichi 474-8522, Japan*

[b]*Tokyo Metropolitan Institute of Gerontology, Japan*

[c]*University of Toronto at Scarborough, Scarborough, Canada*

[d]*University of Rosario, Rosario, Argentina*

ABSTRACT: Past studies including our own have confirmed that chronic administration of deprenyl can prolong life spans of at least four different animal species. Pretreatment with the drug for several weeks increases activities of superoxide dismutase (SOD) and catalase (CAT) in selective brain regions. An up-regulation of antioxidant enzyme activities can also be induced in organs such as the heart, kidney, spleen, and adrenal gland, and all are accompanied by an increase in mRNA levels for SODs in these organs. The effect of deprenyl on enzyme activities has a dose–effect relationship of a typical inverted U shape. A similar inverted U shape also has emerged for the drug's effect on survival of animals. An apparent parallelism observed between these two effects of the drug seems to support our contention that the up-regulation of antioxidant enzymes is at least partially responsible for the life-prolonging effect on animals. Further, when a clinically applied dose of the drug for patients with Parkinson's disease was given to monkeys, SOD and CAT activities were increased in striatum of these monkeys, which suggests potential for the drug's applicability to humans. The drug was also found to increase concentrations of cytokines such as interleukin-1β (IL-1β) and tumor necrosis factor-α (TNF-α) in the above rat organs. Together with past reports demonstrating that deprenyl increases natural killer (NK) cell functions and interferon-γ, and prevents the occurrence of malignant tumors in rodents and dogs, the mobilization of these humoral factors may therefore be included as possible mechanisms of action of deprenyl for its diverse antiaging and life-prolonging effects. The potentials of propargylamines, (−)deprenyl in particular, for human use as antiaging drugs remain worthy of exploration in the future.

KEYWORDS: propargylamines; deprenyl; life span prolongation; antioxidant enzymes; cytokines; rats; monkeys

Address for correspondence: K. Kitani, M.D., National Institute for Longevity Sciences, 36-3, Gengo Morioka-cho, Obu-shi, Aichi 474-8522, Japan. Voice: +81-562450183; fax: +81-562450184.

kitani@nils.go.jp

INTRODUCTION

Aging is a purely biological phenomenon that most organisms undergo. However, the biological mechanism(s) of aging is still poorly understood. The free radical theory of aging was proposed almost half a century ago[1] by Harman and appears to be increasingly supported in recent years. Yet, a direct proof for this theory is still lacking.

Based on the free radical theory of aging, many attempts to intervene in aging by means of administration of chemicals, pharmaceuticals, and nutriceuticals have been performed in the past 50 years.[2,3] However, to date, these types of trials have not achieved a general success. For example, Lipman and coworkers[3] administered five different antioxidants orally to C57BL male mice. They started the administration at the age of 13 months and examined survivals of these animals. None of the five antioxidant-treated groups survived for a longer time than control animals as judged by the 50% survival age.[3] Also, there was no difference between control and treated animals in pathologies as examined after sacrifice of the remaining half of the animals. Thus, the general consensus in experimental gerontology in the last century was (and still is) that the only reliable and reproducible means to extend the life span of animals is "caloric restriction (CR)."[4,5]

Despite these frustrating results in attempts to intervene in aging, several recent attempts by means of pharmaceutical intervention in aging have begun to appear promising. These include propargylamines [(−)deprenyl[6–8] in particular], nitrones starting with α-phenyl-*tert*-butyl-nitrone (PBN),[9,10] and a more recent attempt using a variety of so-called EUKs.[11] Fortunately, in this volume, we have chapters that address the latter two attempts. Accordingly, we attempt here to discuss only the potentials of propargylamines, (−)deprenyl in particular, in intervening in aging and age-associated disorders.

Since we have repeatedly reviewed and discussed results of our own studies as well as those of others in this series,[6–8] the past information relevant to this topic will be only briefly summarized and some new data that may help understand possible mechanisms underlying the pharmacological effects of these drugs will be introduced and their potential clinical relevance as antiaging drugs will be discussed in the present chapter.

HISTORY OF (−)DEPRENYL AS A LIFE SPAN EXTENSION DRUG

(−)Deprenyl was initially developed as an antidepressant.[12] However, when it turned out to be one of the monoamine oxidase (MAO) inhibitors, the clinical application of the drug was soon abandoned. Later, it turned out to be an MAO B inhibitor, and clinical trials as an anti-Parkinson drug have been mostly successful,[13–15] although there are some reports denying the beneficial effect of the drug for this disease.[16]

Birkmayer and coworkers in a retrospective study initially reported that patients with Parkinson's disease who received levodopa and deprenyl lived for a significantly longer period than control patients who received levodopa and placebo.[17]

Many randomized double-blind trials have been done up to now to test its efficacy for patients with Parkinson's disease. To our knowledge, though, there is no report

TABLE 1. Effect of deprenyl on life span of rats

Strain (sex)	Dose	Effect	Authors
Wistar-Logan (M)	0.25 mg/kg, sc (3×/week)[b]	>+100%[a]	Knoll[19]
F344 (M)	0.25 mg/kg, sc (3×/week)[b]	+16%[a]	Milgram et al.[20]
F344 (M)	0.5 mg/kg, sc (3×/week)[c]	+34%[a]	Kitani et al.[21]
F344 (M)	0.5 mg/kg, po (daily)[d]	No significant effect	Bickford et al.[22]
Wistar (M)	0.5 mg/kg, sc (3×/week)[e]	Adverse effect (shortening of life span)	Gallagher et al.[23]

[a]Average life expectancy after 24 months of age.
[b]After 24 months of age.
[c]After 18 months of age.
[d]Between 54 and 118 weeks.
[e]Between 3 and 23 months.

confirming the initial report by Birkmayer and coworkers[17] in terms of life expectancy prolongation. However, the advantage of (−)deprenyl, and possibly related propargylamines, over currently investigated drugs[9–11] is that (−)deprenyl has been used clinically for more than 10 years and the adverse drug effect is confirmed to be very minor, although some studies have cautioned against one side effect of the drug, orthostatic hypotension in particular.[18]

In 1988, Knoll [who had been involved in the development of (−)deprenyl] reported for the first time that male Wistar-Logan cross rats that began receiving the drug (0.25 mg/kg, 3 times a week, sc) at the age of 24 months lived for a significantly longer period than saline-treated control animals, with the average life expectancy at 24 months of age being more than two times greater in treated than control animals.[19] Since then, at least two additional studies,[20,21] including one by ourselves, on male Fischer 344 (F344) rats confirmed the initial results by Knoll, although neither of the two could achieve such a robust effect on the life span of rats as initially reported by Knoll.[19] On the other hand, there are some other studies that did not find any significant increase in remaining life expectancy with the drug.[22,23] Some of the results in rats are summarized in TABLE 1. In mice, the positive effect is more difficult to achieve. The only published study that reported a positive effect in mice in terms of life span extension is that of Archer and Harrison.[24] However, the effect was not so marked as was observed in rats[19–21] and was only marginally significant even in this particular study.[24]

However, this study is the only one that examined the food consumption of deprenyl-fed animals and found that it was not significantly different from that in the control mouse group, thus excluding the indirect effect of the drug of lowering diet consumption.[24] In this connection, we[21] and others[20] have also shown almost identical average body weights for control and (−)deprenyl-treated rats, which also supports the contention that the effect of the drug on life span is not due to CR caused by the drug treatment since no CR paradigm can extend the life span of animals without significantly reducing the body weight of animals.

Ruehl et al.[25] provided convincing evidence that the drug significantly retards the death of aging female beagle dogs, which appears to be largely explained by the significant reduction of the incidence of mammary cancer in treated animals.[25] The antitumorigenic effect of the drug has been recently discussed in relation to immunomodulatory and endocrinological effects of the drug by ThyagaRajan[26] and some additional discussion will be made later in this chapter in relation to our new findings on tumor necrosis factor-α (TNF-α).

FACTORS POSSIBLY CONTRIBUTING TO THE PROLONGATION OF LIFE SPANS OF ANIMALS

Knoll initially reported that a three-week treatment with the drug significantly increased (total) superoxide dismutase (SOD), but not catalase (CAT) activities in striatum of male Wistar-Logan cross rats.[19] Later, however, he could not reproduce this observation of SOD in another strain and cautioned that it may not be a universal effect of the drug.[27] We have extensively worked on this aspect of pharmacology of the drug. Our main observations made in the past 10 years are summarized below:

(1) Not only total SOD, but activities of both species of SODs (Cu, Zn- and Mn-) are significantly increased in brain dopaminergic regions such as s. nigra, striatum, and (to some extent) cerebral cortex, but not in hippocampus, cerebellum, or the liver.[28–31]

(2) Unlike the initial observation by Knoll,[19] we found that CAT, but not glutathione peroxidase (GSHPx) activities are significantly increased by the drug in regions where SOD activities are increased.[28–31]

(3) Very importantly, for the effect of increasing these antioxidant enzyme activities, an optimal dose range exists and, from a certain dose point above this optimal range, the effect becomes less efficient and the drug works adversely, decreasing the activities below physiological levels with an excessive dose[29] (for review, see Refs. 6–8).

(4) An optimal dose range is variable, depending on the sexes and ages of animals. Young F344 male rats have an optimal dose that is 10 times greater than young female rats;[29] however, age affects an optimal dose in opposite directions in male[30] and female[29] rats, decreasing an optimal dose in males, but increasing it in females.

(5) A major cause for the sex difference in an optimal dose in young rats appears to be much more efficient hepatic microsomal cytochrome P-450 enzyme activities in males than in females.[32] Since a big strain difference is known among different strains of even the same sex in P-450 functions in rat livers,[33] an optimal dose may differ among rats of different strains even of the same sex and age. A 2× difference in deprenyl's metabolism has been shown by Yoshida et al.[33] between male rats of different strains. The failure by Knoll in reproducing the same phenomenon observed in his Wistar-Logan cross rats in another strain[27] can be reasonably explained by this mechanism.

(6) In addition to the above factors, the duration of the treatment also determines an optimal effect. In general, the longer the treatment, the narrower

an optimal dose range in increasing antioxidant enzyme activities and the smaller the magnitude of an increase in enzyme activities.[34,35] This effect also depends on the species of animals. Mice are much more susceptible to this effect than rats.[34,35] We suspect that this is one major reason why the significant extension of survival of mice by the drug[6–8] is more difficult to achieve than that of rats.

(7) Recent studies by us have shown that the effect of (–)deprenyl on SOD and CAT activities is shared by other propargylamines such as rasagiline.[36] However, the magnitude of activity increases and the optimal dose range were different, depending on the different propargylamines tested, with the order of efficacy being (–)deprenyl > rasagiline > 2-heptyl-N-methylpropargylamine (HMP) > 2-heptylpropargylamine (HP).[37,38] This observation suggests that the chemical moieties other than the propargylamine are important in determining the magnitude of an increase in antioxidant enzyme activities. Although we have had no occasion to test the effect of desmethyldeprenyl, our experience with HMP and its desmethylated form (HP) suggests that N-methylation appears to strengthen this effect.

(8) Very importantly, we have recently realized that the effect of (–)deprenyl and other propargylamines on antioxidant enzymes is not limited to brain dopaminergic regions. Our studies with rasagiline[36] and (–)deprenyl[37,38] have shown that at least in rats they are effective in significantly increasing SOD and CAT activities in many organs outside of the brain, of primarily catecholaminergic nature. These organs include the heart, kidneys, adrenal glands, and spleen (TABLE 2).

(9) Furthermore, in these organs outside of the brain where SOD and CAT activities were increased, concentrations in humoral factors such as interleukin-1β (IL-1β) and TNF-α were significantly increased (TABLE 3).[37,38]

(10) We have recently examined whether our observations that have been made mainly in rodents and to some extent in dogs[39] can be reproduced in animals evolutionarily closer to humans. We treated young male monkeys (*Macaca fascicularis*) with two different oral doses of (–)deprenyl for 3.5 weeks. A smaller dose of 0.17 mg/kg is roughly equivalent to the clinically prescribed dose of the drug for Parkinson's disease patients (10 mg/day to a patient of 60-kg body weight). Another (higher) dose (1.0 mg/kg) was found to be more effective than lower doses in female beagle dogs.[39] We have found that the smaller dose is more effective than the higher dose in young male monkeys in increasing SOD and CAT activities in s. nigra and striatum and, very importantly, in mononuclear lymphocytes too (FIG. 1). Interestingly, though, the effect in lymphocytes was more marked at 2 weeks after treatment, and at 3.5 weeks after treatment the activity went down (FIG. 1). Further, in lymphocytes, the higher dose was totally ineffective and worked somewhat adversely, decreasing the physiological levels at some time points, suggesting that the higher dose is definitely an excessive dose.[40] The effects of the drug on enzyme activities are compared for rats and monkeys in TABLE 2. In s. nigra and striatum, enzyme activities were significantly increased in both species; however, whereas the rest of the brain regions and organs in rats had enzyme activities that were signifi-

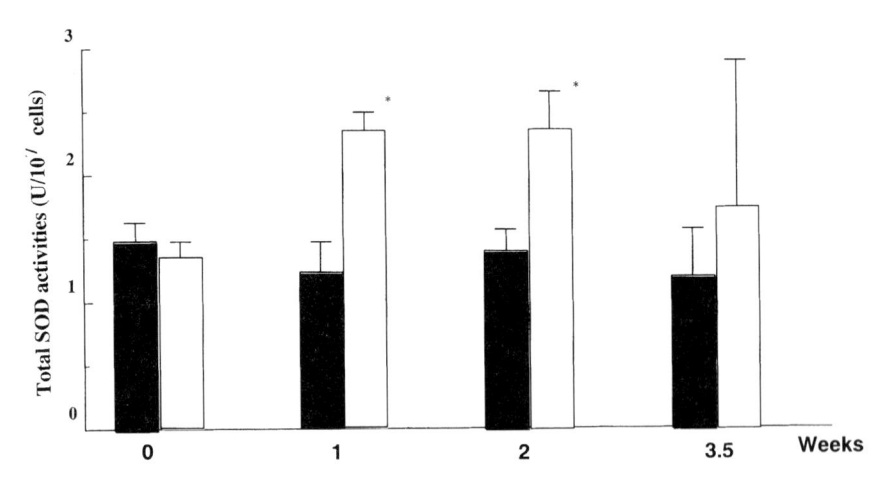

FIGURE 1. The effects of daily oral administration of (−)deprenyl on SOD activities in monkey lymphocytes. *Black bars* indicate control animals given saline solutions and *white bars* indicate experimental animals given a dose of 0.17 mg/kg per day of (−)deprenyl. Values are expressed as mean ± SD (each group, n = 3.) *Significantly different from respective values in control animals ($P < 0.05$).

cantly increased, a significant increase in enzyme activity was not observed in monkeys.[40] Activities here were significantly increased only in ascending aorta[40] (TABLE 2).

DISCUSSION

An Appropriate Dose of Deprenyl Increases the Life Span of Animals

As discussed repeatedly,[6–8] it is obvious that the administration of (−)deprenyl can increase life spans of mice,[24] rats,[19–21] hamsters,[41] and beagle dogs[25] if an appropriate dose is used. In our view, an appropriate dose selection is quite important since lower doses are obviously less effective and a much higher dose is adversely effective,[23,42] shortening life spans of animals. Discrepancies among past studies in terms of this effect of the drug can be explained rather reasonably if this point is taken into account.

For example, the study by Bickford *et al.*[22] used an oral administration of the drug. Since the first-pass effect of the drug by the liver is more than 90% (systemic availability < 10%),[43] the dose used by Bickford *et al.*[22] corresponds to a dose "smaller than 0.05 mg/kg when calculated as a dose by sc injection as adopted by the previous three studies."[19–22] On the other hand, the long-term administration of the drug by Gallagher *et al.*[23] may have become an excessive dose due to possibly rather low efficacy of hepatic microsomal P-450 enzyme activities in the particular strain used versus other strains used successfully.[19–22]

TABLE 2. Comparison of the effects of (−)deprenyl treatment on SOD and CAT activities in different organs and tissues between rats and monkeys

	Total SOD		CAT	
	Rats	Monkeys	Rats	Monkeys
Frontal cortex	↑	−	↑	−
Parietotemporal cortex	↑	−	↑	−
Occipital cortex	↑	−	↑	−
Striatum	⇑	↑	⇑	−
S. nigra	⇑	⇑	⇑	⇑
Cerebellum	−	−	−	−
Thalamus	n.d.	−	n.d.	−
Hippocampus	−	−	−	−
Left ventricle	↑	−	↑	−
Ascending aorta	n.d.	↑	n.d.	↑
Renal cortex	↑	−	↑	↑
Renal medulla	↑	−	↑	↑
Adrenal glands	↑	−	↑	−
Spleen	↑	−	↑	−
Liver	−	−	−	−
Lymphocytes	n.d.	⇑	n.d.	n.d.

NOTE: n.d., not determined; ⇑, marked increase; ↑, significant, but modest increase; −, no significant change.

TABLE 3. The effect of (−)deprenyl treatment on IL-1β and TNF-α concentrations in different organs and tissues in rats

	IL-1β	TNF-α
Striatum	−	−
Heart	−	↑
Renal medulla	↑	↑
Renal cortex	−	↑
Glands	↑	↑
Spleen	−	−

NOTE: ↑, significant increase; −, no significant change.

At present, no convincing data exist to show that the drug prolongs the life span of humans. However, whether the drug can increase the life span of humans should be investigated in the future with this caution in mind since the importance of an optimal dose has never been appreciated in patients treated with the drug and since the optimal dose for humans has never been examined in the past and thus remains totally unknown. However, judging from our recent study in monkeys on SOD and CAT activities,[40] we suspect that the optimal dose for humans, if any, may be much smaller than doses used in rodents and dogs and may be close to the dose used in patients with Parkinson's disease, assuming that effects of the drug on life spans and antioxidant enzyme activities are at least partially causally related, as has been intensively insisted by us.[6–8]

SOD and CAT Activities

The dose dependency is much clearer for the effect of the drug on SOD and CAT activities than for the effect on life spans of animals. The importance of an inverse U-shape effect by the drug has been repeatedly emphasized by us when interpreting studies of various results reported in the past.[6–8,42] From the parallelism of the effects on survivals of animals and on antioxidant enzyme activities, we still maintain the thesis that these two effects of the drug are causally related with each other.

Humoral Factors Possibly Related to Survivals of Animals

Recent observations by ourselves[38] and others have indicated that considerable species of humoral factors are mobilized by the administration of (−)deprenyl. These include neuronal trophic factors and neuronal growth factor (NGF),[44–47] as well as cytokines,[38] especially different species of interleukins. In addition to our observations, IL-2[26] and IL-6[48] have been previously reported to increase in concentration with (−)deprenyl. Further, an activation of natural killer (NK) cells[26,49] and an elevation of interferon-γ[26,49] in serum have been reported.

Recently, the serum levels of insulin-like growth factor-I (IGF-I) in aged rats were reported to recover to that of young rats following deprenyl administration,[50] suggesting that growth hormone secretion may be stimulated by the drug, although no proof for the latter thesis was provided.

The effect of (−)deprenyl on the neuroendocrine axis has been extensively discussed by ThyagaRajan and coworkers.[26] According to their thesis, the drug decreases prolactin concentration in sera of aged animals, thereby decreasing the incidence and progression of breast cancer. In fact, they demonstrated that (−)deprenyl treatment decreases the incidence of spontaneously growing breast cancer in aging female rats as well as of experimentally induced breast cancer in female rats.[26] The effect of (−)deprenyl on serum prolactin levels may possibly explain the earlier observation by Ruehl *et al.* that (−)deprenyl dramatically decreased the incidence of breast cancer in aging female beagle dogs.[25] Further, we have recently observed that concentrations of TNF-α in various visceral organs were raised in rats treated with the drug.[37,38]

We have previously reported that the administration of (−)deprenyl can decelerate the progression of subcutaneous benign tumors in aging male F344 rats.[21] Accordingly, we believe that the drug has a more general antitumorigenic effect than on breast cancer. Our observation on TNF-α and other immunomodulatory effects of deprenyl indicate an antitumorigenic effect.

Apart from antitumorigenic effects, some of these humoral factors mentioned above may beneficially modulate immune functions in aging animals, since it has been previously shown that the drug markedly prolonged the remaining life expectancy of immune-suppressed mice.[51] Accordingly, the effects of the drugs on survivals of animals may involve the neurological, immunological, and endocrine axes of an organism.

Potentials of Propargylamines for Human Use

The advantage of (−)deprenyl over other drugs[9–11] currently investigated for life span extension is that the drug has already been administered for more than 10 years in a large number of patients with Parkinson's disease with very few side effects. Despite the initial favorable observation by Birkmayer *et al.*,[17] recent studies with much larger numbers of patients have not reported a significant prolongation of life expectancies of patients treated with the drug.[13–15] Sano *et al.*,[52] though, reported in a double-blind controlled prospective study that patients with moderate Alzheimer's disease treated with (−)deprenyl had an estimated median survival that was 7 months (>45%) longer than that in placebo-treated control patients (655 days vs. 440 days), although no statistics were presented. It may be that a few months longer median survival in patients with Alzheimer's disease may not be considered to be an advantage of using the drug from a practical point of view. However, from a gerontological point of view, this observation may lend support to our suggestion for future studies utilizing (−)deprenyl for the purpose of extending life spans of healthy humans. In this connection, one study reported the shortening of survival of patients treated with (−)deprenyl.[53] Although this study was repeatedly criticized[54,55] and does not generally agree with results of most other similar studies, the effect of (−)deprenyl on survivals of humans needs to be reexamined taking the following points into account. (−)Deprenyl has been administered to patients with Parkinson's disease for the purpose of retarding the progression of the disease. No consideration has been given for the dose and the duration of the treatment since, once a fixed dose is given, the drug has usually been continuously administered to patients at that same dose.

As is clear from our antioxidant enzyme studies, an excessive dose and too long a treatment period cause a reduction of enzyme activities and possibly the life span of animals. It is possible that humans are not an exception to this rule. One possibility that has not been tested for humans is an "interval" administration of the drug. The problem is how we can judge whether or not the dose and duration are optimal for maintaining SOD (and CAT) activities at higher than pretreatment values, which we believe to be the prerequisite for the purpose of prolonging life spans of animals. It is practically impossible to examine SOD and CAT activities in the brain in living humans. The only possibility is to monitor SOD levels in lymphocytes in patients treated with the drugs. Kushleika and coworkers[56] have reported that SOD activities in lymphocytes in Parkinson's disease patients were significantly higher than those in control subjects and that these activities in patients treated with (−)deprenyl were significantly higher than those in patients without (−)deprenyl treatment.

It has been known in patients with Parkinson's disease that SOD activities are raised in s. nigra and striatum, which may correspond to the observations of Kushleika *et al.*,[56] although there is no way to confirm that SOD activities in the brain and lymphocytes change in parallel with each other. However, it should be worthwhile to examine sequential changes in SOD activities in lymphocytes in patients being treated with the drug. Once the activity becomes lower than values at the pretreatment level, drug withdrawal may be worth trying. Whether this actually occurs in patients with Parkinson's disease has never been looked at to our knowledge. If a long-term treatment with (−)deprenyl downregulates activities of SOD in lymphocytes and possibly in brain regions of dopaminergic nature, the drug may have to be withdrawn in order to recover normal activity levels. The drug can be readministered with some interval, which could be called an "interval deprenyl therapy." This is a suggestion raised from results of animal studies. However, we need to monitor SOD activities in lymphocytes in patients treated with deprenyl and this can be done without difficulty.

It seems possible that an appropriate dose of the drug to maintain SOD activities in humans is even lower than the currently used dose for patients since, in our monkey studies, SOD activities tended to become lower with time even with the lower dose (FIG. 1).

Further, we may need to monitor levels of cytokines in lymphocytes of patients treated with the drug since we have observed a large diversity in the effect of the drug on SOD activities in various organs between rodents and monkeys. It is thus possible that changes in cytokine levels by the drug in various organs differ between rodents and primates, possibly including humans. Whether serum GH levels in old patients are raised with the treatment of the drug should also be examined since the previous study by De la Cruz *et al.* found a significant increase in serum IGF-I levels in old rats, but not in young rats, by (−)deprenyl treatment.[50]

Finally, clinical trials with (−)deprenyl have not been limited to patients with Parkinson's disease and Alzheimer's disease. A recent randomized, double-blind placebo-controlled trial with deprenyl has shown that human immunodeficiency virus–associated cognitive impairment was significantly improved.[57] Such clinical studies may be an excellent occasion to study not only cognitive functions, but also humoral parameters related to immune functions as suggested above.

CONCLUSIONS

Propargylamines, (−)deprenyl in particular, upregulate enzyme activities of SOD and CAT not only in brain regions of dopaminergic nature, but also in visceral organs of primarily catecholaminergic nature in rats. Further, cytokines such as IL-1β and TNF-α are raised in concentration in these organs. Observations continue to support our thesis that up-regulation of SOD and CAT activities by (−)deprenyl is at least a partial mechanism for prolonging life spans of animals. Mobilization of various cytokines as revealed by ourselves and others may also contribute to prolonging the life span of animals by retarding the development and progression of tumors and beneficially modifying immune responses of animals. It remains unanswered whether such effects can be achieved in humans, but it appears to be worth investigating. As a first step toward this purpose, we suggest that patients with Parkinson's disease treated with (−)deprenyl be monitored serially for SOD enzyme activities and other cytokine concentrations in lymphocytes, as well as IGF-I (and growth hormone) levels in serum. This can be easily done. If a down-regulation of enzyme activities is found with the prolonged administration of the drug, we suggest that an interruption of drug treatment may be worthy of consideration. Results from basic animal studies and experiences with humans should now be put together to obtain the benefits of the drug for humans.

ACKNOWLEDGMENTS

Part of this study was supported by a grant in aid from the Ministry of Health and Welfare, Comprehensive Research for Aging and Health (H10-117, H11-008). The skillful secretarial work of T. Ohara is gratefully appreciated.

REFERENCES

1. HARMAN, D. 1956. Aging: a theory based on free radical and radiation chemistry. J. Gerontol. **12:** 257–263.
2. HARMAN, D. 1994. Free-radical theory of aging: increasing the functional life span. Ann. N.Y. Acad. Sci. **717:** 1–15.
3. LIPMAN, R.D., R.T. BRONSON, D. WU et al. 1998. Disease incidence and longevity are unaltered by dietary antioxidant supplementation initiated during middle age in C57BL/6 mice. Mech. Ageing Dev. **103:** 269–284.
4. MASORO, E.J. 1995. Dietary restriction. Exp. Gerontol. **30:** 291–298.
5. YU, B.P. 1996. Aging and oxidative stress: modulation by dietary restriction. Free Radic. Biol. Med. **21:** 651–668.
6. KITANI, K., K. MIYASAKA, S. KANAI, et al. 1996. Upregulation of antioxidant enzyme activities by deprenyl: implications for life span extension. Ann. N.Y. Acad. Sci. **786:** 391–409.
7. KITANI, K., S. KANAI, G.O. IVY, et al. 1998. Assessing the effects of deprenyl on longevity and antioxidant defenses in different animal models. Ann. N.Y. Acad. Sci. **854:** 291–306.
8. KITANI, K., C. MINAMI, T. YAMAMOTO, et al. 2001. Do antioxidant strategies work against aging and age-associated disorders? Propargylamines: a possible antioxidant strategy. Ann. N.Y. Acad. Sci. **928:** 248–260.
9. EDAMATSU, R., A. MORI & L. PACKER. 1995. The spin-trap N-tert-α-phenyl-butyl-nitrone prolongs the life span of the senescence accelerated mouse. Biochem. Biophys. Res. Commun. **211:** 847–849.
10. FLOYD, R.A., K. HENSLEY, M.J. FORSTER, et al. 2002. Nitrones, their value as therapeutics and probes to understand aging. Mech. Ageing Dev. In press.
11. MELOV, S., J. RAVENSCROFT, S. MALIK, et al. 2000. Extension of life-span with superoxide dismutase/catalase mimetics. Science **289:** 1567–1569.
12. KNOLL, J. 1980. Deprenyl (selegiline): the history of its development and pharmaceutical action. Acta Neurol. Scand. Suppl. **95:** 57–80.
13. THE PARKINSON STUDY GROUP. 1989. Effect of deprenyl on the progression of disability in early Parkinson's disease. N. Engl. J. Med. **321:** 1364–1371.
14. THE PARKINSON STUDY GROUP. 1993. Effects of tocopherol and deprenyl on the progression of disability in early Parkinson's disease. N. Engl. J. Med. **328:** 176–183.
15. TETRUD, J.W. & J.W. LANGSTON. 1989. The effect of deprenyl (selegiline) on the natural history of Parkinson's disease. Science **245:** 519–522.
16. BEN-SHLOMO, Y., A. CHURCHYARD, J. HEAD, et al. 1998. Investigation by Parkinson's Disease Research Group of United Kingdom into excess mortality seen with combined levodopa and selegiline treatment in patients with early mild Parkinson's disease: further results of randomized trial and confidential inquiry. Br. Med. J. **316:** 1191–1196.
17. BIRKMAYER, W., J. KNOLL, P. RIEDERER, et al. 1985. Improvement of life expectancy due to L-deprenyl addition to Madopar treatment in Parkinson's disease. J. Neural Transm. **64:** 113–127.
18. CHURCHYARD, A., C.J. MATHIAS, D. PHIL, et al. 1999. Selegiline-induced postural hypotension in Parkinson's disease: a longitudinal study on the effects of drug withdrawal. Movement Disorders **14:** 246–251.
19. KNOLL, J. 1988. The striatal dopamine dependency of life span in male rats: longevity study with (−)deprenyl. Mech. Ageing Dev. **46:** 237–262.

20. MILGRAM, N.W., R.J. RACINE, P. NELLIS, et al. 1990. Maintenance of L-deprenyl prolongs life in aged male rats. Life Sci. **47:** 415–420.
21. KITANI, K., S. KANAI, Y. SATO, et al. 1993. Chronic treatment of (−)deprenyl prolongs the life span of male Fischer 344 rats: further evidence. Life Sci. **52:** 281–288.
22. BICKFORD, P.C., C.E. ADAMS, S.J. BOYSON, et al. 1997. Long-term treatment of male F344 rats with deprenyl: assessment of effects on longevity, behavior, and brain function. Neurobiol. Aging **18:** 309–318.
23. GALLAGHER, I., A. CLOW & V. GLOVER. 1998. Long term administration of (−)deprenyl increases mortality in male Wistar rats. J. Neural Transm. (Suppl.) **52:** 315–320.
24. ARCHER, J.R. & D.E. HARRISON. 1996. L-Deprenyl treatment in aged mice slightly increases life spans, and greatly reduces fecundity by aged males. J. Gerontol. **31A:** B448–B453.
25. RUEHL, W.W., T.L. ENTRIKEN, B.A. MUGGENBURG, et al. 1997. Treatment with L-deprenyl prolongs life in elderly dogs. Life Sci. **61:** 1037–1044.
26. THYAGARAJAN, S. & D.L. FELTON. 2002. Modulation of neuroendocrine-immune signaling by L-deprenyl and L-desmethyldeprenyl in aging and mammary cancer. Mech. Ageing Dev. In press.
27. KNOLL, J. 1989. The pharmacology of selegiline [(−)deprenyl]: new aspects. Acta Neurol. Scand. **126:** 83–91.
28. CARRILLO, M.C., S. KANAI, M. NOKUBO, et al. 1991. Deprenyl induces activities of both superoxide dismutase and catalase, but not of glutathione peroxidase in the striatum of young male rats. Life Sci. **48:** 517–521.
29. CARRILLO, M.C., S. KANAI, M. NOKUBO, et al. 1992. Deprenyl increases activities of superoxide dismutase and catalase in striatum, but not in hippocampus: the sex and age-related differences in the optimal dose in the rat. Exp. Neurol. **116:** 286–294.
30. CARRILLO, M.C., S. KANAI, Y. SATO, et al. 1993. The optimal dosage of (−)deprenyl for increasing superoxide dismutase activities in several brain regions decreases with age in male Fischer 344 rats. Life Sci. **52:** 1925–1934.
31. CARRILLO, M.C., K. KITANI, S. KANAI, et al. 1992. The ability of (−)deprenyl to increase superoxide dismutase activities in the rat is tissue and brain region selective. Life Sci. **50:** 1985–1992.
32. KAMATAKI, T., K. MAEDA, M. SHIMADA, et al. 1985. Age-related alteration in activities of drug-metabolizing enzymes and contents of sex-specific forms of cytochrome P-450 in liver microsomes from male and female rats. J. Pharmacol. Exp. Ther. **233:** 222–228.
33. YOSHIDA, T., T. OGURO & Y. KUROIWA. 1987. Hepatic and extrahepatic metabolism of deprenyl, a selective monoamine oxidase (MAO) B inhibitor of amphetamines in rats: sex and strain differences. Xenobiotica **17:** 957–963.
34. CARRILLO, M.C., K. KITANI, S. KANAI, et al. 1994. The effect of a long term (6 months) treatment with (−)deprenyl on antioxidant enzyme activities in selective brain regions in old female F-344 rats. Biochem. Pharmacol. **47:** 1333–1338.
35. CARRILLO, M.C., K. KITANI, S. KANAI, et al. 1996. Long term treatment with (−)deprenyl reduces the optimal dose as well as the effective dose range for increasing antioxidant enzyme activities in old mouse brain. Life Sci. **59:** 1047–1057.
36. CARRILLO, M.C., C. MINAMI, K. KITANI, et al. 2000. Enhancing effect of rasagiline on superoxide dismutase and catalase activities in the dopaminergic system in the rat. Life Sci. **67:** 577–585.
37. MINAMI, C., T. YAMAMOTO, W. MARUYAMA, et al. 2000. Properties of propargylamines of increasing antioxidant enzyme activities are accompanied by mobilization of cytokines [abstract]. *In* Twenty-fourth Annual Meeting of the Japan Society of Biomedical Gerontology, Osaka, Japan, p. 47.
38. MINAMI, C., T. YAMAMOTO, W. MARUYAMA, et al. 2000. Three different propargylamines share properties of increasing antioxidant enzyme activities in dopaminergic brain regions as well as extra-brain tissues in the rat [abstract]. *In* Twenty-ninth Annual Meeting of the American Aging Association, Boston, p. 39.
39. CARRILLO, M.C., K. KITANI, S. KANAI, et al. 1994. (−)Deprenyl increases activities of superoxide dismutase (SOD) in striatum of dog brain. Life Sci. **54:** 1483–1489.

40. MINAMI, C., H. MAEDA, et al. 2001. A clinically applied dose of (−)deprenyl can increase antioxidant enzyme activities in brain and extra-brain tissues in monkeys [abstract]. *In* Thirtieth Annual Meeting of the American Aging Association (May 31 to June 4, 2001), Madison, pp. 25–26.
41. STOLL, S., U. HAFNER, B. KRAENZLIN, et al. 1997. Chronic treatment of Syrian hamsters with low-dose selegiline increases life span in females, but not males. Neurobiol. Aging **18:** 205–211.
42. CARRILLO, M.C., S. KANAI, K. KITANI, et al. 2000. A high dose of long term treatment with deprenyl loses its effect on antioxidant enzyme activities as well as on survivals of Fischer-344 rats. Life Sci. **67:** 577–585.
43. MAHMOOD, I., D.K. PETERS & W.D. MASON. 1994. The pharmacokinetics and absolute availability of selegiline in the dog. Biopharm. Drug Dispos. **15:** 653–664.
44. KONTKANEN, O. & E. CASTREN. 1999. Trophic effects of selegiline on cultured dopaminergic neurons. Brain Res. **829:** 190–192.
45. LI, X.M., A.V. JUORIO, J. QI, et al. 1998. L-Deprenyl potentiates NGF-induced changes in superoxide dismutase mRNA in PC12 cells. J. Neurosci. Res. **53:** 235–238.
46. TANG, Y.P., Y.L. MA, C.C. CHAO, et al. 1998. Enhanced glial cell line–derived neurotrophic factor mRNA expression upon (−)deprenyl and melatonin treatments. J. Neurosci. Res. **53:** 593–604.
47. SEMKOVA, I., P. WOLZ, M. SCHILLING, et al. 1996. Selegiline enhances NGF synthesis and protects central nervous system neurons from excitotoxic and ischemic damage. Eur. J. Pharmacol. **315:** 19–30.
48. MÜLLER, T., W. KUHN, R. KRUGER, et al. 1996. Selegiline as immunostimulant—a novel mechanism of action? J. Neural Transm. (Suppl.) **52:** 321–328.
49. THYAGARAJAN, S., K.S. MADDEN, J.S. KALVASS, et al. 1998. L-Deprenyl-induced increase in IL-2 and NK cell activity accompanies restoration of noradrenergic nerve fibers in the spleens of old F344 rats. J. Neuroimmunol. **92:** 9–21
50. DE LA CRUZ, C.P., E. REVILLA, J.A. RODRIGUEZ-GOMEZ, et al. 1997. (−)Deprenyl treatment restores serum insulin-like growth factor-I (IGF-I) levels in aged rats to young rat levels. Eur. J. Pharmacol. **327:** 215–220.
51. FREISLEBEN, H.J., A. NEEB, F. LEHR, et al. 1997. Influence of selegiline and lipoic acid on the life expectancy of immunosuppressed mice. Arzneim. Forsch. **47:** 776–780.
52. SANO, M., C. ERNEST, R.G. THOMAS, et al. 1997. A controlled trial of selegiline, α-tocopherol as treatment for Alzheimer's disease. N. Engl. J. Med. **336:** 1216–1222.
53. THOROGOOD, M., B. ARMSTRONG, T. NICHOLAS, et al. 1998. Mortality in people taking selegiline: observation study. Br. J. Med. **317:** 252–254.
54. RIGGS, J.E. 1997. Deprenyl, excess mortality, and epidemiological traps. Clin. Neuropharmacol. **20:** 276–278.
55. GERLACH, M. 1998. Motilatat bei langzeit Applikation von Selegilin. Act. Abt. Neurol. **25:** 5327–5328.
56. KUSHLEIKA, J., H. CHECKOWAY, J.S. WOODS, et al. 1996. Selegiline and lymphocyte superoxide dismutase activities in Parkinson's disease. Ann. Neurol. **39:** 378–381.
57. THE DANA CONSORTIUM ON THE THERAPY OF HV DEMENTIA AND RELATED COGNITIVE DISORDERS. 1998. A randomized, double blind placebo-controlled trial of deprenyl and thioctic acid in human immunodeficiency virus associated cognitive impairment. Neurology **50:** 645–651.

Pharmacological Interventions against Aging through the Cell Plasma Membrane

A Review of the Experimental Results Obtained in Animals and Humans

IMRE ZS.-NAGY

Department of Gerontology (VILEG Hungarian Section), University of Debrecen, Medical and Health Science Center, H-4012 Debrecen, Hungary

ABSTRACT: As was shown in a recent review by this author (Ann. N.Y. Acad. Sci., 928: 187–199, 2001), oxyradicals cannot be considered only as harmful byproducts of the oxidative metabolism, but living cells and organisms implicitly require their production. This idea is supported by numerous facts and arguments, the most important of which is that the complete inhibition of the oxyradical production by KCN (or by any block of respiration) kills the living organisms long before the energy reserves would be exhausted. This new theoretical approach not only helps our understanding of the normal functions of the living organisms, such as the basic memory mechanisms in the brain cells, but also helps in identifying the site-specific, radical-induced damaging mechanisms that represent the undesirable side effects of oxygen free radicals. First of all, these effects make the cell plasma membrane vulnerable and cause a series of intracellular functional disorders, as described by the membrane hypothesis of aging (MHA). The logical way for any antiaging intervention therefore should be to increase the available number of loosely bound electrons inside the plasma membrane that are easily accessible for $OH^{\bullet}$ free radical scavenging. The present review summarizes the available knowledge regarding the theory of the use of membrane-related antiaging pharmaca, like centrophenoxine (CPH), tested in both animal experiments and human clinical trials. A modified, developed version of CPH coded as BCE-001 is also reported.

KEYWORDS: cell plasma membrane; oxyradicals; oxidative metabolism; oxygen free radicals; membrane hypothesis of aging (MHA); antiaging intervention; centrophenoxine (CPH)

INTRODUCTION

Today, one of the most widely accepted ideas regarding the biological aging process is the free radical theory of aging (FRTA) proposed and first tried mainly by Harman,[1–8] and later followed by numerous authors. The basic concept of FRTA is

---

Address for correspondence: University of Debrecen, Medical and Health Science Center, Faculty of Medicine, Department of Gerontology (VILEG Hungarian Section), POB 50, H-4012 Debrecen, Hungary. Voice: +(36-52) 418-470; fax: +(36-52) 418-470.
izsnagy@jaguar.dote.hu

that oxygen free radicals are harmful by-products of aerobic life and as such, are to be considered the main causal factors of aging and numerous diseases.

Although this idea has been widely accepted and implicated in a series of biological phenomena, a deeper analysis has revealed various contradictions, unexplained problems, and paradoxical situations. During the last decade, the present author has formulated the contradictory items of the FRTA,[9–17] and, at the 8th IABG Congress held at Kyongju (South Korea), outlined a new, comprehensive interpretation of the possible biological role of oxygen free radicals in the living state, cell differentiation, and aging.[18] It should be emphasized, however, that although this new concept implicitly contradicts the central dogma of the FRTA just mentioned, it does not obviate the possibility of damaging side effects of these radicals at specific places of the cell structure. The main difference between the FRTA and this new concept is that, according to the latter, the constant flux of oxygen free radicals is an implicit attribute of life, that is, the new concept offers a much wider basis for interpreting the free radical functions.

According to this new concept,[18] the situation in living beings can be compared *mutatis mutandis* to that of electronic devices: in the latter, the supply current is an absolute prerequisite of their function, whereas the very same current may cause breakdowns in some components of the system through undesirable heating, crystal melting, or short-circuiting effects, to name a few. It means that a longer functional "life span" cannot be achieved for electronic devices by eliminating the electric current, but through better circuit design aimed at improving their ability to support the local, undesirable side effects of the current itself. This analogy means that for the living systems the continuous flux of oxygen free radicals always must be maintained during life, and we can only fight against the undesirable side effects of those radicals. In other words, the FRTA can remain valid with the following modifications:

(1) Theoretically, keeping in mind that totally blocking the oxyradical formation has a lethal effect, it is incorrect to propose, in general, eliminating any free radicals as an antiaging strategy.
(2) Recognizing how important the production of oxygen free radicals is for the living state, one has to identify the free radical events that are actually involved in the age-dependent deterioration of brain functions at the cellular level.
(3) Pharmacological interventions against aging have to be aimed at reducing only the really destructive radical effects, which may be possible only through the application of site-specific radical scavengers with well-defined and explored mechanisms of action.

The present review summarizes the available knowledge regarding the effects of a nootropic drug, centrophenoxine (CPH), as one that fulfills the listed criteria, the effects of which may be usefully interpreted in the light of this new approach.

ON THE THEORETICAL BACKGROUND

The theoretical basis of this approach is the membrane hypothesis of aging (MHA).[9–11,13,15,17,19–21] The MHA attributes a leading role in differentiation and aging processes to the plasma membrane, in which inevitable, continuous alterations occur during life. The alterations are due in part to free-radical-induced molecular damage, and also to the "residual heat" formed during each depolarization of the resting potential. These membrane alterations dictate the accumulation of dry mass (i.e., a decrease in the intracellular water content) in the intracellular space, which is a necessary process for the development and maturation, but becomes a rate-limiting factor above a certain physical density of the cell colloids. This statement is supported by the fact that the *in situ* enzyme activities in the cells are all strongly dependent on the density of their microenvironment. MHA is valid mainly for the postmitotic cells, such as neurons and muscle cells, and appears particularly evident as a single cycle in the erythrocytes where *de novo* protein synthesis does not take place. Recent developments in molecular genetics have strongly supported MHA, showing that the great majority of the products of oncogenes or antioncogenes (e.g., gas, ras, kit, fgr, yes, yet, fsv, ros, met, erb, neu, trk, fms oncogenes, senescence-associated gene, schwannomin gene, prohibitin gene, mortalin gene, p53 and p21 gene, statin gene, gerontogenes, etc.) have a more or less close plasma membrane localization.[17,21] These facts confirm the central role of the plasma membrane in the realization of mitotic regulation, cell differentiation, and senescence. Using this approach, one can expect a deeper understanding of the function of the intracellular physicochemical parameters in the cell functions, their governing role in the aging process, and the possibilities of an eventual intervention to prolong the useful life span in both animal and human trials.

DATA ON MEMBRANE-BOUND DRUGS OF ANTIAGING EFFECTS

Early Empirical Data on the Effects of CPH

CPH is an ester of *p*-chlorophenoxyacetic acid (PCPA) and dimethylaminoethanol (DMAE).[22,23] We have reviewed the relevant early literature that considers its *in vitro* and *in vivo* effects.[12] It is important to note that this drug, originally classified as "neuroenergeticum," is today one of the most frequently used types of nootropica in various countries.[12] Nevertheless, in spite of a large number of experimental and clinical studies, the mechanism of CPH's effect on the age-dependent decline of mental performance mostly has been misinterpreted.[12]

In human therapy, a number of beneficial effects of CPH have been observed in cases like cerebral atrophy, brain injury, postapoplectic disorders, chronic alcoholism, and barbiturate intoxications.[24–27]

It has also been observed that prolonged administration of CPH to old animals that are in good health reduced significantly the accumulation of lipofuscin in the brain cells[28] and myocardium (see Ref. 12). Furthermore, the average life span of these CPH-treated animals increased significantly, and the learning ability of the old mice that had received treatment improved as compared to their age-matched controls.[29–32] On the basis of these results, CPH was considered to be a potential antiaging drug.[12]

Ideas About the Mechanism of Action

As regards CPH's mechanism of action, it was suggested that the DMAE moiety of CPH enters the choline synthesis cycle (and consequently improves the brain's acetylcholine supply).[33,34] However, this explanation has been contradicted by others.[34–36] It must be clear that an increase in the supply of choline when a fraction of DMAE from CPH is transformed into choline (which has been shown to take place in the liver; see Ref. 37) cannot be the only explanation for the effect of this drug, since in this case a choline-rich diet alone should have the same effect as CPH has, which is not the case.[35,36] Further data on this problem also have been discussed.[37]

Important information has been revealed by intravenous administration of equimolar doses of ^{14}C-labeled DMAE or CPH in Japan.[38] After this intervention, much higher levels of DMAE were encountered in the brain after CPH treatment than with DMAE alone since, as was the case with earlier assumptions, the esterified form of DMAE with PCPA penetrates the blood-brain barrier much better.[38] CPH was hydrolyzed on both sides of the barrier in its two component parts *in vivo*. However, the DMAE moiety becomes phosphorylated in the brain, yielding phosphoryl-DMAE, which was in turn converted to phosphatidyl-DMAE, apparently the end-metabolite of DMAE in the brain.[38] Phosphatidyl-DMAE is incorporated in nerve cell membranes, and persists in this form for a relatively long time in place of choline.[38] This means that DMAE forms a special class of phospholipids in the brain cell membranes. PCPA moiety is excreted in the urine rather quickly, apparently without any metabolic change.[38] It should be noted that although some amount of DMAE administered either alone or in the form of CPH was found in acid-soluble and lipid cholines in the brain,[38] there is evidence that the trimethylation of DMAE does not occur in the brain, but only in the liver.[38] Therefore, the presence of DMAE in the nerve cell membrane phospholipids had to be considered the starting point of any approach to the mechanism of CPH action.

Evidence of the OH• Radical Scavenger Properties of CPH

Special experiments have been carried out in order to reveal whether the effects of DMAE on brain functions can be interpreted in terms of a local oxyradical protecting effect on the cell membrane components.

Protein Cross-Linking Model

The basic concept of this type of experiment is that the OH• free radicals generated in a Fenton reagent,[39] or by a Co-gamma irradiation,[40] react with the proteins (e.g., bovine serum albumin = BSA), altering their molecular structure. One can detect either a decrease in the protein's water solubility (originally 100% for BSA), and an increase in its average molecular weight, as a result of cross-linking,[39] or an increase in its carbonyl content as a result of protein oxidation.[40] It has been shown in such studies that DMAE efficiently inhibits both the polymerization of BSA induced by the OH• free radicals generated in the Fenton reaction and the radiation-induced oxidation of them.[39,40] These results clearly show that DMAE is an efficient OH• radical scavenger.

Electron Spin Resonance Spectroscopy in Spin-trapping Experiments

The electron spin resonance (ESR) spectroscopy technique applies specially designed compounds (spin traps), the reactions of which with various types of free radicals are well known. The spin trapping experiments demonstrated that the CPH molecule and both of its components display a strong affinity toward the OH• radicals.[41] The reaction-rate constant of DMAE can be estimated to be about 10^9 $M^{-1}s^{-1}$ with OH• free radicals.[41] Since most of the bioorganic compounds react with OH• radicals at a rate of 10^7–10^9 $M^{-1}s^{-1}$,[42] DMAE really may represent an essential protection for numerous cell-membrane components against OH• free radical attacks.

Although these experiments also revealed an OH• radical scavenger capacity of the PCPA moiety of the CPH molecule, PCPA cannot be responsible for the nootropic effects of CPH, since no binding of this compound is known in the brain. It cannot be excluded, however, that this moiety of CPH may have some physiologically meaningful effect in the blood or in some other tissues (e.g., kidney or liver) during its excretion.

It should also be noted that although CPH and both its components display some affinity toward the superoxide radicals, their rate constant is only on the order of magnitude of 10^2 $M^{-1}s^{-1}$, that is, there is no reason to assume that either the components or the CPH molecule itself would represent any efficient protection *in vivo* against superoxide-radical-induced damage.[43]

The Molecular Design of BCE-001

As has been pointed out in a recent review,[44] the reactivity of DMAE with OH• free radicals is most probably due to the trivalent nature of the nitrogen atom in the dimethylamino group of DMAE. This nitrogen atom still has two loosely bound electrons that are able to take part in radical reactions more easily than the other, more strongly bound electrons of the molecule. In order to test this idea, we designed several new molecules during the early 1980s, starting from the concept that a doubling of the loosely bound electrons per molecule may increase the rate constant of the OH• radical scavenging activity of the moiety. Before describing this new molecule, it might be useful to repeat here some conceptual statements from the previous review.[44] It is due to the extremely short lifetime of the OH• free radicals that protection of the neuronal membrane components against OH• radical damage only can be imagined if the following criteria are fulfilled.

(1) The scavenger molecule should have a reaction rate with OH• radicals comparable to that of the target molecule to be protected.
(2) The scavenger should get sufficiently close to the target and remain there as a component part for a sufficiently long time.
(3) The scavenger must not exert any deleterious side effect (toxicity) for the organism in general or in the immediate vicinity of the target molecule.

These criteria suggest that it is most probably a hopeless effort to test various scavengers without having any particular knowledge about their molecular biology, binding sites, and so forth. It should be stressed that so far most of the studies on the dietary antioxidants unfortunately have been performed without having such special information. For example, Weber and Miquel[45] reviewed the available data on the effects of a large number of radical scavenger compounds. Although some antioxidant supplements were indeed capable of extending the life span of experimental animals, the observed effects were not at all consistent when compared with the same drug in various species.[45]

Considering the preceding principles and the results obtained with CPH, we designed a new drug, coded BCE-001. It is basically similar to CPH, the difference being that the PCPA moiety is esterified with 1,3-bis(dimethylamino)-2-propanol (BIDIP) instead of DMAE. Details have been described before,[44] so we will not repeat them here. Nevertheless, it should be pointed out that BIDIP contains two dimethylamino groups, that is, twice as much loosely bound electrons are available in this moiety for the neutralization of OH• radicals. The consequence of this molecular structure was a 1.9-fold increase in the molecule's reaction-rate constant with the OH• free radicals, as measured in spin-trapping experiments, which is quite close to the theoretically expected 2-fold increase. As has been described before,[44] this property of the molecule is biologically meaningful, since it proved to be an efficient nootropic agent of low toxicity *in vivo*, which can be administered orally or even parenterally.[44] To the best of our knowledge, this was the first case of designing a new molecule on the basis of the available knowledge that proved to be efficient in antiaging experiments. This fact is of great importance, apart from the eventual success of this molecule in human antiaging prevention. The development of this molecule for human use is currently under way.

IN VIVO BIOLOGICAL EFFECTS OF CPH AND BCE-001

Animal Experiments

Obviously, neither the presence of DMAE in the brain nerve-cell membranes[38] nor the *in vitro* OH• radical scavenging ability of this compound[41] proves directly that it also acts as an OH• radical scavenger *in vivo*. However, numerous experimental results, listed only briefly below, demonstrate indirectly that the presence of DMAE or BIDIP in the cell membrane is of physiological significance, which can be attributed to their local OH• radical scavenger properties.

Effects on Lipid Fluidity and Protein Molecular-Weight Distribution in Synaptosomal Membranes

Aging causes an increase in microviscosity of the membrane lipids in the synaptosomal membranes. This parameter can be measured by means of fluorescence polarization techniques after diphenyl-hexatriene (DPH) labeling of brain cortical synaptosomal membranes.[46] After treatment of old rats with CPH for 60 days,[46] or with BCE-001 for 20 days (unpublished results), the membrane microviscosity decreased again significantly (to about the same extent after both treatments), as shown by the DPH method.

Spin labeling ESR techniques[47] confirmed the validity of the results obtained by DPH labeling for both drugs (unpublished results). These results show indirectly that BIDIP also reaches the brain synaptosomal membranes, although direct investigations with radiolabeled components have not been carried out. Synaptosomal membranes were well protected by CPH pretreatment against the toxic effect of acute Fe^{2+} overload in the cerebrospinal fluid of young rats *in vivo*;[48] therefore, similar effects also can be expected from BCE-001.

The molecular-weight distribution of the proteins is considerably shifted toward the higher values in the synaptosomes of the rat brain cortex during aging. This is a clear sign of an increased cross-linking of the membrane proteins. Treatment for 60 days with CPH[49] or for 20 days with BCE-001 (unpublished results) reversed this tendency to a significant extent in old rats.

All these results indicate that BCE-001 treatment improves the previously mentioned physicochemical properties of the neuronal membranes about 2–3 times faster than did CPH.

Effects on the Lateral Mobility of Proteins and Lipids in the Cell Membrane

The lateral mobility of membrane proteins and lipids was measured using fluorescence recovery after the photobleaching (FRAP) technique.[50] The lateral diffusion constant of hepatocyte membrane proteins (D_p) displays a characteristic negative linear-age correlation in Fischer 344[50,51] and Wistar[52] rats, in C57BL black mice,[53] in wild mouse strains of considerably different longevity (*Peromyscus leucopus, Mus musculus*),[54] BN/Bi rats,[55] as well as SAM mice.[56] The same finding has been described for the ConA-receptor proteins in the skeletal muscle cells of mice[57] and in the large brain cortical cells of rats.[58] Although it is almost by an order of magnitude faster than D_p, membrane lipid lateral mobility (D_l), showed very similar age-dependence in hepatocyte mernbranes.[59]

The striking fact is that although the absolute values and the rates of age-dependent decays of protein and lipid mobilities in the cell membranes of various tissues are different, they are inversely proportional to the life span of the given strain. In the case of the wild mouse strains mentioned earlier, there exists a 2.6-fold difference in longevity in favor of *P. leucopus*, and the age-related decline of D_p is about 2.5-times slower in the longer-living species.[54]

FRAP experiments on two-year-old Fischer 344 rats pretreated per os through a gastric tube with aqueous solutions of 80 mg/kg CPH or BCE-001 for five weeks revealed a significantly higher value of D_p than in the controls. BCE-001 produced a quantitatively larger increase of the protein diffusion constant using an identical dosage and time of treatment, than did CPH.[60] Another important observation was that the well-known, almost linear body weight loss of the Fischer 344 male rats above the age of two years was slightly inhibited by CPH from the end of the third week of treatment, whereas in the BCE-001-treated group this loss of body weight was almost entirely stopped after one week of treatment.[60] This result indicates that the observed increase in D_p under the effect of CPH or BCE-001 is not only an improvement in the cellular parameter, but it is also meaningful from a general physiological point of view. Inhibition of the body weight loss in these animals is very convincing evidence for the overall improvement of the status of the animals, and is in agreement with the observed life-prolonging effect of BCE-001. It is also noteworthy that caloric restriction experiments on mice also increased the D_p values to an extent that might correspond with the life-prolonging effect of this intervention.[61]

Effects on the Passive Potassium Permeability of the Nerve-cell Membranes

As explained by the MHA, the age-dependent decline of the passive potassium permeability in the nerve cells is a key issue in brain aging. CPH treatment for 60 days (80–100 mg/kg) in old rats reincreased the passive potassium permeability of the neuronal-cell membrane, that is, it decreased the intracellular potassium content and rehydrated the cytoplasm of brain neurons significantly.[62,63] BCE-001 had the same effect, though a lower dose (60 mg/kg) and a shorter period (3–4 weeks) of treatment were sufficient to reach the same level as these improvements in rats (unpublished observations).

These findings indicate that CPH and BCE-001 may be useful in the prevention or therapy of age-dependent brain disorders.

Effects on the Rates of Total and mRNA Synthesis in the Brain Cortex

The rate of synthesis of total, as well as mRNA, was measured using radioisotope methods *in vivo* in rats. An age-dependent decrease in the rates of total and mRNA synthesis was observed in the brain cortex of rats between 1 and 2 years of age (to 40–50% of the young-adult value).[64] The significance of this phenomenon in the age-dependent decrease in protein turnover rates has been clearly shown by MHA to be the main reason for the loss of physiological abilities of all cells and organs.

In vivo treatments with both CPH and BCE-001 reversed this tendency. CPH treatment for 60 days reincreased these rates to 80–90%,[65] whereas BCE-001 resulted in similar increases after 40 days, and values up to 113% were obtained when the drug was applied for 60 days (unpublished results). Therefore, BCE-001 is not only a better OH$^\bullet$ radical scavenger than CPH, but it is able to stimulate more efficiently the *in vivo* rates of brain RNA-synthesis. This fact may be of great significance in the prevention or therapy of human brain disorders like dementias, where decreased RNA and protein synthesis is an obvious reason for the dysfunctions.

Survival Experiments

It has been observed by various authors that CPH treatment prolonged the medium life span of laboratory animals, especially if the treatment started at relatively young ages. It also improved the learning ability of several animal species (see Refs. 63 and 66). In some cases an increase in the medium life span of up to 30% was described in mice, but only if the CPH treatment started at the age of 6 months.

The effect of BCE-001 on the medium life span was studied in one experiment when female CFY rats were treated intraperitoneally (i.p.) from the age of 18 months. The untreated controls displayed a medium life span of 23.6 months, which is a quite usual value for this strain. The BCE-001 treatment increased the medium life span of these rats to 29 months (unpublished results). Per os treatments with BCE-001 increased the medium life span by almost 10 months (unpublished results).

Some Further Animal Experiments

BCE-001 was tested in comparison with CPH in further behavioral and other animal models on the basis of commissions from BIOGAL Pharmaceutical Works, Ltd. (Debrecen, Hungary) in various laboratories in Japan and Hungary. Although the results have not been published, we can mention here briefly the following results: doses of 60–100 mg/kg of BCE-001 administered i.p. for 7–30 days in rats improved the brain functions. It displayed an effect on the neurotransmitters, in particular increasing the 5-HT content in the septum, and improved memory functions through a novel mechanism of action. It was particularly active in the hippocampus and modified its dopaminergic system. It increased the glucose utilization in the brain regions involved in memory and awakening, such as the frontal cortex, nucleus basalis, nucleus lateralis thalami, hippocampus, and reticular formation. BCE-001 exerted a protective action against experimentally induced hypoxia, manifesting itself in a longer survival period. It also inhibited the formation of strokes in spontaneously hypertensive rats. It therefore can be considered to be a cerebrovascular protective agent acting without any prolonged modification of the systemic circulation. Various tests on memory consolidation and retrieval demonstrated that BCE-001 has beneficial effects that are comparable to that of CPH; therefore, the possibility of developing a useful nootropic drug for human use seems to be realistic. It is important to stress here that in comparison to CPH, BCE-001 displayed a more advantageous effect in each of the listed experiments.

Human Experiments with CPH

Several persons around the age of 40, including the author of the present review, started to take CPH (500 mg/day) in 1976, and maintained this experimental treatment until now. Due to the relatively low number of these subjects, this cannot be considered a scientific experiment; nevertheless, all the participants agree that they maintained better physical and mental performance than the untreated persons in their family of similar age. Apart from this observation, it is important to note that the treated persons had no side effects, even after 25 years.

In order to create a basis of comparison for future human applications of BCE-001, specially designed human experiments were performed, and their results are summarized follows. In a double-blind, randomized human clinical trial, CPH treatment for 8 weeks improved the psychometric and behavioral performance in about 50% of patients with a medium level dementia (according to the DSM III, Cat. 1, or ICD No. 299): the placebo group displayed improvement in only 27% of cases.[66] A considerable rehydration of the intracellular mass was observed in the verum group at the expense of the extracellular liquid. Meanwhile, body weight remained unchanged.[67] These data are mentioned here to demonstrate that nootropica, like CPH (and most probably also like BCE-001), also behave in humans in the same predictable way as MHA. Similar human trials will be performed with BCE-001 as soon as the drug achieves human phase II of testing.

CONCLUSIONS AND PERSPECTIVES

The synthetic interpretation of the biological aging phenomena offered by the MHA represents an interdisciplinary approach for describing a cellular mechanism that offers a generally valid explanation for the effects of oxygen free radicals, and that offers a good chance for experimental testing. On the basis of the MHA, the design of a special drug that proves to be efficient could be realized, in good agreement with the theoretical predictions.

The assumption that only site-specific OH• free radical scavengers can be considered seriously as potential preventive antiaging drugs seems to be well supported by the experimental facts. Besides the eventual success or failure of the BCE-001 in future human trials, the most important theoretical message of the reviewed results is that proper improvement of the defense against OH• free radical attacks in the brain cell membrane is beneficial. Following this line, newly designed drugs, which may be helpful in achieving a real breakthrough in geriatric prevention and care, seem to be worth pursuing.

It should be emphasized that even a future life span–prolonging strategy should be based on the FRTA; nevertheless, we have to apply the new concepts outlined in this review. Due to the by now explored properties of the OH• radical reactions, only site-specific, nontoxic, and physicochemically feasible radical protection offer any hope of success. It should also be stressed that in highly evolved living systems, where the natural radical protection is *a priori* much more efficient than in rodents, it is highly probable that only multifactorial radical protection can be successful in improving the natural defence system.

REFERENCES

1. HARMAN, D. 1956. Aging, a theory based on free radical and radiation chemistry. J. Gerontol. **11:** 298–300.
2. HARMAN, D. 1957. Prolongation of the normal life span by radiation protection chemicals. J. Gerontol. **12:** 257–263.
3. HARMAN, D. 1961. Mutation, cancer and aging. Lancet **1:** 200–201.
4. HARMAN, D. 1961. Prolongation of the normal life span and inhibition of spontaneous cancer by antioxidants. J. Gerontol. **16:** 147–154.
5. HARMAN, D. 1981. The aging process. Proc. Natl. Acad. Sci. USA **78:** 7124–7128.
6. HARMAN, D. 1988. Free radical theory of aging, current status. *In* Ipofuscin, State of the Art, I. Zs.-Nagy, Ed.: 3–21. Akadémiai Kiadó. Budapest; Elsevier. Amsterdam.
7. HARMAN, D. 1992. Role of free radicals in aging and disease. Ann. N.Y. Acad. Sci. **673:** 126–141.
8. HARMAN, D. 1994. Free radical theory of aging. Increasing the functional life span. Ann. N.Y. Acad. Sci. **717:** 1–15.
9. ZS.-NAGY, I. 1986. Common mechanisms of cellular aging in brain and liver in the light of the mewbrane hypothesis of aging. *In* Liver and Aging, Liver and Brain, K. Kitani, Ed.: 373–387. Elsevier. Amsterdam.
10. ZS.-NAGY, I. 1987. An attempt to answer the questions of theoretical gerontology on the basis of the membrane hypothesis of aging. Adv. Biosci. **64:** 393–413.
11. ZS.-NAGY, I. 1989. Functional consequences of free radical damage to cell membranes. *In* CRC Handbook of Free Radicals and Antioxidents in Biomedicine, Vol. I, J. Miquel, A.T. Quintanilha, and H. Weber, Eds.: 199–207. CRC Press. Boca Raton, FL.
12. ZS.-NAGY, I. 1989. Centrophenoxine as OH• free radical scavenger. *In* CRC Handbook of Free Radicals and Antioxidants in Biomedicine, Vol. II, J. Miquel, A.T. Quintanilha, and H. Weber, Eds.: 87–94. CRC Press. Boca Raton, FL.
13. ZS.-NAGY, I. 1991. Dietary antioxidants and brain aging: hopes and facts. *In* The Potential for Nutritional Modulation of Aging Processes, D.K. Ingram, G. Baker, and N. Shock, Eds.: 379–399. Food and Nutrition Press. Trumbull, CT.
14. ZS.-NAGY, I. 1992. A proposal for reconsideration of the role of oxygen free radicals in cell differentiation and aging. Ann. N.Y. Acad. Sci. **673:** 142–148.
15. ZS.-NAGY, I. 1994. The Membrane Hypothesis of Aging. CRC Press. Boca Raton, FL.
16. ZS.-NAGY, I. 1995. Semiconduction of proteins as an attribute of the living state: the ideas of Albert Szent-Györgyi revisited in the light of the recent knowledge regarding oxygen free radicals. Exp. Gerontol. **30:** 327–335.
17. ZS.-NAGY, I. 1997. The membrane hypothesis of aging: its relevance to recent progress in genetic research. J. Mol. Med. **75:** 703–714.
18. ZS.-NAGY, I. 2001. On the true role of oxygen free radicals in the living state, aging and degenerative disorders. Ann. N.Y. Acad. Sci. **928:** 187–199.
19. ZS.-NAGY, I. 1978. A membrane hypothesis of aging. J. Theor. Biol. **75:** 189–195.
20. ZS.-NAGY, I. 1979. The role of membrane structure and function in cellular aging: a review. Mech. Ageing Dev. **9:** 237–246.
21. ZS.-NAGY, I. 2001. Membranes, aging and genome. *In* Current Concepts in Experimental Gerontology. Vienna Aging Series, Vol. 6, C. BertoniFreddari and H. Niedermüller, Eds.: 3–14. Facultas. Vienna.

22. PFEIFFER, C., E.H. JENNEY, W. GALLAGHER, et al. 1957. Stimulant effect of 2-dimethylaminoethanol: possible precursor of brain acetylcholine. Science **126**: 610–611.
23. THUILLER, J., P. RUMPF & G. THUILLER. 1959. Derivés des acides regulateurs de croissance des vegetaux. i. proprietés pharmacologiques de lester dimethylaminoethylique de l'Acide *p*-Chlorophenoxyacetique (235 ANP). C.R. Seances Soc. Biol. Fil. **153**: 1914–1918.
24. SCHMIDT, H. & H. BROICHER. 1970. Klinische Erfahrungen bei der Be-handlung von Zustanden zerebraler Insuffizienz mit centrophenoxin (Helfergin). Medsche Welt **33**: 1432–1436.
25. VOJTECHOVSKY, M., B. SOUKUPOVA, V. SAFRATOVA & Z. VOTAVA. 1970. The influence of centrophenoxine (Lucidril) on learning and memory in alcoholics. Int. J. Psychobiol. **1**: 49-56.
26. HERRSCHAFT, H., F. GLEIM & P. DUUS. 1974. Die Wirkung von Centrophenoxin auf die regionale Gehirndurchblutung bei Patienten mit zerebrovascularer Insuffizienz. Dtsch. Med. Wochensch. **99**: 1707–1714.
27. KUGLER, J. 1977. Hirnstoffwechsel and Hirndurchblutung. Berichstband Centrophenoxin-Arbeitstagung, Timmendorfer Strand. Schnetztor Verlag. Konstanz.
28. NANDY, K. & G. BOURNE. 1966. Effects of centrophenoxine on the lipofuscin pigment in the neurons of senile guinea pigs. Nature **210**: 313–314.
29. NANDY, K. 1978. Centrophenoxine: effects on aging mammalian brain J. Am. Geriatr. Soc. **26**: 74–81.
30. HOCHSCHILD, R. 1971. Lysosomes, membranes and aging. Exp. Gerontol. **6**: 153–166.
31. HOCHSCHILD, R. 1973. Effect of dimethylaminoethyl-*p*-chlorophenoxy acetate on the life span of male Swiss Webster albino mice. Exp. Gerontol. **8**: 177–183.
32. HOCHSCHILD, R. 1973. Effect of dimethylaminoethanol on the life span of senile male A/J mice. Exp. Gerontol. **8**: 185–192.
33. LONDON, E.D. & J.T. COYLE. 1978. Pharmacological augmentation of acetylcholine levels in kainate lesioned rat striatum. Biochem. Pharmacol. **27**: 2962–2965.
34. HAUBRICH, D.R., P.F. WANG, D.E. CLODY & P.W. WEDECKING. 1975. Increase in rat brain acetylcholine induced by choline or deanol. Life Sci. **17**: 975–980.
35. ZANISER, N.R., D. CHOU & I. HANIN. 1977. Is 2-dimethylamino-ethanol (deanol) indeed a precursor of brain acetylcholine? A gas chromatographic evaluation. J. Pharmacol. Exp. Ther. **200**: 545–559.
36. JOPE, R.S. & D.J. JENDEN. 1979. Dimethylaminoethanol (deanol) metabolism in rat brain and its effect on acetylcholine synthesis. J. Pharmacol. Exp. Ther. **211**: 472–479.
37. BERTONI-FREDDARI, C., C . GIULI & C. PIERI. 1982. The effect of acute and chronic centrophenoxine treatment on the synaptic plasticity of old rats. Arch. Gerontol. Geriatr. **1**: 365–373.
38. MIYAZAKI, M., K. NAMBU, A.Y. MINAKI, et al. 1976. Comparative studies on the metabolism of beta-dimethylaminoethanol in the mouse brain and liver following administration of beta-dimethylaminoethanol and its *p*-chloro-phenoxyacetate, Meclofenoxate. Chem. Pharm. Bull. **24**: 763–769.
39. ZS.-NAGY, I. & K. NAGY. 1980. On the role of cross-linking of cellular proteins in aging. Mech. Ageing Dev. **14**: 245–251.
40. NAGY, K., G. DAJKÓ, I. URAY & I. ZS.-NAGY. 1994. Comparative studies on the free radical scavenger properties of two nootropic drugs, CPH and BCE-001. Ann. N.Y. Acad. Sci. **717**: 115–121.
41. ZS.-NAGY, I. & R.A. FLOYD. 1984. Electron spin resonance spectroscopic demonstration of the hydroxyl free radical scavenger properties of dimethylaminoethanol in spin trapping experiments confirming the molecular basis for the biological effects of centrophen-oxine. Arch. Gerontol. Geriatr. **3**: 297–310.
42. WALLING, C. 1975. Fenton's reagent revisited. Acc. Chem. Res. **8**: 125–131.
43. SEMSEI, I. & I. ZS.-NAGY. 1985. Superoxide radical scavenging ability of centrophenoxine and its salt dependence in vitro. J. Free Radic. Biol. Med. **1**: 403–408.
44. ZS.-NAGY, I. 1994. A survey of the available data on a new nootropic drug, BCE-001. Ann. N.Y. Acad. Sci. **717**: 102–114.
45. WEBER, H.U. & J. MIQUEL. 1986. Antioxidant supplementation and longevity. *In* Nutritional Aspects of Aging, Vol. I, L.H. Chen, Ed.: 42–49. CRC Press. Boca Raton, FL.

46. NAGY, K., V. ZS.-NAGY, C. BERTONI-FREDDARI & I. ZS.-NAGY. 1983. Alterations of the synaptosomal membrane microviscosity in the brain cortex of rats during aging and centrophenoxine treatment. Arch. Gerontol. Geriatr. **2:** 23–39.
47. NAGY, K., P. SIMON & I. ZS.-NAGY. 1983. Spin label studies on synaptosomal membranes of rat brain cortex during aging. Biochem. Biophys. Res. Commun. **117:** 688–694.
48. NAGY, K., R.A. FLOYD, P. SIMON & I. ZS.-NAGY. 1985. Studies on the effect of iron overload on rat cortex synaptosomal membranes. Biochim. Biophys. Acta **820:** 216–222.
49. NAGY, K. & I. ZS.-NAGY. 1984. Alterations in the molecular weight distribution of proteins in rat brain synaptosomes during aging and centrophenoxine treatment. Mech. Ageing Dev. **28:** 171–176.
50. ZS.-NAGY, I., K. KITANI, M. OHTA, et al. 1986. Age-dependent decrease of the lateral diffusion constant of proteins in the plasma membrane of hepatocytes as revealed by fluorescence recovery after photobleaching in tissue smears. Arch. Gerontol. Geriatr. **5:** 131–146.
51. ZS.-NAGY, I., K. KITANI, M. OHTA, et al. 1986. Age-estimations of rats based on the average lateral diffusion constant of hepatocyte membrane proteins as revealed by fluores-cence recovery after photobleaching. Exp. Gerontol. **21:** 555–563.
52. KITANI, K., I. ZS.-NAGY, S. KANAI, et al. 1988. Correlation between the biliary excretion of ouabain and the lateral mobility of hepatocyte plasma membrane proteins in the rat. The effects of age and spironolactone pretreatment. Hepatology **8:** 125–131.
53. ZS.-NAGY, I., K. KITANI & M. OHTA. 1989. Age dependence of the lateral mobility of proteins in the plasma membrane of hepatocytes in C57BL/6 mice: FRAP studies on liver smears. J. Gerontol. Biol. Sci. **44:** B83–B87.
54. ZS.-NAGY, I., R.G. CUTLER, K. KITANI & M. OHTA. 1993. Comparison of the lateral diffusion constant of hepatocyte membrane proteins in two wild mouse strains of considerably different longevity: FRAP studies on liver smears. J. Gerontol. Biol. Sci. **48:** B86–B92.
55. KITANI, K., S. TANAKA & I. ZS.-NAGY. 1998. Age-dependence of the lateral diffusion coefficient of lipids and proteins in the hepatocyte plasma membrane of BN/BiRijHsd rats as revealed by the smear-FRAP technique. Arch. Gerontol. Geriatr. **26:** 257–273.
56. ZS.-NAGY, I., S. TANAKA & K. KITANI. 2001. Comparison of the lateral diffusion coefficient of hepatocyte plasma membrane proteins in 3 strains of senescence accelerated mouse (SAM). Arch. Gerontol. Geriatr. **32:** 119–137.
57. ZS.-NAGY, I., S. TANAKA & K. KITANI. 1998. Age-dependence of the lateral diffusion coefficient of Con-A-receptor protein in the ske-letal muscle membrane of C57BL/6J mice. Mech. Ageing Dev. **101:** 257–268.
58. ZS.-NAGY, I., S. TANAKA & K. KITANI. 1999. Age-dependence of the lateral diffusion coefficient of Concanavalin-A receptors in the plasma membrane of ex vivo prepared brain cortical nerve cells of BN/BiRijHsd rats. Exp. Brain Res. **124:** 233–240.
59. ZS.-NAGY, I. & K. KITANI. 1996. Age-dependence of the lateral mobility of lipids in hepatocyte plasma membrane of male rats and the effect of life-long dietary restriction. Arch. Gerontol. Geriatr. **23:** 81–93.
60. ZS.-NAGY, I., M. OHTA & K. KITANI. 1989. Effect of centrophenoxine and BCE-001 treatment on the lateral diffusion constant of proteins in the hepatocyte membrane as revealed by fluorescence recovery after photobleaching in rat liver smears. Exp. Gerontol. **24:** 317–330.
61. ZS.-NAGY, I., K. KITANI, M. OHTA & R.G. CUTLER. 1993. The effect of caloric restriction on the lateral diffusion constant of hepatocyte membrane proteins in C57BL/6 male mice of various ages: FRAP studies on liver smears. Mech. Ageing Dev. **71:** 85–96.
62. ZS.-NAGY, I., C. PIERI, C. GIULI & M. DEL MORO. 1979. Effects of centrophenoxine on the monovalent electrolyte contents of the large brain cortical cells of old rats. Gerontology **25:** 94–102.
63. LUSTYIK, GY. & I. ZS.-NAGY. 1985. Alterations of the intracellular water and ion concentrations in brain and liver cells during aging as revealed by energy dispersive X-ray microanalysis of bulk specimens. Scanning Electron Microsc. **1985:** 323–337.

64. SEMSEI, I., F. SZESZÁK & I. ZS.-NAGY. 1982. In vivo studies on the age-dependent decrease of the rates of total and mRNA synthesis in the brain cortex of rats. Arch. Gerontol. Geriatr. **1:** 29–42.
65. ZS.-NAGY, I. & I. SEMSEI. 1984. Centrophenoxine increases the rates of total and mRNA synthesis in the brain cortex of old rats: an explanation of its action in terms of the membrane hypothesis of aging. Exp. Gerontol. **19:** 171–178.
66. PÉK, GY., T. FÜLÖP & I. ZS.-NAGY. 1989. Gerontopsychological studies using NAI ("Nürnberger Alters-Inventar") on patients with organic psychosyndrociie (DSM III, Category 1) treated with centrophenoxine in a double blind, comparative, randomized clinical trial. Arch. Gerontol. Geriatr. **9:** 17–30.
67. FÜLÖP, T., JR., I. WÓRUM, J. CSONGOR, et al. 1990. Effects of centrophenoxine on body composition and some biochemical parameters of demented elderly people as revealed in a double blind clinical trial. Arch. Gerontol. Geriatr. **10:** 239–251.

Nitrones as Neuroprotectants and Antiaging Drugs

ROBERT A. FLOYD,[a,b] KENNETH HENSLEY,[a] MICHAEL J. FORSTER,[c] JUDITH A. KELLEHER-ANDERSON,[d] AND PAUL L. WOOD[d]

[a]*Free Radical Biology and Aging Research Program, Oklahoma Medical Research Foundation, Oklahoma City, Oklahoma 73104, USA*

[b]*Department of Biochemistry and Molecular Biology, University of Oklahoma Health Sciences Center, Oklahoma City, Oklahoma 73104, USA*

[c]*University of North Texas, Fort Worth, Texas 76107-2699, USA*

[d]*Centaur Pharmaceuticals, Inc., Santa Clara, California 95050, USA*

ABSTRACT: Specific nitrones have been used for more than 30 years in analytical chemistry and biochemistry to trap and stabilize free radicals for the purpose of their identification and characterization. PBN (α-phenyl-*tert*-butyl nitrone), one of the more widely used nitrones for this purpose, has been shown to have potent pharmacologic activities in models of a number of aging-related diseases, most notably the neurodegenerative diseases of stroke and Alzheimer's disease. Studies in cell and animal models strongly suggest that PBN has potent antiaging activity. A novel nitrone, CPI-1429, has been shown to extend the life span of mice when administration was started in older animals. It has also shown efficacy in the prevention of memory dysfunction associated with normal aging in a mouse model. Mechanistic studies have shown that the neuroprotective activity of nitrones is not due to mass-action free radical–trapping activity, but due to cessation of enhanced signal transduction processes associated with neuroinflammatory processes known to be enhanced in several neurodegenerative conditions. Enhanced neuroinflammatory processes produce higher levels of neurotoxins, which cause death or dysfunction of neurons. Therefore, quelling of these processes is considered to have a beneficial effect allowing proper neuronal functioning. The possible antiaging activity of nitrones may reside in their ability to quell enhanced production of reactive oxygen species associated with age-related conditions. On the basis of novel ideas about the action of secretory products formed by senescent cells on bystander cells, it is postulated that nitrones will mitigate these processes and that this may be the mechanism of their antiaging activity.

KEYWORDS: nitrones; PBN; DMPO; learning; memory

Address for correspondence: Robert Floyd, University of Oklahoma Health Sciences Center, 825 N.E. 13th Street, Oklahoma City, OK 73104. Voice: 405-271-7580; fax: 405-271-1795.
Robert-Floyd@omrf.ouhsc.edu

Historical Perspective on Nitrones

1957　1969　1975　1985　1990　1998

First Synthesis of PBN (α-phenyl-*tert*-butyl nitrone)[1]

　　Nitrones used to trap free radicals in chemical systems[2]

　　　Nitrones used to trap radicals in biological systems[3]

　　　　Nitrones have pharmaco-protective activity[4]

　　　　　Nitrones have neuro-protective activity[5]

　　　　　　Nitrones have anti-aging activity[6]

FIGURE 1. Important historical events and discoveries pertinent to the antiaging activity of nitrones. Numbers 1–6 denotes relevant references.

INTRODUCTION AND BACKGROUND

One of the most widely known nitrones is PBN (α-phenyl-*tert*-butyl nitrone). FIGURE 1 presents a time sequence of the significant biomedical research discoveries pertinent to nitrones where studies with PBN played an especially prominent role. The compound was first synthesized in 1957.[1] Its widespread use in analytical chemistry was brought about by the pioneering use of it to trap (spin-trap) rapidly reacting free radicals in chemical systems.[2] The more stable nitroxide free radical adduct formed (see FORMULA 1) allowed the characterization of free radical intermediates in many chemical systems where such intermediates were involved.

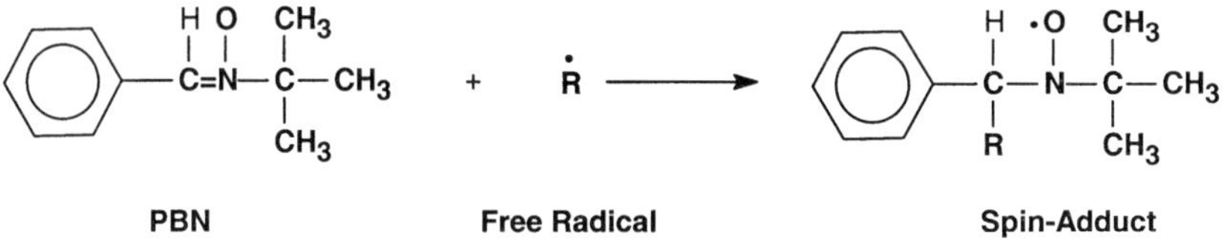

PBN　　　　　Free Radical　　　　　Spin-Adduct

FORMULA 1.

Within six years of the beginning of the use of nitrones in analytical chemistry, they were starting to be used in biochemical systems.[3] Extensive use of PBN, and another spin-trap, DMPO (5,5-dimethyl-1-pyroline-1-oxide), became a prominent method in the 1980s to investigate free radical intermediates in biological systems.

It was during this interval that the pharmacological potential of the nitrones was first noted.[4,5] Novelli *et al.*[4] demonstrated that preadministration of PBN to rats protected them from the shock trauma they experienced caused by placing them in a tumbling mill. The potential of nitrones as neuroprotective agents became clear as a result of our discovery, made in 1988, that administration of PBN protected gerbils from a stroke.[5] The first conclusive demonstration that PBN had antiaging activity was made by Cutler's group in 1998.[6] Earlier observations by Packer's group[7] and Arendash's group[8] made on senescence-accelerated mice and Sprague-Dawley rats, respectively, clearly implicated the antiaging activity of PBN. However, these earlier studies suffered from being done on a mouse model that does not have normal aging characteristics[7] and in the latter case because the experiment was terminated early (i.e., before full life span was completed).[8]

MECHANISTIC BASIS OF THE NITRONE ACTIVITY

A large amount of experimental data has been collected on the neuroprotective activity of nitrones. The following generalizations can be drawn from the studies: (*a*) PBN has been shown to be neuroprotective by a number of laboratories in several models. (*b*) From the limited studies available it is clear that not all nitrones are neuroprotective, that is, neuroprotective activity can vary widely and depends on the specific chemical structure. (*c*) The activity does not depend upon a simple mass action type of mechanism, but appears to reside in nitrone's ability to effectively quell certain exacerbated signal transduction events which are associated with enhanced neuroinflammatory processes common to several neurodegenerative diseases such as stroke, Alzheimer's disease, Parkinson's disease, AIDS-related dementia, and others.[9] (*d*) Nitrones, and especially PBN, have been shown to have potent pharmacological activity in model systems of a wide range of pathological conditions and diseases associated with aging.[10–14]

PBN has become a widely used research tool to explore questions regarding antioxidants and oxidative damage in various research problems. PBN does, in general, lower oxidative stress and oxidative damage, as, for example, in lowering protein oxidative damage in brains of chronically treated old gerbils,[15] yet exactly how it does mitigate oxidative stress and oxidative damage is more complex than the simple concepts normally used to explain antioxidant activity. Instant deductive thought concludes that free radical–trapping explains the mechanistic action of PBN. But many observations and careful analysis of the facts do not support this conclusion. *First*, it is widely observed in classical spin-trapping studies that very high levels (on the order of 50 mM or more) of PBN (and other spin traps) are required to trap significant amounts (50% or more) of the total free radicals being produced in several well-known chemical systems. PBN never reaches very high levels in the target tissue. For instance, administered dosages of 75–150 mg/kg yield brain levels of no more than about 500 μM.[16,17] *Second*, PBN has its action after the highest target tissue free radical flux has occurred. That is, PBN shows neuroprotective activity in "stroked" brains when it is given 30 minutes after the stroke in the case of gerbils,[18,19] and even up to 3 hours after the stroke (brain reperfusion) in the case of the middle cerebral arterial occlusion model in rats.[20] *Third,* in an isolated rat liver microsomal system undergoing rapid lipid peroxidation, PBN is only about 0.01% as effective in ceasing peroxidative activity as is Trolox or butylated hydroxy toluene (BHT) in this system.[21] These three chemicals were tested in head-on comparisons in this system and it required 5 mM of PBN to inhibit 50% of the peroxidation activity but only 40 µM and 6 µM of Trolox and BHT, respectively.

We have concluded that the neuroprotective action of PBN is explained by its ability to prevent the induction of genes, caused by the brain insult brought on by a period of ischemia.[10–12] Some of the induced genes produce products that are toxic to neurons. One such product is nitric oxide and its oxidative products, including peroxynitrite. Brains given a stroke do, within a few hours, show an increase in inducible nitric oxide synthase. In models where strokes are given to transgenic animals lacking this enzyme, or when nitric oxide synthase has been inhibited, significantly less damage was caused by the stroke.[22–25] Microglia and astrocytes, when activated, will mediate the induction of inducible nitric oxide synthase (iNOS), which then produces high levels of nitric oxide, which is much more toxic to neurons than to the glia that produced it. These events represent the basic notions of neuroinflammatory processes and establish a testable notion for examination of the neuroprotective action of PBN and other active nitrones.

The most convincing published research substantiating the notions that the mechanistic action of PBN involves quelling of enhanced signal transduction processes comes from studies in brain cell culture[26,27] and in a few animal model studies.[28] More advanced studies on stroke have shown that certain derivatives of PBN, especially 2,5-disulfonate PBN, (disodium 4-[(*tert*-butylimino)-methyl] benzene-1,3-disulfonate *N*-oxide), protect against brain damage in the rat model of transient occlusive middle cerebral arterial stroke[29] and in the marmoset model of permanent occlusive middle cerebral arterial stroke.[30] In the former model, significant protection was afforded when the drug was administered up to 6 hours after the stroke was initiated.[29] In cell culture studies, signal transduction activation was monitored by p38 map kinase activation in rat brain astrocytes.[26,27] Activation was elicited by hydrogen peroxide or the proinflammation cytokine IL1β. PBN as well as *N*-acetylcysteine at 1 mM suppressed p38 activation by 70–90%. The most direct demonstration of the mechanistic basis of the neuroprotective activity of PBN was shown in kainic acid (KA)–induced epilepsy in rats.[28] PBN given at 150 mg/kg 90 minutes after KA administration significantly protected the rats from seizures and death. Immunohistochemical examination of the CA1 subregion of the hippocampus showed that KA-mediated p38 activation as well as NF-κB activation. Activation of p38 and NF-κB was significantly suppressed by PBN administration 90 minutes after KA was administered.[28] This clearly demonstrates the PBN mediates protection from KA-mediated brain injury, which is closely associated with enhanced signal transduction processes that were significantly suppressed by PBN.

NITRONES IN AGING STUDIES

There are three published reports[6–8] in which PBN was used in mice and rats where life span data clearly indicate the antiaging activity of this compound. The most rigorous study was conducted by Saito *et al.*[6] using C57Bk/6J mice. These mice were administered PBN in the drinking water at 32 mg/kg/day starting when they were 24 months old. PBN significantly increased the mean and maximal life span of these animals from 29.0 to 30.1 months and 31.7 to 33.3 months, respectively.[6] A study by Arendash's group[8] demonstrated that PBN administered 32 mg/kg/day and begun at 24 of months age in Sprague-Dawley rats increased the 50% survivorship from 29.4 to 34.2 months. It also improved memory retention as measured using a Morris water maze.

There are three published reports[31–33] of the effect of PBN on cellular aging under culture conditions. Ames and colleagues demonstrated that PBN caused delay of replicative senescence in cultured human fibroblasts.[31,32] They showed that nitrous-*tert*-butane was a breakdown product of PBN and that it delayed senescence in these cells.[32] Another independent report[33] using human fibroblasts confirmed that PBN increased cellular longevity and decreased rates of telemere shortening.

ANTIAGING ACTIVITY OF A NOVEL NITRONE

A novel nitrone referred to as CPI-1429 (FORMULA 2) has been shown to delay mortality as well as memory impairment in an aging mouse model.[34,35] The results in summary form are presented here.

FORMULA 2.

In this study we evaluated the potential for CPI-1429 to ameliorate or delay progression of the learning and memory deficits associated with normal aging in C57BL/6 mice. Separate groups of young (4–5 month) and old (23–24 month) mice were treated daily (via gavage) with CPI-1429 or vehicle for two weeks prior to testing on a recent memory task motivated by shock avoidance.[34] The daily treatments were maintained for a period of up to 29 weeks, during which the mice were exposed to learning (during weeks 3–8) and retention (after 20 weeks) phases of testing. During the learning phase, the mice were given a series of up to 25 daily sessions during which they could avoid shock by making a correct turn in a T-maze apparatus. Successful avoidance of shock required recall, after a short delay of 1 minute, of information presented at the first trial of each daily session. The retention phase began approximately 12 weeks after the mice had completed the learning phase. During the retention phase, memory capacity of the mice was challenged by requiring them to remember the safe side of the apparatus over longer periods of up to 90 minutes.

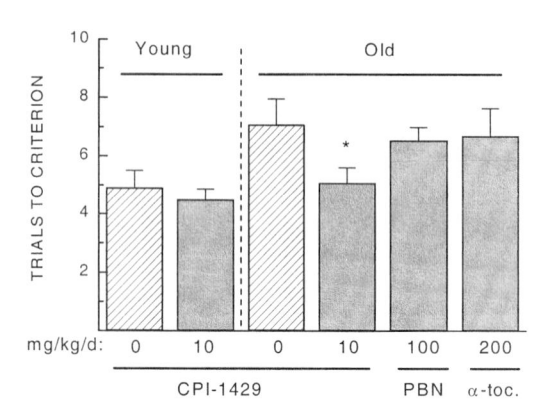

FIGURE 2. Mean number of trials (±SE) for mice to reach a learning criterion of 2 consecutive correct turns to the safe arm under a discriminated avoidance task[36] **as a function of age and treatment regimen.** Young (4–5 mo) and old (23–24 mo) C57BL/6 mice received daily treatment with the vehicle or 10 mg/kg (po) of CPI-1429 for a period of two weeks prior to testing. Results are compared with data from similar studies of α-phenyl-*tert*-butyl nitrone (PBN, 100 mg/kg/d, i.p.) and alpha-tocopheryl acetate (α-toc., 200 mg/kg/day p.o.). *$P = 0.017$ when compared with the old vehicle-treated control group (individual comparison within 1-way ANOVA).

The results of the behavioral studies indicated that performance of vehicle-treated old mice was impaired relative to the younger mice on both learning and retention phases of the test. By contrast, the rate of learning by the old mice treated with 0.1 or 10 mg/kg/day of CPI-1429 was comparable to that of the young mice receiving chronic treatment with the vehicle. The effects of CPI-1429 were particularly prominent on the second session of the learning phase, which involved a "reversal" from the previous session of the safe arm of the maze (FIG. 2). Data from similar studies of the nitrone prototype PBN and vitamin E failed to indicate any significant effects during the avoidance learning phase (FIG. 2).

During the retention phase, when mice were tested for memory under conditions of high demand (after a delay of 90 minutes), the beneficial effect of CPI-1429 was also notable. As indicated in FIGURE 3, performance was more accurate in old mice treated with 0.1 or 10 mg/kg CPI-1429 than in the old vehicle-treated controls.

The treatment regimens were maintained for a significant portion of the life span of the old mice (seven months) in these studies and it was notable that, in addition to improving learning and memory performance, CPI-1429 treatment also resulted in a significant lengthening in the mortality curve of the mice.[34,35] Overall, this pattern of effect on behavior and mortality rate for CPI-1429 is consistent with effects reported for the nitrone prototype, PBN, and is generally supportive of the hypothesized antiaging actions of some nitrones. Nevertheless, the nature of studies performed with CPI 1429 leaves open several possibilities with regard to the exact nature of the beneficial effects. Given the current data, it appears that CPI-1429 could act via any or all of the following mechanisms: (1) a generalized enhancement of cognitive processes; (2) a specific amelioration of age-related brain dysfunctions;

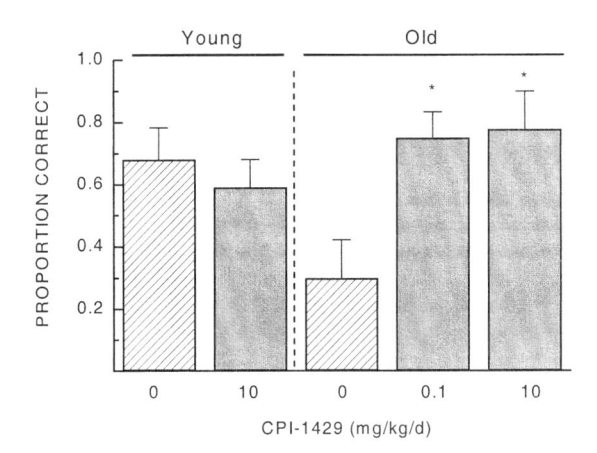

FIGURE 3. Recent memory performance for groups of young and old mice treated for 20 weeks with vehicle or CPI-1429. The figure shows accuracy (mean proportion correct ± SE) over a series of test sessions in which mice could run to the safe side of a T-maze to avoid shock, 90-minutes after the safe side had been first identified.[34] *$P < 0.025$ when compared with the old vehicle-treated control group (individual comparison within 1-way ANOVA).

or (3) an arrest or delay of age-related decline in brain function. That CPI-1429 could enhance maze learning after only two weeks would be difficult to explain in terms of an arrest of age-related decline, but would be consistent with mechanisms 1 or 2. The fact that CPI-1429 dramatically improved performance of the old mice, but was without significant effect on performance of the young mice, suggests an "age-selective" pattern that would tend to support mechanism 2 over mechanism 1. The fact that CPI-1429-treated mice performed in a manner equivalent to young controls after 20 weeks of treatment could have resulted from any of the above mechanisms. Although data are inconclusive, it is much more likely that an arrest of progressive memory decline (3) could have contributed to the superior performance of treated mice after 20 weeks of treatment with CPI-1429.

REFERENCES

1. HAWTHORNE, M.F. & R.D. STRAHM. 1957. Kinetics of the thermal isomeriazation of 2-*tert*-butyl-3-phenyloxazirane. J. Org. Chem. **22:** 1263–1264.
2. JANZEN, E.G. & B.J. BLACKBURN. 1969. Detection and identification of short-lived free radicals by electron spin resonance trapping techniques (spin trapping): photolysis of organolead, -tin, and -mercury compounds. J. Am. Chem. Soc. **91:** 4481–4490.
3. HARBOUR, J.R. & J.R. BOLTON. 1975. Superoxide formation in spinach chloroplasts: Electron spin resonance detection by spin trapping. Biochem. Biophys. Res. Commun. **64:** 803–807.
4. NOVELLI, G.P., P. ANGIOLINI, R. TANI, *et al.* 1985. Phenyl-*t*-butyl-nitrone is active against traumatic shock in rats. Free Radic. Res. Commun. **1:** 321–327.
5. FLOYD, R.A. 1990. Role of oxygen free radicals in carcinogenesis and brain ischemia. FASEB J. **4:** 2587–2597.

6. SAITO, K., H. YOSHIOKA & R.G. CUTLER. 1998. A spin trap, N-*tert*-butyl-α-phenylnitrone extends the life span of mice. Biosci. Biotechnol. Biochem. **62:** 792–794.
7. EDAMATSU, R., A. MORI & L. PACKER. 1995. The spin-trap N-*tert*-α-phenyl-butylnitrone prolongs the life span of the senescence accelerated mouse. Biochem. Biophys. Res. Commun. **211:** 847–849.
8. SACK, C.A., D.J. SOCCI, B.M. CRANDALL, *et al.* 1996. Antioxidant treatment with phenyl-α-*tert*-butyl nitrone (PBN) improves the cognitive performance and survival of aging rats. Neurosci. Lett. **205:** 181–184.
9. FLOYD, R.A. 1999. Neuroinflammatory processes are important in neurodegenerative diseases: an hypothesis to explain the increased formation of reactive oxygen and nitrogen species as major factors involved in neurodegenerative disease development. Free Radic. Biol. Med. **26:** 1346–1355.
10. FLOYD, R.A. & K. HENSLEY. 2000. Nitrone inhibition of age-associated oxidative damage. *In* Reactive Oxygen Species: From Radiation to Molecular Biology. C.C. Chiueh, Ed.: **899:** 222–237. Annals of the NewYork Academy of Sciences. New York.
11. FLOYD, R.A. 1999. Antioxidants, oxidative stress, and degenerative neurological disorders. Proc. Soc. Exp. Biol. Med. **222:** 236–245.
12. FLOYD, R.A. 1997. Protective action of nitrone-based free radical traps against oxidative damage to the central nervous system. Adv. Pharmacol. **38:** 361–378.
13. HENSLEY, K., L. MAIDT, C.A. STEWART, *et al.* 1999. Mitochondrial alteration in aging and inflammation: a possible site of action of nitrone-based free radical traps. *In* Understanding the Process of Aging: The Roles of Mitochondria, Free Radicals, and Antioxidants. E. Cadenas & L. Packer, Eds.: 311–325. Marcel Dekker. New York.
14. HENSLEY, K., J.M. CARNEY, C.A.STEWART, *et al.* 1996. Nitrone-based free radical traps as neuroprotective agents in cerebral ischemia and other pathologies. *In* Neuroprotective Agents and Cerebral Ischaemia. A. R. Green & A. J. Cross, Eds.: 299–317. Academic Press. London.
15. CARNEY, J.M., P.E. STARKE-REED, C.N. OLIVER, *et al.* 1991. Reversal of age-related increase in brain protein oxidation, decrease in enzyme activity, and loss in temporal and spacial memory by chronic administration of the spin-trapping compound N-*tert*-butyl-α-phenylnitrone. Proc.Natl. Acad. Sci. USA **88:** 3633–3636.
16. CHEN, G., *et al.* 1990. Excretion, metabolism and tissue distribution of a spin trapping agent, α-phenyl-N-*tert*-butyl-nitrone (PBN) in rats. Free Radic. Res. Commun. **9:** 317–323.
17. CHENG, H.-Y., T. LIU, G. FEUERSTEIN & F.C. BARONE. 1993. Distribution of spin-trapping compounds in rat blood and brain: In vivo microdialysis determination. Free Radic. Biol. Med. **14:** 243–250.
18. PHILLIS, J.W. & C. CLOUGH-HELFMAN. 1990. Protection from cerebral ischemic injury in gerbils with the spin trap agent *N-tert*-butyl-α-phenylnitrone (PBN). Neurosci. Lett. **116:** 315–319.
19. CLOUGH-HELFMAN, C. & J.W. PHILLIS. 1991. The free radical trapping agent *N-tert*-butyl-α-phenylnitrone (PBN) attenuates cerebral ischaemic injury in gerbils. Free Radic. Res. Commun. **15:** 177–186.
20. ZHAO, Q., K. PAHLMARK, M.-I. SMITH & B.K. SIESJO. 1994. Delayed treatment with the spin trap α-phenyl-*N-tert*-butyl nitrone (PBN) reduces infarct size following transient middle cerebral artery occlusion in rats. Acta Physiol. Scand. **152:** 349–350.
21. JANZEN, E.G., M.S. WEST & J.L. POYER. 1994. Comparison of antioxidant activity of PBN with hindered phenols in initiated rat liver microsomal lipid peroxidation. *In* Frontiers of Reactive Oxygen Species in Biology and Medicine. K. Asada & T. Toshikawa, Eds.: 431–446. Elsevier Science. Amsterdam and New York.
22. IADECOLA, C., F. ZHANG, R. CASEY, *et al.* 1997. Delayed reduction of ischemic brain injury and neurological deficits in mice lacking the inducible nitric oxide synthase gene. J. Neurosci. **17:** 9157–9164.
23. IADECOLA, C., F. ZHANG, S. XU, *et al.* 1995. Inducible nitric oxide synthase gene expression in brain following cerebral ischemia. J. Cereb. Blood Flow Metab. **15:** 378–384.
24. IADECOLA, C., F. ZHANG, R. CASEY, *et al.* 1996. Inducible nitric oxide synthase gene expression in vascular cells after transient focal cerebral ischemia. Stroke **27:** 1373–1380.

25. IADECOLA, C., F. ZHANG & X. XU. 1995. Inhibition of inducible nitric oxide synthase ameliorates cerebral ischemic damage. Am. J. Physiol. **268:** R286–R292.
26. ROBINSON, K.A., C.E. STEWART, Q. PYE, et al. 1999. Basal protein phosphorylation is decreased and phosphatase activity increased by an antioxidant and a free radical trap in primary rat glia. Arch. Biochem. Biophys. **365:** 211–215.
27. ROBINSON, K.A., C.A. STEWART, Q.N. PYE, et al. 1999. Redox-sensitive protein phosphatase activity regulates the phosphorylation state of p38 protein kinase in primary astrocyte culture. J. Neurosci. Res. **55:** 724–732.
28. FLOYD, R. A., K. HENSLEY & G. BING. 2000. Evidence for enhanced neuro-inflammatory processes in neurodegenerative diseases and the action of nitrones as potential therapeutics. J. Neural. Trans. **60:** 337–364.
29. KURODA, S., R. TSUCHIDATE, M.-L. SMITH, et al. 1999. Neuroprotective effects of a novel nitrone, NXY-059, after transient focal cerebral ischemia in the rat. J. Cereb. Blood Flow Metab. **19:** 778–787.
30. MARSHALL, J.W.B., K.J. DUFFIN, A.R. GREEN & R.M. RIDLEY. 2001. NXY-059, A free radical-trapping agent, substantially lessens the functional disability resulting from cerebral ischemia in a primate species. Stroke **32:** 190–198.
31. CHEN, Q., A. FISCHER, J.D. REAGAN, et al. 1995. Oxidative DNA damage and senescence of human diploid fibroblast cells. Proc. Natl. Acad. Sci. USA **92:** 4337–4341.
32. ATAMNA, H., A. PALER-MARTINEZ & B.N. AMES. 2000. N-t-butyl hydroxylamine, a hydrolysis product of α-phenyl-N-t-butyl nitrone, is more potent in delaying senescence in human lung fibroblasts. J.Biol. Chem. **275:** 6741–6748.
33. VON ZGLINICKI, T., R. PILGER & N. SITTE. 2000. Accumulation of single-strand breaks is the major cause of telomere shortening in human fibroblasts. Free Radic. Biol. Med. **28:** 64–74.
34. FORSTER, M. J., Y. WANG, L. NGUYEN & J. KELLEHER-ANDERSON. 1999. Anti-aging actions of novel nitrones [abstract]. American Aging Association (AGE) 28th Annual Meeting. Abstract 60, p. 36.
35. FLOYD, R.A., K. HENSLEY, M.J. FORSTER, et al. 2001. Nitrones, their value as therapeutics and probes to understand aging. Mech. Ageing Devel. In press.
36. FORSTER, M.J. & H. LAL. 1992. Within-subject behavioral analysis of recent memory in aging mice. Behav. Pharmacol. **3:** 337–349.

Therapeutics against Mitochondrial Oxidative Stress in Animal Models of Aging

SIMON MELOV

Buck Institute for Age Research, Novato, California 94945, USA

ABSTRACT: During the course of normal metabolism, reactive oxygen species (ROS) are produced from within the respiratory chain of the mitochondria. These ROS have the capacity to oxidize and damage a variety of cellular constituents including lipids, DNA, and proteins. We have taken a genetic and pharmacological approach in delineating the range of molecular targets that can be oxidatively damaged by mitochondrial ROS. Specifically, we use mice that are lacking the mitochondrial form of superoxide dismutase (*sod 2*$^{-/-}$ mice) to better understand the possible phenotypes that can arise from mitochondrial oxidative stress. *sod 2*$^{-/-}$ mice can be used to test the efficacy of antioxidants, and more generally the efficacy of antioxidants against mitochondrial oxidative stress. We have evaluated superoxide dismutase/catalase mimetics in this mammalian model of mitochondrial oxidative stress, and have shown a high degree of efficacy in protecting against ROS produced within the mitochondria. Similarly, we have employed the nematode *Caenorhabditis elegans* to test the hypothesis that effective antioxidant therapy can prolong the life span of an invertebrate.

KEYWORDS: mitochondria; reacitve oxygen species; oxidative stress; *Caenorhabditis elegans*

INTRODUCTION

The transgenic overexpression in invertebrates of catalytic antioxidant enzymes has illustrated that the endogenous production of reactive oxygen species (ROS) is a major rate-limiting factor of life span.[1–3] As a principle source—and target—of ROS, mitochondria have received considerable attention from molecular gerontologists.[4] In recent work, we have shown that transgenic mice deficient in mitochondrial superoxide dismutase (*sod2* nullizygous mice) die within the first week of life, thereby demonstrating the exceptional toxicity posed by mitochondrial oxidants derived from *normal* cellular metabolism.[5,6] At present, there is not sufficient evidence to make a compelling argument that this mouse model of endogenous oxidative stress is a model of accelerated aging. However, it demonstrates the severe consequences of endogenous mitochondrial oxidative stress to mammalian physiology. It is interesting to contrast mice that are nullizygous for the other isoforms of SOD with that of the SOD2 mouse. In contrast to mice lacking mitochondrial SOD, mice

---

Address for correspondence: Simon Melov, Buck Institute for Age Research, 8001 Redwood Blvd., Novato, CA 94945. Voice: 415-209-2000; fax: 415-209-2232.
smelov@buckinstitue.org

deficient in cytosolic SOD1 or extracellular SOD3 have a very benign phenotype.[7,8] This implies that mitochondrial oxidative stress may be the most important endogenous oxidative stress to neutralize, in order to maximize life span.

As a first step in evaluating this paradigm in mammals, we have recently shown that the mean and maximum life span of the invertebrate *Caenorhabditis elegans* can be increased through chronic catalytic antioxidant treatment.[9] Together, data from transgenic invertebrate models of aging, pharmacological studies with catalytic antioxidants and *C. elegans*, and *sod2* nullizygous mice demonstrate that modulation of *metabolic* ROS can have a profound effect on life span: when mitochondrial ROS are unchecked in mammals, early death ensues,[10,11] and when ROS are decreased throughout the life of invertebrates by genetic or pharmacological approaches, life span is increased. This review will discuss our recent findings about the effects of mitochondrial oxidative stress on both mammalian physiology, and our initial foray into treating this endogenous stress through pharmacological approaches.

REACTIVE OXYGEN SPECIES AND MITOCHONDRIA

Free radicals produced during oxidative phosphorylation, convert about 0.4 to 4% of all oxygen consumed into superoxide ($O_2^{·-}$).[12–15] Although low, this level of ROS generation can have profound pathologic consequences if not detoxified through normal defenses that have evolved within the mitochondria.[5–6] The chief form of defense against mitochondria-generated superoxide is SOD2. Mice lacking SOD2 (*Sod2* nullizygous mice) have a mean life span of 8 days, and at death present with dilated cardiomyopathy, liver dysfunction, metabolic acidosis, a variety of mitochondrial enzymatic abnormalities, and oxidative DNA damage.[5] This demonstrates that mitochondrial oxidative stress can have severe pathological consequences in a variety of organ systems. Treatment of *sod2* nullizygous mice with synthetic SOD mimics (alternatively described as synthetic catalytic antioxidants) increases their life span dramatically, and rescues many of the pathologic phenotypes of the untreated *sod2* mutants.[6] This is accomplished by daily intraperitoneal injection of the synthetic catalytic antioxidant into the mice, or, alternatively, by subcutaneous injections (Melov *et al.*, unpublished observations).

ROS primarily derived from the respiratory chain have the capacity to oxidize proteins, lipids, DNA, and RNA.[16–18] Consequently, eukaryotes have evolved defenses against these toxic byproducts. H_2O_2, which arises from the dismutation of superoxide by SOD, can either diffuse out of the mitochondrion and be converted to water by cytosolic catalase or be converted to water by mitochondrial glutathione peroxidase.[19] The rate of production of ROS by mitochondria is essentially a function of metabolic rate, although ROS production can clearly be altered by respiratory chain architecture and local antioxidant concentration. It has often been speculated that in some genetic mitochondrial diseases, mutations of subunits involved in oxidative phosphorylation may result in an increased propensity for the respiratory chain to generate free radicals and thereby overwhelm the mitochondrion's ability to protect itself from endogenous oxidative stress.[20] However, evidence for this hypothesis is scant at present (Golden and Melov, in press). At present, the clearest example of a disease in which there are hallmarks of mitochondrial oxidative stress is Friedreich's ataxia.[21–23] Although the consequences of mitochondrial oxidative stress to mammalian physiology are now being elucidated, the idea that oxidative stress is a significant component of the aging process goes back decades.

OXIDATIVE STRESS AND AGING

In fact, the hypothesis that oxidative stress is a major factor in the process of senescence has existed for more than 40 years.[24] During this period, much correlative data have been reported, lending support to the idea that cumulative damage inflicted by endogenous prooxidants is deleterious to a cell or organism's ability to maintain homeostasis.[25] For example, a number of interesting findings have recently been reported in relation to specific protein and carbonyl modifications with age.[26,27] In *Drosophila*, carbonyl modifications were found to be associated with life expectancy.[28,29] In addition, specific carbonyl modification of mitochondrial aconitase and the adenine nucleotide translocator (ANT) have been reported with age.[26,27] In addition to model systems such as *Drosophila* and the mouse, protein oxidation has been immunohistochemically described in tissue sections of aged human brain, in association with lipid peroxidation and proteins indicative of stress.[30–33] More recently, results from microarray analysis of skeletal muscle and brains of young vs. old mice, with and without caloric restriction, have been used to argue that a major factor in the efficacy of caloric restriction in retarding age-related changes in the mouse is via oxidative stress and metabolic control.[34] However, these results are difficult to interpret due to inadequate statistical analysis,[35] as well as problems in the production of the microarrays used to generate these data (http://www.affymetrix.com/products/U74productupdate.html).

Some recent compelling arguments that oxidative stresses are a major limiter of life span have come from genetic studies using invertebrates and the mouse.[1,3,5,36,37] Overexpression of genes that are responsible for neutralizing the superoxide free radical have shown that the mean and maximum life span of *Drosophila melanogaster* can be increased, indicating that endogenous superoxide production limits life span in the fly.[1–3] Our recently published studies using synthetic antioxidant compounds to extend life span in *C. elegans* also provide support to the notion that oxidative stress is a major limiter of life span in multicellular organisms, and that appropriate intervention can forestall and extend life span.[9]

Much work has been done correlating the differential production of ROS from mitochondria with life spans of different species.[29,38–42] Although there are broad correlations in the level of ROS produced from isolated mitochondria related to maximum and mean life span, there are a number of notable exceptions to this generalization.[43,44] Pigeons and rats have high metabolic rates that are approximately equivalent, yet pigeons live about 3–5 times longer than the rat. Mitochondria isolated from each species and compared for ROS production do not show equivalence, as might be expected on the basis of metabolic rate.[44] Instead, isolated mitochondria from a variety of tissues of the pigeon have approximately 2–4-fold lower level of ROS production that the rat.[44] Further, recent findings indicate that a contributory factor in preventing oxidative damage in long-lived species is the low level of fatty-acid saturation in membranes.[45] Hence, ROS production and its effects must be taken into account in addition to metabolic rate in testing the free radical theory.

SYNTHETIC ANTIOXIDANTS AND OXIDATIVE STRESS

As there is a credible and substantial body of evidence implicating oxidative stress as a major factor in aging, are there therapeutic approaches that can be used to modulate endogenous oxidative stresses, and thereby further test the free radical theory as well as point towards potential treatments in humans? A variety of studies have been carried out with regard to ameliorating or attenuating aging or the progression of disease by chronic or acute antioxidant treatments.[61-69] The results of these studies are not compelling in terms of either improving specific indicators of the disease, or increasing mean or maximum life span in a robust fashion.[68] Chronic dietary supplementation of antioxidants has either failed, or met with very limited success in extending life span or attenuating the rate of physiological decline, in organisms from *C. elegans* to humans.[63,65-69] The antioxidants used in previous studies (such as vitamin E) are not particularly effective antioxidants, compared to more efficient *catalytic* antioxidants in a number of acute and chronic studies.[70] Hence this may explain the preciousness of previous results that have attempted to manipulate life span through dietary supplementation with antioxidants.[68] Of importance for understanding why potential therapeutics may fail or succeed, it is desirable to know the outcomes of mitochondrial oxidative stress in a variety of animal models.

LIFE SPAN AND ANIMAL MODELS OF OXIDATIVE STRESS

The utility of *C. elegans* for studying aging is well recognized.[46-49] Its small size, rapid life cycle, well-characterized genetics, and defined cell lineage make it an excellent choice of organism for testing hypotheses of aging. In addition, it was the first multicellular organism to have its genome completely sequenced.[50] A number of well-characterized mutants that lengthen life have been identified in *C. elegans*, which by definition implicate the action of these genes in senescence.[46,49,51,52] These genes should not be interpreted as being directly responsible for aging, but rather are one factor that influences mean and maximum life span. An appropriate analogy would be genes that contribute *to* the pathophysiology of heart disease, such as those involved in cholesterol biosynthesis, but are not thought of as being responsible *for* heart disease. Most of the "gerontogenes" in *C. elegans* fall into the dauer pathway, which is an alternate developmental pathway induced by hardship, food scarcity, or overpopulation.[53] Mutations in some genes within this pathway increase the adult life span of *C. elegans* by as much as 100%.

Until recently the emphasis has been on characterizing the genetics of these mutants, rather than the unique physiology that may arise as a result of the mutation.[51] Recent reports demonstrate that at least two of the *age* mutants are perhaps metabolically defective, indicating that the mechanism of extension of life span may be through a reduction in the flux of electrons through the respiratory chain.[54,55] Hence, the effects of *age* mutations may be to yield less ROS from the mitochondria, analogous to an extension of life span by lowering the temperature.[56] A short-lived oxidative stress mutant known as *mev-1* is mutant in the cytochrome *b* subunit of the respiratory chain, which presumably prevents the efficient passage of electrons from complex II to complex III via ubiquinone.[57,58] Phenotypically, this has the effect of reducing the mean life span of these worms by about 25%, and impairing their ability to survive at increased partial pressures of oxygen.[57] Further, *mev-1* mutants have a much greater level of protein carbonylation than wild-type worms as judged by immunoblot assays, consistent with a greater oxidative stress as a result of stalling electrons at complex II within the respiratory chain.[58]

Mouse genetics are also a fruitful tool for studies of aging. In addition to the SOD mutants described above, another mouse mutant of mitochondrial oxidative stress is the adenine nucleotide translocator mutant mouse (ANT1).[59] The ANT protein is responsible for translocating ADP into the mitochondria while exporting ATP out of the mitochondria after oxidative phosphorylation has occurred. Hence, the ANT is responsible for ensuring the availability of substrate for the ATP synthase. As electron flow through the respiratory chain will not occur without phosphorylation of ADP at the ATP synthase, ANT indirectly facilitates passage of electrons through the respiratory chain. Inactivation of the heart/skeletal muscle isoform (ANT1) in mice through homologous recombination results in a mild myopathy, associated with mitochondrial proliferation in the skeletal muscle.[60] Due to the inability of the mitochondria to obtain substrate (ADP), electrons stall throughout the respiratory chain, resulting in the reduction of the electron transport chain. This should increase the propensity for the mitochondria to make superoxide. In concordance with this prediction, an induction of the mRNA level of *sod2* in skeletal muscle is observed in these mice. This is paralleled by an 4–8-fold increase in the production of hydrogen peroxide from isolated mitochondria of the mutant mice compared to controls, presumably as a result of the conversion of superoxide into hydrogen peroxide.[59]

SPECIFIC EFFECTS OF MAMMALIAN MITOCHONDRIAL OXIDATIVE STRESS

We have reported extensively on the biochemical and phenotypic consequences of inactivating the mitochondrial form of superoxide dismutase.[5,6,11] The enzymatic activity of aconitase is directly affected by oxidative stress, with its catalytic activity dependent on a 4Fe-4S tetrameric cluster.[71,72] Superoxide has been shown to oxidize this cluster, resulting in an 3Fe-4S cluster and a decrease in the catalytic activity of the enzyme.[72] Accordingly, we measured mitochondrial aconitase activity from the hearts and brains of *sod2* mutant mice versus controls. We found the activity of aconitase decreased by greater than 90% in the hearts, and by 30–60% in various regions of the brain.[5] This demonstrates a direct effect of mitochondrial oxidative stress on this "gold-standard" marker of superoxide-mediated damage.

To further characterize the metabolic defects of inactivation of *sod2* in mice, we examined the urine organic acids by GC/MS. Large amounts of 3-methylglutaconic, 2-hydroxyglutaric, 3-hydroxy-3-methyl glutaric, and 3-hydroxyisovaleric acids were found in the urine of *sod2* mutant mice and not in controls.[5] This organic acid profile suggested a defect in HMG-CoA lyase, an enzyme involved in ketogenesis and leucine catabolism that is particularly susceptible to oxidative inactivation.[73–75] We therefore measured the catalytic activity of HMG-CoA lyase, and consistent with the finding of organic aciduria, found a 40% decrease in the activity of HMG-CoA lyase when compared to controls.[5]

Also consistent with a lack of protection from mitochondrial oxidative stress, we found an increase in the level of oxidative lesions of total DNA. For our initial studies, we did not have a sufficient number of animals to isolate mitochondrial DNA, which should have the greatest level of oxidative damage due to its proximity to the respiratory chain. However, we isolated total DNA from mutant and control tissues and found 200–300% increases in three specific adducts—5-OH-cytosine, 8-OH-adenosine, and 8-OH-guanine—relative to controls. Again, we saw tissue-specific differences between the brain, heart, and liver, with the brain and heart most affected. This suggests either differential sensitivity to mitochondrial oxidative stress or different metabolic outputs, and hence differing loads of oxidative stress with corresponding variations in tissue damage.[5]

A CATALYTIC ANTIOXIDANT EXTENDS THE LIFE SPAN OF SOD2 MUTANT MICE

We wished to determine whether it was possible to make up for the lack of endogenous mitochondrial *sod* by chronically treating the *sod2* nullizygous mice with synthetic catalytic antioxidants. The first such antioxidant we tested was the SOD-mimetic manganese 5,10,15,20-tetrakis (4-benzoic acid) porphyrin (MnTBAP). By chronically treating the mutant mice with MnTBAP through daily intraperitoneal (i.p.) injection at a dosage of 5 mg/kg, we were able to increase the survival of the *sod* mutant mice from a mean of 8 days of age to 16 days of age.[6]

MnTBPA-TREATED MICE DEVELOP NEUROLOGICAL PATHOLOGY

Not only did MnTBAP treatment of the mutant mice increase the survival of the animals substantially, it also rescued the dilated cardiomyopathy and hepatic lipid accumulation.[6] Interestingly, we observed a pronounced age-related brain disorder in MnTBAP-treated *sod2* mutant mice, starting at about 12 days of age, characterized by a mild tremor accompanied by circling, falling, and barrel-like rolls.[6] By 3 weeks of age, MnTBAP-treated animals were behaviorally compromised, lost the inability to feed due to overt neurological problems, and were therefore sacrificed.[6] The small percentage of untreated *sod2* mutant mice that reached this age (<10%) also developed this neurological disorder.

Our interpretation of these results is that the enhanced survival due to suppression of cardiac pathology by MnTBAP unmasks age-related oxidative brain damage in these mice. Pharmacokinetic studies indicate that MnTBAP does not penetrate the blood–brain barrier. Hence, by preventing the early neonatal death of the *sod2* mutant mice through effective treatment of the heart failure, we allowed the brain sufficient time to develop its own free radical–mediated pathology, a process ultimately due to the endogenous production of mitochondrial free radicals.

Indeed, neuropathological analysis of the brains of the MnTBAP-treated *sod2* mutant mice showed that they develop a severe spongiform encephalopathy in the frontal cortex, and focally within specific regions of the brainstem. The majority of animals showed spongiform changes in the motor nucleus of cranial nerves V and VII, the reticulotegmental nucleus of the pons, and the superior and medioventral periolivary nuclei. Immunohistochemistry carried out with antibodies to glial fibrillary acidic protein (GFAP)—a marker of cellular injury—revealed a variable astrocytic response in areas of vacuolization. GFAP-positive cells were particularly prominent in the trigeminal nucleus in several cases.[6]

This implies that mitochondrial oxidative stress can lead to a loss of cells in the brain. In support of this hypothesis, we identified sporadic cell death in the brains of MnTBAP-treated mice at the ultrastructural level (Melov *et al.*, unpublished observations). We primarily observed these dying cells in frontal cortex of MnTBAP-treated *sod2* mutant mice over 2 weeks of age. There was no widespread pattern of cell death observable by surveying electron micrographs from cortex, brainstem, cerebellum, or striatum in the brains of MnTBAP-treated mutant mice at 12, 14, 16, 18, or 21 days of age.

At the ultrastructural level, the spongiform changes seen in the *sod2* mutant mice are reminiscent of Leigh's disease and Canavan's disease, with a peculiar splitting of the myelin sheaths surrounding neuronal processes, and occasional mitochondria were seen "ballooning" within neurons.[6] Having validated one type of catalytic antioxidant in a mammalian model of mitochondrial oxidative stress, we wished to determine whether this *in vivo* success could be applied to aging itself.

EXTENSION OF LIFE SPAN OF *C. ELEGANS* VIA TREATMENT WITH A CATALYTIC ANTIOXIDANT

Along with our colleagues, we have found that by treating wild-type (N2) *C. elegans* chronically with EUK-134 and EUK-8, two catalytic antioxidants produced by our collaborator Eukarion (Bedford, MA), we can extend the life span of *C. elegans*. These compounds work with a high degree of efficacy in a variety of mammalian models of oxidative stress[70,76–80] and therefore demonstrate the broad-spectrum efficacy of these compounds in widely divergent species. Given that the life span of *C. elegans* can be extended through *appropriate* antioxidant treatment to a magnitude roughly equivalent to single gene AGE mutants (for example *age-1*), we wished to determine whether antioxidant treatment would also be beneficial in an oxidative stress mutant in *C. elegans*. The *mev-1* mutant of *C. elegans* can be argued to be analogous to the *sod2* mutant mice, due to the elevated levels of ROS within the mitochondria, and the defect in complex II of the respiratory chain. Hence we tested the efficacy of a catalytic antioxidant on the *mev-*1 mutants. Untreated *mev-1* mutants live about 25% shorter than controls[57] (see above). We were able to normalize the life span of the *mev-*1 mutants by treating them with EUK-134.[9] These data argue that this class of compounds is capable of rescuing cells from the effects of mitochondrial dysfunction due to oxidative stress, and subsequently extending life span.

Our results in extending the mean and maximum life span of *C. elegans* using the Eukarion compounds raises the possibility that chronic treatment of mammals with *effective* catalytic antioxidants may prolong both the mean and maximum life span of a mammal. Significantly, the compounds we used in extending the life span of the invertebrate *C. elegans* have already proven efficacious in preventing many disorders of endogenous and exogenous stress in mammals, and hence it is of great interest to see whether the results we obtained in *C. elegans* with this type of compound will translate to mammals.

REFERENCES

1. PARKES, T.L. *et al.* 1998. Extension of *Drosophila* lifespan by overexpression of human SOD1 in motorneurons. Nat. Genet. **19:** 171–174.
2. ORR, W.C. & R.S. SOHAL. 1994. Extension of life-span by overexpression of superoxide dismutase and catalase in *Drosophila melanogaster.* Science **263:** 1128–1130.
3. SUN, J. & J. TOWER. 1999. FLP recombinase-mediated induction of Cu/Zn-superoxide dismutase transgene expression can extend the life span of adult *Drosophila melanogaster flies.* Mol. Cell. Biol. **19:** 216–228.
4. SOHAL, R.J. & R. WEINDRUCH. 1996. Oxidative stress, caloric restriction, and aging. Science **273:** 59–63.
5. MELOV, S. *et al.* 1999. Mitochondrial disease in superoxide dismutase 2 mutant mice. Proc. Natl. Acad. Sci. USA **96:** 846–851.
6. MELOV, S. *et al.* 1998. A novel neurological phenotype in mice lacking mitochondrial manganese superoxide dismutase. Nat. Genet. **18:** 159–163.
7. REAUME, A.G. *et al.* 1996. Motor neurons in Cu/Zn superoxide dismutase-deficient mice develop normally, but exhibit enhanced cell death after axonal injury. Nat. Genet. **13:** 43–47.
8. CARLSSON, L.M. *et al.* 1995. Mice lacking extracellular superoxide dismutase are more sensitive to hyperoxia. Proc. Natl. Acad. Sci. USA **92:** 6264–6268.
9. MELOV, S. *et al.* 2000. Extension of life-span with superoxide dismutase/catalase mimetics. Science **289:** 1567–1569.
10. LEBOVITZ, R.M. *et al.* 1996. Neurodegeneration, myocardial injury, and perinatal death in mitochondrial superoxide dismutase-deficient mice. Proc. Natl. Acad. Sci. USA **93:** 9782–9787.
11. LI, Y. *et al.* 1995. Dilated cardiomyopathy and neonatal lethality in mutant mice lacking manganese superoxide dismutase. Nat. Genet. **11:** 376–381.
12. BOVERIS, A., 1984. Determination of the production of superoxide radicals and hydrogen peroxide in mitochondria. Methods Enzymol. **105:** 429–435.
13. CHANCE, B., H. SIES & A. BOVERIS. 1979. Hydroperoxide metabolism in mammalian organs. Physiol. Rev. **59:** 527–605.
14. TURRENS, J.F. & A. BOVERIS. 1980. Generation of superoxide anion by the NADH dehydrogenase of bovine heart mitochondria. Biochem. J. **191:** 421–427.
15. HANSFORD, R.G., B.A. HOGUE & V. MILDAZIENE. 1997. Dependence of H_2O_2 formation by rat heart mitochondria on substrate availability and donor age. J. Bioenerg. Biomembr. **29:** 89–95.
16. BECKMAN, K.B. & B.N. AMES. 1999. Endogenous oxidative damage of mtDNA. Mutat. Res. **424:** 51–58.
17. HALLIWELL, B. & S. CHIRICO. 1993. Lipid peroxidation: its mechanism, measurement, and significance. Am. J. Clin. Nutr. (Suppl.) **57:** 715S–724S [discussion 724S–725S].
18. STADTMAN, E.R. 1995. Role of oxidized amino acids in protein breakdown and stability. Meth. Enzymol. **258:** 379–393.
19. PANFILI, E., G. SANDRI & L. ERNSTER. 1991. Distribution of glutathione peroxidases and glutathione reductase in rat brain mitochondria. FEBS Lett. **290:** 35–37.
20. ROBINSON, B.H. 1998. Human complex I deficiency: clinical spectrum and involvement of oxygen free radicals in the pathogenicity of the defect. Biochim. Biophys. Acta **1364:** 271–286.
21. PANDOLFO, M. 1998. Molecular genetics and pathogenesis of Friedreich ataxia. Neuromusc. Disord. **8:** 409–415.
22. ROTIG, A. *et al.* 1997. Aconitase and mitochondrial iron-sulphur protein deficiency in Friedreich ataxia. Nat. Genet. **17:** 215–217.
23. PUCCIO, H. *et al.* 2001. Mouse models for Friedreich ataxia exhibit cardiomyopathy, sensory nerve defect and Fe-S enzyme deficiency followed by intramitochondrial iron deposits. Nat. Genet. **27:** 181–186.
24. HARMAN, D. 1956. Aging: a theory based on free radical and radiation chemistry. J. Gerontol. **11:** 298–300.
25. BECKMAN, K.B. & B.N. AMES. 1998. The free radical theory of aging matures. Physiol. Rev. **78:** 547–581.

26. YAN, L.J. & R.S. SOHAL. 1998. Mitochondrial adenine nucleotide translocase is modified oxidatively during aging. Proc. Natl. Acad. Sci. USA **95:** 12896–12901.
27. YAN, L.J., R.L. LEVINE & R.S. SOHAL. 1997. Oxidative damage during aging targets mitochondrial aconitase. Proc. Natl. Acad. Sci. USA **94:** 11168–11172.
28. AGARWAL, S. & R.S. SOHAL. 1995. Differential oxidative damage to mitochondrial proteins during aging. Mech. Ageing Dev. **85:** 55–63.
29. SOHAL, R.S. et al. 1993. Protein oxidative damage is associated with life expectancy of houseflies. Proc. Natl. Acad. Sci. USA **90:** 7255–7259.
30. SMITH, C.D. et al. 1991. Excess brain protein oxidation and enzyme dysfunction in normal aging and in Alzheimer disease. Proc. Natl. Acad. Sci. USA **88:** 10540–10543.
31. SMITH, M.A. & G. PERRY. 1995. Free radical damage, iron, and Alzheimer's disease. J. Neurol. Sci. (Suppl.) **134:** 92–94.
32. SMITH, M.A. & G. PERRY. 1996. Oxidative stress and protein modification in neurodegenerative disease. In Free Radicals in Brain Physiology and Disorders. L. Packer, M. Hiramatsu, and T. Yoshikawa, Eds.: 287–292. Academic Press. San Diego, CA.
33. SMITH, M.A. et al. 1997. Iron accumulation in Alzheimer disease is a source of redox-generated free radicals. Proc. Natl. Acad. Sci. USA **94:** 9866–9868.
34. LEE, C.K. et al. 1999. Gene expression profile of aging and its retardation by caloric restriction. Science **285:** 1390–1393.
35. HAN, E. & S.G. HILSENBECK. 2001. Array-based gene expression profiling to study aging. Mech. Ageing Dev. **122:** 999–1018.
36. LARSEN, P.L. 1993. Aging and resistance to oxidative damage in Caenorhabditis elegans. Proc. Natl. Acad. Sci. USA **90:** 8905–8909.
37. VANFLETEREN, J.R. 1993. Oxidative stress and ageing in Caenorhabditis elegans. Biochem. J. (Pt.2) **292:** 605–608.
38. SOHAL, R.S., B.H. SOHAL & W.C. ORR. 1995. Mitochondrial superoxide and hydrogen peroxide generation, protein oxidative damage, and longevity in different species of flies. Free Radic. Biol. Med. **19:** 499–504.
39. SOHAL, R.S. & A. DUBEY. 1994. Mitochondrial oxidative damage, hydrogen peroxide release, and aging. Free Radic. Biol. Med. **16:** 621–626.
40. SOHAL, R.S. & W.C. ORR. 1992. Relationship between antioxidants, prooxidants, and the aging process. Ann. N.Y. Acad. Sci. **663:** 74–84.
41. MIQUEL, J., R. BINNARD & J.E. FLEMING. 1983. Role of metabolic rate and DNA-repair in Drosophila aging: implications for the mitochondrial mutation theory of aging. Exp. Gerontol. **18:** 167–171.
42. PEREZ-CAMPO, R. et al. 1998. The rate of free radical production as a determinant of the rate of aging: evidence from the comparative approach. J. Comp. Physiol. [B] **168:** 149–158.
43. BARJA, G. et al. 1994. Low mitochondrial free radical production per unit O_2 consumption can explain the simultaneous presence of high longevity and high aerobic metabolic rate in birds. Free Radic. Res. **21:** 317–327.
44. KU, H.H. & R.S. SOHAL. 1993. Comparison of mitochondrial pro-oxidant generation and anti-oxidant defenses between rat and pigeon: possible basis of variation in longevity and metabolic potential. Mech. Ageing Dev. **72:** 67–76.
45. PAMPLONA, R. et al. 2000. Double bond content of phospholipids and lipid peroxidation negatively correlate with maximum longevity in the heart of mammals. Mech. Ageing Dev. **112:** 169–183.
46. JOHNSON, T.E. 1990. Increased life-span of age-1 mutants in Caenorhabditis elegans and lower Gompertz rate of aging. Science **249:** 908–912.
47. JOHNSON, T.E. & G.J. LITHGOW. 1992. The search for the genetic basis of aging: the identification of gerontogenes in the nematode Caenorhabditis elegans. J. Am. Geriatr. Soc. **40:** 936–945.
48. JOHNSON, T.E. 1997. Genetic influences on aging. Exp. Gerontol. **32:** 11–22.
49. HSIN, H. & C. KENYON. 1999. Signals from the reproductive system regulate the lifespan of C. elegans [see comments]. Nature **399:** 362–366.
50. 1998. Genome sequence of the nematode C. elegans: a platform for investigating biology. The C. elegans Sequencing Consortium. Science **282:** 2012–2018.

51. KENYON, C. et al. 1993. A *C. elegans* mutant that lives twice as long as wild type [see comments]. Nature **366**(6454): 461-464.
52. LIN, K. et al. 1997. daf-16: an HNF-3/forkhead family member that can function to double the life-span of *Caenorhabditis elegans* [see comments]. Science **278**: 1319–1322.
53. RIDDLE, D.L. et al., Eds. 1997. *C. Elegans* II.: 1222. Cold Spring Harbor Laboratory Press. Cold Spring Harbor, NY.
54. VAN VOORHIES, W.A. & S. WARD. 1999. Genetic and environmental conditions that increase longevity in *Caenorhabditis elegans* decrease metabolic rate. Proc. Natl. Acad. Sci. USA **96**: 11399–11403.
55. JONASSEN, T., P.L. LARSEN & C.F. CLARKE. 2001. A dietary source of coenzyme Q is essential for growth of long-lived *Caenorhabditis elegans* clk-1 mutants. Proc. Natl. Acad. Sci. USA **98**: 421–426.
56. RAGLAND, S.S. & R.S. SOHAL. 1975. Ambient temperature, physical activity and aging in the housefly, *Musca domestica*. Exp. Gerontol. **10**: 279–289.
57. ISHII, N. et al. 1990. A methyl viologen-sensitive mutant of the nematode *Caenorhabditis elegans*. Mutat. Res. **237**: 165–171.
58. ISHII, N. et al. 1998. A mutation in succinate dehydrogenase cytochrome *b* causes oxidative stress and aging in nematodes. Nature **394**: 694–697.
59. ESPOSITO, L.A. et al. 1999. Mitochondrial disease in mouse results in increased hydrogen peroxide production and mitochondrial DNA damage. Proc. Natl. Acad. Sci. USA **96**: 4820–4825.
60. GRAHAM, B.H. et al. 1997. A mouse model for mitochondrial myopathy and cardiomyopathy resulting from a deficiency in the heart/muscle isoform of the adenine nucleotide translocator. Nat. Genet. **16**: 226–234.
61. BEHL, C. 1999. Alzheimer's disease and oxidative stress: implications for novel therapeutic approaches. Progr. Neurobiol. **57**: 301–323.
62. GEY, K.F. 1995. Cardiovascular disease and vitamins. Concurrent correction of "suboptimal" plasma antioxidant levels may, as important part of "optimal" nutrition, help to prevent early stages of cardiovascular disease and cancer, respectively. Bibl. Nutr. Dieta **52**: 75–91.
63. HALLER, J. et al. 1996. Mental health: minimental state examination and geriatric depression score of elderly Europeans in the SENECA study of 1993. Eur. J. Clin. Nutr. **50 (Suppl 2)**: S112–S116.
64. PERRIG, W.J., P. PERRIG & H.B. STAHELIN. 1997. The relation between antioxidants and memory performance in the old and very old. J. Am. Geriatr. Soc. **45**: 718–724.
65. GALE, C.R., C.N. MARTYN & C. COOPER. 1996. Cognitive impairment and mortality in a cohort of elderly people. Br. Med. J. **312**: 608–611.
66. MIQUEL, J., J. FLEMING & A.C. ECONOMOS. 1982. Antioxidants, metabolic rate and aging in *Drosophila*. Arch. Gerontol. Geriatr. **1**: 159–165.
67. HARRINGTON, L.A. & C.B. HARLEY. 1988. Effect of vitamin E on lifespan and reproduction in *Caenorhabditis elegans*. Mech. Ageing Dev. **43**: 71–78.
68. LIPMAN, R.D. et al. 1998. Disease incidence and longevity are unaltered by dietary antioxidant supplementation initiated during middle age in C57BL/6 mice. Mech. Ageing Dev. **103**: 269–284.
69. JAMA, J.W. et al. 1996. Dietary antioxidants and cognitive function in a population-based sample of older persons: The Rotterdam Study. Am. J. Epidemiol. **144**: 275–280.
70. DOCTROW, S.R. et al. 1997. Salen-manganese complexes: combined superoxide dismutase/catalase mimics with broad pharmacological efficacy. Adv. Pharmacol. **38**: 247–269.
71. GARDNER, P.R., D.D. NGUYEN & C.W. WHITE. 1994. Aconitase is a sensitive and critical target of oxygen poisoning in cultured mammalian cells and in rat lungs. Proc. Natl. Acad. Sci. USA **91**: 12248–12252.
72. GARDNER, P.R. 1997. Superoxide-driven aconitase FE-S center cycling. Biosci. Rep. **17**: 33–42.
73. HRUZ, P.W. & H.M. MIZIORKO. 1992. Avian 3-hydroxy-3-methylglutaryl-CoA lyase: sensitivity of enzyme activity to thiol/disulfide exchange and identification of proximal reactive cysteines. Protein Sci. **1**: 1144–1153.

74. ROBERTS, J.R. *et al.* 1994. 3-Hydroxy-3-methylglutaryl-CoA lyase: expression and isolation of the recombinant human enzyme and investigation of a mechanism for regulation of enzyme activity. J. Biol. Chem. **269:** 17841–17846.
75. CULLINGFORD, T.E. *et al.* 1998. Molecular cloning of rat mitochondrial 3-hydroxy-3-methylglutaryl-CoA lyase and detection of the corresponding mRNA and of those encoding the remaining enzymes comprising the ketogenic 3-hydroxy-3-methylglutaryl-CoA cycle in central nervous system of suckling rat. Biochem. J. **329:** 373–381.
76. PONG, K. *et al.* 2001. Attenuation of staurosporine-induced apoptosis, oxidative stress, and mitochondrial dysfunction by synthetic superoxide dismutase and catalase mimetics in cultured cortical neurons. Exp. Neurol. In press.
77. JUNG, C. *et al.* 2001. Synthetic superoxide dismutase/catalase mimetics reduce oxidative stress and prolong survival in a mouse amyotrophic lateral sclerosis model. Neurosci. Lett. **304:** 157–160.
78. RONG, Y. *et al.* 1999. EUK-134, a synthetic superoxide dismutase and catalase mimetic, prevents oxidative stress and attenuates kainate-induced neuropathology. Proc. Natl. Acad. Sci. USA **96:** 9897–9902.
79. BAKER, K. *et al.* 1998. Synthetic combined superoxide dismutase/catalase mimetics are protective as a delayed treatment in a rat stroke model: a key role for reactive oxygen species in ischemic brain injury. J. Pharmacol. Exp. Ther. **284:** 215–221.
80. MALFROY, B. *et al.* 1997. Prevention and suppression of autoimmune encephalomyelitis by EUK-8, a synthetic catalytic scavenger of oxygen-reactive metabolites. Cell. Immunol. **177:** 62–68.

A Unified Mechanism in the Initiation of Cancer

ERCOLE L. CAVALIERI AND ELEANOR G. ROGAN

Eppley Institute for Research in Cancer and Allied Diseases, University of Nebraska Medical Center, Omaha, Nebraska 68198-6805, USA

ABSTRACT: Estrogens are involved in the initiation of breast, prostate, and other kinds of human cancer. In this process, the endogenous estrogens, estrone and estradiol, are metabolized to 2-catechol estrogens (2-CE, major) and 4-CE (minor). If the 4-CEs are further oxidized to CE-3,4-quinones, they may react with DNA to form depurinating adducts at N-7 of guanine and N-3 of adenine, and generate apurinic sites. Similarly, the carcinogenic synthetic estrogen hexestrol, a hydrogenated derivative of diethylstilbestrol, is metabolized to its quinone, which reacts with DNA to form analogous depurinating adducts. This could be the primary critical event leading to oncogenic mutations and then initiation of cancer. Evidence supporting this hypothesis has been obtained from the human breast and animal models susceptible to estrogen-induced tumors, including the Syrian golden hamster kidney, ACI rat mammary gland, and Noble rat prostate. The oxidation of phenols to catechols and then to quinones is not only a mechanism of tumor initiation for natural and synthetic estrogens, but also for the leukemogen benzene. In fact, catechol, one of the metabolites of benzene, when oxidized to its quinone, reacts with DNA to form N7guanine and N3adenine depurinating adducts. Thus, a unifying mechanism, namely formation of catechol quinones and reaction with DNA, could initiate not only cancer by oxidation of specific endogenous estrogen metabolites, but also leukemia by oxidation of benzene.

KEYWORDS: catechol estrogens; catechol quinones. depurinating DNA adducts; 1,4-Michael addition

Exposure to estrogens is a risk factor for cancer of the breast, prostate, and other organs in humans. Initiation of these kinds of cancer has been hypothesized to result from reaction of specific estrogen metabolites with DNA to generate mutations in critical genes that modulate cell growth and death. These include oncogenes and tumor suppressor genes, which give rise to transformation and abnormal cell prolifer-

---

ABBREVIATIONS: Ade, adenine; BP, benzo[*a*]pyrene; CE, catechol estrogen(s); CE-Q, catechol estrogen quinone(s); COMT, catechol-*O*-methyltransferase; CYP, cytochrome P450; DB[*a,l*]P, dibenzo[*a,l*]pyrene; DMBA, 7,12-dimethylbenz[*a*]anthracene; E_1, estrone; E_2, estradiol; Gua, guanine; GSH, glutathione; H, Harvey; OHE$_2$, hydroxyestradiol; PAH, polycyclic aromatic hydrocarbon(s).

Address for correspondence: Ercole L. Cavalieri, 986805 Nebraska Medical Center, Omaha, NE 68198-6805. Voice: 402-559-7237; fax: 402-559-8068.
  ecavalie@unmc.edu

TABLE 1. Correlation of depurinating adducts with H-*ras* mutations in mouse skin papilomas papillomas and in mouse skin

		H-ras Mutations	
Compound	Major DNA Adducts[a]	No. of mutations[b] / No. of mice	Codon
Skin papillomas			
DMBA	N7Ade (79%)	4/4 CAA → CTA	61
DB[*a,l*]P	N7Ade (32%) N3Ade (49%)	10/12 CAA → CTA	61
BP	C8Gua + N7Gua (46%) N7Ade (25%)	10/20 GGC → GTC 5/20 CAA → CTA	13 61
Skin			
E_2-3,4-Q	N7Gua (49%) N3Ade (51%)	5/29 A → G	not at 13 or 61

[a]DNA adducts were determined in a treated area of dorsal skin 4 hr after treatment with PAH[3,4] or 1 hr after treatment with E_2-3,4-Q.[16]

[b]Mutations were determined in DNA isolated from individual papillomas induced by the PAH on mouse skin.[4] For E_2-3,4-Q-treated mouse skin, mutations were determined in DNA isolated from mouse skin 6 hr after treatment with E_2-3,4-Q. The mutations were analyzed in 29 plasmids containing the H-*ras* insert. Each mutation was at a different point in exons 1 and 2 of the H-*ras* gene.[16]

ation.[1] Understanding the origin of these mutations opens the door to strategies for controlling and preventing cancer.

GENOTOXICITY: STABLE AND DEPURINATING CARCINOGEN–DNA ADDUCTS

Chemical carcinogens covalently bind to DNA to form two types of DNA adducts: stable ones that remain in DNA unless removed by repair and depurinating ones that are released from DNA by destabilization of the glycosyl bond.[2,3] Depurinating adducts are obtained when carcinogens covalently bind at the N-3 or N-7 of adenine (Ade) or the N-7 or sometimes C-8 of guanine (Gua), whereas stable adducts are formed when carcinogens react with the exocyclic N^6 amino group of Ade or N^2 amino group of Gua. The loss of Ade or Gua by depurination leads to formation of apurinic sites that can generate the mutations leading to tumor initiation.

There is a correlation between the identities and levels of depurinating adducts and oncogenic mutations in mouse skin treated with carcinogenic polycyclic aromatic hydrocarbons (PAH), suggesting that these adducts are the primary culprits in the tumor initiating pathway.[3–5] The depurinating DNA adducts formed in mouse skin by dibenzo[*a,l*]pyrene (DB[*a,l*]P), 7,12-dimethylbenz[*a*]anthracene (DMBA), and benzo[*a*]pyrene (BP) determine the mutations in the Harvey (H)-*ras* oncogene in mouse skin papillomas initiated by these three PAHs (TABLE 1). This pattern of *ras* mutations suggests that the oncogenic mutations in mouse skin papillomas induced by these PAHs are generated by misrepair of the apurinic sites derived from loss of the depurinating adducts.[5] Repair of apurinic sites induced by PAH might be expected, since thousands of apurinic sites are formed by cells each day.[6] The level of apurinic sites arising from treatment with these PAHs is, however, 15–120 times higher than those formed spontaneously, suggesting that this large increase in apurinic sites could lead to misrepair.[5,7] Thus, apurinic sites can generate the mutations that play the critical role in the initiation of cancer, and formation of depurinating adducts has become the common denominator for recognizing the potential of a chemical to initiate cancer.

FORMATION, METABOLISM, CONJUGATION, AND DNA ADDUCTS OF ESTROGENS

The natural estrogens, estrone (E_1) and estradiol (E_2), induce tumors in various hormone-dependent and independent organs of several animal species and strains.[8–10] Following the approach used to understand how PAHs generate oncogenic mutations, the ability of estrogen metabolites to form DNA adducts that can initiate carcinogenesis has been studied.[11] Catechol estrogens (CE) are among the major metabolites of E_1 and E_2. If these metabolites are oxidized to the electrophilic CE quinones (CE-Q), they may react with DNA. Specifically, the carcinogenic 4-CE[12–14] are oxidized to CE-3,4-Q, which reacts with DNA to form depurinating adducts.[11,15] These adducts generate apurinic sites that induce mutations (TABLE 1) and may lead to tumor initiation.[5,7,16]

Metabolic Activation and Deactivation of Estrogens

The estrogens E_1 and E_2 are obtained by aromatization of 4-androsten-3,17-dione and testosterone, respectively, catalyzed by cytochrome P450 (CYP)19, aromatase (FIG. 1), and are biochemically interconvertible by the enzyme 17β-estradiol dehydrogenase. E_1 and E_2 are metabolized via two major pathways: formation of CE and, to a lesser extent, 16α-hydroxylation (not shown in FIGURE 1). Estrogen metabolism can be viewed as activating or deactivating (protective) in terms of forming metabolites, CE-Q, that can react with DNA. The first activating step is formation of CE, the 2- and 4-hydroxylated estrogens. The major 4-hydroxylase in extrahepatic tissues is CYP1B1.[17–19] In general, the CE are inactivated by conjugating reactions such as glucuronidation and sulfation, especially in the liver (not shown in FIGURE 1). The most common pathway of conjugation in extrahepatic tissues, however, occurs by O-methylation catalyzed by the ubiquitous catechol-O-methyltransferase (COMT).[20]

A reaction that competes with the conjugation of CE is their catalytic oxidation to CE-semiquinones and CE-Q (FIG. 1). The semiquinones and CE-Q can be neutralized by conjugation with glutathione (GSH). A second inactivating pathway for CE-Q is their reduction to CE by quinone reductase and/or cytochrome P450 reductase.[21,22] If these two inactivating processes are insufficient, CE-Q may react with DNA to form stable and depurinating adducts (FIG. 1).[23] The carcinogenic 4-CE[12–14] are oxidized to form predominantly the depurinating adducts 4-OHE$_1$(E$_2$)-1-N3Ade and 4-OHE$_1$(E$_2$)-1-N7Gua.[11,15,24] The weakly carcinogenic 2-CE[14] are oxidized to form predominantly stable adducts, 2-OHE$_1$(E$_2$)-6-N^{6}dA and 2-OHE$_1$(E$_2$)-6-N^{2}dG, but also depurinating adducts to a much lesser extent.[24–26]

Reaction of Catechol Estrogen Quinones with DNA

To determine whether DNA adducts can be formed in biological systems, E$_2$-3,4-Q or enzymatically activated 4-hydroxyestradiol (4-OHE$_2$) was reacted with DNA for 2 hr at 37 EC.[11,15] The stable adducts were quantified by the ^{32}P-postlabeling method,[25] and the depurinating adducts were analyzed by HPLC interfaced with an electrochemical detector.[27] When E$_2$-3,4-Q reacted with DNA, almost the same amount of the depurinating adducts 4-OHE$_2$-1-N3Ade and 4-OHE$_2$-1-N7Gua were obtained, and the amount of stable adducts was 0.02% of the depurinating ones. The same two depurinating adducts were obtained in equal amounts when 4-OHE$_2$ was activated with tyrosinase or phenobarbital-induced rat liver microsomes. Activation of 4-OHE$_2$ by horseradish peroxidase yielded higher levels of the N7Gua and N3Ade adducts, whereas the mammalian lactoperoxidase produced a similar amount of N3Ade adduct, but about 50% more N7Gua adduct. In all cases, the level of stable adducts was 0.02% or less compared to the depurinating adducts (Cavalieri *et al.*, unpublished results).

DNA adducts were also observed *in vivo* in rat mammary gland and mouse skin after treatment of the animals with E$_2$-3,4-Q or 4-OHE$_2$. Female ACI rats, which are susceptible to E$_2$-induced mammary tumors,[28] were treated by intramammillary injection of E$_2$-3,4-Q or 4-OHE$_2$ (200 nmol in 20 μL DMSO/gland at four teats) for 1 hr. The mammary tissue was excised, extracted, and analyzed for stable and depurinating adducts. N3Ade and N7Gua adducts from both 4-OHE$_2$ and 4-OHE$_1$ were detected in the range of 100–300 μmol/mol DNA-P, but the level of stable adducts was not above the low level detected in untreated mammary tissue (Cavalieri *et al.*, unpublished results).

Female SENCAR mice were treated topically on a shaved area of dorsal skin with E$_2$-3,4-Q [200 nmol in 50 FL acetone/DMSO (9:1)] for 1 hr.[16] The treated area of skin was excised, extracted, and analyzed for stable and depurinating adducts. Equal amounts of 4-OHE$_2$-1-N3Ade and 4-OHE$_2$-1-N7Gua, approximately 12 μmol/mol DNA-P, were detected, and the amount of stable adducts was 0.02% of the depurinating adducts. Detection of these adducts in rats and mice demonstrates that the depurinating CE-DNA adducts are formed *in vivo*, leaving apurinic sites in the DNA that could generate oncogenic mutations.

THE BALANCE BETWEEN ESTROGEN ACTIVATION AND DEACTIVATION

The CE-DNA adducts are formed *in vivo* only if the deactivating (protective) metabolism of estrogens is overwhelmed by activating steps. Several factors could unbalance estrogen homeostasis, namely, the equilibrium between activating and deactivating metabolic pathways with the scope of averting the reaction of endogenous CE-Q with DNA (FIG. 1). First, excessive synthesis of E$_2$ by overexpression of aromatase, CYP19, in target tissues[29–33] and/or the presence of excess sulfatase that converts stored E$_1$ sulfate to E$_1$[34] could increase the concentrations of E$_1$ and E$_2$. The

TABLE 2. Selected estrogen metabolites, conjugates, and adducts formed in hamsters treated with E_2 or E_2 plus BSO[a]

	\multicolumn{4}{c}{Tissue(nmol/g)}
	\multicolumn{2}{c}{Kidney}	\multicolumn{2}{c}{Liver}
Metabolites/conjugates[b]/adducts	E_2	E_2 + BSO	E_2	E_2 + BSO
2-OHE$_2$(E$_1$)	2.66	1.02	4.75	10.27
4-OHE$_2$(E$_1$)	0.29	0.14	0.44	1.04
2-OCH$_3$E$_2$(E$_1$)	1.13	0.42	4.16	4.46
E$_2$(E$_1$)-2,3-Q conjugates[b]	1.36	0.21	0.63	0.13
E$_2$(E$_1$)-3,4-Q conjugates[b]	0.30	0.09	0.06	0.01
E$_2$(E$_1$)-3,4-Q N7Gua adducts	<0.01	0.27	<0.01	<0.01

[a]Data are from Cavalieri et al.[35] BSO: L-buthionine (SR)-sulfoximine.
[b]Conjugates include all compounds produced by reaction of CE-Q with GSH and detected as GSH, cysteine, or N-acetylcysteine conjugates.

observation that breast tissue can synthesize E_2 *in situ* suggests that much more E_2 is present in some sites of target tissues than would be predicted from plasma concentrations.[33]

Second, the presence of high levels of 4-CE due to overexpression of CYP1B1, which converts E_2 predominantly to 4-OHE$_2$ (FIG. 1),[17–19] could unbalance estrogen homeostasis. A relatively large amount of 4-CE could lead to more extensive oxidation to CE-3,4-Q, with increased likelihood of damaging DNA.

Third, a lack or low level of COMT activity could leave CE unprotected. If this enzyme is insufficient, either through a low level of expression or its low activity allele, 4-CE will not be effectively methylated, facilitating their oxidation to the ultimate carcinogenic metabolites CE-3,4-Q (FIG. 1).

Fourth, a low level of GSH and/or low levels of quinone reductase and/or cytochrome P450 reductase[21,22] could leave available a higher level of CE-Q that may react with DNA. The effects of some of these factors have already been observed in model studies with Syrian golden hamsters,[35] transgenic knock-out mice[36] and male Noble rats,[37] as well as in human breast tissue samples.[38]

Model Studies in Syrian Golden Hamsters

The hamster provides an excellent model for studying activation and deactivation (protection) of estrogen metabolites in relation to formation of CE-Q. Implantation of E_1 or E_2 in male Syrian golden hamsters induces renal carcinomas in 100% of the animals, but does not induce liver tumors.[39] Comparison of the profiles of estrogen metabolites, conjugates, and DNA adducts in the two organs should provide information concerning the imbalance in estrogen homeostasis generated by treatment with E_2. To study this, hamsters were treated for 2 hr with 8 μmol of E_2 per 100 g body weight, and liver and kidney extracts were analyzed for 31 estrogen metabolites, conjugates, and depurinating DNA adducts by HPLC interfaced with an electrochemical detector.[35] Neither the liver nor the kidney contained 4-methoxyCE, presumably due to the known inhibition of COMT by 2-CE.[40] More *O*-methylation

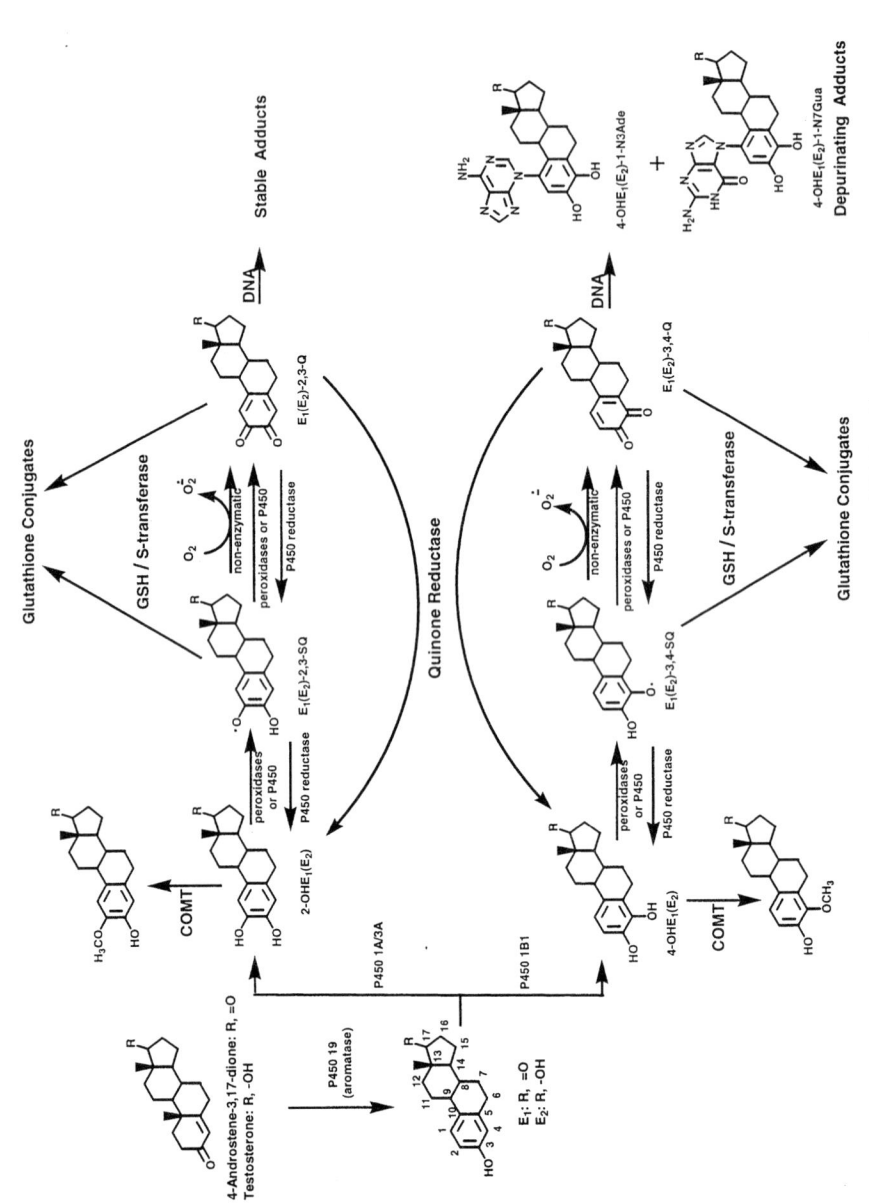

FIGURE 1. Formation, metabolism, conjugation, and DNA adducts of estrogens.

of 2-CE was observed in the liver, whereas more formation of CE-Q was detected in the kidney (TABLE 2).[35] These results suggest less protective methylation of 2-CE and more pronounced oxidation of CE to CE-Q in the kidney.

To further investigate the rationale behind this interpretation, hamsters were pretreated with *L*-buthionine (*SR*)-sulfoximine, an inhibitor of GSH synthesis, to deplete GSH levels. Then the hamsters were treated with E_2 for 2 hr. Very low levels of CE and methoxyCE were observed in the kidney compared to the liver, suggesting little protective reduction of CE-Q to CE in the kidney (TABLE 2). Most significantly, the 4-OHE$_2$(E$_1$)-1-N7Gua depurinating adducts, arising from reaction of CE-3,4-Q with DNA, were detected in the kidney, but not in the liver (TABLE 2).[35] From these results, it seems that tumor initiation in the kidney occurs because of poor methylation of CE, which favors the competitive oxidation of CE to CE-Q, and poor reductase activity to remove CE-Q. A combination of these two effects leads to a large amount of CE-Q, which can react with biological nucleophiles, including those in DNA.

Studies in the Estrogen Receptor-α Knockout (ERKO)/Wnt-1 Mouse Model

A novel model for breast cancer was established by crossing mice carrying the *Wnt-1* transgene (100% of adult females develop spontaneous mammary tumors) with the ERKO mouse line, in which the mice lack estrogen receptor-α. Mammary tumors develop in these mice despite the lack of functional estrogen receptor-α.[41] To begin investigating whether estrogen metabolite-mediated genotoxicity plays a critical role in the initiation of mammary tumors, the pattern of estrogen metabolites and conjugates was analyzed in ERKO/Wnt-1 mice. Extracts of hyperplastic mammary tissue and mammary tumors were analyzed by HPLC interfaced with an electrochemical detector.[36] Picomole amounts of the 4-CE were detected, but their methoxy conjugates were not. Neither 2-CE nor 2-methoxyCE was detected. 4-CE-GSH conjugates or their hydrolytic products (conjugates of cysteine and *N*-acetylcysteine) were detected in picomole amounts in both tumors and hyperplastic mammary tissue, demonstrating the formation of CE-3,4-Q. These preliminary findings indicate that estrogen homeostasis is unbalanced in the mammary tissue; that is, the normally minor 4-CE metabolites were detected in the mammary tissue, but not the normally predominant 2-CE. In addition, methylation of CE was not detected, but formation of 4-CE-GSH conjugates was. These results are consistent with the hypothesis that mammary tumor development is primarily initiated by metabolism of estrogens to CE-3,4-Q, which may react with DNA to induce oncogenic mutations.

Studies in the Noble Rat Prostate

The male Noble rat provides an excellent model for the study of prostate cancer. Treatment of these rats with testosterone plus E_2 induces ductal adenocarcinoma of the prostate in 100% of the animals, whereas treatment with testosterone alone causes prostate cancer in only 40%.[42] The carcinomas arise in the dorsolateral and periurethral regions of the prostate, but not in the ventral or anterior prostate. We hypothesize that estrogens initiate prostate cancer via formation of endogenous CE-3,4-Q, while testosterone promotes tumor development.

To study the role of estrogens in the initiation of prostate tumors, rats were treated with 6 μmol of 4-OHE$_2$ or E$_2$-3,4-Q/100 g body weight for 90 min. The prostates were then excised, separated into the four regions, extracted and analyzed for estrogen metabolites and conjugates by HPLC with electrochemical detection.[37] After treatment with 4-OHE$_2$, the two regions of the prostate in which tumors do not develop (ventral and anterior prostate) had higher levels of 4-methoxyCE than the two areas in which carcinomas are induced by treatment with E$_2$ and testosterone (dorsolateral and periurethral prostate). This finding suggests that the protective enzyme COMT is more effective in the ventral and anterior prostate than in the other two regions. In addition, the level of GSH conjugates was higher in the nonsusceptible ventral and anterior prostate than in the susceptible dorsolateral and periurethral prostate. This could mean that the two nonsusceptible regions of the prostate metabolize 4-CE to CE-3,4-Q more efficiently than the susceptible regions or that the protection by GSH is more abundant in the ventral and anterior prostate than in the susceptible regions.

These possibilities and the protection provided by reduction of CE-Q to CE in the various regions of the prostate were investigated in the rats treated with E$_2$-3,4-Q.[37] In these rats, the total CE-3,4-Q conjugates were more abundant in the nonsusceptible ventral and anterior regions of the prostate than in the susceptible dorsolateral and periurethral prostate regions, suggesting that the level of protection by GSH in the susceptible areas is lower. This result implies that the dorsolateral prostate and periurethral prostate conjugate relatively less CE-Q, increasing the likelihood of the CE-3,4-Q reacting with DNA. The level of 4-methoxyCE in the nonsusceptible regions was higher than in the susceptible regions, indicating that the protective action of COMT is more abundant in the non-susceptible regions of the prostate.

In summary, these experiments reveal that the two regions of the Noble rat prostate not susceptible to cancer induction, the ventral and anterior prostate, are better protected than the susceptible dorsolateral and periurethral prostate regions at the CE level by methylation and at the CE-Q level by better conjugation with GSH and more effective reduction to CE.[37]

Estrogen Analysis in Human Breast Tissue

Imbalances in estrogen homeostasis were also observed in women with breast carcinoma compared to women without breast cancer (TABLE 3).[38] Breast tissue specimens obtained from women undergoing breast biopsy or surgery were analyzed for 31 estrogen metabolites, conjugates, and depurinating DNA adducts by HPLC with electrochemical detection. In women without breast cancer, a larger amount of 2-CE than 4-CE was observed. In women with breast carcinoma, the 4-CE were 3.5 times more abundant than the 2-CE and were 4 times higher than in the women without breast cancer. Furthermore, a statistically lower level of methylation was observed for the CE in cancer cases compared to controls. Finally, the level of CE-Q conjugates in women with cancer was 3 times that in controls, suggesting a larger probability for the CE-Q to react with DNA in the breast tissue of women with carcinoma. These data suggest that initiation of human breast cancer is due to imbalances in estrogen homeostasis that result in excessive formation of the electrophilic CE-Q. In particular, the CE-3,4-Q can react with DNA to generate

TABLE 3. Estrogen metabolites and conjugates in breast tissue from women with and without breast cancer

Breast Tissue	4-OHE$_1$(E$_2$)	2-OHE$_1$(E$_2$)	4-OHE$_1$(E$_2$) / 2-OHE$_1$(E$_2$)	4-OCH$_3$E$_1$(E$_2$)	2-OCH$_3$E$_1$(E$_2$)	4-OCH$_3$E$_1$(E$_2$)+ 2-OCH$_3$E$_1$(E$_2$)	CE-Q conjugates
Controls[a]	3.6 ± 2.1 (10)[b]	6.9 ± 6.1 (25)	0.52	4.9 ± 1.8 (24)	3.6 ± 2.3 (16)	8.5	2.6 ± 1.3 (29)
Breast cancer cases[a]	14.7 ± 11.5 (53)	4.2 ± 4.6 (46)	3.5	3.1 ± 2.3 (39)	1.7 ± 1.0 (29)	4.8	8.2 ± 6.4 (57)
p[c]	0.047	n.s.[d]		0.049	0.050		0.003

[a]Controls include 18 women with benign breast tissue and 31 with benign fibrocystic changes for a total of 49 women. Breast cancer cases include 28 women with carcinoma of the breast.
[b]Number in parentheses indicates the percentage of specimens in which the compound was detected.
[c]P was calculated by the Student's t-test.
[d]n.s.: not significant.

successively depurinating adducts, apurinic sites, and oncogenic mutations leading to breast cancer.

UNIFIED MECHANISM IN THE INITIATION OF CANCER

Synthetic Estrogens

Oxidation of catechols to semiquinones and quinones has been proposed as a pathway to initiate cancer by endogenous estrogens, as well as synthetic estrogens such as the human carcinogens diethylstilbestrol[43] and its hydrogenated derivative hexestrol. These two compounds are also carcinogenic in the kidney of Syrian golden hamsters,[39,44] and the major metabolites are their catechols.[44–47] These catechols may be metabolized to catechol quinones. The catechol quinone of hexestrol has chemical and biochemical properties similar to those of CE-3,4-Q, namely, it specifically forms N7Gua and N3Ade adducts by 1,4-Michael addition after reaction with dG or Ade, respectively, as well as DNA (FIG. 2) (Ref. 48 and Cavalieri et al., unpublished results). These results suggest that the hexestrol catechol quinone is involved in tumor initiation by hexestrol. Furthermore, they support the hypothesis that CE-3,4-Q may be the major endogenous tumor initiators.

Benzene

In addition to being a mechanism of tumor initiation for natural and synthetic estrogens, oxidation of phenols to catechols and then to semiquinones and quinones could also be the mechanism of tumor initiation for the leukemogen benzene (FIG. 2). In fact, when the benzene metabolite catechol is oxidized to catechol quinone, it reacts with dG and Ade to form the depurinating adducts catechol-4-N7Gua and catechol-4-N3Ade in high yields, respectively.[49,50] Oxidation of catechol catalyzed by horseradish peroxidase, tyrosinase, or phenobarbital-induced rat liver microsomes in the presence of DNA yielded the catechol-4-N7Gua adduct, while the catechol-4-N3Ade adduct was obtained only with tyrosinase.[50] These initial results suggest that reaction of catechol quinone with DNA to form specific depurinating adducts may initiate the process leading to benzene-induced leukemia.

SUMMARY

The carcinogenicity of estrogens in animal models suggested that estrogen metabolites could react with DNA and lead to mutations initiating cancer. The electrophilic CE-3,4-Q can, indeed, react with DNA by 1,4-Michael addition to form specific depurinating adducts bonded at the N-7 of Gua and N-3 of Ade.[11,15] These adducts are thought to play a very important role in the oncogenic mutations leading to cancer.[11,16] This specific reaction with DNA has been observed with both natural estrogens and carcinogenic synthetic estrogens such as hexestrol. Metabolic formation of the hexestrol catechol and further oxidation to its catechol quinone lead to formation of analogous specific depurinating adducts at the N-7 of Gua and N-3 of Ade.[48] In addition, the catechol quinone metabolite of the leukemogen benzene binds to DNA to form N7Gua and N3Ade adducts.[50]

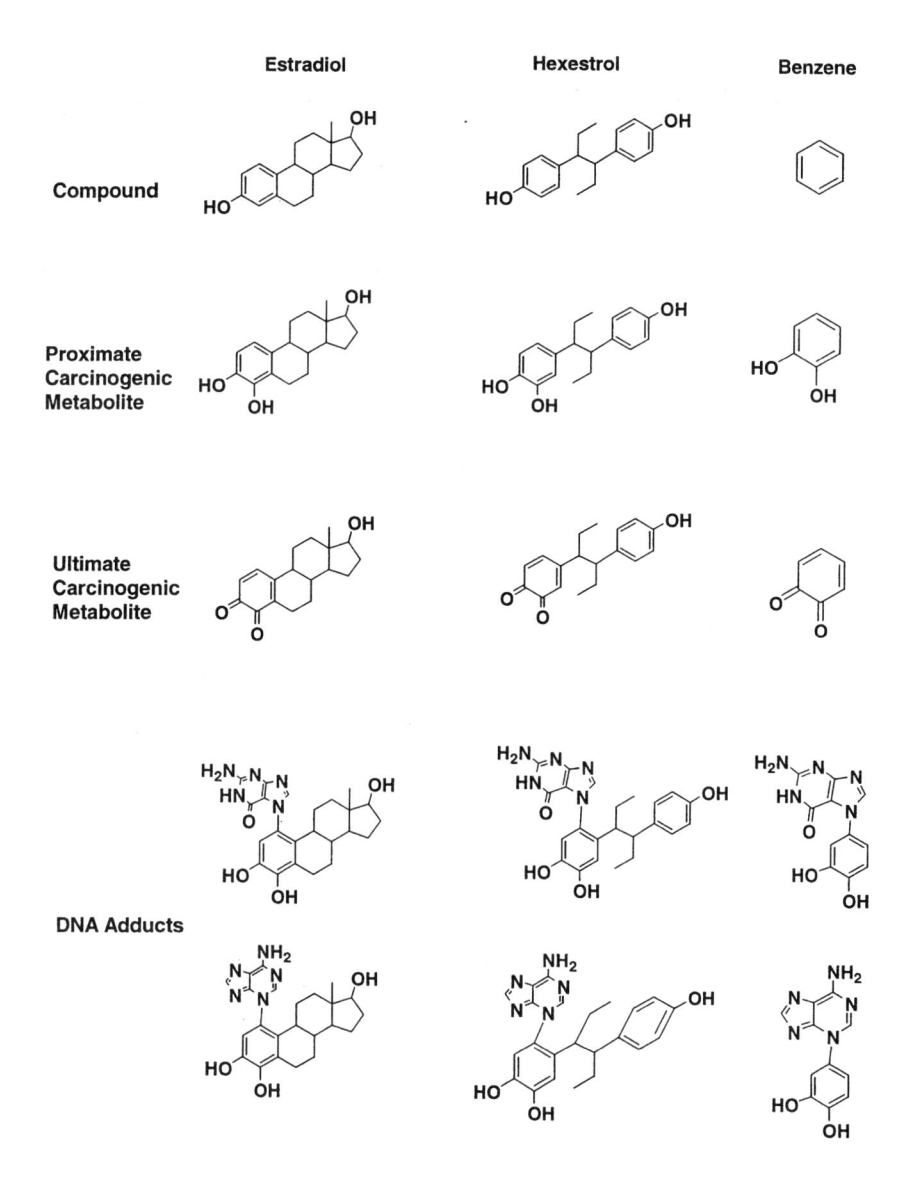

FIGURE 2. A unifying mechanism of activation and formation of DNA adducts for natural and synthetic estrogens, and benzene.

Thus, a unifying mechanism, namely, formation of catechol quinones and reaction with DNA by 1,4-Michael addition to yield depurinating adducts could be at the origin of cancers induced by oxidation of endogenous and synthetic estrogens and leukemia by oxidation of benzene. This proposed unifying mechanism in the initiation of cancer lays the groundwork for developing strategies for cancer risk assessment and prevention.

ACKNOWLEDGMENTS

Preparation of this article was supported by U.S. Public Health Service Grants P01 CA49210 and R01 CA49917 from the National Cancer Institute. Core support to the Eppley Institute is provided by Grant P30 CA36727 from the National Cancer Institute.

REFERENCES

1. WEINBERG, R.A. 1996. How cancer arises. Sci. Am. **275:** 62–77.
2. CAVALIERI, E.L. & E.G. ROGAN. 1992. The approach to understanding aromatic hydrocarbon carcinogenesis: the central role of radical cations in metabolic activation. Pharmacol. Ther. **55:** 183–199.
3. CAVALIERI, E.L. & E.G. ROGAN. 1998. Mechanisms of tumor initiation by polycyclic aromatic hydrocarbons in mammals. In The Handbook of Environmental Chemistry: PAHs and Related Compounds, Vol. 3J. A.H. Neilson, Ed.: 81–117. Springer. Heidelberg, Germany.
4. CHAKRAVARTI, D., J.C. PELLING, E.L. CAVALIERI & E.G. ROGAN. 1995. Relating aromatic hydrocarbon-induced DNA adducts and c-Harvey-*ras* mutations in mouse skin papillomas: the role of apurinic sites. Proc. Natl. Acad. Sci. USA **92:** 10422–10426.
5. CHAKRAVARTI, D., P. MAILANDER, E.L. CAVALIERI & E.G. ROGAN. 2000. Evidence that error-prone DNA repair converts dibenzo[*a,l*]pyrene-induced depurinating lesions into mutations, clonal proliferation and regression of initiated cells carrying H-*ras* oncogene mutations in early preneoplasia. Mutat. Res. **456:** 17–32.
6. LINDAHL, T. & B. NYBERG. 1972. Rate of depurination of native deoxyribonucleic acid. Biochemistry **11:** 3610–3618.
7. CHAKRAVARTI, D., P. MAILANDER, J. FRANZEN, *et al.* 1998. Detection of dibenzo[*a,l*]pyrene-induced H-*ras* codon 61 mutant genes in preneoplastic SENCAR mouse skin using a new PCR-RFLP method. Oncogene **16:** 3203–3210.
8. INTERNATIONAL AGENCY FOR RESEARCH ON CANCER. 1974. Evaluation of Carcinogenic Risks to Humans, Sex hormones. Vol. **6:** 99–132. Lyon, France.
9. INTERNATIONAL AGENCY FOR RESEARCH ON CANCER. 1979. Evaluation of Carcinogenic Risks to Humans, Sex hormones (II). Vol. **21:** 279–362. Lyon, France.
10. INTERNATIONAL AGENCY FOR RESEARCH ON CANCER. 1987. Overall evaluations of carcinogenicity: an updating of IARC monographs volumes 1 to 42. IARC Monographs on the Evaluation of Carcinogenic Risks to Humans. Suppl. **7:** 272–310. Lyon, France.
11. CAVALIERI, E.L., D.E. STACK, P.D. DEVANESAN, *et al.* 1997. Molecular origin of cancer: catechol estrogen-3,4-quinones as endogenous tumor initiators. Proc. Natl. Acad. Sci. USA **99:** 10937–10942.
12. LIEHR, J.G., W.F. FANG, D.A. SIRBASKU & A. ARI-ULUBELEN. 1986. Carcinogenicity of catecholstrogens in Syrian hamsters. J. Steroid Biochem. **24:** 353–356.
13. LI, J.J. & S.A. LI. 1987. Estrogen carcinogenesis in Syrian hamster tissue: role of metabolism. Fed.Proc. **46:** 1858–1863.
14. NEWBOLD, R.R. & J.G. LIEHR. 2000. Induction of uterine adenocarcinoma in CD-1 mice by catechol estrogens. Cancer Res. **60:** 235–237.

15. LI, K.M., P.D. DEVANESAN, E.G. ROGAN & E L. CAVALIERI. 1998. Formation of the depurinating 4-hydroxyestradiol (4-OHE$_2$)-1-N7Gua and 4-OHE$_2$-1-N3Ade adducts by reaction of E$_2$-3,4-quinone with DNA. Proc. Am. Assoc. Cancer Res. **39:** 636.
16. CHAKRAVARTI, D., P. MAILANDER, K.-M. LI, et al. 2001. Evidence that a burst of DNA depurination in SENCAR mouse skin induces error-prone repair and forms mutations in the H-*ras* gene. Oncogene **20:** 7945–7953.
17. SPINK, D.C., C.L. HAYES, N.R. YOUNG, et al. 1994. The effects of 2,3,7,8-tetrachlorodibenzo-*p*-dioxin on estrogen metabolism in MCF-7 breast cancer cells: Evidence for induction of a novel 17ß-estradiol 4-hydroxylase. J. Steroid Biochem. Mol. Biol. **51:** 251–258.
18. HAYES, C.L., D.C. SPINK, B.C. SPINK, et al. 1996. 17β-Estradiol hydroxylation catalyzed by human cytochrome P450 1B1. Proc. Natl. Acad. Sci. USA **93:** 9776–9781.
19. SPINK, D.C., B.C. SPINK, J.Q. CAO, et al. 1998. Differential expression of CYP1A1 and CYP1B1 in human breast epithelial cells and breast tumor cells. Carcinogenesis **19:** 291–298.
20. MÄNNISTÖ, P.T. & S. KAAKOLA. 1999. Catechol-*O*-methyltransferase (COMT): biochemisty, molecular biology, pharmacology and clinical efficacy of the new selective COMT inhibitors. Pharmacol. Rev. **51:** 593–628.
21. 1987. DT diaphorase: a quinone reductase with special functions in cell metabolism and detoxication. *In* Chemica Scripta. L. Ernester, R. W. Estabrook, P. Hochstein & S. Orrenius, Eds.: 27A.
22. ROY, D. & J.G. LIEHR. 1988. Temporary decrease in renal quinone reductase activity induced by chronic administration of estradiol to male Syrian hamsters. J. Biol. Chem. **263:** 3646–3651.
23. CAVALIERI, E., K. FRENKEL, J.G. LIEHR, et al. 2000. Estrogens as endogenous genotoxic agents: DNA adducts and mutations. *In* JNCI Monograph 27: Estrogens as Endogenous Carcinogens in the Breast and Prostate. E. Cavalieri & E. Rogan, Eds.: 75–93. Oxford Press. Washington, DC.
24. STACK, D.E., J. BYUN, M.L. GROSS, et al. 1996. Molecular characteristics of catechol estrogen quinones in reactions with deoxyribonucleosides. Chem. Res. Toxicol. **9:** 851–859.
25. DWIVEDY, I., P. DEVANESAN, P. CREMONESI, et al. 1992 Comparison of DNA adducts formed by the quinones *versus* horseradish peroxidase-activated catechol estrogens. Chem. Res. Toxicol. **5:** 828–833.
26. VAN AERDEN C., L. DEBRAUWER, J.C. TABET & A. PARIS. 1998. Analysis of nucleoside-estrogen adducts by LC-ESI-MS-MS. Analyst **123:** 2677–2680.
27. DEVANESAN, P., R. TODOROVIC, J. ZHAO, et al. 2001. Catechol estrogen conjugates and DNA adducts in the kidney of male Syrian golden hamsters treated with 4-hydroxyestradiol: potential biomarkers for estrogen-initiated cancer. Carcinogenesis **22:** 489–497.
28. SHULL, J.D., T.J. SPADY, M.C. SNYDER, et al. 1997. Ovary intact, but not ovariectomized, female ACI rats treated with 17β-estradiol rapidly develop mammary carcinoma. Carcinogenesis **18:** 1595–1601.
29. MILLER, W.R. & J. O'NEILL. 1987. The importance of local synthesis of estrogen within the breast. Steroids **50:** 537–548.
30. SIMPSON, E.R., M.S. MAHENDROO, G.D. MEANS, et al. 1994. Aromatase cytochrome P450, the enzyme responsible for estrogen biosynthesis. Endocrine Rev. **15:** 342–355.
31. YUE, W., J.P. WANG, C.J. HAMILTON, et al. 1998. In situ aromatization enhances breast tumor estradiol levels and cellular proliferation. Cancer Res. **58:** 927–932.
32. YUE, W., R.J. SANTEN, J.P. WANG, et al. 1999. Aromatase within the breast. Endocrine-Related Cancer **6:** 157–164.
33. JEFCOATE, C.R., J.G. LIEHR, R.J. SANTEN, et al. 2000. Tissue-specific synthesis and oxidative metabolism of estrogens. *In* JNCI Monograph 27: Estrogens as Endogenous Carcinogens in the Breast and Prostate. E. Cavalieri & E. Rogan, Eds.: 95–112. Oxford Press.Washington, DC.
34. REED, M. J.& A. PUROHIT. 1997. Breast cancer and the role of cytokines in regulating estrogen synthesis: an emerging hypothesis. Endocr. Rev. **18:** 701–715.

35. CAVALIERI, E.L., S. KUMAR, R. TODOROVIC, et al. 2001. Imbalance of estrogen homeostasis in kidney and liver of hamsters treated with estradiol: implications for estrogen-induced initiation of renal tumors. Chem. Res. Toxicol. **14:** 1041–1050.
36. DEVANESAN, P, R.J. SANTEN, W.P. BOCCHINFUSO, et al. 2001. Catechol estrogen metabolites and conjugates in mammary tumors with hyperplastic tissue from estrogen receptor-α knock-out (ERKO)/Wnt-1 mice: implications for initiation of mammary tumors. Carcinogenesis **22:** 1573–1576.
37. CAVALIERI, E.L., P. DEVANESAN, M. C. BOSLAND, et al. 2002. Catechol estrogen metabolites and conjugates in different regions of the prostate of Noble rats treated with 4-hydroxyestradiol: implications for estrogen-induced initiation of prostate cancer. Carcinogenesis **23:** 329–333.
38. BADAWI, A.F., P.D. DEVANESAN, J.A. EDNEY, et al. 2001. Estrogen metabolites and conjugates: biomarkers of susceptibility to human breast cancer. Proc. Am. Assoc. Cancer Res. **42:** 664.
39. LI, J.J., S.A. LI, J.K. KLICKA, et al. 1983. Relative carcinogenic activity of various synthetic and natural estrogens in the Syrian hamster kidney. Cancer Res. **43:** 5200–5204.
40. ROY, D., J. WEISZ & J. G. LIEHR. 1990. The O-methylation of 4-hydroxyestradiol is inhibited by 2-hydroxyestradiol: Implications for estrogen-induced carcinogenesis. Carcinogenesis **11:** 459–462.
41. BOCCHINFUSO, W.P., W.P. HIVELY, J.F. COUSE, et al. 1999. A mouse mammary tumor virus-*Wnt*-1 transgene induces mammary gland hyperplasia and tumorigenesis in mice lacking estrogen receptor-α. Cancer Res. **59:** 1869–1876.
42. BOSLAND, M.C., H. FORD & L. HORTON. 1995. Induction at high incidence of ductal prostate adenocarcinomas in NBL/Cr and Sprague-Dawley Hsd:SD rats treated with a combination of testosterone and estradiol-17β or diethylstilbestrol. Carcinogenesis **16:** 1311–1317.
43. HERBST, A.L., H. ULFELDER & D.C. POSKANZER. 1971. Adenocarcinoma of the vagina: association of maternal stilbestrol therapy with tumor appearance in young women. N. Engl. J. Med. **284:** 878–881.
44. LEHR, J.G., A.M. BALLATORE, B.B. DAGUE & A.A. ULUBELEN. 1985. Carcinogenicity and metabolic activation of hexestrol. Chem.-Biol. Interactions **55:** 157–176.
45. HAAF, H. & M. METZLER. 1985. *In vitro* metabolism of diethylstilbestrol by hepatic, renal and uterine microsomes of rats and hamsters. Biochem. Pharmacol. **34:** 3107–3115.
46. BLAICH, G., M. GÄTTLICHER, P. CIKRYT & M. METZLER. 1996. Effects of various inducers on diethylstilbestrol metabolism, drug-metabolizing enzyme activities and the aromatic hydrocarbon (Ah) receptor in male Syrian golden hamster livers. J. Steroid Biochem. **35:** 201–204.
47. METZLER, M. & J.A. MCLACHLAN. 1981. Oxidative metabolism of the synthetic estrogens hexestrol and dienestrol indicates reactive intermediates. Adv. Exp. Med. Biol. **136A:** 829–837.
48. JAN, S.-T., P. DEVANESAN, D. STACK, et al. 1998. Metabolic activation and formation of DNA adducts of hexestrol, a synthetic non-steroidal carcinogenic estrogen. Chem. Res. Toxicol. **11:** 412–419.
49. BALU, N., K.-M. LI, E. ROGAN & E. CAVALIERI. 1999. A unifying mechanism in the reaction of catechol-, catecholamine- and catechol estrogen-quinones with nucleophilic sites in DNA. Proc. Am. Assoc. Cancer Res. **40:** 46.
50. CAVALIERI, E.L., K.-M. LI, N. BALU, et al. 2002. Catechol ortho-quinones: the electrophilic compounds that form depurinating DNA adducts and could initiate cancer and other diseases. Carcinogenesis. In press.

Coenzyme Q_{10} Protects the Aging Heart against Stress

Studies in Rats, Human Tissues, and Patients

FRANKLIN L. ROSENFELDT, SALVATORE PEPE, ANTHONY LINNANE, PHILIP NAGLEY, MICHAEL ROWLAND, RUCHONG OU, SILVANA MARASCO, WILLIAM LYON, AND DONALD ESMORE

Cardiac Surgical Research Unit, Alfred Hospital and Baker Institute, Prahran 3181, Australia

Centre for Molecular Biology and Medicine, Epworth Hospital, Melbourne, Australia

Department of Biochemistry and Molecular Biology, Monash University, Melbourne, Australia

ABSTRACT: With aging of the population, increasing numbers of elderly patients are presenting for cardiac surgery. However, the results in the elderly are inferior to those in the young. A likely contributing factor is an age-related reduction in cellular energy production in the myocardium during surgery, which is known to induce aerobic and ischemic stress. The lipophilic antioxidant and mitochondrial respiratory chain redox coupler, coenzyme Q_{10} (CoQ_{10}), has the potential to improve energy production in mitochondria by bypassing defective components in the respiratory chain as well as by reducing the effects of oxidative stress. We hypothesized that CoQ_{10} pretreatment prior to stress could improve the recovery of the myocardium after stress.

KEYWORDS: cardiovascular surgery; contractile function; energy metabolism; mitochondria; aging; coenzyme Q_{10}

BACKGROUND

Cardiovascular disease, especially cardiac failure, is a major cause of mortality and morbidity in the elderly.[1] With aging of the population, increasing numbers of elderly patients are presenting for interventional cardiac treatment, such as angioplasty, thrombolysis, and cardiac surgery.[2] However, the results of these interventions in the elderly are inferior to those in the young. The mortality rate for cardiac surgery in the patient over 70 is two to three times greater than in younger counterparts.[3] A likely contributing factor is an age-related reduction in cellular energy production in the myocardium during interventions that induce aerobic or ischemic stress. Coenzyme Q_{10} is a lipid soluble antioxidant and a key component of the res-

Address for correspondence: Assoc. Prof. Franklin Rosenfeldt, CJOB Cardiothoracic Unit, The Alfred Hospital, P.O. Box 315, Prahran 3181, Australia. Voice: +61-3-9276-3684; fax : +61-3-9276-2317.

f.rosenfeldt@alfred.org.au

piratory chain. It is found in highest concentrations in organs with high rates of oxygen consumption, such as the heart and the brain. CoQ_{10} has the potential to improve energy production in mitochondria by bypassing defective components in the respiratory chain as well as by reducing the effects of oxidative stress. We hypothesized that CoQ_{10} pretreatment prior to stress could improve the recovery of the myocardium after stress. We investigated this hypothesis in three studies. In the first study, isolated hearts taken from senescent or mature rats treated with CoQ_{10} were subjected to rapid electrical pacing.[4] In the second study, human atrial tissue was obtained at the time of open heart surgery and subjected to simulated ischemia in the organ bath after incubation with CoQ_{10}.[5] In the third study, a clinical trial of CoQ_{10} was performed in patients undergoing cardiac surgery.

COENZYME Q_{10} TREATMENT OF SENESCENT RATS IMPROVES TOLERANCE TO AEROBIC STRESS

Introduction

The aim of this study was to investigate whether CoQ_{10} improves the functional recovery of senescent and young rat hearts after aerobic stress, produced by rapid pacing with or without CoQ_{10} pretreatment of the whole animal.

Methods

Young (4.8 ± 0.1 months) and senescent (35.3 ± 0.2 months) rats were given daily intraperitoneal injections of CoQ_{10} (4 mg/kg) or vehicle for 6 weeks. Their isolated working hearts were rapidly paced at 510 bpm for 120 min to induce aerobic stress without ischemia.

Results

In untreated senescent hearts, prepacing cardiac work was 74% ($P<0.05$) and oxygen consumption (MVO_2) 66% of that in young hearts. In senescent hearts, CoQ_{10} treatment increased cardiac work by 28% compared to untreated hearts ($P<0.01$). After pacing, the untreated senescent hearts, compared to young, showed reduced recovery of prepacing work (16.8 ± 4.3 vs. $44.5 \pm 7.4\%$, $P<0.01$) and MVO_2 (61.3 ± 4.0 vs. $74.1 \pm 5.0\%$, $P = 0.06$). CoQ_{10} treatment in senescent hearts improved recovery of work (48.1 ± 4.1 vs. $16.8 \pm 4.3\%$, $P<0.0001$), MVO_2 (82.1 ± 2.8 vs. $61.3 \pm 4.0\%$, $P<0.01$), and efficiency ($61.4 \pm 12.0\%$ vs 25.7 ± 6.5, $P<0.05$) in treated versus untreated hearts, respectively. Postpacing levels of these parameters in CoQ_{10}-treated senescent hearts were as high as in young hearts.

Conclusions

Senescent rat hearts have reduced baseline function and reduced tolerance to aerobic stress compared to young hearts. Pretreatment with CoQ_{10} improves baseline function of the senescent heart and its tolerance to aerobic stress.

COENZYME Q_{10} *IN VITRO* NORMALIZES IMPAIRED POSTISCHEMIC CONTRACTILE RECOVERY OF AGED HUMAN MYOCARDIUM

Introduction

The aim of this study was to test whether the reduced capacity of aging human myocardium to recover preischemic contractile function, compared to younger tissue, is improved by pretreatment with the lipophilic antioxidant and mitochondrial respiratory chain redox coupler, coenzyme Q_{10} (CoQ_{10}). Since patients aged 70 years and over represent a high-risk group for cardiac surgery, atrial trabeculae were grouped according to whether they were taken from patients aged 70 years or over or less than 70 years.

Methods

Young and aged human right atrial pectinate trabeculae were obtained at surgery. After 30 min treatment with either CoQ_{10} (400 µM) or vehicle, trabeculae were paced at 1 Hz in oxygenated Ringer's solution (37°C), and then subjected to 60 min simulated ischemia (humidified N_2, perfusate free). Postischaemic recovery of developed force (DF) after 30 min was expressed as a percentage of prestress values. Extracted muscle CoQ_{10} content was measured by HPLC.

Results

Postischaemic trabeculae from the ≥70-yo group (76.4 0.8 yo) displayed less contractile recovery compared to the <70-yo group (57.6±1.7 yo), but this difference was abolished by CoQ_{10}. CoQ_{10} content was lower in the ≥70-yo group versus the <70-yo group. CoQ_{10} treatment elevated CoQ_{10} content twofold in those <70 yo and sevenfold in those ≥70 years old.

TABLE 1.

	Percent Recovery of DF		CoQ_{10} content (µg/mg protein)	
Age	<70 yo	≥70 yo	<70 yo	≥ 70 yo
Control (*n*)	63.4 ± 3.4(30)	53.0 ± 2.9(21)	13.8 ± 1.7(6)	3.9 ± 0.7(6)[b]
CoQ_{10} (*n*)	71.5 ± 3.3(29)	74.6 ± 3.5(19)[a]	29.2 ± 1.5(6)[a]	27.7 ± 2.9(6)[a]

$P < 0.05$: [a] vs. control, [b] vs. <70 yo.

Conclusions

CoQ_{10} pretreatment *in vitro* raises CoQ_{10} content and overcomes the reduced capacity of aged trabeculae to recover contractile function after ischemia compared to younger tissue. CoQ_{10} content is decreased in aged atrial trabeculae, which may contribute to the reduced recovery of contractile function in aged myocardium observed after cardiac surgery.

IMPROVED OUTCOMES IN CORONARY ARTERY BYPASS GRAFT SURGERY WITH PREOPERATIVE COENZYME Q_{10}: A RANDOMIZED, DOUBLE-BLIND PLACEBO CONTROLLED TRIAL

Introduction

On the basis of our previous studies we believed that CoQ_{10} should have a beneficial effect in patients undergoing cardiac surgery, especially those aged 70 years and over. We therefore set out to test in cardiac surgical patients whether oral CoQ_{10} therapy (1) increases CoQ_{10} content in atrial trabeculae and mitochondria, (2) improves mitochondrial respiration, (3) protects the myocardium against posthypoxic contractile dysfunction, and (4) attenuates operative myocardial injury and improves postoperative recovery.

Methods

Patients were randomized to receive orally either CoQ_{10} (300 mg/day) or placebo for seven days prior to elective cardiac surgery. Trabeculae were excised and mitochondria were isolated from discarded right atrial appendages. Biochemical and clinical parameters were measured postoperatively.

Results

Compared to placebo, therapy increased CoQ_{10} content of trabeculae (21 ± 4 to 40 ± 5 μg/g w.w., $P < 0.001$) and isolated mitochondria (5.7 ± 0.8 to 11.2 ± 0.9 μg CoQ_{10}/mg protein, $P < 0.0001$). Mitochondrial respiration was more efficient after CoQ_{10} pretreatment (ADP:O, CoQ_{10} vs. placebo: 4.2 ± 0.2 vs. 2.9 ± 0.4, $P<0.05$). After 30 min hypoxia, CoQ_{10}-treated trabeculae exhibited a greater recovery of developed force compared to placebo ($64.0 \pm 18\%$ vs. $46.2 \pm 28\%$, $P < 0.01$). CoQ_{10} patients had a lower release of TnI than placebo patients (39.4 ± 8.5 vs. 64.5 ± 4.1 μg/L, $P<0.001$) and a shorter length of hospital stay (6.8 ± 0.7 vs. 8.7 ± 2.1 days, $P < 0.05$).

Conclusions

Preoperative oral CoQ_{10} therapy (1) increases CoQ_{10} content in atrial trabeculae and cardiac mitochondria, (2) improves efficiency of mitochondrial energy production, (3) improves posthypoxic myocardial contractile function, and (4) reduces myocardial damage and shortens the hospital stay.

DISCUSSION

We have reported the findings of two laboratory studies and one clinical trial, all of which showed the consistent finding that CoQ_{10} improved recovery of the heart after stress. There were two findings common to the laboratory studies: first, that the aging myocardium had reduced tolerance to stress either ischemic or aerobic, and second, that CoQ_{10} improves the tolerance of the aging heart to both types of stress. These laboratory findings gave us confidence to proceed with the clinical trial because a large proportion of cardiac surgery patients fall into the elderly age group, and also because the stresses used in the laboratory studies were models of those occurring in cardiac surgery. The heart experiences aerobic (oxygen demanding) stress in the postoperative period due to tachyarrhythmias, such as atrial fibrillation and the use of positive inotropic drugs. Hypoxia is a part of global ischemia during cardioplegic arrest used during surgery and also occurs not infrequently in the postoperative period due to pulmonary complications, such as basal atelectasis after weaning from mechanical ventilation.

The findings in the clinical trial from the mitochondrion to the whole patient, showed a consistent benefit of CoQ_{10} therapy. CoQ_{10} improved the efficiency of mitochondrial energy production, which meant that more cellular energy was available for contractile function in the postoperative period. CoQ_{10} improved the functional recovery of myocardial strips from hypoxia, especially in the aged (70 years and older) patients. This should contribute to improved cardiac function in the postoperative period. Improved myocardial recovery was evident by greater cardiac pump function in response to cardiac filling in the CoQ_{10}-treated groups. Reduced myocardial damage was evidenced by reduced release of troponin I, which is well accepted as an index of improved outcomes after cardiac surgery.[6]

The antioxidant action of CoQ_{10} could reduce myocardial injury from cardioplegia and thus decrease troponin I release. The sum total of the beneficial effects of CoQ_{10} at various levels, both cellular and whole organ, would be expected to contribute to more rapid patient recovery and thus a shorter stay in the hospital. Our findings are in accordance with the majority of previous clinical studies of CoQ_{10} in cardiac surgery. From 1982 to 1996 six trials of CoQ_{10} in cardiac surgery were reported.[7] Of these, five showed a beneficial effect at a cellular or a whole patient level. In the one showing no effect, CoQ_{10} was administered only 12 hours before surgery, which would be expected to be too short to achieve adequate tissue levels of CoQ_{10}.

We conclude that CoQ_{10} administration can improve recovery of the mitochondrion and the cardiac myocyte from stress. When given for one week prior to cardiac surgery, CoQ_{10} can accelerate cardiac recovery and lead to earlier discharge of the patient from the hospital.

REFERENCES

1. KELLY, D.T. 1997. Our future society. A global challenge. Circulation **95:** 2459–2464.
2. EDWARDS, F.H., R.E. CLARK & M. SCHWARTZ. 1994. Coronary artery bypass grafting: The Society of Thoracic Surgeons National database experience. Ann. Thorac. Surg. **57:** 12–19.
3. TU, J.V., S. JAGLAL & C.D. NAYLOR. 1995. Multicenter validation of a risk index for mortality, intensive care unit stay, and overall hospital length of stay after cardiac surgery. Circulation **91:** 677–684.
4. ROWLAND, M.A., P. NAGLEY, A.W. LINNANE & F.L. ROSENFELDT. 1998. Coenzyme Q_{10} treatment improves the tolerance of the senescent myocardium to pacing stress in the rat. J. Cardiovasc. Res. **40:** 165–173.
5. ROSENFELDT, F.L., S. PEPE, R. OU, et al. 1999. Coenzyme Q_{10} improves the tolerance of the senescent myocardium to aerobic and ischemic stress: studies in rats and in human atrial tissue. BioFactors **9:** 291–299.
6. GREENSON, N., J. MACOVIAK, P. KRISHNASWAMY, et al. 2001. Usefulness of cardiac troponin I in patients undergoing open heart surgery. Am. Heart J. **141:** 447–455.
7. LANGSJOEN, P.H. & A.M. LANGSJOEN. 1998. Coenzyme Q_{10} in cardiovascular disease with emphasis on heart failure and myocardial ischaemia. Asia Pac. Heart J. **7:** 160–168.

The Maillard Hypothesis on Aging: Time to Focus on DNA

JOHN W. BAYNES

Department of Chemistry and Biochemistry, University of South Carolina, Columbia, South Carolina 29208, USA

ABSTRACT: Aging is the outcome of the contest between chemistry and biology in living systems. Chronic, cumulative chemical modifications compromise the structure and function of biomolecules throughout the body. Proteins with long life spans serve as cumulators of exposure to chemical damage, which is detectable in the form of advanced glycation and lipoxidation end products (AGEs, ALEs); amino acids modified by reactive oxygen, chlorine, and nitrogen species; and deamidated and racemized amino acids. Not all of these modifications are oxidative in nature, although oxidative reactions are an important source of age-related damage. Measurements of AGEs and ALEs in proteins are useful for assessing the rate and extent of Maillard reaction damage, but it is the damage to the genome that undoubtedly has the greatest effect on the viability of the organism. The extent of genomic damage represents a balance between the rate of modification and the rate and fidelity of repair. Damage to DNA accumulates not in the form of modified nucleic acids, but as chemically "silent" errors in repair—insertions, deletions, substitutions, transpositions, and inversions in DNA sequences—that affect the expression and structure of proteins. These mutations are random, vary from cell to cell, and are passed forward from one cell generation to another. Although they are not detectable in DNA by conventional analytical techniques, purines and pyrimidines modified by Maillard reaction intermediates may be detectable in urine, and studies on these compounds should provide insight into the role of Maillard reactions of DNA in aging and disease.

KEYWORDS: advanced glycation end product (AGE); advanced lipoxidation end product (ALE); collagen; DNA; glycation; lipid peroxidation; Maillard reaction; oxidation; oxidative stress; pentosidine

INTRODUCTION

The Maillard reaction is a complex set of nonenzymatic protein browning and cross-linking reactions, originally observed during the heating of foods in the presence of reducing sugars. This reaction yields a broad range of products that contribute to the brown color, texture, taste, and aroma of cooked foods. Biological interest in the Maillard reaction began with the observation in the late 1970s that hemoglobin contained glucose bound nonenzymatically to valine residues at the

Address for correspondence: John W. Baynes, Department of Chemistry and Biochemistry, University of South Carolina, Columbia, SC 29208. Voice/fax: 803-777-7272.
baynes@mail.chem.sc.edu

TABLE 1. Chemical modifications that accumulate in proteins with age

AGEs	AGEs/ALEs	Amino acids
Crosslines	CML	MetSO
Fluorolink	CEL	o- & m-Tyr
Pentosidine	GOLD	dityrosine
Vesperlysines	MOLD	racemization, deamidation

NOTE: AGE, advanced glycation end product; ALE, advanced lipoxidation end product; CEL, N^ε-(carboxyethyl)lysine; CML, N^ε-(carboxymethyl)lysine; GOLD, glyoxal-lysine dimer, an imidazolium salt cross-link formed on reaction of glyoxal with lysine; MetSO, methionine sulfoxide; MOLD, methylglyoxal-lysine dimer, an imidazolium salt cross-link formed on reaction of methylglyoxal with lysine; ROS, reactive oxygen species.

amino terminus of its β-chains, that the extent of glycation of hemoglobin increased with the age of the red cell, and that the mean level of glycated hemoglobin was increased in proportion to the degree of hyperglycemia in diabetes. Glycation, the formation of the Amadori (ketoamine) adduct of a sugar to an amino group on protein, was already recognized as an early step in the Maillard reaction in food chemistry, suggesting that the later, browning stages of the reaction might also occur in living systems. Indeed, during the next 25 years, a large number of Maillard reaction products, known as advanced glycation end products (AGEs), were identified in tissue proteins.[1,2] Many of these AGEs increase with age in long-lived tissue proteins, such as collagens and crystallins (TABLE 1, column 1).

THE MAILLARD THEORY OF AGING

In the 1980s, Monnier[3] and Cerami[4] proposed a glucose or Maillard theory of aging, hypothesizing that chronic formation and accumulation of Maillard products in biomolecules was a determinant of the rate of aging of species. The argument for this hypothesis was based on the observed increase in browning and fluorescence of crystallins and collagens with age, the age-dependent accumulation of AGEs in these proteins, and the age-dependent increase in cross-linking and insolubility of these proteins. However, the acceptance of the Maillard hypothesis has been hampered by two major problems: (1) AGEs are present at only trace concentrations in tissue proteins, so it has been difficult to argue on quantitative grounds that they have a significant effect on protein structure and function and on the viability of mammalian species; (2) the levels of AGEs are generally lower in collagens from short-lived, versus long-lived, animals at the same fraction of their maximum life span, arguing that the accumulation of AGEs is not a relevant determinant of the rate of aging.

The first objection is commonly addressed by invoking the "tip of the iceberg" corollary to the AGE hypothesis, that is, that the known AGEs represent only a small fraction of total AGEs, the majority of which are labile to acidic or basic conditions used for the hydrolysis of proteins to measure AGEs. This argument is reasonable because known AGEs often account for only a small fraction of modified lysine residues in proteins browned by reducing sugars *in vitro*. New AGEs are also being characterized at the rate of 1–2 per year, and many of these compounds are labile to acid and/or base hydrolysis, so they are identified only after exhaustive proteolysis of the protein. It has also become clear that carbohydrates are not the only compounds involved in chemical modification of proteins, either during cooking or in tissues. Transition metal ions, primarily iron and copper released from proteins during cooking or denaturation, catalyze the peroxidation of polyunsaturated fatty acids, leading to chemical modification of proteins by lipid-derived, advanced lipoxidation end products (ALEs)[2] (TABLE 1, column 2). Some compounds, such as N^ε-(carboxymethyl)lysine (CML) and N^ε-(carboxyethyl)lysine (CEL), are best described as AGEs/ALEs or EAGLEs (either advanced glycation or lipoxidation end products) because they may be formed from both carbohydrates and lipids.[2,5]

Maillard reactions of carbohydrates and lipids also produce reactive oxygen species (ROS), for example, hydrogen peroxide, which cause oxidation of amino acids in proteins in parallel with the formation of AGEs and ALEs during the Maillard reaction. Thus, methionine sulfoxide (MetSO) and o-tyrosine accumulate in parallel with AGEs during reaction of glucose with collagen *in vitro*[6] and MetSO is formed during metal-catalyzed oxidation of lipoproteins.[7] Chemicals that prevent the increase in AGEs and ALEs in the proteins, including chelators, antioxidants, and reducing agents, also inhibit the formation of MetSO. Other chemical modifications of protein derived from enzymatic oxidative chemistry, including *o*- and *m*-tyrosine, chlorotyrosine, nitrotyrosine, and dityrosine, are also commonly detected in proteins at sites of formation of AGEs and ALEs,[8] and some of these also accumulate in long-lived proteins with age (TABLE 1, column 3).

In summary, although the known chemical modifications account for only a small fraction of amino acids in protein, there is increasing evidence for a broader spectrum of AGEs in proteins and evidence that AGEs are only one aspect of the chemical modification of proteins during the Maillard reaction. In addition to AGEs, ALEs, and oxidized amino acids, other nonoxidative modifications also increase in proteins with age, for example, racemized and deamidated amino acids (TABLE 1). Whether the currently characterized compounds are the tip of the *iceberg* or the tip of the *ice cube* is not yet clear, but it is apparent that a wide range of chemical modifications increase with age in tissue proteins and could contribute to fundamental mechanisms of aging.

The second objection to the Maillard hypothesis is also quantitative, that is, that the level of Maillard products in proteins of old, short-lived animals is not comparable to the levels of these compounds in tissues of old, long-lived animals. As shown in TABLE 2, for example, the levels of CML, CEL, and pentosidine in skin from a middle-aged, Sprague-Dawley rat are only about 10% of those in a middle-aged human. Sell *et al.*[9] also noted that maximum levels of the AGE pentosidine in skin collagen differed significantly among different species of animals with similar life spans. This problem also exists within a species, as illustrated in TABLE 2 by the comparison of levels of AGEs in skin collagen of Sprague-Dawley and Zucker (lean) rats, animals with similar life spans, but with significantly different levels of AGEs. In much earlier studies, Harrison *et al.*[10] found no clear relationship between cross-linking of collagen, measured as tail tendon breaking time, and life span of various strains of mice. In general, because of the lack of a clear relationship between AGEs or cross-links in long-lived proteins and the maximum strain or species life span, it is difficult to argue that the accumulation of AGEs (and/or other chemical modifications of proteins) is a significant determinant of the rate of aging.

TABLE 2. Comparative levels of AGEs/ALEs in skin collagen of rats and humans

Species	Biomarker		
	CML (mmol/mol Lys)	CEL (mmol/mol Lys)	Pentosidine (µmol/mol Lys)
Human	0.4	0.12	8
Rat (Sprague-Dawley)	0.057	0.02	0.58
Rat (Zucker, lean)	0.45	0.13	0.02

NOTE: Levels of biomarkers in 30-year-old humans and 9-month-old rats (unpublished), representing approximately 25% of the life span of these species.

Recent observations by Verzijl et al.[11] suggest that differences in the rate of protein turnover may explain differences in levels of AGEs among old animals with different life spans, as well as differences among species or strains of animals with similar life spans. These authors observed that levels of CML, CEL, and pentosidine were ~3 times higher in human articular collagen, compared to skin collagen, of the same age. The chronological ages of these collagens were estimated from their content of D-aspartate (D-Asp), which accumulates in proteins as a linear function of protein age. When the levels of AGEs were normalized for the D-Asp content of the collagens, it became clear that AGEs were formed at comparable rates in articular and skin collagen, but that articular collagen turned over more slowly than skin collagen, with estimated half-lives of 120 and 15 years, respectively. By a similar analogy, the lower levels of AGEs in skin collagen of old rats, compared to old humans, as well as differences in maximal levels of AGEs in skin collagen among species with similar life span, may be explained by differences in the rate of turnover of skin collagen among species. Because the level of AGEs represents a steady state between the rates of AGE formation and turnover of tissue protein, the absolute level of AGEs is not a determinant of life span.

In summary, it seems that the accumulation of AGEs and other chemical modifications of proteins correlates with age, but does not determine life span. This is not to say that AGEs, ALEs, and other modifications are unimportant in aging and life span. In long-lived species such as humans, the gradual accumulation of these compounds may alter the structure and function of proteins and may contribute to the development of pathology in age-related diseases, such as diabetes and atherosclerosis. AGEs may also contribute to oxidative stress and inflammation associated with neurodegenerative and musculoskeletal diseases of aging.

MAILLARD REACTIONS INVOLVING DNA

If Maillard reactions of proteins are not critical to the process of aging, what then is the role of the Maillard reaction in aging? I would like to propose that the critical target of the Maillard reaction is not protein, but DNA. Indeed, Maillard reactions of proteins may be described as an assault of electrophiles on the nucleophilic groups in proteins. The electrophiles include ROS themselves, as well as carbonyl, dicarbonyl, and activated carbonyl species, such as hydroxyaldehydes and ketones, alkenals, and hydroxyalkenals. The nucleophilic targets in proteins include the amino, sulfhydryl, guanidino, and imidazole side chains of amino acids. DNA also has nucleophilic groups, for example, the amino groups of adenine and guanine. Although nuclear DNA is well protected by a shield of nucleophilic histones and polyamines, it is clear that some electrophiles reach their target, for example, the wide range of carcinogenic alkylating agents. The detection of Amadori adducts and CML in histones also indicates that Maillard intermediates have access to the nucleosome.[12] AGEs/ALEs have also been detected in mitochondria,[13] and mitochondrial DNA, which lacks a histone shield, may be even more susceptible to Maillard reaction damage, consistent with recent emphasis on mitochondrial theories of aging.[14] Several methylglyoxal-DNA adducts are formed during glycation of DNA by glucose[15] and in cells exposed to the AGE/ALE precursor methylglyoxal at nontoxic doses *in vitro*.[16] Jacobson and colleagues[17] have also reported increased levels of carbonyl compounds in histones of cells exposed to alkylating agents and oxidative stress. These stresses commonly cause single-strand breaks in DNA and lead to increases in the synthesis and turnover of poly-ADP-ribose and in the intracellular pool of ADP-ribose monomer. ADP-ribose is a potent protein glycating agent and may be a source of AGEs in DNA in response to chemical and physical stresses. Oxidative stress, induced by glycation and/or AGEs/ALEs, may also catalyze the production of ROS, enhancing oxidative damage to DNA.[18]

THE NATURE OF DAMAGE TO DNA

Despite the evidence that DNA should be an accessible target for the Maillard reaction, studies in this area *in vivo* are hampered by the fact that damage to DNA does not accumulate, at least from the viewpoint of an analytical chemist seeking chemical biomarkers of damage. As summarized in TABLE 3, damage to DNA is "silent". Modified bases are excised and replaced, so chemical damage does not accumulate in DNA, as it does in protein. Further, the rate of the Maillard reaction is slow, so levels of modified bases are also low. There are, to my knowledge, no published reports on the detection of Maillard-modified nucleobases either in tissue DNA or in urine. At the same time, repair processes, although they work with high efficiency and fidelity, are not error-free. Thus, Maillard reactions, like other nucleophilic modifications of DNA, will lead to a gradual loss in the integrity of the genome, resulting from accumulated mutations, expressed in the form of altered sequence, rather than altered composition of DNA (TABLE 3). Chronic changes to the structure of DNA contribute to the loss of cells by apoptosis and necrosis in aging and chronic disease, and also to the increasing rate of appearance of cancer in the population with age. It is not essential that the rate of the Maillard reaction be increased, but only that repair be less efficient in shorter-lived species, as appears to be the case.[19] In summary, the Maillard reaction may be seen as one of a range of environmental chemical and physical factors that chronically assault the structure of the genome. Although this reaction contributes to aging, it is the efficiency and fidelity of repair of damage to DNA that sets limits on the life span of species.

TABLE 3. Nature of age-related Maillard reaction damage to DNA

Random	Occurring at random sites in the genome
Variable	Oxidative and nonoxidative chemistry
Unique	Damage is specific to each cell
Cumulative	Increases with cell and organism age
Stable	Transferred to daughter cells
Sequential	Alterations in nucleotide sequence
Silent	Nucleotide structure is unchanged

PROTECTIVE MECHANISMS

Long-lived species have evolved a number of mechanisms for protection against the Maillard reaction. These include transport and storage proteins that restrict the availability of free metal ion catalysts of Maillard reactions; metabolic pathways that reduce, oxidize, or otherwise inactivate or detoxify reactive intermediates; and antioxidant systems that limit the propagation of oxidative damage induced by the Maillard reaction. In addition, mammals have metabolic pathways that limit the free concentrations of reactive sugars. The evolutionary selection of glucose as blood sugar has been ascribed to the fact that glucose, among all sugars, exists to the greatest extent in the cyclic conformation, so it is the least reactive with proteins (and DNA) and is also the most resistant to oxidative degradation to more reactive species.[20] The concentrations of metabolic intermediates, such as sugar phosphates and dehydroascorbate, which are more reactive than glucose with protein, are also maintained at micromolar, rather than millimolar, concentrations in cells. A large fraction of these metabolites may exist primarily in protein-bound forms, focusing their nonenzymatic reactivity on enzymes with relatively rapid turnover and restricting their reactivity with DNA. A special level of protection is afforded to eukaryotic DNA, in addition to its histone and polyamine shields, by the fact that it is localized in the nucleus, shielded from Maillard reaction intermediates and ROS by cytoplasmic proteins and membranes. The protection of DNA in the cell nucleus may have been important in the evolution of rapidly dividing, short-lived prokaryotes to more slowly dividing, long-lived eukaryotic species. Limiting the influx of glucose into cells by development of insulin resistance, either with age or in diabetes, may also be a mechanism for limiting Maillard reaction damage to the DNA of postmitotic cells in long-lived organisms.

FUTURE DIRECTIONS

For the last 20 years, studies on the Maillard reaction *in vivo* have focused almost exclusively on the chemical modification of proteins. DNA has been a less attractive subject for study because Maillard adducts do not increase in this biopolymer with age or in disease. However, with the availability of exquisitely sensitive, high-resolution technologies, such as microbore HPLC and capillary electrophoresis interfaced to electrospray ionization tandem mass spectrometry, it should now be possible to detect modified nucleotides formed during the Maillard reaction, certainly in urine and in cells *in vitro*, but possibly also in tissues. Studies on Maillard reaction damage to DNA and the effects of AGE/ALE inhibitors on the modification of DNA will provide critical information for assessing the role of the Maillard reaction in aging.

ACKNOWLEDGMENTS

This work was supported by Research Grant No. DK-19971 from the National Institutes of Diabetes, Digestive, and Kidney Diseases.

REFERENCES

1. BAYNES, J.W. & S.R THORPE. 1999. Glycation and advanced glycation reactions. *In* Diabetes in the New Millennium, pp. 337–350. Endocrinology and Diabetes Research Foundation. Sydney, Australia.
2. BAYNES, J.W. & S.R THORPE. 2000. Glycoxidation and lipoxidation in atherogenesis. Free Radical Biol. Med. **28:** 1708–1716.
3. MONNIER, V.M. 1989. Toward a Maillard reaction theory of aging. Prog. Clin. Biol. Res. **304:** 1–22.
4. ULRICH, P. & A. CERAMI. 2001. Protein glycation, diabetes, and aging. Recent Prog. Horm. Res. **56:** 1–21.
5. THORPE, S.R., T.J. LYONS & J.W. BAYNES. 2000. Glycation and glycoxidation in diabetic vascular disease. *In* Oxidative Stress and Vascular Disease, pp. 259–283. Kluwer Academic. Norwell, MA.
6. WELLS-KNECHT, M.C., T.J. LYONS, D.R. MCCANCE, *et al.* 1997. Age-dependent increase in *ortho*-tyrosine and methionine sulfoxide in human skin collagen is not accelerated in diabetes: evidence against a generalized increase in oxidative stress in diabetes. J. Clin. Invest. **100:** 839–846.
7. GARNER, B., P.K. WITTING, A.R. WALDECK, *et al.* 1998. Oxidation of high density lipoproteins: I. Formation of methionine sulfoxide in apolipoproteins AI and AII is an early event that accompanies lipid peroxidation and can be enhanced by alpha-tocopherol. J. Biol. Chem. **273:** 6080–6087.
8. BAYNES, J.W. & S.R THORPE. 1996. Role of the Maillard reaction in diabetes mellitus and diseases of aging. Drugs Aging **9:** 69–77.
9. SELL, D.R., M.A. LANE, W.A. JOHNSON, *et al.* 1996. Longevity and the genetic determination of collagen glycoxidation kinetics in mammalian senescence. Proc. Natl. Acad. Sci. U.S.A. **93:** 485–490.
10. HARRISON, D.E., J.R. ARCHER, G.A. SACHER & F.M. BOYCE. 1978. Tail collagen aging in mice of thirteen different genotypes and two species: relationship to biological age. Exp. Gerontol. **13:** 63–73.
11. VERZIJL, N., J. DEGROOT, S.R. THORPE, *et al.* 2000. Effect of collagen turnover on the accumulation of advanced glycation end products. J. Biol. Chem. **275:** 39027–39031.
12. GUGLIUCCI, A. & M. BENDAYAN. 1995. Histones from diabetic rats contain increased levels of advanced glycation end products. Biochem. Biophys. Res. Commun. **212:** 56–62.
13. LING, X., N. SAKASHITA, M. TAKEYA, *et al.* 1998. Immunohistochemical distribution and subcellular localization of three distinct specific molecular structures of advanced glycation end products in human tissues. Lab. Invest. **78:** 1591–1606.
14. KOWALD, A. 2001. The mitochondrial theory of aging. Biol. Signals Recept. **10:** 162–175.
15. SEIDEL, W. & M. PISCHETSRIEDER. 1998. Immunochemical detection of N^2-[1-(1-carboxy)ethyl]guanosine, an advanced glycation end product formed by the reaction of DNA and reducing sugars or L-ascorbic acid *in vitro*. Biochim. Biophys. Acta **1425:** 478–484.

16. VACA, C.E., J.A. NILSSON, J.L. FANG & R.C. GRAFSTROM. 1998. Formation of DNA adducts in human buccal epithelial cells exposed to acetaldehyde and methylglyoxal *in vitro*. Chem. Biol. Interact. **108:** 197–208.
17. WONDRAK, G.T., D. CEREVANTES-LAUREAN, E.L. JACOBSON & M.K. JACOBSON. 2000. Histone carbonylation *in vivo* and *in vitro*. Biochem. J. **351:** 769–777.
18. CERIELLO, A. 2000. Oxidative stress and glycemic regulation. Metabolism **49**(suppl. 1): 27–29.
19. CORTOPASSI, G.A. & E. WANG. 1996. There is substantial agreement among interspecies estimates of DNA repair activity. Mech. Ageing Dev. **91:** 211–218.
20. BUNN, H.F. & P.J. HIGGINS. 1981. Reaction of monosaccharides with proteins: possible evolutionary significance. Science **213:** 222–224.

Oxidative Stress and Programmed Cell Death in Diabetic Neuropathy

ANDREA M. VINCENT,[a] MICHAEL BROWNLEE,[b] AND JAMES W. RUSSELL[a]

[a]*Department of Neurology, University of Michigan, Ann Arbor, Michigan 48109, USA*
[b]*Diabetes Research Center, Albert Einstein College of Medicine, Bronx, New York 10461, USA*

ABSTRACT: Recent evidence in both animal models and human sural nerve biopsies indicates an association with oxidative stress, mitochondrial (Mt) membrane depolarization (MMD), and induction of programmed cell death (PCD). In streptozotocin (STZ)–treated diabetic rats, hyperglycemia induces typical apoptotic changes as well as swelling and disruption of the Mt cristae in diabetic dorsal root ganglion neurons (DRG) and Schwann cells (SC), but these changes are only rarely observed in control neurons. In human sural nerve biopsies, from patients with diabetic sensory neuropathy, there is transmission electromicrograph evidence of swelling and disruption of the Mt and cristae compared to patients without peripheral neuropathy. In human SH-SY5Y neurons, rat sensory neurons, and SC, *in vivo*, there is an increase in reactive oxygen species (ROS) after exposure to 20 mM added glucose. In parallel, there is an initial Mt membrane hyperpolarization followed by depolarization (MMD). In turn, MMD is coupled with cleavage of caspases. Various strategies aimed at inhibiting the oxidative burst, or stabilizing the $\Delta\Psi_M$, block induction of PCD. First, growth factors such as NGF can block induction of ROS and/or stabilize the $\Delta\Psi_M$. This, in turn, is associated with inhibition of PCD. Second, reduction of ROS generation in neuronal Mt prevents neuronal PCD. Third, up-regulation of uncoupling proteins (UCPs), which stabilize the $\Delta\Psi_M$, blocks induction of caspase cleavage. Collectively, these findings indicate that hyperglycemic conditions observed in diabetes mellitus are associated with oxidative stress–induced neuronal and SC death, and targeted therapies aimed at regulating ROS may prove effective in therapy of diabetic neuropathy.

KEYWORDS: oxidative stress; diabetes; apoptosis; mitochondria; neuropathy

INTRODUCTION

Increasing evidence indicates that mitochondria (Mt) are intimately associated with initiation of programmed cell death (PCD) in neurons (see Ref. 1 for review) and that Mt membrane depolarization (MMD) is associated with induction of reactive oxygen species (ROS) and initiation of PCD. Cells use free radical scavengers

Address for correspondence: James Russell, M.D., M.S., Department of Neurology, University of Michigan, 200 Zina Pitcher Place, 4414 Kresge III, Ann Arbor, MI 48109-0588. Voice: 734-763-7276; fax: 734-763-7275.
jruss@umich.edu

to detoxify superoxide and hydroxyl radicals and thereby prevent cellular injury due to oxidative stress. Detoxification of H_2O_2 occurs primarily in the Mt, where it is reduced by glutathione. Reduction of H_2O_2 generates an oxidized glutathione disulfide that, in turn, must be reduced by NADPH to regenerate glutathione. With hyperglycemia, glucose flux generates sorbitol, which is converted to fructose and depletes the NADPH needed for regenerating glutathione, thus resulting in Mt dysfunction.[2] Increased metabolic flux in the Mt due to high glucose results in increased formation of ROS such as superoxides, peroxinitrites, and highly reactive hydroxyl radicals.[3] These ROS are associated with membrane lipid peroxidation, nitration of proteins (including tyrosine residues), and degradation of DNA, all of which are associated with induction of apoptosis.[4] In neurons, accumulation of NADH coupled with failure of the Mt creatine phosphate pump to regenerate ATP from ADP also results in disruption of the Mt electron transfer chain and depletion of ATP associated with apoptosis.[1] Although ROS has been associated with animal models of diabetes, it is unclear if oxidative stress is also important in human diabetic neuropathy. Further, the mechanisms linking oxidative stress to PCD and ultimately dorsal root ganglion (DRG) neuronal and Schwann cell (SC) loss in diabetic neuropathy are essentially unknown and will be discussed below.

METHODS

Dissociated embryonic DRGs from Harlan Sprague-Dawley rats were aseptically plated on air-dried, collagen-coated ACLAR dishes in the presence of serum- and insulin-free media and 10 ng/mL nerve growth factor (NGF) as previously described.[5,6] SH-SY5Y human neuroblastoma cells were grown in DMEM with 10% calf serum at 37°C in a humidified atmosphere containing 10% CO_2 as previously described.[7] In experiments, cells were subcultured in DMEM alone with the experimental condition. SC were cultured as previously described.[8] SH-SY5Y neurons and SC do not normally require NGF for survival.

To obtain tissue samples, animals were perfused prior to death with Trump's fixative (4% paraformaldehyde and 1% glutaraldehyde in 0.1 M phosphate buffer) by intracardiac infusion.[6] The whole vertebral column was removed and a 4- to 5-mm strip of bone was excised from the dorsal roof of the vertebral column as previously described.[6] In cell culture, neurons were fixed for 15 min in 4% paraformaldehyde. Human sural nerve biopsies were obtained from four subjects with moderately severe diabetic neuropathy or from four subjects of similar age after traumatic amputation (two) or with connective tissue disease and sensory symptoms (two) as previously described.[9]

To detect caspase-3 staining, DRG neurons or tissue sections (10 μm) were stained with 0.1 μg/mL CM1 antibody (kindly provided by A. Srinivasan, IDUN Pharm, La Jolla, CA) and 7.5 μg/mL rhodamine-conjugated goat anti-rabbit antibody (Vector, Burlingame, CA) for 1 h as previously described.[6,10] The nuclear chromatin was counterstained with 1 μg/mL bisbenzamide in PBS. Neurons were considered to have active caspase-3 if staining could be clearly localized to the neuronal or SC cytosol on sequential sections using both DIC and immunofluorescence. To determine if staining is specific for cleaved caspase-3, the antibody was pre-immunoabsorbed with peptide in sections[10] to indicate cleaved (active) caspase-3.

TdT-mediated dUTP-biotin nick end labeling (TUNEL) staining was used to detect apoptotic neurons. For staining of apoptotic nuclei in cell cultures, cells are grown on ACLAR dishes and fixed in 4% paraformaldehyde. Samples are labeled with digoxigenin-dUTP and then stained with FITC-conjugated antidigoxigenin antibody as previously described.[6] Transmission electron microscopy (TEM) of DRG neurons and SC was performed as previously described.[5,6]

A caspase-3 fluorometric assay kit (Pharmingen, San Diego, CA) was used to determine caspase-3 activation in SH-SY5Y neurons and SC. The assay was conducted according to the manufacturer's instructions and in conjunction with an Epics Elite flow cell sorting (FACS-Coulter Cytometry, Hialeah, FL) using excitation at 380 nm and emission at 440 nm.[8] All experiments were conducted with the following controls: cell lysate alone, Ac-DEVD-AMC alone, nonapoptotic cells, and positive apoptotic controls. Caspase cleavage was gated in live cells with propidium iodide (PI) exclusion (18 μg/mL). The mean of the peak caspase-3 level and the percent of neurons expressing cleaved caspase-3 were measured. Changes in the Mt membrane potential ($\Delta\Psi_M$) in SC were determined by incubating with 5 μg/mL rhodamine 123 (Rh123) for 30 min at 37°C followed by FACS. Alternatively, DRGs were incubated in 2.5 mg/mL JC-1 for 30 min at 37°C, and 590:530 ratios were measured using a fluorometer (Fluoroskan Ascent, Labsystems, Helsinki, Finland) and confirmed by confocal microscopy.

Adenovirus (Ad) constructs for uncoupling protein-1 (UCP1) and green fluorescent protein (GFP) were purified in the University of Iowa Viral Core. For DRG neurons, we obtained a 95–100% infection rate at 24 h with an MOI of 1000. Adenoviral constructs showed no intrinsic toxicity to DRG neurons. NGF p75 receptor function blocking antibody (p75NTR FBA) was kindly provided by Louis Reichardt (University of California, San Francisco).

Immunoblotting for caspase-9 was performed in lysates of whole 12-month streptozotocin (STZ) diabetic rat nerves (kindly provided by Douglas Zochodne, University of Calgary) with caspase-9 Ab (Santa Cruz, CA) at 1:1000 for 2 h. The secondary antibody was a horseradish peroxidase conjugate, applied for 1 hour, and visualized with enhanced chemiluminescence reagents (Amersham, MA).[8]

RESULTS

Hyperglycemia Is Associated with Oxidative Stress in Diabetic Neuropathy Models

In human neuronal (SH-SY5Y) cells exposed to high glucose, there is an increase in ROS generation that peaks at 2–3 h (FIG. 1) and then declines corresponding to increased cell death.[11] Increased ROS generation is associated with Mt depolarization and enlargement.[11] Swelling of Mt has been confirmed in STZ diabetic and acutely hyperglycemic rats, where the DRG neurons contain ballooned Mt with disrupted cristae.[6] Although, at very high magnification, lysosomal integrity is maintained, frequent large vacuoles measuring from 0.25 to 1 μm in diameter are observed evenly distributed throughout the cytoplasm.[6] At high magnification, these vacuoles are seen to occur in Mt that are ballooned and have disruption of the inner

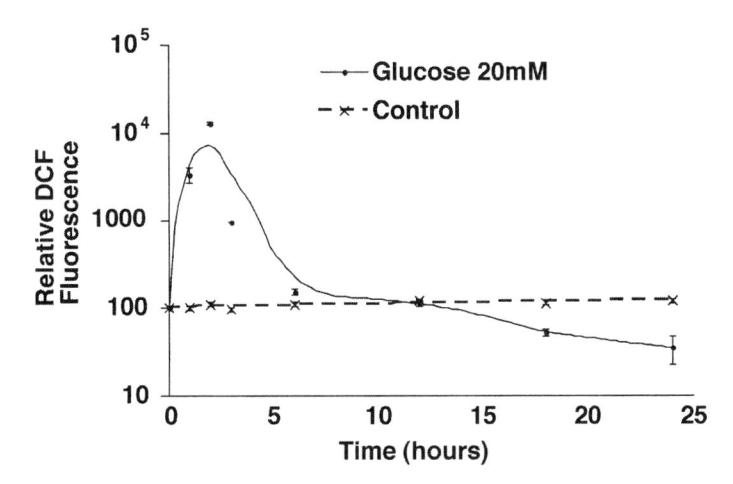

FIGURE 1. Glucose induces production of ROS in SH-SY5Y human neurons. SH-SY5Y neurons were cultured up to 24 h in control serum-free media ± 20 mM added glucose, treated with 2 μM CM-H$_2$DCFDA, and analyzed with FACS to determine changes in oxidative stress. Experiments were standardized against control values at 0 h. With addition of 20 mM added glucose, there was an initial threefold increase in the mean relative DCF fluorescence that peaked at 2 h ($P < 0.0001$) and then declined, corresponding to increased neuronal death. Plotted values represent the mean relative DCF fluorescence as a percent of control at 0 h (100%) ± SEM. Data were obtained from three separate experiments.

cristae structure. Although occasional vacuolization is observed in DRG cells from control animals, the Mt structure appears normal.

In human SC, there is also clear evidence of Mt enlargement and disruption of the normal cristae structure (FIG. 2). Whereas SC from nondiabetic subjects have normal Mt and rough endoplasmic reticulum, those from subjects with moderately severe diabetic neuropathy show formation of frequent vacuoles of variable size ranging up to 300 nm in diameter. While many of the vacuoles lack specific organellar structure, several enlarged Mt with still visible cristae structures are observed (FIG. 2C), consistent with increased oxidative damage to the Mt structure.

Hyperglycemia Results in Mt Swelling and Dysregulation of the Inner Mt Membrane Potential

Based on the findings of induction of oxidative stress and Mt damage in the peripheral nervous system (PNS), we next looked at the changes in the Mt membrane potential in neurons and SC. In DRG neurons exposed to increased concentrations of glucose, there is an initial hyperpolarization (more negative $\Delta\Psi_M$) followed by depolarization (less negative $\Delta\Psi_M$), as seen in FIGURE 3A. DRG neurons were treated with 20 mM added glucose for a period of 6 h, and changes in the $\Delta\Psi_M$ were measured using the potentiometric dye, JC-1. JC-1 exists as an aggregate at very negative membrane potentials ($\Delta\Psi_M < -100$ mV) with a red fluorescence at 590 nm, and as a monomer with green fluorescence at 530 nm with less negative potentials ($\Delta\Psi_M >$

FIGURE 2. *See following page for legend.*

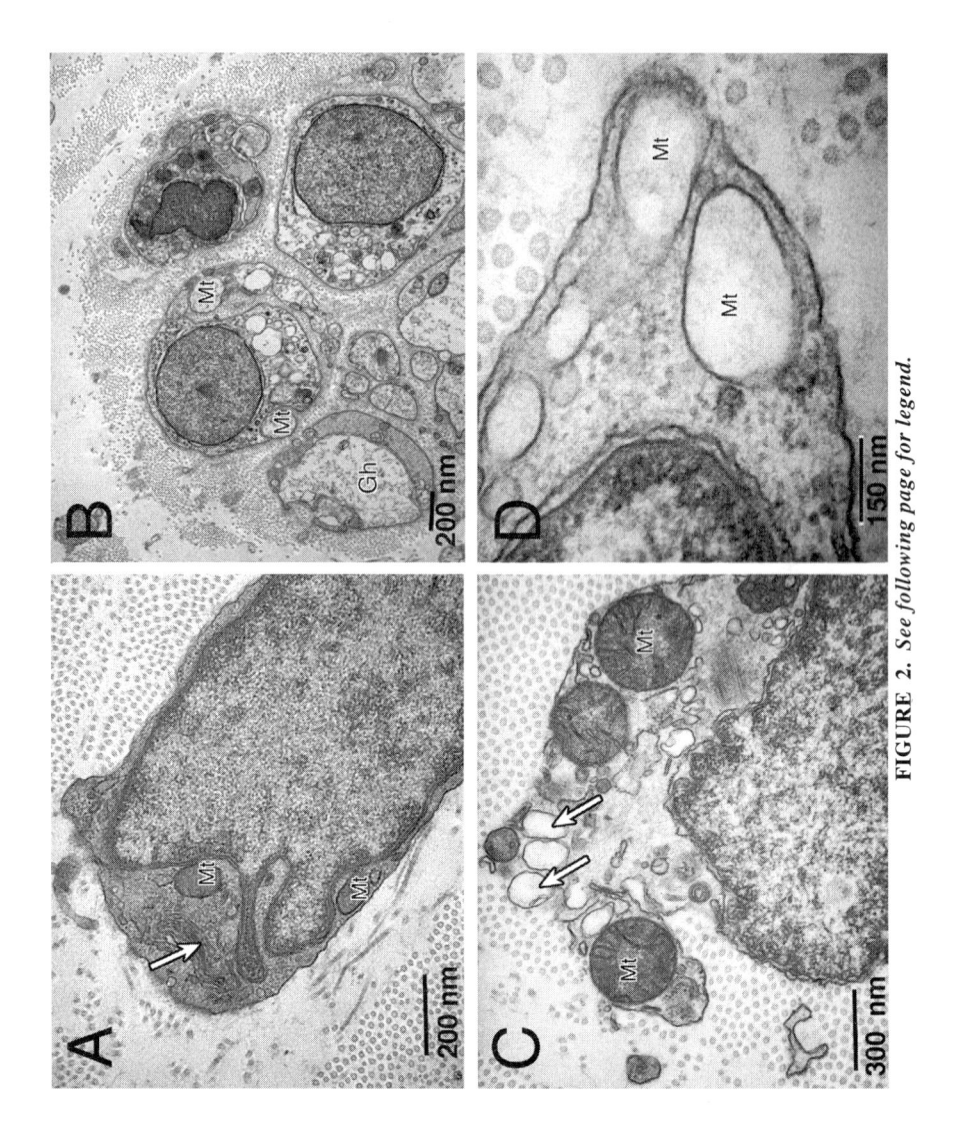

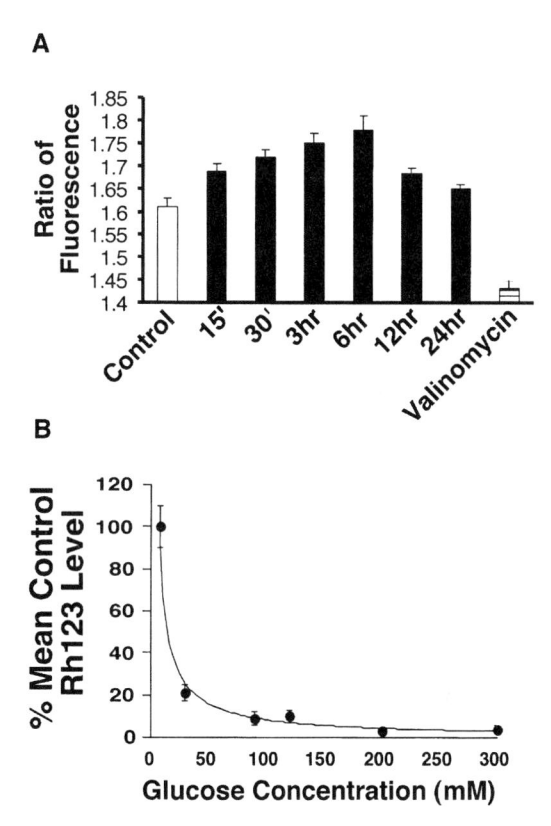

FIGURE 3. In neurons and SC, hyperglycemia is associated with disturbance of Mt polarization. (**A**) Dorsal root ganglion (DRG) neurons were incubated in JC-1 dye, and the 590 nm (aggregate) to 530 nm (monomer) ratio was measured to determine the $\Delta\Psi_M$ under control and 20 mM added glucose conditions at time points of 15 min to 12 h. There is initial hyperpolarization on exposure to glucose followed by depolarization starting between 3 and 6 h. Complete depolarization is observed with valinomycin or oligomycin controls. (**B**) SC were cultured for 24 h with increasing glucose, followed by FACS analysis with Rh123. The data were plotted as a percent of the corresponding control value at the same time point. Even with 20 mM added glucose, the $\Delta\Psi_M$ was significantly reduced compared to control after 24 h ($P < 0.0001$).

−100 mV). Equal numbers of neurons were used at each time point and the ratio was standardized against protein levels. There was an increase in the 590:530 ratio with glucose exposure from 15 min to 3–6 h, followed by a decline in the ratio consistent with depolarization, which persists to at least 24 h. With valinomycin or oligomycin

---

FIGURE 2. In human SC, there is swelling and disruption of the Mt and of the rough endoplasmic reticulum (**RER**). SC TEMs were from normal human controls and patients with moderately severe diabetic neuropathy. (**A**) Control SC: normal Mt and RER (*white arrow*). (**B, C, D**) Diabetic SC: There are multiple enlarged Mt within the SC with disruption of the normal cristae structure and formation of cytoplasmic vacuoles (*white arrows*).

(not shown), complete depolarization was observed. Similar results are obtained using Rh123 and TMRM, although evidence of depolarization is usually observed by 6 h using these cell-permeant dyes (data not shown). TMRM has the advantage of reducing fluorescent quenching sometimes observed with JC-1. In SC exposed to high concentrations of glucose, there is a dose-dependent decline in the $\Delta\Psi_M$ consistent with MMD. With 20 mM added glucose, the mean Rh123 measured using FACS decreased to 20% of control ($P < 0.001$), with almost complete loss of the $\Delta\Psi_M$ with 300 mM glucose (FIG. 3B).

Hyperglycemia Is Associated with PCD in Diabetic Neuropathy Models and Human Disease

Recent observations from our own and other laboratories indicate that apoptosis is one of the underlying causes of diabetic neuropathy.[6,8,12–14] Clear pathological changes of apoptosis occur in DRG neurons and SC in STZ-treated diabetic rats.[6,8] Hyperglycemia induces caspase-3 cleavage in DRG cultures and a significant number of neurons are TUNEL-positive in STZ-treated rats after 1 month of hyperglycemia, indicating extensive and regular DNA fragmentation associated with apoptosis. The percent of apoptotic neurons in diabetic animals closely correlates with the serum glucose levels ($R^2 > 0.9$), indicating that hyperglycemia is a likely trigger for apoptosis. In addition to the Mt dysfunction and apoptosis, our previously published data demonstrate a loss of neurons in rats after 3 months of diabetes. Using counting corrections for split nuclei, we estimated that the DRG number was 164 ± 16 in STZ diabetic animals, and 128 ± 19 in control animals, with a reduction in mean DRG area from 1110.3 ± 81.2 in control animals to 906.8 ± 51.3 μm^2 in diabetics.[6]

In tissue from C57BL/6 mice made acutely hyperglycemic with slow peritoneal infusion of 50% dextrose (mean serum glucose = 311.2 ± 13.4 mg/dL, $n = 5$) and control animals (mean serum glucose = 161.8 ± 7.3 mg/dL, $n = 5$), there is an increase in caspase-3 staining in DRG and, to a lesser extent, in SC (FIG. 4). Animals were sacrificed 24 h after attaining maximal hyperglycemia. Cytosolic caspase-3 cleavage was coupled with evidence of nuclear chromatin condensation, although this was a less sensitive measure of neuronal injury. In addition to cleavage of caspase-3 in both neurons and SC,[8] there is also evidence of caspase-9 cleavage in nerves from 12-month STZ diabetic rats. Although minimal cleavage of caspases is observed in most tissue that is removed from live animals and processed, there was a 40% increase in caspase-9 cleavage in sural nerve from the diabetic animals (FIG. 4E).

Changes in animal models of diabetes are reproduced in human SC (FIG. 5). Compared to normal human SC with diffuse chromatin staining, there is increased chromatin condensation (FIG. 5B), with shrinkage of the SC cytosol. Eventually, there is loss of the SC nucleus and cytosol with preservation of the plasma membrane and supporting collagen, forming ghost cells. These changes are consistent with single cell deletion observed in apoptosis, but rarely in necrosis. No inflammatory infiltrates were observed in the affected nerves, such as might be seen with necrosis of the peripheral nerve.

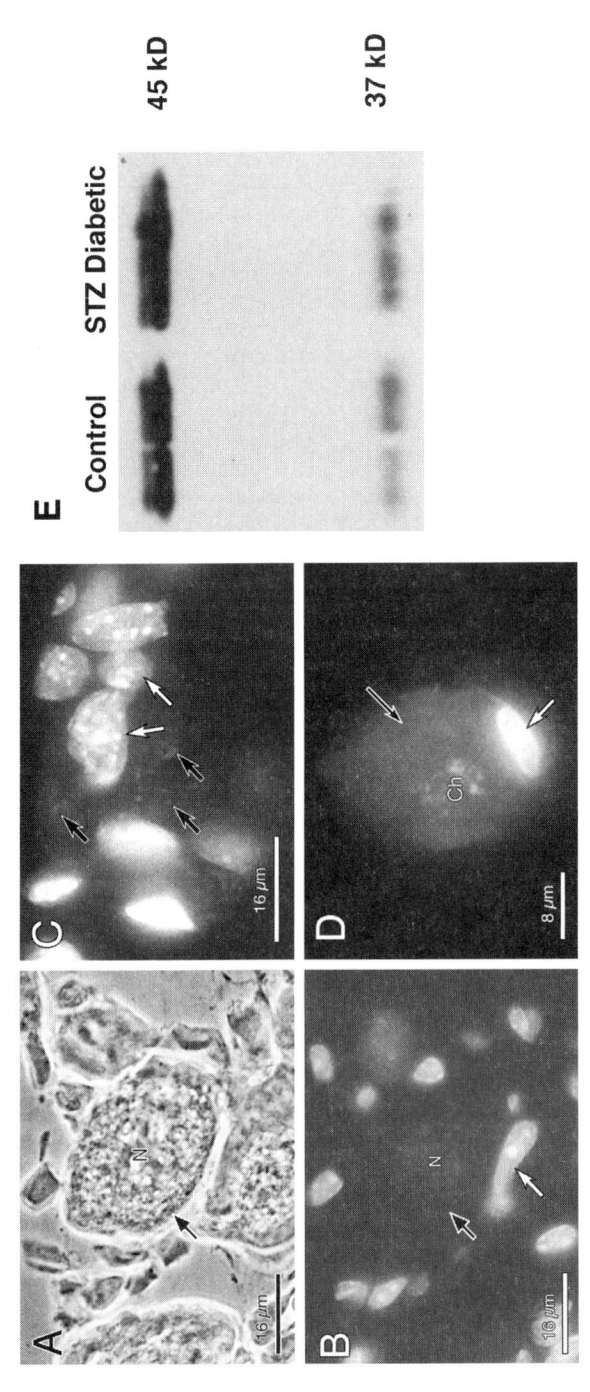

FIGURE 4. Cleavage of caspases in the mouse and rat peripheral nervous system. (A–D) In DRG from acutely hyperglycemic C57BL/6J mice, there is an increase in neuronal staining for cleaved caspase-3. Mice were given a constant glucose infusion for 6 h in order to induce acute apoptotic changes in SC. Sections were costained with CM1 antibody to indicate cleaved (active) caspase-3 and with 1 µg/mL bisbenzamide to indicate nuclear chromatin. **(A)** Phase-contrast image showing normal DRG neuron (*black arrow*) and nucleus (N). **(B)** Immunofluorescent image showing normal pale diffuse nuclear staining (N) in the neuron (*black arrow*). Several SC (*white arrow*) with lobular dark chromatin (contrast with the neuronal nucleus) are seen around the neurons. **(C)** Cleaved caspase-3 in the cytoplasm (*black arrows*) with degeneration of neuronal perikaryon. Several normal SC are seen surrounding the degenerating neurons (*white arrows*). **(D)** High magnification of a single DRG neuron showing punctate diffuse CM1 staining (cleaved caspase-3) in the cytoplasm (*black arrow*), with chromatin clumping consistent with dissolution of the nucleus (Ch). The *white arrow* indicates chromatin condensation in a Schwann cell. **(E)** Caspase-9 cleavage is increased in chronic diabetic rat nerve. Immunoblotting of whole 12-month STZ diabetic rat nerves for caspase-9 showed a 40% increase in the 37-kDa cleavage product, using densitometry, compared to control.

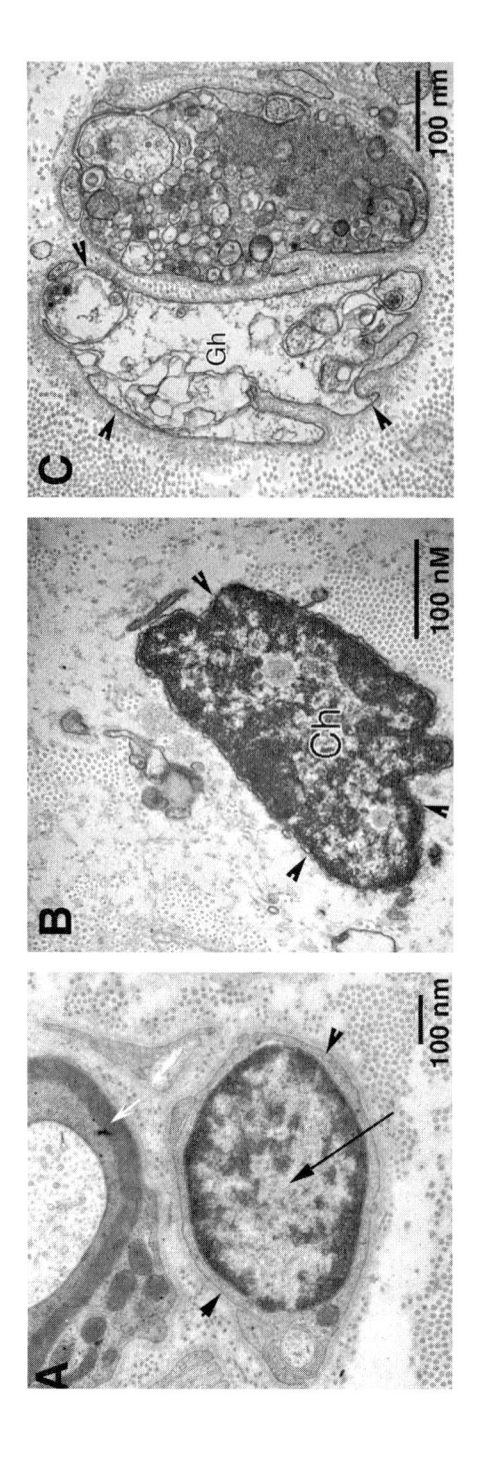

FIGURE 5. Apoptosis and single cell deletion in human SC from patients with diabetic neuropathy. (A) SC from a patient without diabetes. There is diffuse chromatin staining in the nucleus (*black arrow*), an intact perikaryon and basal lamina (*black arrowheads*), and myelinated axon. (B) SC from a subject with diabetic neuropathy. There is chromatin condensation in the nucleus with cytoplasmic shrinkage (*black arrowheads*). (C) Two SC from a subject with diabetic neuropathy, showing loss of normal cytoplasm and nuclear structure. In one SC only, the plasma membrane remains, forming a ghost (*black arrowheads*).

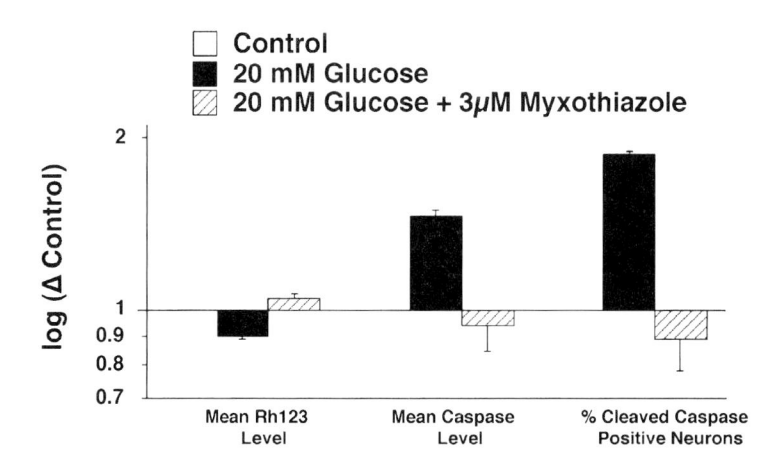

FIGURE 6. Myxothiazole, an inhibitor of the Mt respiratory chain, reduces MMD and cleavage of caspase-3 in SH-SY5Y neurons exposed to high glucose. The graph indicates the change from control as 1.0 on a log scale. SH-SY5Y neurons were cultured for 6 h in 20 mM added glucose, and the $\Delta\Psi_M$ was measured using Rh123 and FACS. There is a decrease in the $\Delta\Psi_M$ at 6 h with 20 mM added glucose, which is blocked by addition of 3 μM myxothiazole. The mean level of cleaved caspase-3 and the percent of caspase-3-positive neurons are increased in the presence of 20 mM added glucose and reduced by myxothiazole.

Regulation of Glucose-induced Oxidative Stress and Mt Membrane Potential Inhibits PCD

Glucose oxidation in the Mt increases the supply of electrons to the electron transfer chain, leading to increased proton pumping from the Mt and resulting in initial hyperpolarization of the $\Delta\Psi_M$. Ultimately, increased electron loss from the electron transfer chain induces formation of superoxide anions and other ROS. This can be blocked by treatment with electron transfer inhibitors such as myxothiazole. In neurons cultured under control conditions, a reduction in electron transfer along the chain by myxothiazole would lead to a reduction in the $\Delta\Psi_M$. Myxothiazole inhibits the Mt respiratory chain at cytochrome b-c$_1$.[15] In control neurons, addition of 3 μM myxothiazole results in mild depolarization, whereas it maintains the $\Delta\Psi_M$, which is usually decreased, in the presence of high glucose (FIG. 6). In Mt treated with high glucose that are biochemically compromised, oligomycin induces rapid depolarization consistent with Mt dependence on ATP synthase (data not shown). In high glucose states, myxothiazole is able to regulate generation of superoxides and prevent MMD. Coupled with this, myxothiazole blocks an increase in the mean level of caspase-3 cleavage and in the percentage of caspase-3-positive neurons (FIG. 6).

A further approach to regulating the $\Delta\Psi_M$ in the presence of high glucose is with growth factors. Growth factors such as NGF may also serve as antioxidants and this function may contribute to their role as possible therapeutic entities in diabetic neuropathy.[16–18] At 24 h, exposure to increased glucose results in MMD that is blocked by a physiological concentration of NGF (FIG. 7). By contrast, pretreatment with 50 μg/mL p75NTR FBA blocks the effect of NGF on the $\Delta\Psi_M$. These results

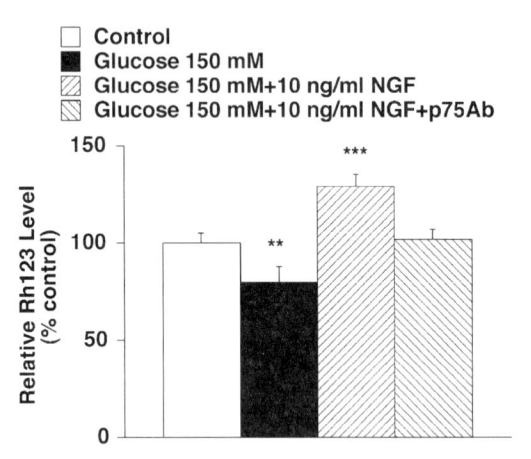

FIGURE 7. NGF prevents MMD in SC exposed to high glucose using FACS. The mean Rh123 level is decreased at 24 h, in the presence of high glucose, but maintained by addition of a physiological concentration of NGF (10 ng/mL). NGF inhibition of MMD is blocked by 50 μg/mL p75NTR FBA.

indicate that NGF mediates some of its Mt stabilizing effects through the p75NTR. High glucose induces dose-dependent cleavage of caspases in SC (FIG. 8). SC were cultured for 6 h in increasing glucose, and caspase-3 cleavage was measured. Caspase-3 cleavage was increased by 6 h with 20–50 mM glucose and blocked by 10 ng/mL NGF or the caspase-3 inhibitor, DEVD-CHO. A similar inhibition of apoptosis, measured with TUNEL, was seen with 10 ng/mL NGF, but was reversed by pretreatment with p75NTR FBA (FIG. 8B). These results show that NGF inhibits SC apoptosis through the p75NTR.

The UCPs are inner Mt membrane proteins that can dissipate the proton-electrochemical gradient; that is, they uncouple Mt electron transfer from oxidative phosphorylation.[19] UCPs share considerable amino acid sequence homology to one another, suggesting that they all possess an uncoupling function. However, the UCPs also have frequent homology to Mt transporters, as well as displaying typical Mt energy transfer protein signatures, suggesting that they may be Mt carriers.[20,21] This function will help regulate the $\Delta\Psi_M$ with hyperglycemic Mt injury and will prevent initial hyperpolarization. UCP1 is a classical UCP that is not normally expressed in neurons. In the presence of 20 mM added glucose, there is an increase in cleavage of caspase-3 and TUNEL-positive DRG neurons (FIG. 9). Cleavage of caspases is blocked at 6 h by overexpression of UCP1 (FIG. 9), and induction of apoptosis is blocked at 24 h ($P < 0.001$).

DISCUSSION

Recent evidence suggests that oxidative stress is responsible for the development and progression of neuropathy.[22] Blocking oxidative stress in the diabetic animal prevents the development of neuropathy[22] and restores sciatic and saphenous nerve

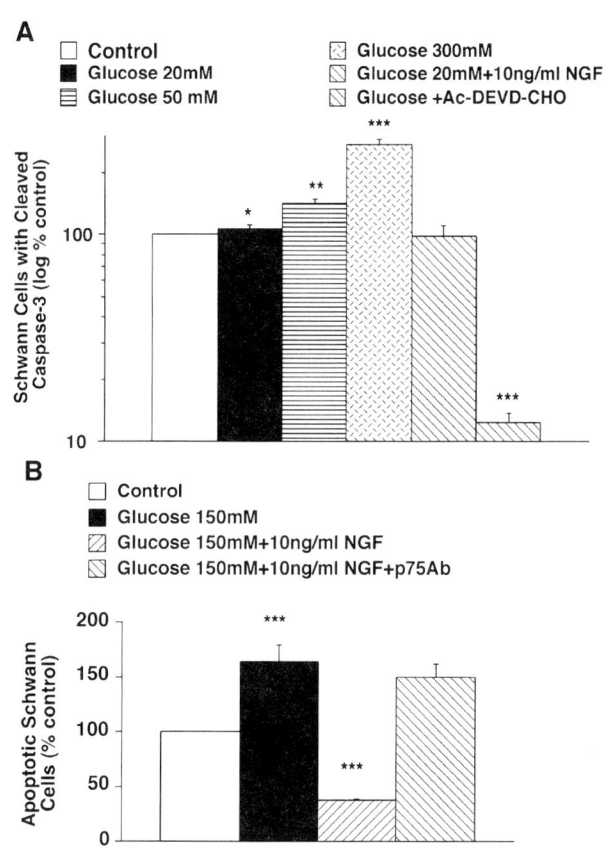

FIGURE 8. NGF inhibition of glucose-induced apoptosis is blocked by p75NTR FBA. (**A**) Cleavage of caspase-3 is increased in SC exposed to high glucose in a dose-dependent fashion. The percent of SC with cleavage of caspase-3 was determined at 6 h using increasing concentrations of glucose ± 10 ng/mL NGF or DEVD-CHO, and is expressed as a log scale. (**B**) Apoptosis in SC is inhibited by addition of NGF. SC apoptosis was determined at 24 h using PI and FACS analysis. Treatment with 50 µg/mL p75NTR FBA blocked NGF neuroprotection. *$P < 0.05$, **$P < 0.01$, ***$P < 0.001$ compared to control.

conduction velocities in STZ diabetic rats.[23,24] Our data indicate that increased concentrations of glucose rapidly induce production of ROS. This can be modulated by reducing electron flux along the electron transfer chain and generation of superoxide anions using myxothiazole. In turn, myxothiazole is able to reduce MMD seen with high glucose and to block induction of caspase cleavage. This most likely results from the ability of myxothiazole to reduce generation of ROS and to stabilize the $\Delta\Psi_M$.

In DRG and SC exposed to high glucose, both *in vivo* and *in vitro*, there is Mt swelling and ultimately a decrease in the $\Delta\Psi_M$, an event that in other paradigms initiates PCD.[1] It has previously been shown that release of cytochrome c into the

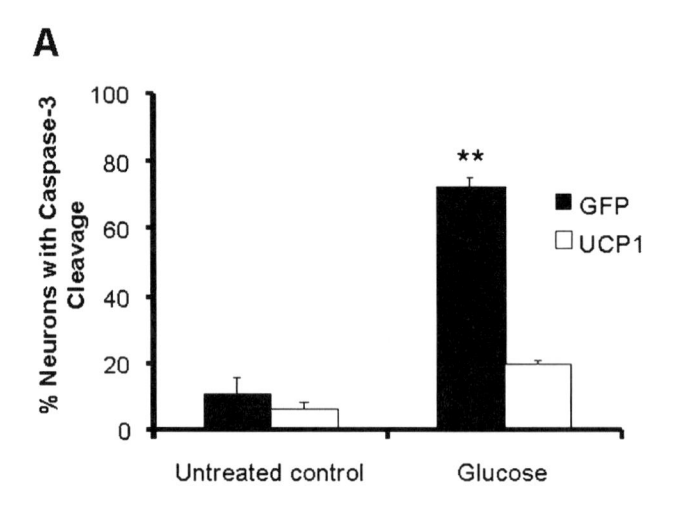

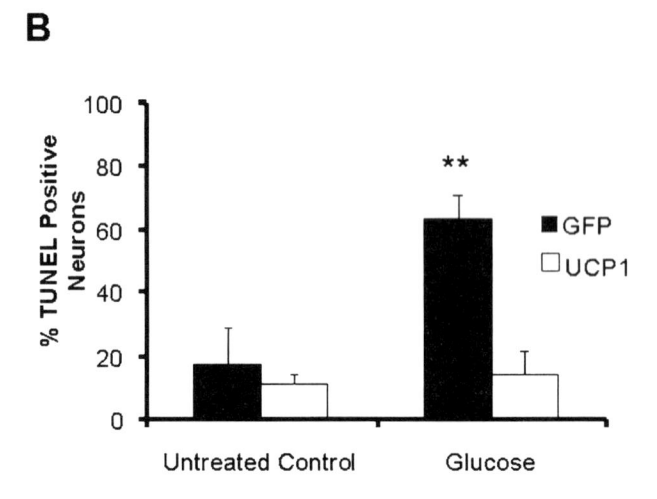

FIGURE 9. Adenovirus-mediated UCP1 expression prevents glucose-induced neuronal PCD. DRG neurons were infected with adenoviral constructs coding for either green fluorescent protein (GFP) as control or UCP1. (**A**) Caspase-3 cleavage was measured at 6 h and was increased with 20 mM added glucose and reduced by infection with UCP1. (**B**) Neurons were fixed 24 h following exposure to control media or 20 mM added glucose. The fragmentation of genomic DNA was then assessed by TUNEL staining. **$P < 0.01$ compared to control.

cytosol is associated with formation of a cytochrome c/caspase-9/Apaf-1 complex (the apoptosome) and cleavage of downstream effector caspases such as caspase-3 and caspase-7.[1] In human and rat neurons, hyperglycemia induces Mt dysfunction and apoptosis,[6,14] and similar changes are observed in another important cell in the PNS—namely, the SC. In nerve from 12-month diabetic rats, there is an increase in caspase-9 cleavage, and caspase-3 cleavage is seen in cultured SC exposed to high glucose. Similar to changes in rat neurons, human SC show evidence of both Mt swelling and apoptosis.

Impaired trophic support, such as reduced NGF levels seen in diabetic neuropathy, results in increased peroxinitrite formation and cleavage of caspases.[17] By contrast, we show that administration of NGF regulates MMD and blocks PCD. NGF may prevent PCD by blocking cell death signaling through the p75NTR[25] and by up-regulating PCD threshold proteins such as Bcl-xL and Bcl-2.[17,26] While chronic diabetes in humans may be associated with down-regulation of UCPs, up-regulation of UCP1 is clearly mediated through increased expression of p85α-phosphatidyl-inositol 3-kinase (PI-3K) or mitogen-activated protein kinase (MAPK)/MAP-extracellular signal–regulated kinase (MEK). These signal transduction molecules are critical intermediates of several growth factors including NGF and insulin-like growth factor (IGF-I).[27,28] Growth factor regulation of the $\Delta\Psi_M$ by UCPs, especially UCP2 and UCP3, expressed in DRG neurons,[29] would reduce generation of ROS and prevent induction of PCD, and ultimately may ameliorate diabetic neuropathy.

CONCLUSIONS

These observations in the PNS have led to our proposing the following model for regulation of glucose-induced oxidative stress and PCD in neuropathy. Glucose induction of ROS is critical to the pathogenesis of diabetic neuropathy. Loss of electrons from the Mt electron transfer chain, coupled with initial hyperpolarization of the $\Delta\Psi_M$, results in generation of excess ROS in the Mt. In turn, there is increased Mt injury, MMD, and swelling with release of apoptosis-inducing factors from the Mt into the cytosol, leading to formation of an apoptosome. Growth factors upregulate UCPs in the Mt and Bcl PCD threshold proteins like Bcl-2/Bcl-xL, stabilize the $\Delta\Psi_M$, and block formation of ROS and induction of PCD. Further understanding of these mechanisms will be useful in developing potential therapeutic strategies in diabetic neuropathy.

ACKNOWLEDGMENTS

This work was supported by grants from the NIH (Nos. NS 01938, NS 42056, and NIDDK 5P60DK-20572), The Juvenile Diabetes Research Foundation Center for the Study of Complications in Diabetes, VA Merit Review, funds from the Ann Arbor Geriatric Research and Clinical Center (GRECC), and the Program for Understanding Neurological Diseases (PFUND).

We also would like to thank Judy Boldt for secretarial support, and Eva Feldman, Mila Blaivas, Kelli Sullivan, and Catherine Delaney at the University of Michigan for their helpful discussions and assistance with this work; Douglas Zochodne at the University of Calgary for providing tissue from 12-month diabetic rats; the Michigan Imaging Analysis Laboratory (MIL) for assistance with electron microscopy; and the University of Michigan Core Flow Cytometry for assistance with FACS (supported in part by the UM-Comprehensive Cancer Center [NIH CA46592], the UM-Multipurpose Arthritic Center [NIH AR20557], and the UM-BRCF Core Flow Cytometry Facility).

REFERENCES

1. GREEN, D.R. & J.C. REED. 1998. Mitochondria and apoptosis. Science **281:** 1309–1312.
2. FELDMAN, E.L., M.J. STEVENS & D.A. GREENE. 1997. Pathogenesis of diabetic neuropathy. Clin. Neurosci. **4:** 365–370.
3. GREENE, D.A., I. OBROSOVA, M.J. STEVENS & E.L. FELDMAN. 2000. Pathways of glucose-mediated oxidative stress in diabetic neuropathy. *In* Antioxidants in Diabetes Management, pp. 111–119. Dekker. New York.
4. FUJIMURA, M., Y. MORITA-FUJIMURA, M. KAWASE, *et al.* 1999. Manganese superoxide dismutase mediates the early release of mitochondrial cytochrome c and subsequent DNA fragmentation after permanent focal cerebral ischemia in mice. J. Neurosci. **19:** 3414–3422.
5. RUSSELL, J.W., H-L. CHENG & D. GOLOVOY. 2000. Insulin-like growth factor-I promotes myelination of peripheral sensory axons. J. Neuropathol. Exp. Neurol. **59:** 575–584.
6. RUSSELL, J.W., K.A. SULLIVAN, A.J. WINDEBANK, *et al.* 1999. Neurons undergo apoptosis in animal and cell culture models of diabetes. Neurobiol. Dis. **6:** 347–363.
7. VAN GOLEN, C.M. & E.L. FELDMAN. 2000. Insulin-like growth factor I is the key growth factor in serum that protects neuroblastoma cells from hyperosmotic-induced apoptosis. J. Cell. Physiol. **182:** 24–32.
8. DELANEY, C.L., J.W. RUSSELL, H-L. CHENG & E.L. FELDMAN. 2001. Insulin-like growth factor-I and over-expression of Bcl-xL prevent glucose-mediated apoptosis in Schwann cells. J. Neuropathol. Exp. Neurol. **60:** 147–160.
9. RUSSELL, J., J. KARNES & P. DYCK. 1996. Sural nerve myelinated fiber density differences associated with meaningful changes in clinical and electrophysiological measurements. J. Neurol. Sci. **135:** 114–117.
10. SRINIVASAN, A., K.A. ROTH, R.O. SAYERS, *et al.* 1998. *In situ* immunodetection of activated caspase-3 in apoptotic neurons in the developing nervous system. Cell Death Differ. **5:** 1004–1016.
11. FELDMAN, E.L., J.W. RUSSELL, K.A. SULLIVAN & D. GOLOVOY. 2000. New insights into the pathogenesis of diabetic neuropathy. Curr. Opin. Neurol. **12:** 553–563.
12. SRINIVASAN, A., M.J. STEVENS & J.W. WILEY. 2000. Diabetic peripheral neuropathy: evidence for apoptosis and associated mitochondrial dysfunction. Diabetes **49:** 1932–1938.
13. RUSSELL, J.W., C. DELANEY, A.R. BERENT, *et al.* 2001. Diabetes and impaired glucose tolerance induce axonal neuropathy and programmed cell death (PCD) in the obese Zucker rat. Endocr. Soc. Abstr. **P1-363:** 226.
14. RUSSELL, J.W. & E.L. FELDMAN. 1999. Insulin-like growth factor-I prevents apoptosis in sympathetic neurons exposed to high glucose. Horm. Metab. Res. **31:** 90–96.
15. VANDEN HOEK, T.L., L.B. BECKER, Z. SHAO, *et al.* 1998. Reactive oxygen species released from mitochondria during brief hypoxia induce preconditioning in cardiomyocytes. J. Biol. Chem. **273:** 18092–18098.
16. PAN, Z., D. SAMPATH, G. JACKSON, *et al.* 1997. Nerve growth factor and oxidative stress in the nervous system. Adv. Exp. Med. Biol. **429:** 173–193.
17. PARK, D.S., E.J. MORRIS, L. STEFANIS, *et al.* 1998. Multiple pathways of neuronal death induced by DNA-damaging agents, NGF deprivation, and oxidative stress. J. Neurosci. **18:** 830–840.
18. LIEBERTHAL, W., V. TRIACA, J.S. KOH, *et al.* 1998. Role of superoxide in apoptosis induced by growth factor withdrawal. Am. J. Physiol. **275**(5, pt. 2): F691–F702.
19. NISHIKAWA, T., D. EDELSTEIN, X.L. DU, *et al.* 2000. Normalizing mitochondrial superoxide production blocks three pathways of hyperglycaemic damage. Nature **404:** 787–790.
20. BOSS, O., S. SAMEC, A. PAOLONI-GIACOBINO, *et al.* 1997. Uncoupling protein-3: a new member of the mitochondrial carrier family with tissue-specific expression. FEBS Lett. **408:** 39–42.
21. BAIROCH, A. 1993. The PROSITE dictionary of sites and patterns in proteins: its current status. Nucleic Acids Res. **21:** 3097–3103.

22. STEVENS, M.J., I. OBROSOVA, X. CAO, et al. 2000. Effects of DL-alpha-lipoic acid on peripheral nerve conduction, blood flow, energy metabolism, and oxidative stress in experimental diabetic neuropathy. Diabetes **49:** 1006–1015.
23. LOW, P.A., K.K. NICKANDER & H.J. TRITSCHLER. 1997. The roles of oxidative stress and antioxidant treatment in experimental diabetic neuropathy. Diabetes **46**(suppl. 2): S38–S42.
24. CAMERON, N.E. & M.A. COTTER. 1997. Metabolic and vascular factors in the pathogenesis of diabetic neuropathy. Diabetes **46**(suppl. 2): S31–S37.
25. BREDESEN, D.E. & S. RABIZADEH. 1997. p75NTR and apoptosis: Trk-dependent and Trk-independent effects. Trends Neurosci. **20:** 287–290.
26. MULLER, Y., K. TANGRE & J. CLOS. 1997. Autocrine regulation of apoptosis and bcl-2 expression by nerve growth factor in early differentiating cerebellar granule neurons involves low affinity neurotrophin receptor. Neurochem. Int. **31:** 177–191.
27. VALVERDE, A.M., M. LORENZO, P. NAVARRO & M. BENITO. 1997. Phosphatidylinositol 3-kinase is a requirement for insulin-like growth factor I–induced differentiation, but not for mitogenesis, in fetal brown adipocytes. Mol. Endocrinol. **11:** 595–607.
28. TERUEL, T., A.M. VALVERDE, P. NAVARRO, et al. 1998. Inhibition of PI 3-kinase and RAS blocks IGF-I and insulin-induced uncoupling protein 1 gene expression in brown adipocytes. J. Cell. Physiol. **176:** 99–109.
29. VINCENT, A.M., C. GONG, M. BROWNLEE & J.W. RUSSELL. 2001. Glucose induced neuronal programmed cell death is regulated by manganese superoxide dismutase and uncoupling protein-1. Endocr. Soc. Abstr. **P1-289:** 210.

Alzheimer's Disease: Role of Aging in Pathogenesis

DENHAM HARMAN

Department of Medicine, University of Nebraska College of Medicine, Omaha, Nebraska 68198-4635, USA

ABSTRACT: Alzheimer's disease (AD) is characterized by intraneuronal fibrillary tangles, plaques, and cell loss. Brain lesions in both sporadic AD (SAD) and familial AD (FAD) are the same, and in the same distribution pattern, as those in individuals with Down syndrome (DS) and in smaller numbers in nondemented older individuals. Dementia onset is around 40 years for DS, 40–60 years for FAD, and usually over 60 years for SAD. The different categories of AD may be due to processes that augment to different degrees the innate cellular aging rate, that is, mitochondrial superoxide radical (SO) formation. Thus, they increase the rate of accumulation of AD lesions. This lowers the age of onset into the dementia ranges associated with DS, FAD, and SAD, and concomitantly shortens life spans. Faster aging lowers AD onset age by decreasing the onset age for neurofibrillary tangle formation and neuronal loss, and the age when brain intercellular H_2O_2 can activate microglial cells. The early AD onset in DS is attributed to a defective mitochondrial complex 1. The proteins associated with FAD and their normal counterparts undergo proteolytic processing in the endoplasmic reticulum (ER). The mutated compounds increase the ratio of βA_{42} to βA_{40} and likely also down-regulate the ER calcium (Ca^{2+}) buffering activity. Decreases in ER Ca^{2+} content should increase the mitochondrial Ca^{2+} pool, thus enhancing SO formation. SAD may be due to increased SO formation caused by mutations in the approximately 1000 genes involved in mitochondrial biogenesis and function. The hypothesis suggests measures to prevent and treat.

KEYWORDS: aging; mutations; free radicals; Alzheimer's disease; dementia pugilistica

INTRODUCTION

Alzheimer's disease (AD) is the chief cause of dementia.[1] It is a systemic disorder whose major manifestations are in the brain.[2–4] The majority of cases[5] (90–95%) are sporadic (SAD). The remaining 5–10% are familial (FAD).[5] Most FAD cases are caused by mutations in the gene for presenilin 1 (PS1) on chromosome 14,[5,6] some by mutations in the gene for presenilin 2 (PS2) on chromosome 1,[7] while a few have mutations in the gene for the amyloid precursor protein (APP) on chromosome 21.[7,8]

Address for correspondence: Denham Harman, M.D., Department of Medicine, University of Nebraska College of Medicine, 984635 Nebraska Medical Center, Omaha, NE 68198-4635. Voice: 402-559-4416; fax: 402-559-7330.

AD is characterized by intraneuronal fibrillary tangles, plaques, and cell loss;[1,2,9–12] major steps in pathogenesis have been summarized.[4] Plaques contain βA peptides (mainly $βA_{42}$), formed by proteolysis of APP, that have aggregated into fibrils. Most peptides are in plaques that are not recognized by the usual Congo Red and thioflavin methods, that is, preamyloid plaques, also termed diffuse or amorphous plaques. The minor peptide fraction, formed by the action of free radicals on the fibrillary form of the βA peptide present in preamyloid,[13] is in plaques recognized by Congo Red, that is, amyloid plaques. Amyloid formation is generally associated with the clinical manifestations of AD.

The brain lesions in both SAD and FAD are the same, and in the same distribution pattern, as those seen in individuals with Down syndrome (DS)[1,14] and in smaller numbers in nondemented older individuals.[15,16]

Dementia onset is around age 40 for DS,[14] 40–60 years for FAD,[5] and usually over 60 years for SAD.[5] Lower dementia onset ages are associated with shorter life spans.

Extensive studies of AD have yet to result in a generally accepted hypothesis on pathogenesis.[17–20] Major emphasis has been placed on the role of amyloid,[19–24] the neurotoxin formed by the action of free radicals on preamyloid.[12,13]

HYPOTHESIS ON PATHOGENESIS OF ALZHEIMER'S DISEASE

The frequent presence of AD lesions in normal older persons, coupled with the association between lower dementia onset ages and shorter life spans, prompted the hypothesis that the different categories of AD are the result of processes that augment to different degrees the innate cellular aging rate, that is, mitochondrial superoxide radical (SO) formation. Thus, they increase the rate of accumulation of AD lesions. This lowers the age of onset into the dementia ranges associated with DS, FAD, and SAD, and concomitantly shortens life spans.

Aging

Aging is the accumulation of diverse deleterious changes in the cells and tissues that increase the risk of disease and death.[25,26] Many theories have been advanced to account for aging. No theory is generally accepted. The free radical theory of aging[27,28] (FRTA) is a promising hypothesis; the subsequent discussion is based on the assumption that it is correct. The FRTA postulates that aging changes are caused by free radical reactions. Those responsible for the innate cellular aging process largely stem from the superoxide radicals (SO) formed by the mitochondria at an increasing rate with age in the course of normal metabolism. These, plus the free radicals arising from suboptimal living conditions,[29] cause "aging."

Involvement of the aging process in formation of the characteristic lesions of AD:

(1) Intraneuronal fibrillary tangles: The progressive oxidative stress with age due to SO should eventually cause sustained elevation of calcium concentrations in the intracellular compartments;[4] this leads to disruption of the cytoskeleton and activation of calcium-dependent catabolic enzymes. Some neurons may be expected to undergo apoptosis and die; in others,

activation of kinases such as CaMK may be expected to progressively phosphorylate tau and thereby decrease the strength of its binding with microtubules. The latter permits phosphorylated tau to self-assemble and form paired helical filaments and, in turn, neurofibrillary tangles, while concomitantly the destabilized microtubules break down. Cells with neurofibrillary tangles eventually die.

(2) Neuritic plaques: The progressive increase in cellular SO formation with age[30,31] should be reflected in rising intercellular levels of H_2O_2 in the brain. At some age and in some locations, these levels could begin to exceed the threshold for the activation of microglia cells in a manner akin to the upregulation of the synthesis of cytokines IL-8 and TNF-α by dendritic cells.[32] Then, free radicals formed by activated microglia could serve to catalyze the oxidative conversion of preamyloid in the microglia area to amyloid, and simultaneously initiate the inflammation[19,33] involved in neuritic plaque formation and neuronal cell loss.

Thus, increasing mitochondria SO production lowers AD onset age by decreasing the onset age of AD lesions. How apolipoprotein E4 lowers AD onset age is not known. The O_2-mediated interaction between apoE4[34] and βA4 suggests a possible explanation: reaction of tissue O_2 with apoE4 may serve as a catalyst for the slow oxidative compaction of preamyloid, a process that results eventually in formation of amyloid. Therefore, when H_2O_2-induced microglia activation occurs, less time is required to complete the compaction. Hence, the age of onset of clinical symptoms of AD is decreased—and more so the longer the period of apoE4-associated compaction.

Augmentation of the Innate Aging Rate

Sporadic AD

Increases in mitochondrial SO formation in SAD are attributed[4] to accumulating free radical–induced mutation(s) in one or more of the approximately 1000 mtDNA and nucDNA genes involved in mitochondrial biogenesis and function.[35] This should decrease the age when the normally accumulating AD lesions increase into the AD dementia onset ages associated with SAD, and concomitantly shortens life span.

In view of the above, it is not surprising that efforts to find the gene(s) responsible for sporadic AD have been inconclusive.[19,36–38] This disorder could be initiated by one or more of a large number of combinations of mutations of the genes associated with mitochondrial function, for example, those influencing cytochrome oxidase.[39] Identification of the initiating mutation(s) would be expected to be made progressively more difficult with time by the continuing accumulation of mutations throughout life.

Familial AD

APP, PS1, and PS2, as well as their mutated forms, undergo proteolytic processing in the endoplasmic reticulum (ER) membrane.[19] These compounds are ubiquitously expressed transmembrane proteins; APP has a single transmembrane domain, while PS1 and PS2 have 6–9.[40] The turnover time of normal APP is short (20–30 min).[40,41] Turnover times of PS1 and PS2 are also short, about 15 min;[42] that of the complex formed from the N- and C-terminal fragments is apparently greater than 12 hours.[43] Mutations in the APP and presenilins should further shorten turnover times.[44]

Cleavage of APP by α- or β-secretase produces, respectively, membrane-bound 83- and 99-residue C-terminal fragments. These fragments are cleaved by γ-secretase, apparently formed[45] from the N- and C-terminal fragments of either PS1 or PS2; the products of the C99 cleavage include the βA_{40} and βA_{42} peptides. Mutants of the presenilins increase the fraction of βA_{42} and increase it further with mutated APP.[19]

The calcium-buffering activity of the ER is modulated by the ATPase calcium pumps,[46–48] located in the ER membrane,[49,50] and by the associated Ca^{2++} release channels.[51,52] Many compounds influence ER calcium content, including (1) phospholamban;[53–55] (2) the ganglioside GM1 and GM3;[56,57] (3) 6-gingerol[58] and ellagic acid;[58] (4) procaine,[49] caffeine,[49] thapsigargin,[49] and dantrolene;[49] and (5) the erythrocyte isoenzyme of acylphosphatase[59]—this enzyme inhibits the Ca^{2+} pump by hydrolyzing the phosphointermediate formed during the catalytic cycle of the calciumATPase.

It seems very likely that mutations in APP or the presenilins decrease ER calcium buffering in a manner akin to that of one or more of the substances known to influence it, resulting in compensatory increases in other calcium pools, particularly in mitochondria. The foregoing is strongly supported by studies with cultured neurons.[60–62] Increases in mitochondrial calcium content enhance SO formation[63] and, in turn, lower the AD onset age.

Clinical manifestations of FAD, and death, occur at significantly lower ages than for those with SAD. This can be attributed to a combination of one or more of the following: (1) mitochondrial SO formation is increased secondary to the increased O_2 consumption associated with increased turnover of the mutated forms of APP and of the presenilins; (2) increased formation of the more amyloidogenic forms of Aβ, that is, $A\beta_{42}$; (3) downregulation of the calcium-buffering activity of the ER leading to increased mitochondrial SO formation; (4) amyloid-associated inflammatory responses.

Down Syndrome

Individuals with this disorder have three copies of chromosome 21 rather than the normal two. Chromosome 21 codes for both superoxide dismutase (SOD) and APP; these gene products are increased in the cells of individuals with DS.[64] Persons with this disorder display premature aging;[64,65] manifestations include rapid aging of the skeletal system and skin, early menopause, short life span, and AD-like pathology[14] after about age 40. The first indication of the latter is generally apathy[64] and recent memory loss.[66]

The early onset of AD in individuals with DS is attributed to an enhanced rate of neuronal SO formation,[67,68] probably a result of a defect in complex 1 of the respiratory chain.[67] Thus, the early appearance of AD in individuals with DS, as with SAD and FAD, may be largely caused by a higher than normal rate of increase with age of SO.

Dementia Pugilistica (DP): An AD-Related Disorder

A blow(s) to the head is a risk factor for AD.[69] Repeated blows are associated with DP—the punch-drunk syndrome.[70,71] The severity of the syndrome correlates with the length of the boxing career and total number of bouts, and has an overall incidence of about 17% in professional boxers that rises with age.[70,71]

There are numerous neurofibrillary tangles in the cerebral cortex, particularly in the temporal lobe.[70,71] In contrast to AD, neuritic plaques are few, while diffuse preamyloid plaques[70] are abundant; the diffuse plaques can form within days after head injury.[72] Most cases show evidence of past brain hemorrhage.[73]

The initiating steps in pathogenesis of DP may be similar to those of SAD. Extracellular iron, for example, in the form of heme, may disrupt calcium homeostasis by increasing the influx of calcium through the neuronal membrane by (1) catalyzing oxidative alterations in the membrane and (2) increasing intracellular H_2O_2 concentrations (by catalyzing the aggregation rate of extracellular βA peptides to form amyloid; this in turn perturbs the neuronal membrane so as to activate an NADPH oxidase[74]). Increasing neuronal calcium concentration in the foregoing manner should result in neurofibrillary tangle formation.[4]

The relative paucity of neuritic plaques in boxers is probably due to the fact that their brain intercellular levels of H_2O_2, like those of the average person, are below the level needed to induce activation of microglial cells.

PREVENTION AND TREATMENT

The above discussion, as well as previous ones,[4,75] suggests measures to prevent and treat AD. The suggested treatments include some that are currently being used,[76] for example, antioxidants and antiinflammatory compounds.

Alzheimer's Disease

The age of onset of all categories of AD should be increased by measures to delay conversion of preamyloid to amyloid (TABLE 1, item 2).

Sporadic AD

Prevention: The incidence may be decreased by efforts to minimize free radical reactions involved in the initiation of this disorder. In particular, women who wish to become pregnant should increase their daily intake of antioxidants by consuming (1) a diet rich in high antioxidant–containing fruits and vegetables and (2) antioxidant supplements at intake levels deemed "safe" during pregnancy.

Treatment: Presented in TABLE 1.

Familial AD

Chromosomes 1 and 14

Prevention:

(1) Possibly in the future with gene therapy.

TABLE 1. Treatment of sporadic AD

Rate of progression may be slowed by a combination of the following:[26,29,77]

(1) Decrease free radical initiation rates: (a) lower caloric intake to an acceptable level; (b) add compounds to the diet that can compete with O_2 for electrons from the mitochondrial respiratory chain;[29] spin-traps, for example, nitrones or nitroso compounds, can apparently do so.

(2) Supplement the diet with antioxidants such as vitamin E and selegiline.[78] Specifically, increase the brain concentration of substances that may be able to minimize the expected rise of tissue H_2O_2 in the brain—possibly, lipoic acid,[79] ascorbic acid (dehydroascorbic acid),[80] propofol hemisuccinate,[81] and measures to increase metallothionein-III[82,83] (could this be the unknown normal[82] function of this readily oxidized metallothionein-III?).

(3) Dietary supplementation with compounds employed to improve mitochondrial function; for example, riboflavin,[84] menadione,[85] and (in particular) coenzyme Q_{10}.[86]

(4) Compounds to depress inflammatory reactions associated with senile plaques,[87–89] for example, indomethacin.[87]

(5) Estrogen treatment in postmenopausal women.[90]

(6) Possibly by (a) immunization with amyloid-β,[91] (b) selective inhibition of Alzheimer's γ-secretase activity,[92] and (c) peptides that bind to Aβ's and prevent β-sheet formation.[93]

---

(2) Measures, for example, procaine or dantrolene, that may help to maintain normal calcium-buffering activity of the ER during pregnancy.

Treatment: Same as (2) above, plus measures employed for sporadic SDAT.

Chromosome 21

Prevention and treatment: Same as for chromosomes 1 and 14.

Down Syndrome

Prevention: This disorder is caused by the failure of the two homologues of chromosome 21 to separate during the nuclear division of the maturing oocyte in meiosis I. This failure increases with age, which suggests that free radical reactions may be involved. If so, the measures suggested above for the prevention of SAD may be beneficial.

Treatment: If detected during pregnancy, the disorder may be ameliorated by decreasing the level of more-or-less random free radical reactions: for example, decrease caloric intake to an acceptable level or increase consumption of antioxidants by diet and/or supplements at levels deemed safe. After birth, treatment similar to that for SAD should be beneficial.

Dementia Pugilistica

Prevention: Measures to prevent injuries to the head.
Treatment: As with SAD. Use of iron chelators.

TABLE 2. Processes that augment to different degrees the innate cellular aging process (mitochondrial SO formation), lower the age when the normally accumulating AD lesions increase into the dementia ranges associated with SAD, FAD, and DS

AD category	Processes
SAD	Accumulation of free radical–induced mutation(s) in one or more of the approximately 1000 mtDNA and nucDNA genes involved in mitochondrial biogenesis and function.
FAD	Mutations in APP or the presenilins that down-regulate ER calcium-buffering capacity. This increases mitochondrial calcium levels, resulting in enhanced SO formation.
DS	Defective complex 1 of the mitochondrial respiratory chain. This increases SO formation.

TESTING THE HYPOTHESIS

Sporadic AD

Examine pregnancy records of the mothers of AD patients, for example, in Sweden. They may show the presence of conditions that could predispose to mutations in the developing embryo, for example, obesity, smoking, alcohol consumption, and antioxidant-poor diet.

Familial AD

The life span of affected individuals, as well as of transgenic mice expressing mutant APP or PS genes, may be increased by the following:

(i) antioxidants capable of passing the blood-brain barrier, to lower brain intracellular concentrations of H_2O_2, thus delaying the conversion of preamyloid to amyloid;

(ii) efforts to maintain normal cellular calcium levels, for example, administration of procaine to slow release of calcium from the ER.

Down Syndrome

(a) Onset of AD should be delayed by slowing the increase with age of the intracellular concentration of H_2O_2 in the brain; see above.

(b) Examine the pregnancy records of mothers with DS children. They may suggest that the embryo was under increased oxidative stress.

(c) Supplement the diet of DS female mice (Jackson Laboratories, Bar Harbor, Maine: designated B6EIC38, stock number 001924) with antioxidants. This treatment may decrease the incidence of DS.

COMMENT

The brain lesions of SAD, FAD, and those seen after about age 40 in individuals with DS, and in older nondemented persons, are the same and have the same distribution, but differ in the age of onset and the degree of involvement. The foregoing prompted the hypothesis that the different categories of AD are the result of processes (TABLE 2) that augment to different degrees the innate cellular aging rate, that is, the rate of mitochondrial SO formation. These lower AD dementia onset ages to those associated with DS, FAD, and SAD, and concomitantly shorten life spans.

The age of the appearance of neurofibrillary tangles and of that for neuritic plaques are not necessarily the same.

The innate aging process serves as the final common pathway for AD.

REFERENCES

1. KATZMAN, R. 1986. Alzheimer's disease. N. Engl. J. Med. **314:** 964–973.
2. KATZMAN, R. & T. SAITOH. 1991. Advances in Alzheimer's disease. FASEB J. **5:** 278–286.
3. BAKER, A.C., L-W. KO & J.P. BLASS. 1988. Systemic manifestations of Alzheimer's disease. Age **11:** 60–65.
4. HARMAN, D. 1995. Free radical theory of aging: Alzheimer's disease pathogenesis. Age **18:** 97–119.
5. GOEDERT, M., J. STRITTMATTER & A.D. ROSES. 1994. Risky apolipoprotein in brain. Nature **372:** 45–46.
6. SCHELLENBERG, G.D., T.D. BIRDD, E.M. WIJSMAN, et al. 1992. Genetic linkage evidence for a familial Alzheimer's disease locus on chromosome 14. Science **258:** 668–671.
7. LEVY-LAHAD, E.W., E.M. WIJSMAN, E. NEMENS, et al. 1995. A familial Alzheimer's disease locus on chromosome 1. Science **269:** 970–973.
8. GOATE, A., M-C. CHARTIER-HARLIN, M. MULLAN, et al. 1991. Segregation of a missense mutation in the amyloid precursor protein gene with familial Alzheimer's disease. Nature **349:** 704–706.
9. KATZMAN, R. & J.E. JACKSON. 1991. Alzheimer disease: basic and clinical advances. J. Am. Geriatr. Soc. **39:** 516–525.
10. MCKEE, A.C., K.S. KOSIK & N.W. KOWALL. 1991. Neuritic pathology and dementia in Alzheimer's disease. Ann. Neurol. **30:** 156–165.
11. TERRY, R.D. 1978. Ultrastructural alterations in senile dementia. In Alzheimer's Disease: Senile Dementia and Related Disorders, pp. 375–382. Raven Press. New York.
12. TERRY, R.D., E. MASLIAK & L.A. HANSEN. 1994. Structural basis of the cognitive alterations. In Alzheimer Disease, pp. 179–196. Raven Press. New York.
13. DYRKS, T., E. DYRKS, T. HARTMANN, et al. 1992. Amyloidogenicity of βA4-bearing amyloid protein precursor fragments by metal-catalyzed oxidation. J. Biol. Chem. **267:** 18210–18217.
14. MANN, D.M.A. & M.M. ESIRI. 1989. The pattern of acquisition of plaques and tangles in the brains of patients under 50 years of age with Down's syndrome. J. Neurol. Sci. **89:** 169–179.
15. CRYSTAL, H., D. DICKSON, P. FULD, et al. 1988. Clinico-pathologic studies in dementia: nondemented subjects with pathologically confirmed Alzheimer's disease. Neurology **38:** 1682–1687.
16. ARRIAGADA, P.V., K. MARZLOFF & B.T. HYMAN. 1992. Distribution of Alzheimer-type pathologic changes in nondemented elderly individuals matches the pattern in Alzheimer's disease. Neurology **42:** 1681–1688.
17. EDITORIAL. 1998. Amyloid and Alzheimer's disease. Nat. Med. **4:** 745.

18. GASPARINI, L., M. RACCHI, G. BINETTI, et al. 1998. Peripheral markers in testing pathophysiological hypotheses and diagnosing Alzheimer's disease. FASEB J. **12:** 17–34.
19. SELKOE, D.J. 1999. Translating cell biology into therapeutic advances in Alzheimer's disease. Nature **399**(suppl.): A23–A31.
20. YANKNER, B.A. 1996. Mechanisms of neuronal degeneration in Alzheimer's disease. Neuron **16:** 921–932.
21. HARDY, J.A. & G.A. HIGGINS. 1992. Alzheimer's disease: the amyloid cascade hypothesis. Science **256:** 134–184.
22. YANKNER, B.A. 1996. New clues to Alzheimer's disease: unraveling the roles of amyloid and tau. Nat. Med. **2:** 850–852.
23. SELKOE, D.J. 1997. Alzheimer's disease: genotypes, phenotypes, and treatments. Science **275:** 630–631.
24. DICKSON, D.W. 1997. The pathogenesis of senile plaques. J. Neuropathol. Exp. Neurol. **56:** 321–338.
25. HARMAN, D. 1998. Aging: phenomena and theories. Ann. N.Y. Acad. Sci. **850:** 1–7.
26. HARMAN, D. 1994. Aging: prospects for further increases in the functional life span. Age **17:** 119–146.
27. HARMAN, D. 1956. Aging: a theory based on free radical and radiation chemistry. J. Gerontol. **11:** 298–300.
28. HARMAN, D. 1992. Free radical theory of aging: history. In Free Radicals and Aging, pp. 1–10. Birkhäuser. Basel.
29. HARMAN, D. 1999. Free radical theory of aging: increasing the average life expectancy at birth and the maximum life span. J. Anti-Aging Med. **2:** 199–208.
30. SOHAL, R.S. & B.H. SOHAL. 1991. Hydrogen peroxide release by mitochondria increases during aging. Mech. Ageing Dev. **57:** 187–202.
31. OZAWA, T. 1998. Mitochondrial DNA mutations and age. Ann. N.Y. Acad. Sci. **854:** 128–154.
32. VERHASSELT, V., M. GOLDMAN & F. WILLEMS. 1998. Oxidative stress up-regulates IL-8 and TNF-α synthesis by human dendritic cells. Eur. J. Immunol. **28:** 3886–3890.
33. LUE, L-F., L. BRACHOVA, W.H. CIVIN & J. ROGERS. 1996. Inflammation, Aβ deposition, and neurofibrillary tangle formation as correlates of Alzheimer's disease neurodegeneration. J. Neuropathol. Exp. Neurol. **55:** 1083–1088.
34. STRITTMATTER, W.J., K.H. WEISGRABER, D.Y. HUANG, et al. 1993. Binding of human apolipoprotein E to synthetic amyloid β peptide: isoform-specific effects and implications for late-onset Alzheimer's disease. Proc. Natl. Acad. Sci. USA **90:** 8098–8102.
35. LARSSON, N-G. & R. LUFT. 1999. Revolution in mitochondrial medicine. FEBS Lett. **455:** 199–202.
36. BONILLA, E., K. TANJI, M. HIRANO, et al. 1999. Mitochondrial involvement in Alzheimer's disease. Biochim. Biophys. Acta **1410:** 171–182.
37. BROWN, M.D., J.M. SHOFFNER, Y.L. KIM, et al. 1996. Mitochondrial DNA sequence analysis of four Alzheimer's and Parkinson's disease patients. Am. J. Med. Genet. **61:** 283–289.
38. BLACKER, D. & R.E. TANZI. 1998. The genetics of Alzheimer's disease: current status and future prospects. Arch. Neurol. **55:** 294–296.
39. DAVIS, R.E., S. MILLER, C. HERRNSTADT, et al. 1997. Mutations in mitochondrial cytochrome c oxidase genes segregate with late-onset Alzheimer's disease. Proc. Natl. Acad. Sci. USA **94:** 4526–4531.
40. HARDY, J. 1997. Amyloid, the presenilins, and Alzheimer's disease. Trends Neurosci. **20:** 154–159.
41. STOREY, E., T. SPURCK, J. PICKETT-HEAPS, et al. 1996. The amyloid precursor protein of Alzheimer's disease is found on the surface of static, but not actively motile portions of neurites. Brain Res. **735:** 59–66.
42. YU, G., F. CHEN, G. LEVESQUE, et al. 1998. The presenilin 1 protein is a component of a high molecular weight intracellular complex that contains β-catenin. J. Biol. Chem. **273:** 16470–16475.
43. JACOBSEN, H., D. RESINHARDT, M. BROCKHAUST, et al. 1999. The influence of endoproteolytic processing of familial Alzheimer's disease presenilin 2 on Aβ42 amyloid peptide formation. J. Biol. Sci. **274:** 35233–35239.

44. MARZELLA, L. & H. GLAUMANN. 1987. Autophagy, micro-autophagy, and crinophagy as mechanisms for protein degradation. *In* Liposomes: Their Role in Protein Breakdown, pp. 319–366. Academic Press. New York.
45. KIMBERLY, W.T., W. XIA, T. RAHMATI, *et al.* 2000. The transmembrane aspartates in presenilin 1 and 2 are obligatory for γ-secretase activity and amyloid β-protein generation. J. Biol. Chem. **275:** 3173–3178.
46. ZHANG, P., C. TOYOSHIMA, K. YONEKURA, *et al.* 1998. Structure of the calcium pump from sarcoplasmic reticulum at 8-Å resolution. Nature **392:** 835–839.
47. AUER, M., G.A. SCARBOROUGH & W. KUHLBRANDT. 1998. Three-dimensional map of the plasma membrane H+-ATPase in the open conformation. Nature **392:** 840–843.
48. MACLENNAN, D.H., W.J. RICE & N.M. GREEN. 1997. The mechanism of Ca^{2+} transport by sarco(endo)plasmic reticulum Ca^{2+}-ATPases. J. Biol. Chem. **272:** 28815–28818.
49. MILLER, R.J. 1991. The control of neuronal Ca^{2+} homeostasis. Prog. Neurobiol. **37:** 255–285.
50. BERRIDGE, M.J. & R.F. IRVINE. 1989. Inositol phosphates and cell signalling. Nature **341:** 197–205.
51. MESZAROS, L.G., I. MINAROVIC & A. ZAHRADNIKOVA. 1996. Inhibition of the skeletal muscle ryanodine receptor calcium channel by nitric oxide. FEBS Lett. **380:** 49–52.
52. XU, L., J.P. EU, G. MEISSNER & J.S. STAMLER. 1998. Activation of the cardiac calcium release channel (ryanodine receptor) by poly-*S*-nitrosylation. Science **279:** 234–237.
53. KIMURA, Y., K. KURZYDLOWSKI, M. TADA & D.H. MACLENNAN. 1996. Phospholamban regulates the Ca^{2+}-ATPase through intramembrane interactions. J. Biol. Chem. **271:** 21726–21731.
54. HUGHES, G., A.P. STARLING, R.P. SHARMA, *et al.* 1996. An investigation of the mechanism of inhibition of the Ca^{2+}-ATPase by phospholamban. Biochem. J. **318:** 973–979.
55. LEVINE, B.A., V.B. PATCHELL, R. SHARMA, *et al.* 1999. Sites on the cytoplasmic region of phospolamban involved in interaction with calcium-activated ATPase of the sarcoplasmic reticulum. Eur. J. Biochem. **264:** 905–913.
56. WANG, L.H., Y.P. TU, X.Y. YANG, *et al.* 1996. Effect of ganglioside GM3 on the activity and conformation of reconstituted Ca^{2+}-ATPase. FEBS Lett. **388:** 128–130.
57. WANG, Y., Z. TSUI & F. YANG. 1999. Antagonistic effect of ganglioside GM1 and GM3 on the activity and conformation of sarcoplasmic reticulum Ca^{2+}-ATPase. FEBS Lett. **457:** 144–148.
58. ANTIPENKO, A.Y., A.I. SPIELMAN & M.A. KIRCHABERAGER. 1999. Interactions of 6-gingerol and ellagic acid with the cardiac sarcoplasmic reticulum Ca^{2+}-ATPase. J. Pharmacol. Exp. Ther. **290:** 227–234.
59. LIGURI, G., C. CECCHI, L. LATORRACA, *et al.* 1996. Alteration of acylphosphatase levels in familial Alzheimer's disease fibroblasts with presenilin gene mutations. Neurosci. Lett. **210:** 153–156.
60. MATTSON, M.P., H. ZHU, J. YU & M.S. KINDY. 2000. Presenilin-1 mutation increases neuronal vulnerability to focal ischemia *in vivo* and to hypoxia and glucose deprivation in cell culture: involvement of perturbed calcium homeostasis. J. Neurosci. **20:** 1358–1364.
61. GUO, Q., S. CHRISTAKOS, N. ROBINSON & M.P. MATTSON. 1998. Calbindin D28k blocks the proapoptotic actions of mutant presenilin 1: reduced oxidative stress and preserved mitochondrial function. Proc. Natl. Acad. Sci. USA **95:** 3227–3232.
62. GUO, Q., L. SEBASTIAN & B.L. SOPHER. 1999. Increased vulnerability of hippocampal neurons from presenilin-1 mutant knock-in mice to amyloid β-peptide toxicity: central roles of superoxide production and caspase activation. J. Neurochem. **72:** 1019–1029.
63. RICHTER, C., V. GOGVADZE & R. LAFFRANCHI. 1995. Oxidants in mitochondria: from physiology to diseases. Biochim. Biophys. Acta **1271:** 67–74.
64. OLIVER, C. & A.J. HOLLAND. 1986. Down's syndrome and Alzheimer's disease: a review. Psychol. Med. **16:** 307–322.
65. RUMBLE, B., R. RETALLACK, C. HILBICH, *et al.* 1988. Amyloid A4 protein and its precursor in Down's syndrome and Alzheimer's disease. N. Engl. J. Med. **320:** 1446–1452.

66. WISNIEWSKI, K.E., A.L. HILL & H.M. WISNIEWSKI. 1992. Aging and Alzheimer's disease in people with Down's syndrome. *In* Advances in Medical Care, pp. 167–183. Wiley-Liss. New York.
67. SCHUCHMANN, S. & U. HEINEMANN. 2000. Increased mitochondrial superoxide generation in neurons from trisomy 16 mice: a model of Down's syndrome. Free Radic. Biol. Med. **28:** 235–250.
68. BUSCIGLIO, J. & B.A. YANKNER. 1995. Apoptosis and increased generation of reactive oxygen species in Down's syndrome neurons *in vitro*. Nature **378:** 776–779.
69. GRAVES, A.B., E. WHITE, T.D. KOEPSELL, *et al.* 1990. The association between head trauma and Alzheimer's disease. Am. J. Epidemiol. **131:** 491–501.
70. ROBERTS, G.W., D. ALLSOP & C. BRUTON. 1990. The occult aftermath of boxing. J. Neurol. Neurosurg. Psychiatry **53:** 373–378.
71. GUTERMAN, A. & R.W. SMITH. 1987. Neurological sequelae of boxing. Sports Med. **4:** 194–210.
72. ROBERTS, G.W., S.M. GENTLEMEN, A. LYNCH & D.I. GRAHAM. 1991. βA4 amyloid protein deposition in brain after head trauma. Lancet **338:** 1422–1423.
73. ADAMS, C.W.M. & C.J. BRUTON. 1989. The cerebral vasculature in dementia pugilistica. J. Neurol. Neurosurg. Psychiatry **52:** 600–604.
74. BEHL, C., J.B. DAVIS, R. LESLEY & D. SCHUBERT. 1994. Hydrogen peroxide mediates amyloid β protein toxicity. Cell **77:** 817–827.
75. HARMAN, D. 2000. Alzheimer's disease: a hypothesis on pathogenesis. J. Am. Aging Assoc. **23:** 147–161.
76. EMILIEN, G., K. BEYREUTHER, C.L. MASTERS & J-M. MALOTEAUX. 2000. Prospects for pharmacological intervention in Alzheimer's disease. Arch. Neurol. **57:** 454–459.
77. HARMAN, D. 1999. Aging: minimizing free radical damage. J. Anti-Aging Med. **2:** 15–36.
78. SANO, M., C. ERNESTO, R.G. THOMAS, *et al.* 1997. A controlled trial of selegiline, alpha-tocopherol, or both as treatment for Alzheimer's disease. N. Engl. J. Med. **336:** 1216–1222.
79. PACKER, L., H.T. TRITSCHLER & K. WESSEL. 1997. Neuroprotection by the metabolic antioxidant α-lipoic acid. Free Radic. Biol. Med. **22:** 359–378.
80. AGUS, D., S.S. GAMBHIR, W.M. PARDRIDGE, *et al.* 1997. Vitamin C crosses the blood-brain barrier in the oxidized form through the glucose transporters. J. Clin. Invest. **100:** 2842–2848.
81. SAGARA, Y., S. HENDLER, S. KHOH-REITER, *et al.* 1999. Propofol hemisuccinate protects neuronal cells from oxidative injury. J. Neurochem. **73:** 2524–2530.
82. PALMITER, R.D. 1998. The elusive function of metallothioneins. Proc. Natl. Acad. Sci. USA **95:** 8428–8430.
83. ERICKSON, J.C., A.K. SEWELL, L.T. JENSEN, *et al.* 1994. Enhanced neurotrophic activity in Alzheimer's disease cortex is not associated with down-regulation of metallothionein-III (GIF). Brain Res. **649:** 297–304.
84. ARTS, W.F.M., H.R. SCHOLTE, J.M. BOGAARD, *et al.* 1983. NADH-CoQ reductase deficient myopathy: successful treatment with riboflavin. Lancet **2:** 581–582.
85. ELEFF, S., N.G. KENNAWAY, N.R.M. BUIST, *et al.* 1984. ^{31}P NMR study of improvement in oxidative phosphorylation by vitamin K_3 and C in a patient with a defect in electron transport at complex III in skeletal muscle. Proc. Natl. Acad. Sci. USA **81:** 3529–3533.
86. OGASAHARA, S., Y. NISHIKAWA, S. YORIFUJI, *et al.* 1986. Treatment of Kearns-Sayre syndrome with coenzyme Q_{10}. Neurology **36:** 45–53.
87. ROGERS, J., L.C. KIRBY, S.R. HEMPEIMAN, *et al.* 1993. Clinical trial of indometachin in Alzheimer's disease. Neurology **43:** 1609–1611.
88. BREITNER, J.C.S., B.A. GAU, K.A. WELSH, *et al.* 1994. Inverse association of anti-inflammatory treatments and Alzheimer's disease: initial results of a co-twin control study. Neurology **44:** 227–232.
89. ROGERS, J., S. WEBSTER, L-F. LUE, *et al.* 1996. Inflammation and Alzheimer's disease pathogenesis. Neurobiol. Aging **17:** 681–686.
90. TANG, M-X., D. JACOBS, Y. STERN, *et al.* 1996. Effect of oestrogen during menopause on risk and age at onset of Alzheimer's disease. Lancet **348:** 429–432.

91. SCHENK, D., R. BARBOUR, W. DINN, *et al.* 1999. Immunization with amyloid-β attenuates Alzheimer-disease-like pathology in the PDAPP mouse. Nature **400:** 173–177.
92. WOLFE, M.S., M. CITRON, T.S. DIEHL, *et al.* 1998. A substrate-based difluoro ketone selectively inhibits Alzheimer's γ-secretase activity. J. Med. Chem. **41:** 6–9.
93. SOTO, C., M. KINDY, M. BAUMANN & B. FRANGIONE. 1996. Inhibition of Alzheimer's amyloidosis by peptides that prevent β-sheet conformation. Biochem. Biophys. Res. Commun. **226:** 672–680.

Human Aging and Global Function of Coenzyme Q$_{10}$

ANTHONY W. LINNANE,[a] CHUNFANG ZHANG,[a] NATALIA YAROVAYA,[a] GEORGE KOPSIDAS,[a] SERGEY KOVALENKO,[a] PENNY PAPAKOSTOPOULOS,[a] HAYDEN EASTWOOD,[a] STEPHEN GRAVES,[b] AND MARTIN RICHARDSON[c]

[a]*Centre for Molecular Biology and Medicine, Epworth Medical Centre, Richmond, Victoria 3121, Australia*

[b]*Royal Melbourne Hospital, Orthopaedic Department, Gratten Street, Parkville, Victoria 3052, Australia*

[c]*Epworth Medical Centre, 173 Lennox Street, Richmond, Victoria 3121, Australia*

ABSTRACT: In this paper, we review two parts of our recent work on human skeletal muscle. The first part mainly describes changes occurring during aging, whereas the second part discusses the functions of coenzyme Q$_{10}$ (CoQ$_{10}$), particularly in relation to the aging process. During the lifetime of an individual, mtDNA undergoes a variety of mutation events and rearrangements. These mutations and their consequent bioenergenic decline, together with nuclear DNA damage, contribute to the reduced function of cells and organs, especially in postmitotic tissues. In skeletal muscle, this functional decline can be observed by means of changes with age in fiber type profile and the reduction in the number and size of the muscle fibers. In addition to the functions of coenzyme Q$_{10}$ as an electron carrier in the respiratory chain and as an antioxidant, CoQ$_{10}$ has been shown to regulate global gene expression in skeletal muscle. We hypothesize that this regulation is achieved via superoxide formation with H$_2$O$_2$ as a second messenger to the nucleus.

KEYWORDS: human aging; skeletal muscle; mtDNA mutations; coenzyme Q$_{10}$; gene expression; vastus lateralis

INTRODUCTION

This paper reviews part of our continuing studies on the human aging process, particularly as related to skeletal muscle.[1–4,6,7] We have earlier proposed that damage to tissue cells, as exemplified by mitochondrial DNA in cells, is of a stochastic nature,[2] whereby cells within a single tissue would suffer from various degrees of damage. During the aging process, a "damage mosaic" develops where, in different individuals, different tissues in the same individual, different cells in the same tissue, and different organelles in the same cell have undergone a range of changes. The sys-

---

Address for correspondence: Anthony W. Linnane, Centre for Molecular Biology and Medicine, Epworth Medical Centre, 185-187 Hoddle Street, Richmond, Victoria 3121, Australia. Voice: +61-3-9426-4200; fax: +61-3-9426-4201.
tlinnane@cmbm.com.au

tem is a dynamic one with repair and ongoing damage in a finely tuned equilibrium, which with age tilts increasingly towards damage and cell loss. The whole process is affected by the individual's genetic makeup and environmental factors also have an impact.

This paper is organized into two parts: the first part mainly describes changes occurring during aging. In the second part, we will discuss the functions of coenzyme Q_{10} (CoQ_{10}), particularly in relation to the aging process.

PART 1: CHANGES DURING THE AGING PROCESS

Changes in Mitochondrial DNA and Consequent Decline in Bioenergy Capacity in Human Tissues

It was proposed by Linnane and colleagues[1] that during one's lifetime, numerous mtDNA mutations occur and accumulate in tissues and that accumulation of such mutations makes a significant contribution to the aging process. This idea has gained significant support. Data from a number of laboratories has confirmed that various mutations of mtDNA occur with age in postmitotic tissues (for review, see Refs. 2 and 5). Our laboratory has applied the technique of extra-long PCR (XL-PCR) to analyze the mtDNA genome extracted from human *vastus lateralis* muscle of individuals of different ages. We have shown that the amount of full-length mtDNA that could be amplified by XL-PCR is decreased with age and that multiple heterogenous mtDNA deletions appear in skeletal muscle of older individuals. The decrease in the amount of full-length mtDNA and the appearance of numerous mtDNA deletions seem to be associated with a decreased activity of cytochrome *c* oxidase (COX), the complex IV of the electron transport chain.[6] To be able to correlate the changes in mtDNA with age with the age-related decline in bioenergetic capacity of the tissue, we have performed XL-PCR on isolated single skeletal muscle fibers of predetermined COX activity. All COX-positive muscle fibers isolated from tissues of individuals of different ages were shown to contain full-length mtDNA as well as a small number of mtDNA deletions. By contrast, muscle fibers negative for COX activity did not contain a detectable amount of full-length mtDNA but had multiple heterogeneous mtDNA species that were different in different muscle fibers of the same individual. These data lead us to the conclusion that there is a link between the amount of full-length mtDNA and the bioenergic capacity of the tissue, measured through the activity of COX.[7]

Muscle Fiber Types and Muscle Aging

An important aspect of muscle physiology is the recognition that skeletal muscle consists of two major fiber groups: type I and type II. Type I fibers have greater oxidative capacity and contain more mitochondria per cell and preferentially use oxidative phosphorylation for their bioenergy metabolism. Type II fibers, which can be further subgrouped into IIa, IIb, and IIx/d fibers, have fewer mitochondria per cell and are more glycolytic with respect to energy requirements. Fiber type and, consequently, the energy metabolism of muscle fiber, are determined by the myosin heavy chain, which is expressed by the fiber. The proportion of fiber types varies among different muscles and among the same muscle of different subjects.

Fiber type composition of some muscles has been reported to change with advanced age. Early studies on aging and muscle fiber type profile have shown that type I fiber percentage increases from 39% to 66% in skeletal muscle of men aged 20 to 70.[8] However, other researchers have observed much smaller changes in the percentage of type I fibers with age (from 49% to 52%) or no statistically significant changes in fiber type proportion with age.[9,10] The loss of muscle mass and changes of fiber type during aging may be secondary to age-related denervation of muscle fibers. During the aging process, preferential denervation of type II muscle fibers occurs that can lead to their atrophy. Some type II fibers may be reinnervated by type I motor neurons, which leads to the transition of type II fibers into type I fibers. As a result of these processes, the proportion of type I fibers in the elderly is higher, and the proportion of type II fibers lower, than in younger persons. It should also be noted that the aging profile is different in various muscles. The above-mentioned phenomenon of the increase in the number of type I fibers and the decrease in the number of type II fibers with age has been reported, for example, for limb muscle including *vastus lateralis*. Other muscles, for example, human jaw muscles, exhibit the inverse change in fiber type profile with advanced age.[11]

Organ Cell Loss with Age

Another important aspect of skeletal muscle aging studies is the recognition of a gradual loss of muscle fibers throughout the life of the organism. It is considered that the muscle cell loss in humans is minimal before the age of 50 years. Thereafter, the loss accelerates and reaches about 5% per decade. The number of muscle fibers in one study has been shown to decrease by 39% in *vastus lateralis* muscle of old men (80+ years old) compared to young men (20–30 years old).[12]

Earlier studies of age-related changes in the central nervous system (CNS) have shown a similar rate of cell loss for CNS neurons. It has been reported that approximately 25% of CNS neurons are lost between the ages of 50 and 90 years, with an attrition rate of about 0.5% per year.[13,14] Later studies of the age-related cell loss in CNS have shown that the cell loss is unequal in different parts of the brain, with some areas showing a slow, gradual loss of neurons with age and others not showing significant changes in neuron numbers. For brain areas exhibiting cell loss, the rate of fallout was estimated at about 10% over decades.[15] For human cardiomyocytes, the cell loss between the ages of 18 and 90 years was estimated to reach 38 million cells per year in the left ventricle and 14 million cells per year in the right ventricle.[16] It is also of great interest that the age-related cell loss is generally accompanied by considerable hypertrophy of remaining cells that may be necessary to compensate for the decrease in cell numbers.[15,16]

We suggest that cell loss is the quintessential characteristic of the aging process of postmitotic tissues. By contrast, in mitotic tissues such as liver, cells are being continually replaced over one's lifetime, so that the organ function is well maintained; thus, age-associated systemic degeneration of liver function is an uncommon phenomenon.

Dual COX/SDH Histochemistry to Follow Muscle Fiber Loss with Age

As human aging is a gradual process taking place over decades, age-related changes observed at any one particular time point cannot be expected to be large relative to some earlier time. We have used a dual COX and SDH (succinate dehydrogenase) enzyme histochemistry assay to visualize the aforementioned age-associated muscle fiber loss. The COX enzyme complex of the electron transport chain (complex IV) comprises 13 subunits; the three catalytic subunits of the COX enzyme complex are encoded by mtDNA. The loss of COX activity in some muscle fibers with age has been widely reported,[17,18] and its loss coincides with nonfunctional mtDNA and mitochondrial energy loss.[6,7] COX negative fibers are extremely rare in young persons, but are readily detected in skeletal muscle of persons over 50 years of age.[17,18] The SDH enzyme complex (complex II) is a nuclear-encoded complex of the electron transport chain; therefore, negative SDH activity is a reflection of nuclear genome mutations.

We have used dual COX/SDH enzyme histochemistry to estimate the number of COX- and/or SDH-deficient fibers in vastus lateralis muscle of individuals of different age groups; thus, a large number of muscle fibers were examined for their COX and SDH reactivity (TABLE 1). The large majority of the fibers (97–99%) were COX and SDH positive. About 0–2%, however, were either of low COX activity or COX negative; more rarely and only in some patients, fibers that were both COX negative and SDH negative were detected (FIG. 1). We interpret the COX-negative fibers as severely damaged, probably progressing to death. On the other hand, the dual COX/SDH-negative fibers represent muscle cells that are either dead or in the process of dying and removal from the muscle mass as they represent cells whose mitochondrial and nuclear genomes have undergone extensive damage. These fibers exemplify the attrition rate of the tissue. Although only a low number of such fibers are seen at any one time over decades from the age of 50 to 80 years, it is suggested that such fibers could account for the overall loss of muscle mass and decrease in muscle function.

Gene Expression in Skeletal Muscle during Aging

There has long been a need for a global approach to the study of the aging process with its multiplicity of seemingly both related and unrelated random and nonrandom progression. Studies of identical twins separated early in life have demonstrated that even individuals with such closely related genomes can age very differently, emphasizing the key role played by an individual's physical and metabolic environment. It is then obvious that there will be a wide range of gene expressions in the tissues of individual subjects, some directly relevant, some irrelevant to the aging process.

About 5000–8000 particular genes can be estimated to determine an individual major cell type making up an organ such as skeletal muscle. The putative genes are largely unknown, and human gene microarrays are still in their developmental infancy. The results herein are too preliminary to comment upon except in a very generalized way, but they can serve to illustrate the direction in which future studies of the aging process will develop.

To begin the necessary studies, which will take many years to eventually detail and comprehend, we have applied microarray technology in order to study the role of changes in gene expression in muscle deterioration with age. Eight subjects were

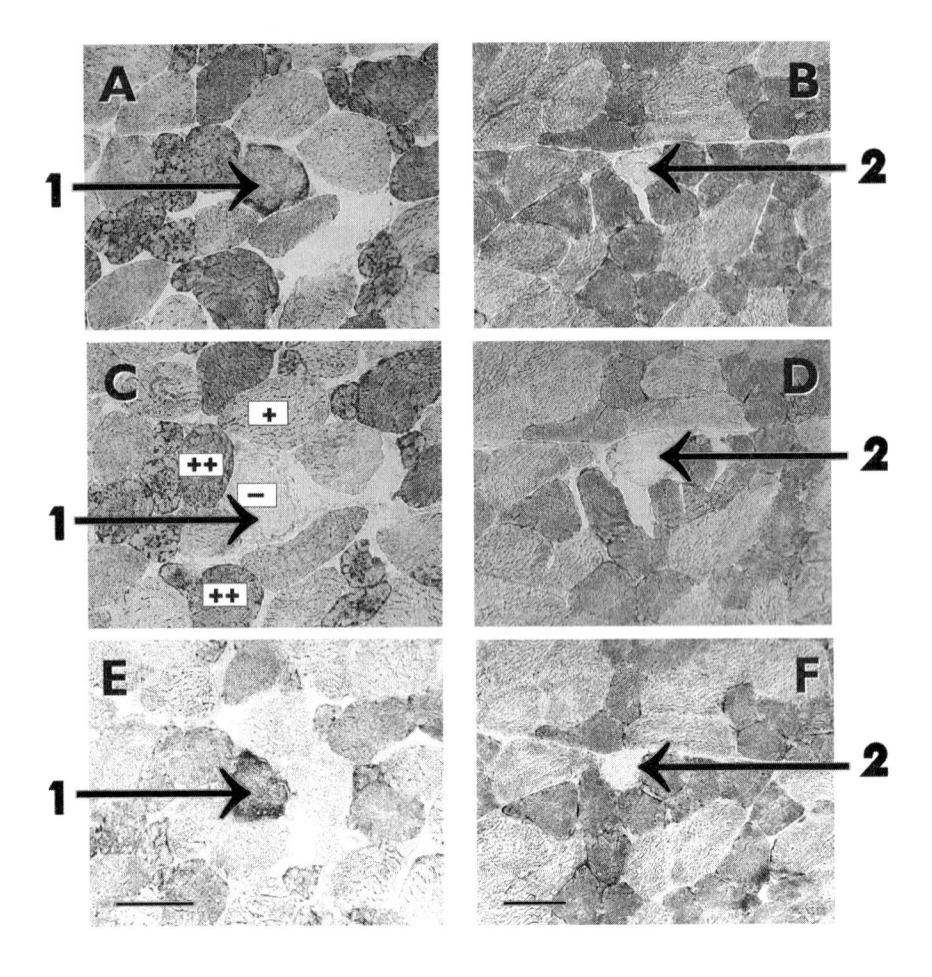

FIGURE 1. Dual COX/SDH activity histochemical staining of human vastus lateralis muscle. Serial sections of two quadriceps muscle samples (*left and right panels*) were stained either for COX activity (**C, D**), SDH activity (**E, F**), or for both activities on the same section (**A, B**). A small number of both COX-deficient and COX-negative fibers occurs in skeletal muscle of aged individuals (*arrows*). The large majority of COX-defective fibers are still positive for SDH activity ("1"); however, a very low number of fibers (less than 1%) defective in both enzymes ("2") is observed. "1" indicates a COX-negative/SDH-positive muscle fiber. "2" indicates a COX-negative/SDH-negative muscle fiber. ++, heavy staining of COX activity; +, weak staining of COX activity; −, no staining of COX activity. Bar indicates 100 µm.

TABLE 1. Human quadriceps muscle fiber analysis: COX/SDH activity

Age (years)	COX-positive Total	COX-positive % of total	COX trace/SDH-positive Total	COX trace/SDH-positive % of total	COX-negative/SDH-positive Total	COX-negative/SDH-positive % of total	COX-/SDH-negative Total	COX-/SDH-negative % of total
30	879	100	0	0	0	0	0	0
57	1954	99.95	0	0	1	0.05	0	0
63	828	100.00	0	0	0	0	0	0
69	1817	99.73	3	0.16	2	0.11	0	0
70	1126	99.1	7	0.6	3	0.3	0	0
75	1050	98.9	5	0.47	7	0.66	0	0
84	629	98.4	6	0.94	4	0.6	0	0
87	642	98.00	8	1.25	5	0.76	0	0
88	1748	97.22	34	1.89	16	0.89	0	0
89	846	99.06	3	0.35	5	0.59	0	0
56	622	96.14	5	0.77	3	0.46	17	2.63
58	3310	99.55	4	0.12	7	0.21	4	0.12
79	1708	99.13	9	0.52	5	0.29	1	0.06
86	760	96.45	21	2.66	4	0.51	3	0.38

NOTE: The percentage of COX-positive, COX trace/SDH-positive, COX-negative/SDH-positive, COX-negative/SDH-negative muscle fibers was determined as a percentage of the total number of fibers counted from particular individuals.

TABLE 2. Microarray analysis of gene expression in skeletal muscle — comparison of young and old human subjects

Category	Differential expression (fold)	Array 1 (30/85 years)	Array 2 (56/84 years)	Array 3 (22/81 years)	Array 4 (22/77 years)
Young > old	≥2	9	14	32	41
	1.5–1.9	27	49	89	102
Old > young	≥2	8	7	9	22
	1.5–1.9	38	161	39	210

TABLE 3. Number of genes consistently changed expression levels between young and old subjects (with a cut off point of 1.5-fold)

Category	Consistent in all 4 arrays	Consistent in any 3 arrays	Consistent in any 2 arrays
Young > Old	2	14	49
Old > young	1	1	39

arbitrarily assigned to four pairs, each consisting of a young subject and an old one. The ages of the individuals in the four pairs were 30/85, 56/84, 22/81, and 22/77 years. Messenger RNA (mRNA) was extracted, converted to cDNA, and labeled with the fluorescent dyes Cy-3 (for the young) and Cy-5 (for the old). The two fluorescently labeled samples (young and old) in each pair were mixed and used to hybridize a UniGEM V cDNA microarray (Incyte) containing 7000 genes and expressed sequence tags (ESTs). The hybridized array was then scanned, and the different intensities of the two fluorescent dyes were used as an indication of differential expression of particular genes.

A differential expression of a number of genes was seen in samples obtained from young and old subjects in each pair, as shown in TABLE 2. When the cutoff point was set at a twofold or greater difference, the number of genes showing higher expression in the young sample was 9, 14, 32, and 41 in the four pairs of samples. Eight, 7, 9, and 22 genes had higher expression in the old in the same four pairs of samples.

The differentially expressed genes were then compared between the four pairs of samples (TABLE 3). With 1.5-fold or greater difference as the cutoff point, only three genes changed expression consistently in all four pairs: two down-regulated and one up-regulated with age. Fifteen genes were consistent in any three pairs, and 88 genes consistent in any two pairs.

Among the genes with altered expression, the most prominent was the one encoding mitochondrial superoxide dismutase, which was down-regulated in old subjects in all four pairs, with an average 4.6-fold decrease in the old. Reactive oxygen species have been implicated in the aging process.[19,20] Superoxide is particularly damaging to macromolecules, and superoxide dismutase is an essential enzyme to convert superoxide to the less toxic hydrogen peroxide, which can then be further detoxified. The downregulation of gene expression of this enzyme with age is particularly pertinent to the aging process. Indeed, overexpression of cytosolic superoxide dismutase (together with catalase) has been reported to delay the aging process in the fly *Drosophila melanogaster*,[21] and treatment of the worm *Caenorhabditis elegans* with small synthetic superoxide dismutase/catalase mimetics increased the organism's mean lifespan.[22]

While our results are of a preliminary nature, they illustrate the power of these technologies for the study of the aging process. It can be readily envisioned that detailed gene expression and proteomic atlases of individual tissues of various ages will be a major future activity of many laboratories.

PART 2: EFFECTS OF CoQ_{10} IN SKELETAL MUSCLE OF AGED INDIVIDUALS

We have earlier reported on the re-energizing effect of CoQ_{10} and some of its analogues on skeletal muscle and isolated submitochondrial particles of aged rats.[23–25] There are also a large number of anecdotal reports of the beneficial effects of CoQ_{10} for the treatment of a variety of apparently unrelated clinical syndromes, as diverse as congestive heart failure,[26] muscular dystrophy,[27] chronic fatigue syndrome,[28] breast cancer,[29] and primary biliary cirrhosis.[30] It has also been suggested as an amelioration therapy, such as support for AIDS patients treated with AZT[31] with improved immune function.[32] However, the mechanism for these beneficial effects remains unclear.

In order to explore the wide-ranging effects of CoQ_{10} on human tissues, we have set up a clinical trial on the effects of CoQ_{10} on human vastus lateralis muscle. Human test subjects about to undergo hip replacement surgery received 300 mg CoQ_{10} per day for 25–30 days before surgery, whereas control subjects received placebo treatment. At the time of surgery, samples of vastus lateralis muscle were taken from the same region, and gene and protein expression patterns and muscle fiber type profiles were compared between placebo and CoQ_{10}-treated subjects. We report here that CoQ_{10} regulates the expression of numerous genes and proteins. Furthermore, a dramatic change in muscle fiber types towards profiles of young people was observed in subjects treated with CoQ_{10}. We conclude that CoQ_{10} can function as a gene regulator, which may account for its wide-ranging effects.

Effects of CoQ_{10} on Gene Expression in Skeletal Muscle of Aged Individuals Studied by Microarray Analysis

As we have earlier reported,[3] we assessed the effects of CoQ_{10} on gene expression in human skeletal muscle of aged individuals by gene microarray analysis. Skeletal muscle samples of three CoQ_{10} subjects (aged 70, 75, and 76 years) and two placebo subjects (aged 63 and 79 years) were studied. Total RNA isolated from each muscle sample obtained at surgery was used, after appropriate labeling, to hybridize a human U95A oligonucleotide array (Affymetrix) containing 12,000 annotated genes. We then compared the gene expression levels between each of the three CoQ_{10}-treated persons and each of the two placebo subjects, generating a total of six comparisons. Many genes showed differential expression between the two samples in each comparison. Differentially expressed genes consistent in all six comparisons

TABLE 4. Number of proteins resolved in each gel

	Gel pH 4-7		Gel pH 7-10		
Patient	Fraction 1 (soluble)	Fraction 2 (sediment)	Fraction 1 (soluble)	Fraction 2 (sediment)	Total
Placebo 1	660	539	667	188	2054
Placebo 2	749	661	560	174	2144
Placebo 3	830	596	772	176	2374
Placebo 4	620	459	447	211	1737
CoQ_{10} 1	727	442	587	181	1937
CoQ_{10} 2	697	688	524	160	2069
CoQ_{10} 3	765	538	707	160	2170

were then identified. At a cutoff point of 1.8-fold, there were 115 genes consistently differentially expressed in all six comparisons, with 47 genes up-regulated and 68 down-regulated in the CoQ_{10}-treated subjects.

Examples of the up-regulated genes include the following: the glutamate receptor protein GluR5, which has a function in neuronal transmission and synapsis development;[33] guanylyl cyclase, which is the receptor for nitric oxide signaling[34] and is redox sensitive;[35] fibroblast growth factor receptor N-SAM is essential for muscle growth and development; and a number of protein kinases that are involved in cell cycle control and cell signaling. The down-regulated genes include TTF-1 interacting peptide 20, which is important in transcription termination; and the TR3 orphan receptor, which is a steroid hormone receptor involved in apoptosis.[36,37] Several transcription factors and the gene regulator hZFH helicase[38] were also down-regulated, as was the major group Rhinovirus receptor, which is an adhesion molecule essential for cold virus infection.[39] It is difficult to interpret these changes for a variety of reasons, and no attempt is made to do so, but the conclusion that can be reached is that CoQ_{10} modulates gene expression.

Effects of CoQ_{10} on Skeletal Muscle Proteome

In order to determine whether the regulation of gene expression by CoQ_{10} is also reflected at the protein level, the high-abundance proteome of vastus lateralis muscle samples from four placebo and three CoQ_{10}-treated individual were analyzed with the aim of identifying proteins potentially regulated by CoQ_{10}. By overlaying and matching the seven 2D gels in each of two pH ranges (pH 4–7 and pH 7–10), individual proteins could be identified and categorized into one of three groups: (a) specific proteins that only appear in the CoQ_{10} samples or at least three of the four placebo samples; (b) common proteins that appear in at least six of the seven samples; or (c) nonmatched proteins that appear in five or fewer samples nonspecifically between the treated and placebo samples.

Approximately 2000 proteins were visualized in each of the samples (TABLE 4). The results of protein matching are summarized in TABLE 5. Of the proteins detected, the expression of 229 proteins appear to be induced by CoQ_{10}, whereas the expres-

TABLE 5. Protein matching of coenzyme Q10 vs placebo vastus lateralis muscle samples—average gel results

Protein	Gel pH 4-7 Fraction 1 (soluble)	Gel pH 4-7 Fraction 2 (sediment)	Gel pH 7-10 Fraction 1 (soluble)	Gel pH 7-10 Fraction 2 (sediment)
Placebo	116	31	58	31
CoQ$_{10}$	91	61	57	20
Common	460	369	127	155
Nonmatched	75	60	338	11

sion of 236 appears to be repressed by the treatment. Although of a preliminary nature, these results suggest that CoQ$_{10}$ treatment is modulating muscle protein expression. Current work is concerned with the expansion of the number of samples in both the treated and placebo groups, and the characterization of specific proteins by MALDI-TOF mass spectroscopy.[40]

Change of Fiber Type Composition of Vastus Lateralis Muscle upon CoQ$_{10}$ Treatment

Skeletal muscle is a highly heterogenous tissue consisting of a few different muscle fiber types that vary in their energy profile. The type of the muscle fiber is determined by the type of myosin heavy chain it expresses; some fibers express only one myosin heavy chain ("pure" fibers), whereas others may co-express two or more myosin heavy chains ("hybrid" fibers). Myofibrillar actomyosin adenosine triphosphatase (mATPase) histochemistry analysis is one of the most common procedures used for the delineation of muscle fiber types.[41] This method is based on the observation that fast and slow myosins have different alkaline and acid stabilities. Histochemically, fast muscle fibers display high mATPase activity under alkaline conditions and low activity under acid conditions, whereas slow muscle fibers exhibit the inverse. Routine mATPase histochemistry allows delineation of the following fiber types: I, IIa, IIab, IIb, Ic, IIc, and IIac. The last three fiber types are intermediate in their staining characteristics between type I and type IIa fibers and are often referred to as C-fibers or IM (intermediate) fibers.

It is well known that aging results in a gradual loss of muscle function. This loss is due to the age-associated changes in the number and size of muscle fibers, and also to the age-related changes in the muscle fiber type composition. Type I fibers seem to be little affected by aging. Numerous studies have failed to show any significant changes in cross-sectional area of type I fibers with age,[10,42,43] whereas type II fibers have been reported to decrease in size by about 25% from age 20 to 80.[12] Changes in size for both type IIa and IIb muscle fibers have been documented.[44]

It should be emphasized that analysis of the quadriceps fiber type composition in humans is complicated because of the high variability of the muscle profile in different individuals. In addition, the proportion of fiber types varies significantly in different portions of the muscle, with a higher number of type I fibers in the medial part of the quadriceps and a lower number in the lateral part. Thus, for comparative

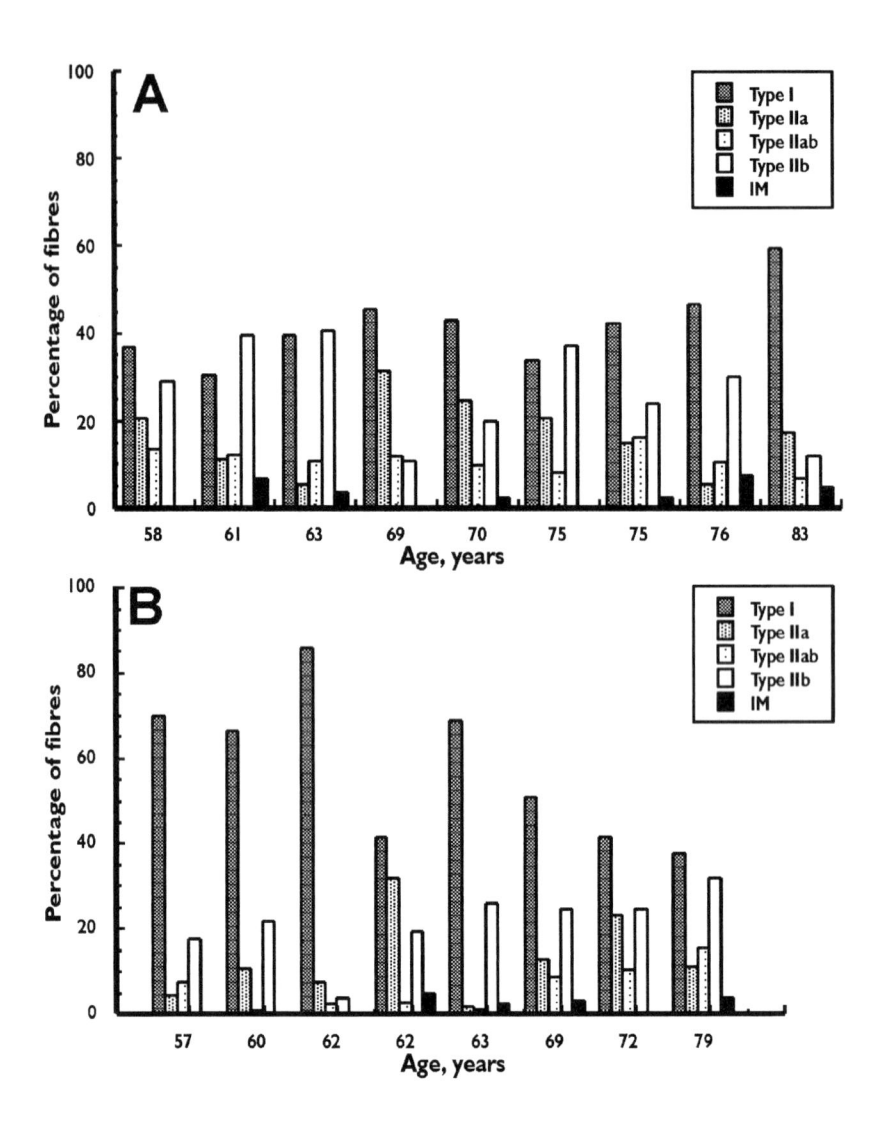

FIGURE 2. Fiber type composition of vastus lateralis muscle from CoQ_{10}-treated (A) and placebo (B) patients. Indicated is the proportion of each of the common fiber types found in quadriceps muscle samples from nine individuals treated with CoQ_{10} (**A**) and eight individuals treated with placebo (**B**). The different fiber types in muscle sections can be distinguished by evaluation of myofibrillar ATPase activity of muscle fibers. The procedure is based on the observation that fast (type II) and slow (type I) myosins have different alkaline and acid stability. This classical histochemical technique allows the recognition of the following fiber types: I, IIa, IIab, IIb, Ic, IIc, and IIac. To simplify the analysis, all C fibers (Ic, IIc, and IIac) were pooled together (IM = intermediate fibers).

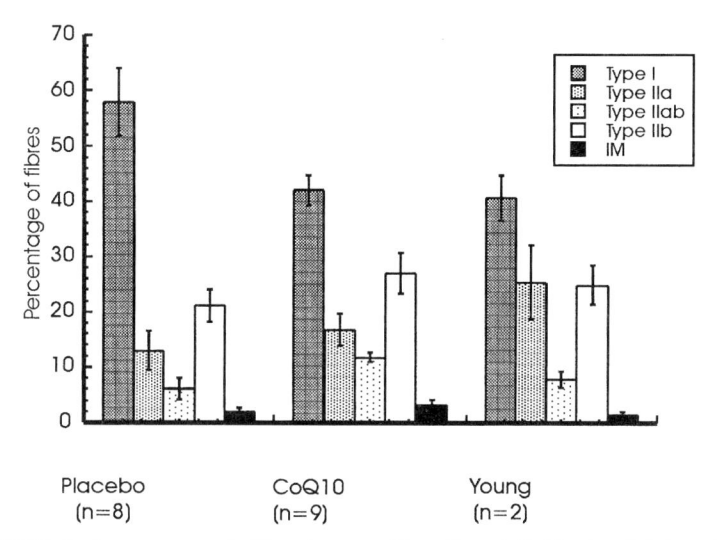

[Bar chart showing percentage of fibres for Placebo (n=8), CoQ10 (n=9), and Young (n=2) groups, with Type I, Type IIa, Type IIab, Type IIb, and IM fiber types.]

FIGURE 3. Average muscle fiber type profiles of aged CoQ_{10}-treated ($n = 9$) and aged placebo-treated ($n = 8$) individuals compared to an average muscle fiber type profile of young (<50 yr) males ($n = 2$).

analyses, it is important that the muscle tissue is collected from the same portion of the muscle in different subjects.

In our study, we have analyzed fiber type profiles of quadriceps muscles of 17 male subjects older than 57 years, eight receiving the placebo (mean age 65.5 ± 2.6) and nine receiving the CoQ_{10} supplementation (mean age 70.4 ± 2.7). Despite large variations in fiber type composition both among placebo and CoQ_{10} subjects, it was clear that the placebo and CoQ_{10} samples were different in their fiber type composition. The number of type I fibers in vastus lateralis muscle of eight out of nine CoQ_{10}-treated subjects was less than 50%, whereas five out of nine placebo samples showed the proportion of type I fiber type higher than 50% (FIG. 2). The difference in the number of type I fibers between placebo and CoQ_{10} patients was found to be statistically significant ($P < 0.05$). CoQ_{10}-treated samples generally had a higher proportion of type II fibers (IIa, IIab, IIb), but the difference was statistically significant ($P < 0.05$) for type IIab fibers only (FIG. 3). The results obtained suggest that the patients receiving CoQ_{10} have an altered fiber type composition more reflective of younger muscle than the group receiving the placebo.

CONCLUSION

It is important to recall that the human organism ages to death over decades, so that deleterious aging effects on a yearly basis will be small. The number of cells of postmitotic tissues slowly decreases in late life, compensated for commonly by cellular hypertrophy and fibrous tissue expansion to maintain mass or even increase organ size. The tissues are in a dynamic equilibrium: Macromolecular damage and repair are finely balanced, with the equilibrium gradually shifting towards damage.

During a person's lifetime, mtDNA undergoes a variety of mutations and rearrangements. These mutations and the consequent bioenergenic decline, especially in postmitotic tissues, are among the factors contributing to the reduced function of cells and organs. Fiber type profiles of skeletal muscle change during aging, and the number and size of the muscle fibers are reduced. The COX/SDH double-negative fibers represent both mtDNA mutation and nuclear DNA damage in those cells, and these fibers are considered to be in the process of death and elimination.

In this paper we have asked the question whether CoQ_{10} can ameliorate the rate of tissue aging. The results suggest that this may indeed be possible. The data presented here indicate that CoQ_{10} functions as a major skeletal muscle gene regulator and modulates cellular metabolism. CoQ_{10}, as demonstrated by microarray gene expression analysis, affects the expression of a number of genes. Proteome analysis reflects the global response of CoQ_{10} supplementation on the protein expression profile of the muscle tissue. In addition, skeletal muscle fiber types were shown to change as a result of CoQ_{10} administration to human subjects towards the muscle fiber profile of younger subjects.

How can CoQ_{10} have such wide-ranging effects and act as a gene regulator when it is membrane localized? The wide-ranging effects of CoQ_{10} may be explained by its broad-based cellular redox function. It has been proposed that CoQ_{10} plays a key role in manipulating the redox potential poise, thereby affecting subcellular membrane potential changes, resulting in the differential regulation of subcellular membrane activities and compartments.[3] Different subcellular redox poises and their modulation would lead to wide-ranging metabolic changes. Furthermore, superoxide anions generated by reactions involving CoQ_{10} would reflect specific redox poise and would play a major role in cellular regulation. H_2O_2 produced from superoxide would act as a second messenger in the regulation of gene and proteome expression.

In deriving these concepts, the following facts were considered: It has been reported that the relative oxidation/reduction level of plastoquinone regulates chloroplast DNA transcription and the specific products of transcription. It was hypothesized that mitochondrial transcription may be similarly regulated.[45] Through the Q cycle, CoQ_{10} is involved in determining mitochondrial membrane potential and, in turn, energy synthesis and mitochondrial substrate utilization. CoQ_{10} has also been shown to be an essential cofactor of the uncoupling proteins that act to downregulate mitochondrial membrane potential.[46] The occurrence of a lysosomal CoQ_{10} oxido-reductase system, which establishes a proton gradient across the membrane, has recently been demonstrated.[47] Such a system would contribute to the regulation of metabolite movement in and out of the lysosome. Crane and colleagues have extensively reported on the properties of a CoQ_{10} NADH oxido-reductase enzyme complex in the plasma membrane, which again will contribute to redox potential poise and substrate movement.[48] Furthermore, Crane et al.[49] have made a preliminary report on a CoQ_{10} oxido-reductase localized in the Golgi membrane complex. Based on these observations, we have proposed that further studies may show that the CoQ_{10} located in other membrane systems reflects undiscovered oxido-reductase systems that will contribute to the determination of individual membrane potentials.[3]

CoQ_{10} has been shown to function as a proton/electron donor through which sulfhydryl/disulfide intraprotein crosslinks are converted, and, in part, it determines protein conformations.[50] Finally, CoQ_{10} not only acts as an antioxidant, but also as a prooxidant, continually giving rise to superoxide anion, which is converted to H_2O_2 by superoxide dismutase. Because H_2O_2 has been shown to function as a mitogen and is involved in the regulation of gene expression,[51,52] the regulation of gene expression by CoQ_{10} may be achieved using H_2O_2 as a second messenger.[3]

REFERENCES

1. LINNANE, A.W. et al. 1989. Mitochondrial DNA mutations as an important contributor to ageing and degenerative diseases. Lancet **1:** 642–645.
2. KOPSIDAS, G. et al. 2000. Tissue mitochondrial DNA change: a stochastic system. Ann. N.Y. Acad. Sci. **908:** 226–243.
3. LINNANE, A.W. et al. 2001. Cellular redox activity of coenzyme Q_{10}: effect of CoQ_{10} supplementation on human skeletal muscle. Free Radic. Res. In press.
4. LINNANE, A.W. 2000. Human skeletal muscle aging; a lifestyle determinant. Proc. Fifth Shizuoka Forum on Health and Longevity: 43–52. Shizuoka Perpetual Government, Japan.
5. NAGLEY, P. & C. ZHANG. 1998. Mitochondrial DNA mutations in aging. In Mitochondrial DNA Mutations in Aging, Disease and Cancer. K.K. Singh, Ed.: 205–238. Springer-Verlag and R.G. Landes. Georgetown, TX.
6. KOVALENKO, S.A. et al. 1998. Tissue-specific distribution of multiple mitochondrial DNA rearrangements during human aging. Ann. N.Y. Acad. Sci. **854:** 171–182.
7. KOPSIDAS, G. et al. 1998. An age-associated correlation between cellular bioenergy decline and extensive mtDNA rearrangements in human skeletal muscle. Mutat. Res. **421:** 27–36.
8. LARSSON, L., B. SJODOIN & J. KARLSSON. 1978. Histochemical and biochemical changes in human skeletal muscle with age in sedentary males age 22–65 years. Acta Physiol. Scand. **103:** 31–39.
9. LEXELL, J. et al. 1983. Distribution of different fibre types in human skeletal muscles: effect of aging studied in whole muscle cross-sections. Muscle Nerve **6:** 588–593.
10. ANIANSSON, A. et al. 1981. Muscle morphology, enzyme activity, and muscle strength in elderly men and women. Clin. Physiol. **1:** 75–86.
11. MONEMI, M. et al. 1999. Adverse changes in fibre type and myosin heavy chain compositions of human jaw muscle vs. limb muscle during ageing. Acta. Physiol. Scand. **167:** 339–345.
12. LEXELL, J., C.C. TAYLOR & M. SJOSTROM. 1988. What is the cause of the ageing atrophy? Total number, size and proportion of different fibre types studied in whole vastus lateralis muscle from 15- to 83-year old men. J. Neurol. Sci. **84:** 275–294.
13. BYRNE, E. & X. DENNETT. 1992. Respiratory chain failure in adult muscle fibers: relationship with ageing and possible implications for the neuronal pool. Mutat. Res. **275:** 125–131.
14. BROOKS, S.V. & J.A. FAULKNER. 1994. Skeletal muscle weakness in old age: underlying mechanisms. Med. Sci. Sports Exerc. **26:** 432–439.
15. MORRISON, J.H. & P.R. HOF. 1997. Life and death of neurons in the aging brain. Science **278:** 412–419.
16. OLIVETTI, G. et al. 1991. Cardiomyopathy of the aging human heart. Myocyte loss and reactive cellular hypertrophy. Circ. Res. **68:** 1560–1568.
17. MÜLLER-HÖCKER, J. 1990. Cytochrome c oxidase deficient fibers in the limb muscle and diaphragm of man without muscular disease: an age-related alteration. J. Neurol. Sci. **100:** 14–21.
18. NAGLEY, P. et al. 1992. Mitochondrial DNA mutation associated with aging and degenerative disease. Ann. N.Y. Acad. Sci. **673:** 92–102.
19. HARMAN, D. 1956. Role of free radical and radiation chemistry. J. Gerontol. **11:** 298–300.

20. HARMAN, D. 1983. Free radical theory of aging: consequences of mitochondrial aging. Age **6:** 86–94.
21. ORR, W.C. & R.S. SOHAL. 1994. Extension of life-span by overexpression of superoxide dismutase and catalase in *Drosophila melanogaster*. Science **263:** 1128–1130.
22. MELOV, S. *et al.* 2000. Extension of life-span with superoxide dismutase/catalase mimetics. Science **289:** 1567–1569.
23. LINNANE, A.W. *et al.* 1995. The universality of bioenergetic disease and amelioration with redox therapy. Biochim. Biophys. Acta **1271:** 191–194.
24. ROSENFELDT, F.L. *et al.* 1999. Coenzyme Q_{10} improves the tolerance of the senescent myocardium to aerobic and ischemic stress: studies in rats and in human atrial tissue. Biofactors **9:** 291–299.
25. ROWLAND, M.A. *et al.* 1998. Coenzyme Q_{10} treatment improves the tolerance of the senescent myocardium to pacing stress in the rat. Cardiovasc. Res. **40:** 165–173.
26. LANGSJOEN, H. *et al.* 1994. Usefulness of coenzyme Q_{10} in clinical cardiology: a long-term study. Mol. Aspects Med. **15**(Suppl.): s165–s175.
27. FOLKERS, K. & R. SIMONSEN. 1995. Two successful double-blind trials with coenzyme Q_{10} (vitamin Q_{10}) on muscular dystrophies and neurogenic atrophies. Biochim. Biophys. Acta **1271:** 281–286.
28. WERBACH, M.R. 2000. Nutritional strategies for treating chronic fatigue syndrome. Alt. Med. Rev. J. Clin. Ther. **5:** 93–108.
29. LOCKWOOD, K. *et al.* 1995. Progress on therapy of breast cancer with vitamin Q_{10} and the regression of metastases. Biochem. Biophys. Res. Commun. **212:** 172–177.
30. WATSON, J.P. *et al.* 1999. Case report: oral antioxidant therapy for the treatment of primary biliary cirrhosis: a pilot study. J. Gastroenterol. Hepatol. **14:** 1034–1040.
31. TANNER, H.A. 1992. Energy transformations in the biosynthesis of the immune system: their relevance to the progression and treatment of AIDS. Med. Hypoth. **38:** 315–321.
32. FOLKERS, K., M. MORITA & J. McREE JR. 1993. The activities of coenzyme Q_{10} and vitamin B6 for immune responses. Biochem. Biophys. Res. Commun. **193:** 88–92.
33. DINGLEDINE, R. & P.J. CONN. 2000. Peripheral glutamate receptors: molecular biology and role in taste sensation. J. Nutr. **130**(Suppl.): 1039S–1042S.
34. KOESLING, D. 1999. Studying the structure and regulation of soluble guanylyl cyclase. Methods **19:** 485–493.
35. DIERKS, E.A. & J.N. BURSTYN. 1998. The deactivation of soluble guanylyl cyclase by redox-active agents. Arch. Biochem. Biophys. **351:** 1–7.
36. LI, H. *et al.* 2000. Cytochrome c release and apoptosis induced by mitochondrial targeting of nuclear orphan receptor TR3. Science **289:** 1159–1164.
37. UEMURA, H. & C. CHANG. 1998. Antisense TR3 orphan receptor can increase prostate cancer cell viability with etoposide treatment. Endocrinology **139:** 2329–2334.
38. AUBRY, F., M.G. MATTEI & F. GALIBERT. 1998. Identification of a human 17p-located cDNA encoding a protein of the Snf2-like helicase family. Eur. J. Biochem. **254:** 558–564.
39. BELLA, J. & M.G. ROSSMANN. 2000. ICAM-1 receptors and cold viruses. Pharm. Acta Helv. **74:** 291–297.
40. WALSH, B.J., M.P. MOLLOY & K.L WILLIAMS. 1998. The Australian Proteome Analysis Facility (APAF): assembling large scale proteomics through integration and automation. Electrophoresis **19:** 1883–1890.
41. BROOKE, M.H. & K.K. KAISER. 1970. Muscle fibre types: how many and what kind? Arch. Neurol. **23:** 369–379.
42. LEXELL, J. & C.C. TAYLOR. 1991. Variability in muscle fibre areas in whole human quadriceps muscle: effects of increasing age. J. Anat. **174:** 239–249.
43. JAKOBSSON, F., K. BORG & L. EDSTROM. 1990. Fibre type composition, structure and cytoskeletal protein location of fibres in anterior tibialis muscle: comparison between young adults and physically active aged humans. Acta Neuropathol. **80:** 459–468.
44. COGGAN, A.R. *et al.* 1992. Histochemical and enzymatic comparison of the gastrocnemius muscle of young and elderly men and women. J. Gerontol. **47:** B71–B76.

45. PFANNSCHMIDT, T., A. NILSSON & J.F. ALLEN. 1999. Photosynthetic control of chloroplast gene expression. Nature **397**: 625–628.
46. VAN BELZEN, R. *et al.* 1997. The iron-sulfur clusters 2 and ubisemiquinone radicals of NADH:ubiquinone oxidoreductase are involved in energy coupling in submitochondrial particles. Biochemistry **36**: 886–893.
47. GILLE L. & H. NOHL. 2000. The existence of a lysosomal redox chain and the role of ubiquinone. Arch. Biochem. Biophys. **375**: 347–354.
48. MORRE, D.J. *et al.* 1993. NADH oxidase activity of rat liver plasma membrane activated by guanine nucleotides. Biochem. J. **292**: 647–653.
49. CRANE, F.L. *et al.* 1984. Coenzyme Q in Golgi apparatus membrane redox activity and proton uptake. *In* Biomedical and Clinical Aspects of Coenzyme Q. Vol. 4. K. Folkers & Y. Yamamura, Eds.: 77–85. Elsevier. Amsterdam.
50. GLOCKSHUBER, R. 1999. Where do the electrons go? Nature **401**: 30–31.
51. RUSNAK F. & T. REITER. 2000. Sensing electrons: protein phosphatase redox regulation. Trends Biochem. Sci. **25**: 527–529.
52. SMITH, J., E. LADI, *et al.* 2000. Redox state is a central modulator of the balance between self-renewal and differentiation in a dividing glial precursor cell. Proc. Natl. Acad. Sci. USA **97**: 10032–10037.

Mitochondrial DNA Deletion Mutations and Sarcopenia

JUDD AIKEN, ENTELA BUA, ZHENGJIN CAO, MARISOL LOPEZ, JON WANAGAT, DEBBIE McKENZIE, AND SUSAN McKIERNAN

*Department of Animal Health and Biomedical Sciences,
University of Wisconsin—Madison, Madison, Wisconsin 53706, USA*

> ABSTRACT: This manuscript summarizes our studies on mitochondrial DNA and enzymatic abnormalities that accumulate, with age, in skeletal muscle. Specific quadricep muscles, rectus femoris in the rat and vastus lateralis in the rhesus monkey, were used in these studies. These muscles exhibit considerable sarcopenia, the loss of muscle mass with age. The focal accumulation of mtDNA deletion mutations and enzymatic abnormalities in aged skeletal muscle necessitates a histologic approach in which every muscle fiber is examined for electron transport system (ETS) enzyme activity along its length. These studies demonstrate that ETS abnormalities accumulate to high levels within small regions of aged muscle fibers. Concomitant with the ETS abnormalities, we observe intrafiber atrophy and, in many cases, fiber breakage. Laser capture microdissection facilitates analysis of individual fibers from histologic sections and demonstrates a tight association between mtDNA deletion mutations and the ETS abnormalities. On the basis of these results, we propose a molecular basis for skeletal muscle fiber loss with age, a process beginning with the mtDNA deletion event and culminating with muscle fiber breakage and loss.
>
> KEYWORDS: mitochondrial DNA deletion mutations; sarcopenia; rectus femoris; vastus lateralis; electron transport system

MITOCHONDRIAL HYPOTHESIS OF AGING

The concept of mitochondrial DNA abnormalities being a causative factor in the aging process was proposed almost 20 years ago.[1,2] The circular 16-kb mitochondrial DNA molecule encodes 22 tRNAs, 2 rRNAs, and 13 polypeptides of the electron transport system (ETS). Each mitochondrion contains two to ten copies of the genome. The mitochondrial genome is susceptible to mutation damage due to a number of factors, including the following: (1) its close proximity to the source of reactive oxygen species generation; (2) the lack of protecting histone proteins; and (3) limitations of the mtDNA repair pathways. In addition, the compactness of the genetic information increases the likelihood that alterations of the genome would have a negative impact on the enzymatic activity.

Address for correspondence: Judd M. Aiken, 1656 Linden Dr., Madison, WI 53706. Voice: 608-262-7362; fax: 608-262-7420.

aiken@ahabs.wisc.edu

Direct evidence for the age-associated accumulation of mtDNA abnormalities required the development of the polymerase chain reaction (PCR), a technology that provided the sensitivity necessary to identify these low-abundance changes. Initial studies focused on human tissues and identified an age-associated increase in a specific 4977-bp mtDNA deletion mutation, often termed the "common deletion."[3,4] Subsequent studies identified multiple mtDNA deletion mutations in a variety of species, including humans,[5] rhesus monkeys,[6] mice,[7-10] and rats.[11-13] These studies, largely based on the analysis of tissue homogenates, demonstrated that mtDNA deletion mutations increase in frequency with age. Accurate estimates of the abundance of these abnormalities required the design of experiments that considered a focal (and not homogeneous) distribution of these abnormalities.

FOCAL ACCUMULATION OF mtDNA ABNORMALITIES

Initially, we characterized age-associated mtDNA abnormalities by examining whole-tissue homogenates of rodent and primate skeletal muscle of diverse ages. A PCR-based approach was employed to identify mtDNA deletion mutations. Primers were positioned ~8 kb apart, within the major arc of the mitochondrial genome, and amplification conditions were designed to selectively amplify smaller than wild-type products (i.e., deletion mutations). The number of mtDNA deletion products increased with age. The different deletion products were also variable in size and location, suggesting that different mtDNA genes had been lost. As mentioned above, the necessity of using PCR to identify these changes indicated that, in tissue homogenates, which contain tens of thousands of muscle fibers, the abundance of an individual deletion product (compared to wild-type mtDNA) was exceedingly low. Homogenate studies are, however, premised upon the assumption that the molecular events being analyzed (in this case, mtDNA deletion mutations) are distributed evenly in every cell or muscle fiber. Using *in situ* hybridization, Müller-Höcker[14] demonstrated that deletion mutations in human skeletal muscle were not distributed homogeneously but rather in a mosaic manner. Through the molecular analysis of defined numbers of muscle fibers from aged primates, we determined that the number of deletion products observed increased with the number of fibers assayed.[15] mtDNA deletion mutations were rarely observed when 10 fibers were used for PCR, whereas all 75 fiber samples contained numerous mtDNA deletion mutations. Furthermore, the calculated abundance of the individual mtDNA deletion product was inversely proportional to the number of fibers in the assay. The abundance of the mtDNA deletion mutations identified in the 10 fiber samples dramatically increased from the abundance calculated from the 75 fiber or tissue homogenate samples.[15] In summary, both histological and biochemical analyses argued the inappropriateness of homogenate studies for the characterization of age-associated mtDNA deletion mutations.

Although it was clear that mtDNA deletion mutations accumulated, with age, to high levels in individual muscle fibers, questions remained as to whether these changes resulted in an observable phenotype and whether they had any potential deleterious consequences. *In situ* hybridization studies[14,16,17] revealed that mitochondrial ETS abnormalities were concomitant with the mtDNA deletion mutation. Age-associated defects of mitochondrial respiratory function are known to accumulate in skeletal muscle of humans, rhesus monkeys, and rodents.[13,16–19] Two ETS enzyme activities are typically and conveniently studied: cytochrome c oxidase (COX, complex IV) and succinate dehydrogenase (SDH, complex II). Histological analysis of these two ETS enzyme activities can provide an initial indication of the integrity of the mitochondrial genomes present in a cell. Complex IV comprises 10 subunits, three of which are encoded by the mtDNA. Loss or disruption of any of the mitochondrially encoded COX subunits would result (if the mutant mtDNA accumulates to sufficient levels) in an overt decline in COX activity. Complex II, on the other hand, being entirely nuclear encoded, would not be directly affected. A common ETS-abnormal phenotype observed in aging skeletal muscle is the complete loss of detectable COX activity (COX^-) concomitant with SDH hyperreactivity (SDH^{++}). The SDH^{++} phenotype results from a dramatic increase in the number of mitochondria in the affected region, presumably due to a nuclear response to the decline in COX and/or an energy deficit in the muscle fiber. The number of muscle fibers containing ETS abnormalities was found to increase with age in both rats and rhesus monkeys. In the rhesus monkey, due to the diverse ages of animals studied, a relative comparison of

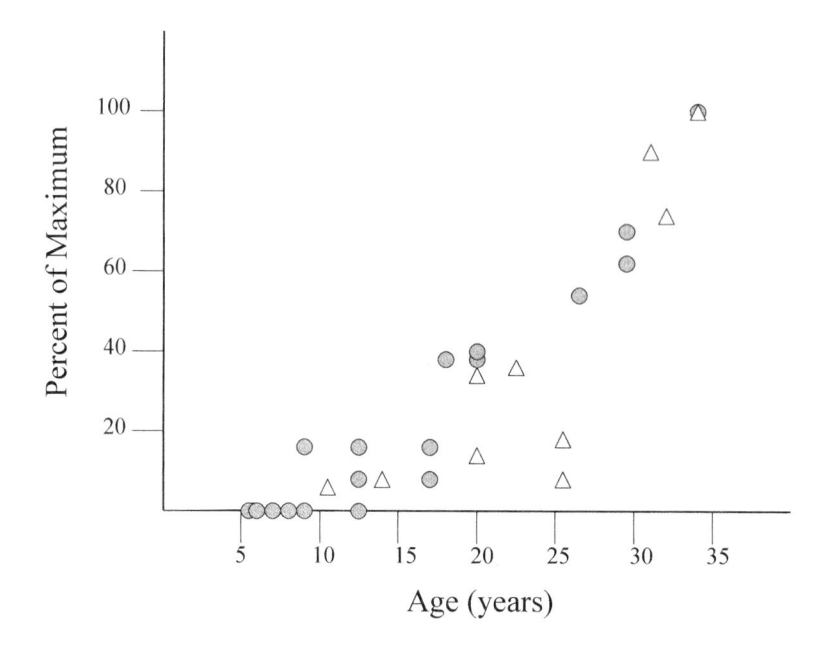

FIGURE 1. Correlation of mitochondrial DNA deletion mutations with ETS abnormalities in rhesus monkeys. The number of mtDNA deletion mutations (*gray circles*) and the number of ETS abnormalities (*open triangles*) are presented as a percent of the maximum number of each observed. mtDNA deletion mutations were determined by analysis of vastus lateralis muscle by PCR, using mitochondrial DNA-specific primers. ETS abnormalities were determined by histologic staining of several sections of the vastus lateralis muscle for COX and SDH activities. A fiber was considered to be abnormal if the enzymatic phenotype was COX^-/SDH^{++}.

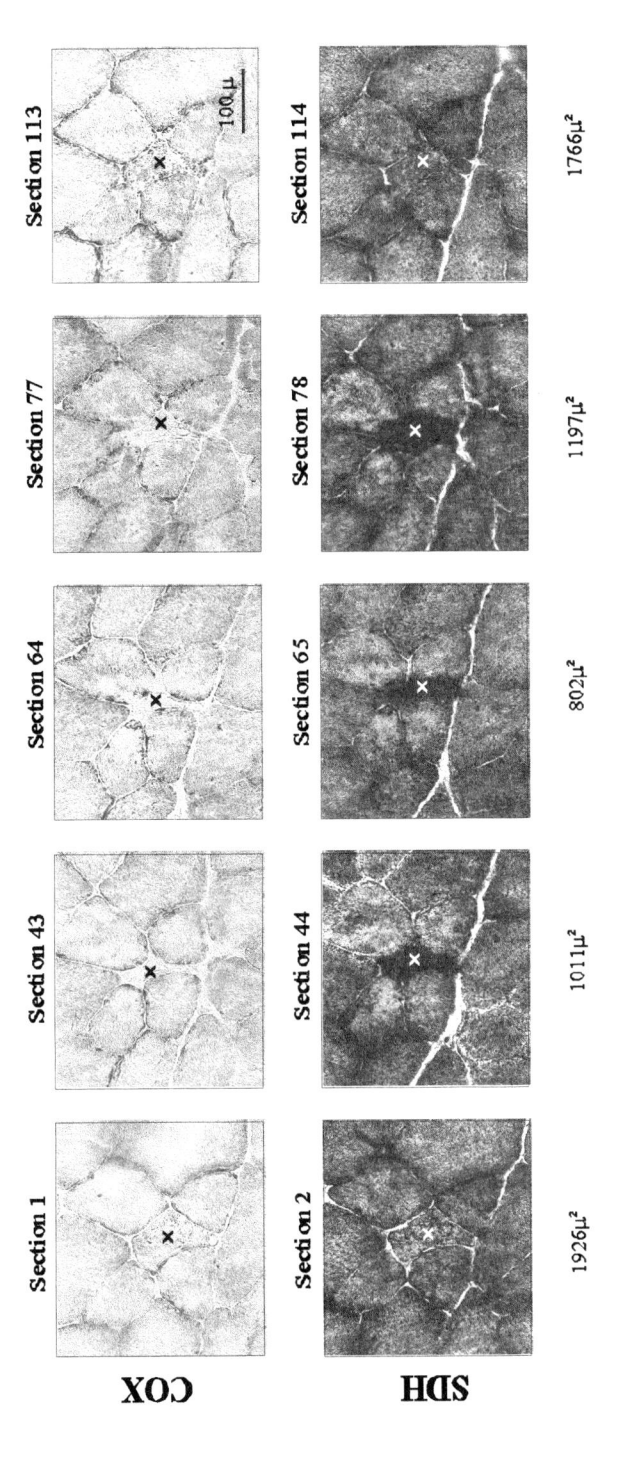

FIGURE 2. Identification and characterization of ETS-abnormal fibers in rectus femoris muscle. Adjacent serial sections, 70 microns apart, from rat rectus femoris muscle were stained with COX and SDH, respectively. The fiber that displays the ETS abnormality is marked with an "x." The cross-sectional area of the highlighted fiber is indicated below the pairs of sections.

the accumulation of the genomic and enzymatic abnormalities can be made. The number of mtDNA deletion mutations (primers to the major arc region, ~8 kb apart) from tissue homogenates and the number of ETS abnormalities from rhesus monkey vastus lateralis muscle of diverse ages were plotted as a percentage of the maximum value (FIG. 1). The age-associated increase in the number of amplification products coincides temporally with the increase in ETS abnormalities with age.

Although ETS abnormalities and mtDNA deletion mutations increase in abundance with age, the determination of the total number of fibers containing these linked abnormalities required an extensive histologic analysis of muscle fibers along their length. This is because the ETS abnormalities do not extend throughout the length of the affected muscle fiber but rather are localized to a small region or segment of the fiber. This phenomenon is illustrated in FIGURE 2; muscle fibers from old rats were stained for COX and SDH and followed along their length. One fiber (indicated with an "x") exhibits normal COX and SDH staining in the first set of slides analyzed. By slide 43 (430 microns from the initial sections), a COX^-/SDH^{2+} phenotype was evident. The fiber remained ETS abnormal through slides 64, 65 and 77, 78, returning to a normal COX and SDH phenotype by slides 113 and 114, respectively. Thus, because of this segmental distribution, individual fibers should be followed along their length for an accurate estimate of the abundance of ETS-abnormal fibers.

Rat rectus femoris muscle (one of the quadricep muscles) was dissected from young (5 month, $n = 6$), middle-aged (18 months, $n = 9$), and old (36 and 38 months, $n = 11$) Fisher 344 × Brown Norway F1 hybrid rats. Each muscle was weighed, bisected at the midbelly, and embedded in OCT. One hundred consecutive frozen serial sections were obtained. Slide 1 was stained with hemotoxylin and eosin (H&E), slide 2 for COX activity, and slide 3 for SDH activity. This pattern was repeated on slides 8, 9, 10…15, 16, 17…etc, through the 100 consecutive sections obtained. In this manner, we characterized ETS enzyme phenotypes and their abnormalities throughout the 1 mm of tissue sectioned with a resolution of 70 microns. Fiber number was determined by directly counting the number of fibers present in an H&E-stained section from the midbelly for each dissected muscle.

Considerable sarcopenia was evident in the rat rectus femoris muscle. A significant muscle mass loss was observed in the muscle obtained from old rats (FIG. 3a). Between 18 months and 36–38 months, a 45% decline in muscle weight occurred. Fiber number also declined tremendously during this period, with an average of 10,358 fibers being present at the midbelly of rectus femoris muscle in 18-month-old rats and only 7606 fibers remaining in the old animals (FIG. 3b).

Every muscle fiber was followed through the 1000 microns of tissue sectioned. Abnormal COX and SDH phenotypes were noted. None of the 5-month-old muscle fibers (62,000 fibers examined) harbored a COX^-/SDH^{++} phenotype (FIG. 4). One fiber (90,000 fibers examined) in the 18-month-old rectus femoris displayed this ETS abnormality. The 36- and 38-month-old rats, however, showed a significant increase in the number of COX^-/SDH^{++}-containing fibers (FIG. 4). At 36 months, 65 ETS abnormalities were observed in 45,000 fibers examined. In the 38-month-old animals, a total of 127 COX^-/SDH^{++} fibers were observed (39,000 fibers characterized). Thus, in rectus femoris, a muscle that undergoes considerable muscle mass and fiber loss with age, significant increases in the abundance of ETS abnormalities occur.

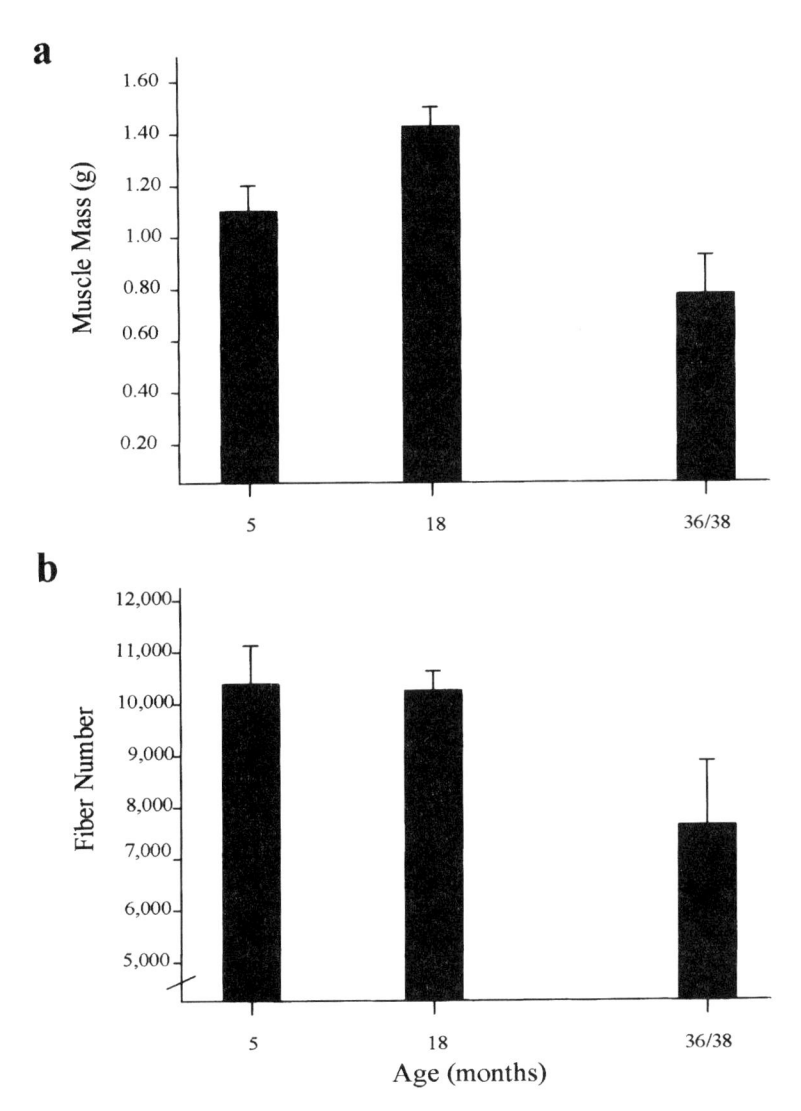

FIGURE 3. Sarcopenia in rat rectus femoris muscle. (a) Muscle mass of rectus femoris from 5- ($n = 6$), 18- ($n = 9$), and 36/38-month-old ($n = 11$) rats. (b) Fiber number from the same muscle and age groups as described in (a). Numbers were determined by counting fibers of a histochemically stained section from the midbelly of the muscle.

A similar approach was used for the characterization of vastus lateralis muscle from rhesus monkeys of diverse ages. In this study, muscle biopsies were obtained, and OCT embedded and sectioned. All the fibers present in the biopsy were followed for a length of 1600 microns.[17] An age-associated increase in abundance of ETS abnormalities was identified. One can estimate, based on the known length of a rhesus

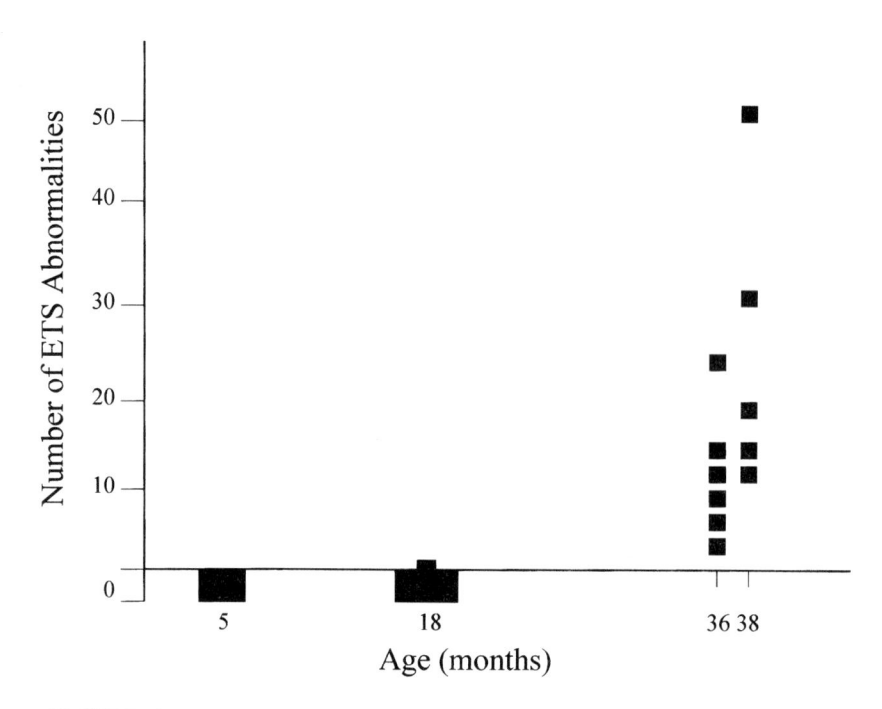

FIGURE 4. Age-associated accumulation of ETS abnormalities in the rectus femoris of rats. The number of ETS abnormalities was determined by histologic staining of the rectus femoris for COX and SDH activities; fibers were considered ETS abnormal if the staining pattern for a specific fiber was COX$^-$/SDH^{++}. Six animals were analyzed in the 5-month-old age group, nine animals in the 18-month-old age group, six in the 36-month-old group, and five in the 38-month-old group.

monkey vastus lateralis muscle fiber, the percentage of muscle fibers containing ETS abnormalities. These calculations indicate that ~60% of the muscle fibers present in rhesus monkeys >30 years of age contain an ETS abnormality somewhere along their length.[17] The diversity of ages studied, combined with the histological approaches employed, allowed us to compare the maximum length of the ETS abnormalities with age (FIG. 5). Some caution, however, must be employed in interpreting these results. First, many of the ETS abnormalities in the older animals extended beyond the length of muscle sectioned. Secondly, the increased number of ETS abnormalities present in the muscle of older animals could result in a broader range of lengths. Given these caveats, however, our data suggest that ETS abnormalities are being generated throughout the life of the animal. In addition, these abnormalities, with time, compose a larger and larger proportion of the muscle fiber. Given that ETS abnormalities were first observed in animals in their early teens, yet the maximum lengths of the abnormalities were not observed until the monkeys were in their early 30s, this expansion may, in the rhesus monkey, take years to develop.

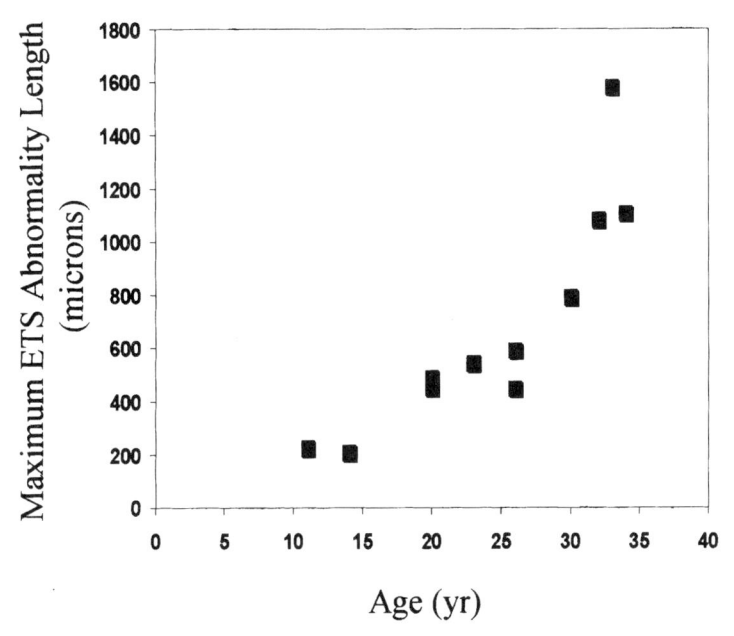

FIGURE 5. Maximum ETS abnormality length in different ages of rhesus monkeys. The maximum length of the ETS abnormalities found was determined by the longitudinal analysis of serial sections from the vastus lateralis of rhesus monkeys of different ages.

MITOCHONDRIAL ABNORMALITIES, INTRAFIBER ATROPHY, AND FIBER LOSS

The question still remained whether the mitochondrial abnormalities have a physiological impact on the affected skeletal muscle fibers. The examination of muscle fibers along their length clearly demonstrates intrafiber atrophy and fiber breakage to be concomitant with the COX$^-$/SDH^{++} regions of fibers. The longer the ETS-abnormal region, the greater the likelihood that the abnormal fiber would display fiber atrophy and fiber breakage. An example of this phenomenon is presented in FIGURE 2. The highlighted fiber is COX$^-$/SDH^{++}, and, as it is followed along its length, it dramatically declines in cross-sectional area. This intrafiber atrophy is present within the ETS-abnormal regions of muscle fibers; the adjacent ETS-normal region of the same fiber does not exhibit the atrophy.[13,17] Cross-sectional area was obtained using ImagePro software to quantitate the digital images of individual muscle fibers. The initial sections of the muscle fiber highlighted in FIGURE 2 are normal with respect to COX and SDH activities. Further along the fiber, 420 microns from the initial sections, the enzymatic activities of the fiber change to COX$^-$/SDH^{++}, and a 48% decline in cross-sectional area is observed. Moving 210 microns further along the length, the affected fiber remains COX$^-$/SDH^{++}, and the cross-sectional area is reduced 58% compared to the initial slides. Finally, 490 microns further along the muscle, the fiber exhibits normal COX and SDH activities again, and its cross-sectional area is similar to the first set of slides. With many fibers, the ETS-abnormal region declined in size to a point it no longer could be followed. We are interpreting this as evidence of fiber breakage. These data suggest a process by which an ETS-abnormal region develops, extends along the length of muscle fiber, becomes atrophic with time, and, eventually, breaks.

LASER CAPTURE MICRODISSECTION: DEFINING mtDNA ABNORMALITIES IN ETS-ABNORMAL REGIONS OF SINGLE MUSCLE FIBERS

In situ hybridization studies identified the presence of mtDNA deletion mutations in the majority of ETS-abnormal regions of muscle fibers. In rhesus monkey, for example, 90% of the COX^-/SDH^{++} fibers analyzed by *in situ* hybridization, using mtDNA probes from five different regions of the mitochondrial genome, did not react with one or more of the probes, indicating the presence of deletion mutations within those fibers. These studies do not permit precise determination of the breakpoints in the mtDNA, nor could we conclude that mtDNA deletion mutations were absent in the 10% of the ETS-abnormal fibers that reacted with all five probes (deletion events located between the probes would not be detected). Laser capture microdissection (LCM) allows us to directly address these questions. LCM facilitates the precise isolation and subsequent molecular characterization of individual cells or portions of cells from histologic samples. Individual skeletal muscle fiber sections were microdissected using a PixCell II laser capture microscope (Arcturus). Both COX^-/SDH^{++} and ETS-normal fibers, from the 10-micron sections of aged rat muscle, were captured by LCM. The samples were incubated in a DNA isolation buffer and amplified by PCR using mtDNA-specific primers.[20] The primers were specific to the control region of the rat mtDNA, and the amplification conditions employed (long extension PCR) facilitated amplification of the entire mitochondrial genome. Of the 29 ETS-abnormal regions analyzed by PCR, *all* produced smaller than wild-type amplification products.[20] Wild-type amplification products (16 kb) were not observed. Not only does this suggest the presence of high levels of deletion mutations within the ETS-abnormal region, but also the inability to amplify detectable levels of wild-type products indicates that the wild-type genome is either absent or present at very low levels. In contrast, amplification of 10 ETS-normal fibers and of regions adjacent to the ETS-abnormal region resulted in only wild-type product.[20] Sequence analysis of the deletion products precisely defined the size and breakpoints of the deletion mutations. All of the mtDNA deletion mutations were large, ranging in size from 4.4 to 9.7 kb, corresponding to mtDNAs of 6.6–11.9 kb. The deletions all occurred within the major arc region of the rat mtDNA (FIG. 6). Direct repeat sequences were not present at the mtDNA deletion breakpoints. These repeated sequences, which are present at the breakpoints of mtDNA deletion mutations associated with some mitochondrial myopathies, are often found at the breakpoints of age-associated mtDNA deletions in rhesus monkeys[6,21] and humans.[22] It has been argued that direct repeat sequences are important in mtDNA deletion formation. This would appear not to be a factor in deletion formation in the rat.

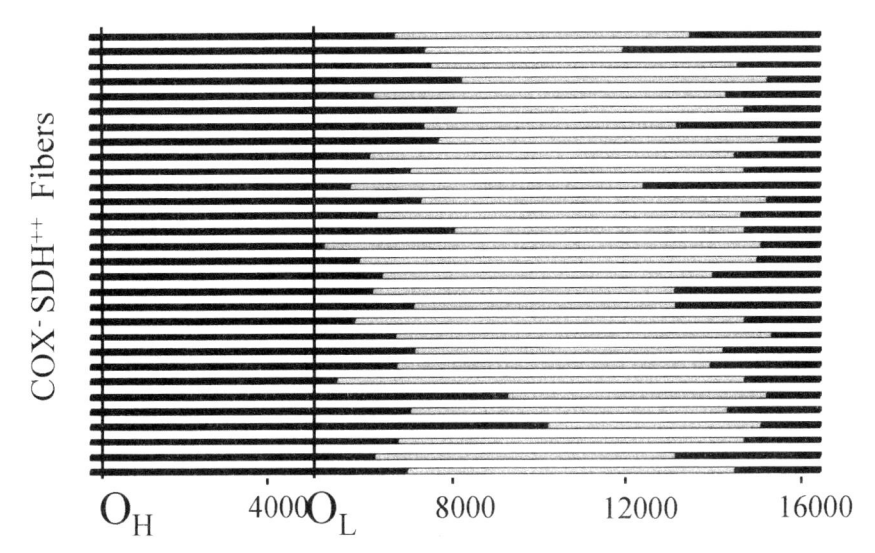

FIGURE 6. COX⁻/SDH⁺⁺-abnormal regions of a fiber were isolated using laser capture microscopy, and the DNA isolated and amplified, using conditions specific for whole mitochondrial genome amplification.[20] The region from O_H to O_L is the minor arc; the region from O_L to 16,000 kb is the major arc. The light bars represent the deleted sequences.

LCM was also used to capture the same fiber within and outside of the ETS-abnormal region. Smaller than wild-type amplification products were not observed in the ETS-normal regions of the fiber. Sampling the ETS-abnormal region from two different sections identified the same mtDNA deletion mutation, demonstrating the clonality of the deletion mutation within a given fiber.[20]

A MOLECULAR BASIS FOR AGE-ASSOCIATED FIBER LOSS

These studies have led us to propose the following mechanism for muscle fiber loss with age (FIG. 7). An early event is a mtDNA replication error that results in the deletion of a large region of the mitochondrial genome. This small genome apparently out-replicates the wild-type genome, becoming the predominant species in an expanding region of the muscle fiber. The high abundance of the deletion mutation in a specific region of a muscle fiber results in a focal decline in COX activity. The nuclear response to this decline in ETS efficiency appears to result in nuclear upregulation of mitochondrial biogenesis, further exacerbating the problem and producing the COX⁻/SDH⁺⁺ phenotype. This process expands along the length of the muscle fiber until the resulting energy deficit triggers the fiber atrophy and, eventually, fiber breakage. This fiber breakage produces the fiber loss observed with age.

MtDNA Deletion Mutation
↓
Accumulation of Deleted Genome
↑↓
ETS Abnormalities
↓
Intrafiber Atrophy
↓
Fiber Loss

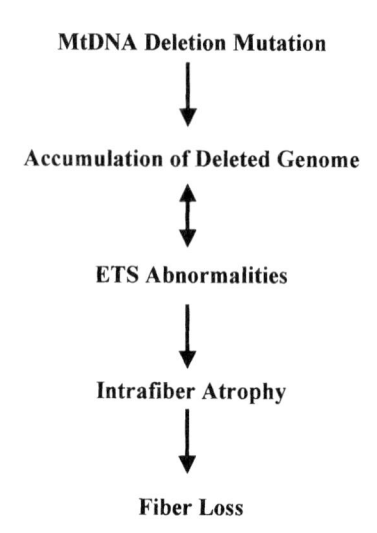

FIGURE 7. Schematic representation of the cascade of events initiated by an mtDNA deletion mutation.

ACKNOWLEDGMENTS

This work was supported by Grants RO1 AG11604, AG17543, P01 AG11915, and T32 AG00213 from the National Institutes of Health. We wish to thank Aubrey de Grey for his suggestion that we consider comparing maximum ETS length with age (FIG. 5).

REFERENCES

1. FLEMING, J.E., J. MIQUEL, S. COTTRELL, *et al.* 1982. Is cell aging caused by respiration-dependent injury to the mitochondrial genome? Gerontology **28:** 44–53.
2. HARMAN, D. 1983. Free radical theory of aging: consequences of mitochondrial aging. Age **6:** 86–94.
3. LINNANE, A.W., S. MARZUKI, T. OZAWA & M. TANAKA. 1989. Mitochondrial DNA mutations as an important contributor to ageing and degenerative diseases. Lancet. **1:** 642–645.
4. CORTOPASSI, G.A. & N. ARNHEIM. 1990. Detection of a specific mitochondrial DNA deletion in tissues of older humans. Nucleic Acids Res. **18:** 6927–6933.
5. ZHANG, C., A. BAUMER, R.J. MAXWELL, *et al.* 1992. Multiple mitochondrial DNA deletions in an elderly human individual. FEBS Lett. **297:** 34–38.
6. LEE, C.M., S. CHUNG, J.M. KACKOWSKI, *et al.* 1993. Multiple mitochodrial DNA deletions asssociated with age in skeletal muscle of rhesus monkeys. J. Gerontol. **48:** B201–B205.
7. CHUNG, S.S., R. WEINDRUCH, S.R. SCHWARZE, *et al.* 1994. Multiple age-associated mitochondrial DNA deletions in skeletal muscle of mice. Aging (Milano). **6:** 193–200.
8. BROSSAS, J.-Y., E. BARREAU, Y. COURTOIS & J. TRETON. 1994. Multiple deletions in mitodhondrial DNA are present in senescent mouse brain. Biochem. Biophys. Res. Commun. **202:** 654–659.

9. TANHAUSER, S.M. & P.J. LAIPIS. 1995. Multiple deletions are detectable in mitochondrial DNA of aging mice. J. Biol. Chem. **270:** 24769–24775.
10. EIMON, P.M., S.S. CHUNG, C.M. LEE, et al. 1996. Age-associated mitochondrial DNA deletions in mouse skeletal muscle: comparison of different regions of the mitochondrial genome. Dev. Genet. **18:** 107–113.
11. VAN TUYLE, G.C., J.P. GUDIKOTE, V.R. HURT, et al. 1996. Multiple, large deletions in rat mitochondrial DNA: evidence for a major hot spot. Mutat. Res. **349:** 95–107.
12. ASPNES, L.E., C.M. LEE, R. WEINDRUCH, et al. 1997. Caloric restriction reduces fiber loss and mitochondrial abnormalities in aged rat muscle. FASEB J. **11:** 573–581.
13. WANAGAT, J., Z. CAO, P. PATHARE & J.M. AIKEN. 2001. Mitochondrial DNA deletion mutations colocalized with segmental electron transport system abnormalities, muscle fiber atrophy, fiber splitting, and oxidative damage in sarcopenia. FASEB J. **15:** 323–332.
14. MÜLLER-HÖCKER, J., P. SEIBEL, K. SCHNEIDERBANGER & B. KADENBACH. 1993. Different *in situ* hybridization patterns of mitochondrial DNA in cytochrome *c* oxidase-deficient extraocular muscle fibres in the elderly. Virchows Arch. A Pathol. Anat. Histopathol. **422:** 7–15.
15. SCHWARZE, S.R., C.M. LEE, S.S. CHUNG, et al. 1995. High levels of mitochondrial DNA deletions in skeletal muscle of old rhesus monkeys. Mech. Ageing Devel. **83:** 91–101.
16. LEE, C.M., M.E. LOPEZ, R. WEINDRUCH & J.M. AIKEN. 1998. Association of age-related mitochondrial abnormalities with skeletal muscle fiber atrophy. Free Radic. Biol. Med. **25:** 964–972.
17. LOPEZ, M.E., N.L. VAN ZEELAND, D.B. DAHL, et al. 2000. Cellular phenotypes of age-associated skeletal muscle mitochondrial abnormalities in rhesus monkeys. Mutat. Res. **452:** 123–138.
18. MÜLLER-HÖCKER, J. 1989. Cytochrome-*c*-oxidase deficient cardiomyocytes in the human heart—an age-related phenomenon. A histochemical ultracytochemical study. Am. J. Pathol. **134:** 1167–1173.
19. MÜLLER-HÖCKER, J. 1990. Cytochrome *c* oxidase deficient fibres in the limb muscle and diaphragm of man without muscular disease: an age-related alteration. J. Neurol. Sci. **100:** 14–21.
20. CAO, Z., J. WANAGAT, S.H. MCKIERNAN & J.M. AIKEN. 2001. Mitochondrial DNA deletions mutations are concomitant with ragged red regions of individual aged muscle fibers: analysis by laser capture microdissection. Nucleic Acids Res. **29:** 4502–4508.
21. LEE, C.M., P. EIMON, R. WEINDRUCH & J.M. AIKEN. 1994. Direct repeat sequences are not required at the breakpoints of age-associated mitochondrial DNA deletions in rhesus monkeys. Mech. Ageing Dev. **75:** 69–79.
22. WANAGAT, J., M. LOPEZ & J.M. AIKEN. 2001. Alterations of the mitochondrial genome. *In* Handbook of the Biology of Aging. E. Masoro, Ed.: 114–139. Academic Press. New York.

Involvement of Mitochondria and Other Free Radical Sources in Normal and Abnormal Fetal Development

ALAN G. FANTEL AND RICHARD E. PERSON

Birth Defects Research Laboratory, Division of Genetics and Development, Department of Pediatrics, University of Washington, Seattle, Washington 98195, USA

ABSTRACT: Shepard and Mackler have documented quantitative increases in mitochondrial cristae between gestational days 10 and 14 in rats accompanied by decreased glucose utilization and increased NADH oxidase activity. Findings show a shift from glycolytic to oxidative metabolism starting at around the time of implantation. Exposure to many substances that cause transient uteroplacental hypoperfusion, including cocaine, phenytoin, calcium channel blockers, and nitric oxide synthase (NOS) inhibitors, induce limb and central nervous system (CNS) malformations while sparing the heart. We have reported that isolated electron transport particles prepared from sensitive tissues show reduced NADH oxidase activities compared with insensitive heart. They also have significantly greater superoxide formation in association with significantly reduced superoxide dismutase activities. NOS inhibitors induce severe limb reductions in late gestation. Exposure is associated with hemorrhage and nitrotyrosine (NT) formation shortly after treatment. Hemorrhage, malformations, and NT formation can be significantly reduced by coadministration of PBN, allopurinol, or aminoguanidine. On the basis of these findings, we have proposed a role for the formation of reactive oxygen species (ROS) and reactive nitrogen species (RNS) in the genesis of limb reduction defects. It is important to note that limb reduction defects occur in humans (~0.22/1000) and have been associated with the agents listed above.

KEYWORDS: free radicals; mitochondria; reactive oxygen species; reactive nitrogen species; teratogenesis; ischemia/reperfusion

INTRODUCTION

This paper reviews research on mitochondrial development and the role of other free radical sources in embryonic and fetal development. The changing morphology of mitochondria during embryogenesis has been the focus of research conducted by Dr. Tom Shepard, while concurrent changes in mitochondrial enzymes concerned with terminal electron transport and oxidative phosphorylation were studied by Dr. Bruce Mackler. As mitochondria are a primary source of reactive oxygen species

---

Addresss for correspondence: Alan G. Fantel, Department of Pediatrics, Box 356320, University of Washington, Seattle, Washington 98195-6320. Voice: 206-543-3373; fax: 206-543-3184.
agf@u.washington.edu

(ROS), the work by these pioneers in the fields of teratology and bioenergetics has provided a foundation for our recent studies of free radicals in normal and abnormal fetal development. All studies reported here were performed in the rat.

The rat embryo undergoes profound changes presumably related to the availability and utilization of oxygen between gestational days 10 and 14. Concomitantly, this is the period of major organogenesis and greatest sensitivity to environmental teratogens.

MITOCHONDRIAL MATURATION, OXYGENATION, AND EMBRYONIC DEVELOPMENT

Conventionally, the prenatal period is divided into embryonic and fetal stages. In the former, tissues and organs are specified and form, while in the latter most organs grow and begin to perform their "adult" functions. Thus, organogenesis takes place during the embryonic stage. During early development, profound changes occur in the availability and utilization of oxygen. These changes take place during the period of organogenesis, when the conceptus is at its peak of teratogenic vulnerability. Significantly, studies from the laboratory of New indicated clearly that normal development occurs only within a dynamic but narrow range of oxygen tensions.[2] To perform these studies, New[2] developed techniques for growing rat embryos *ex utero* in culture medium. Although data are lacking for the normal oxygen tensions of embryonic tissues *in utero*, the ability to vary culture conditions enabled New to demonstrate the importance of oxygen tensions for development.

Gestation in Sprague-Dawley rats lasts for 21 days, if the day after successful mating is designated as gestational day 0 (gd-0). During preimplantation through early postimplantation stages, rats and mice are largely dependent on their "inverted" yolk sac placenta for the transfer of metabolic precursors, oxygen, and waste products. This membrane has a relatively simple relationship with maternal uterine tissue and remains the predominant transfer membrane until later postimplantation stages beginning on and after gd-12. At these later stages, the labyrinthine architecture of the chorioallantoic placenta brings the fetal and maternal blood streams into close apposition utilizing countercurrent flow.

Shepard *et al.*[3,4] have reported a sequence of morphologic changes in the mitochondria between gd-10 and -12 in rats. Most evident are changes in shape from round to elongated. At the same time, the cristae increase in number and change from a vesicular to a laminar shape. With Tanimura,[5] Shepard also demonstrated the Pasteur effect, in which glucose utilization by embryonic tissue decreases significantly during this period while the production of lactate declines. These findings suggest increased utilization of the Krebs cycle and oxidative phosphorylation. During a similar period in rats, Mackler[6] showed significant increases in NADH oxidase activity as illustrated in FIGURE 1 without comparable changes in the activities of other mitochondrial enzymes, including mtATPase, succinic oxidase, or cytochrome oxidase.

The oxygen requirements of rodent embryos in culture change from early to later stages. In rats, culture on gd-9 requires 5% O_2; on gd-10, 20% O_2; and on gd-11, 40–90% O_2. All later cultures require 95% O_2. Neurulation appears to be especially vulnerable to inappropriate oxygenation, with abnormalities developing when early em-

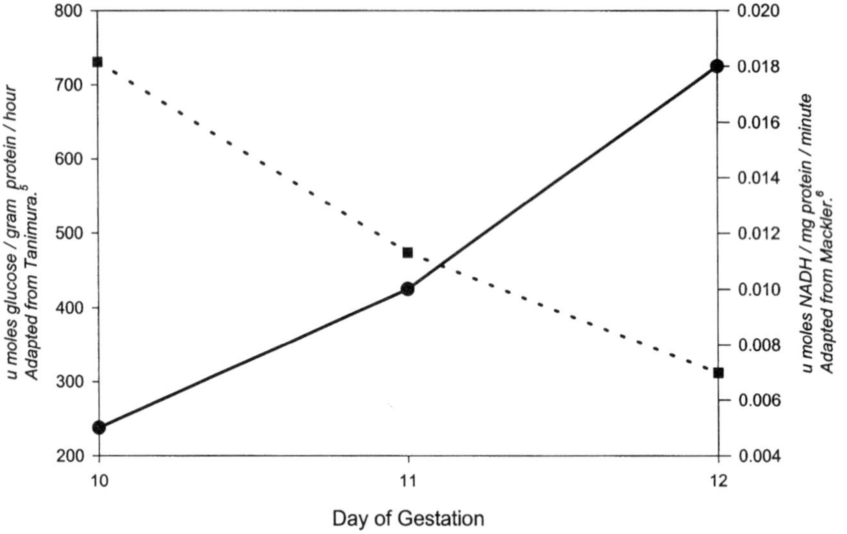

FIGURE 1. Glucose utilization (*dotted line*) and NADH oxidase activity (*solid line*) in the rat embryo at various days of gestation.

bryos were cultured in hyperoxic conditions.[1] Closure of the neural tube is a major organogenetic event. It is a complex process that essentially begins medially, extending to the anterior and posterior ends of the embryo. If closure fails, the brain case fails to close, leading to anencephaly. This condition is invariably fatal, usually prenatally. If closure fails at the posterior end, the embryo, fetus, or newborn will have a meningomyelocele or spina bifida. In these cases, varying degrees of paralysis result from exposure of the spinal cord. Children can survive with this condition with antibiotic treatment. There are varying degrees of these defects from small isolated and covered lesions through spinal dysraphia, in which the entire length of the CNS is exposed.

Mitochondrial morphology also showed a clear relationship to oxygen tension in culture. Thus, the mitochondria of gd-10 embryos could be made to resemble those of gd-12 embryos by culture in 20 or 40% O_2, the same concentration that resulted in abnormal neurulation. Correspondingly, Mackler[6] showed that NADH oxidase activities could be significantly increased from levels measured in submitochondrial particles prepared from gd-11 rat embryos to those of gd-14 preparations by permitting gravidas to breath 85% O_2 (plus 0.4% CO_2) from gd-8. On the other hand, hyperoxia from gd-11 had no detectable effect on NADH oxidase activities on gd-14.

From these studies, it can be concluded that there is a sequence of morphologic and biochemical development of mitochondria and that this sequence is regulated, at least in part, by embryonic oxygenation. Additionally, normal development, including neurulation, requires oxygenation that is appropriate to gestational age. This suggests that placental maturation may play a crucial role in normal and abnormal development.

TABLE 1. Exposures associated with limb reduction defect

Uterine vascular clamping
Calcium channel blockers
Phenytoin
Cocaine
Nitric oxide synthase inhibitors
Chorionic villus sampling

FREE RADICAL PERTURBATION AND FETAL DEVELOPMENT

Numerous exposures to drugs or physical treatment (TABLE 1) have been shown to induce limb and central nervous system (CNS) defects in developing rats when the exposure occurs during fetal stages. Although a chemically and physically diverse group is shown in the table, exposure to each of the chemicals or events that have been studied has been found to have vasoactive or cardioactive consequences that result in transient uteroplacental hypoperfusion. The prototypical exposure involves transient clamping of the uterine vasculature reducing or eliminating the transport of materials including oxygen to and from the fetus. A study published by Leist and Grauweiler[7] reported that clamping for periods of 30–90 minutes on a single day between gd-14 and -16 resulted in transverse limb reduction malformations in which digits appeared amputated or missing. Examination within hours of exposure revealed extensive hemorrhage and edema concentrated in the distal limb regions that later showed defects.

Exposure to a number of things has been associated with limb and CNS defects in human pregnancy. These include the antiseizure medication phenytoin,[8,9] chorionic villus sampling,[10–13] (performed for prenatal diagnostic purposes), and cocaine abuse.[14] In order to examine the teratogenicity of cocaine in late gestation, Webster and Brown-Woodman[15] exposed rat fetuses to two intraperitoneal injections of cocaine separated by one or more hours on various gestational days. They found that fetuses were highly sensitive on gestational days 16–19, with abnormalities appearing in limbs, heads, tails and genital tubercles. Limb reduction anomalies common at term were preceded by limb hemorrhages that could be documented as soon as 2 hours after the second cocaine injection. Immediate and term changes were comparable to those induced by uterine vascular clamping.

Because cocaine is a well-recognized vasoconstrictor, we became interested in the question of whether cocaine is directly fetotoxic or whether its limb toxicity results from changes it induces in conceptal oxygenation.[16] A fetal culture system was developed that enabled us to model the *in vivo* study of Webster and Brown-Woodman, carefully manipulating both oxygen and drug concentrations. It must be kept in mind that rat cultures require 95% O_2 (termed normoxia) after gd-11, while gd-14 fetuses require continuous gassing throughout the period of culture. Even with this and other adaptations, gd 14-15 represents the last interval that is amenable to culture.

Gravidas were anesthetized and fetuses removed from the uteri and placed in sterile culture flasks containing Earle's balanced salt solution supplemented with 25%

TABLE 2. Survival and limb defects[a]

	N	% Survival	% Defects
Control 74	74	73	0
1 Cocaine (2×)	21	52	0
2 Hypoxia (2×)	37	27	8
3 Coc + hyp (2×)	15	0	–
4 Hypoxia (1×)	74	40	11

[a]Adapted from Fantel.[17]

heat-inactivated, immediately centrifuged, rat serum. After a two-hour preculture period, the fetuses were randomly placed in one of five flasks (one control and four experimental). Control fetuses were exposed to 95% O_2 for the next 18 hours. Experimental groups included: (1) 2–30-min exposures to cocaine (25 µM) separated by 30 minutes in normal medium; (2) 2–30-min exposures to hypoxia (20% O_2) separated by 30 min of normoxia; (3) 2–30-min exposures to combined hypoxia and cocaine separated by 30 min of normal medium and normoxia; (4) a single 90-min period of hypoxia. At the end of the final exposure period, fetuses were returned to normal culture conditions for the remainder of the culture period.

The external anatomy of control and cocaine-exposed fetuses was normal for gestational age while those exposed to a single period of hypoxia had reduced limb size. No fetuses survived the combination of cocaine plus hypoxia. Fetuses exposed to two episodes of hypoxia had severe reduction anomalies (TABLE 2).[17] In order to investigate the possibility that reactive oxygen species were formed on reperfusion, the experiment was repeated with the addition of a superoxide anion radical, 3-[4,5-dimethylthiazol-2-yl]-2,5-diphenyltetrazolium bromide (MTT) added to the medium. MTT enters cells, but when reduced by superoxide, forms a colored formazan precipitate. Formazan staining was detected only in the limbs and yolk sacs of fetuses exposed to two episodes of hypoxia, suggesting a role for ROS formation and toxicity in limb reduction malformations associated with cocaine exposure. We then examined rates of superoxide anion radical formation in sensitive and insensitive fetal (limb and CNS vs. heart) and adult (muscle, heart and brain) tissue.[18] These experiments were carried out by spectrophotometric monitoring of the reduction of cytochrome c by homogenates prepared from various tissues. When azide was omitted from these preparations, only fetal limb and CNS demonstrated superoxide formation. When azide was added, these two tissues formed significantly greater amounts of superoxide that did the others (TABLE 3).

The next issue we considered was the basis of apparent vulnerability of two tissues, limbs, and CNS to vasoactive agents and of their heightened capacity to form superoxide. No differences were detected in NADH oxidase activities in sensitive and insensitive tissues. On the other hand, significant differences were measured in overall superoxide dismutase (SOD) activities (TABLE 4). Specifically, SOD activities were significantly lower in homogenates prepared from fetal brain and limb than they were in the adult or the insensitive fetal tissue.[19] The difference between fetal and adult tissues was not surprising since numerous studies have reported that

TABLE 3. Superoxide production in adult and fetal tissues[a]

Tissue	Azide Inhibited	Azide Uninhibited
Heart, adult	0.19	0
Muscle, adult	0.64	0
Brain, adult	0.34	0
Heart, ave. GD[b]-14, 15, 16, 18	0.51	0
Limb bud, ave. GD-14, 15, 16	0.75	0.28
Brain, GD-16	0.87	0.21

Superoxide production in mM/min/nM aa_3

[a]Adapted from Fantel.[18]
[b]Gestational day.

TABLE 4. Superoxide dismutase activities in fetal and adult tissues[a]

Tissue	Superoxide dismutase activity nM / min / mg protein
Heart, adult	41
Muscle, adult	14
Brain, adult	16
Heart, GD-16	22
Limb bud, GD-16	6.4
Brain, GD-16	3.3

[a]Adapted from Mackler.[19]

antioxidant activities remain depressed in fetal tissues until just prior to parturition.[20–23] It appears that prenatal tissues exist in a relatively reduced state and that this condition is required for normal differentiation.

In addition to its low antioxidant activities, there are other features of fetuses that may be responsible for their apparently heightened capacity to form ROS. First, implantation places the fetus in increasing proximity to the maternal blood supply. Preimplantation and early postimplantation rat embryos are largely dependent on the unique, inverted yolk sac placenta to meet their transfer requirements. This structure, although well vascularized, lacks the intimate relationship with the maternal vasculature of the chorioallantoic placenta that develops rapidly after gd-13. This latter structure develops a highly efficient countercurrent relationship with the maternal blood flow. At the same time, vasculogenesis and angiogenesis are occurring throughout the fetus. Increasing hemoglobin and iron stores provide transition metal for reduction of peroxides to the highly reactive hydroxyl radical via Fenton chemistry.

TABLE 5. Effect of L-NAME and PBN on term limb defects[a]

Treatment	Percent abnormal
Control	0
PBN 50 mg/kg	0
L-NAME 25 mg/kg	72
L-NAME 25 mg/kg plus PBN 50 mg/kg	49
L-NAME 50 mg/kg	100
L-NAME 50 mg/kg plus PBN 50 mg/kg	99

[a]Adapted from Fantel.[28]

TABLE 6. Amelioration of L-NAME–induced limb hemorrhage and nitrotyrosine by allopurinol and aminoguanidine[a]

Treatment	Percent abnormal	Nitrotyrosine/tyrosine peak ratio
L-NAME 50 mg/kg	100	0.13
L-NAME 50 mg/kg plus allopurinol	10	0.02
L-NAME 50 mg/kg plus aminoguanidine	9	0.02

[a]Adapted from Fantel.[28]

LIMB TOXICITY OF L-NAME

The final section of this paper reviews studies of the fetotoxicity of N^G-nitro-L-arginine methyl ester (L-NAME), a nonspecific inhibitor of nitric oxide synthase (NOS). Several investigators have reported that oral treatment of gravidas with L-NAME on or after gd-14 results in limb reduction malformations.[24–27] We found that intraperitoneal dosing on gd-16 resulted in dose-responsive incidences of limb reduction ranging to 100% of fetuses treated with doses of 50 mg/kg.[28] When gravidas were cotreated with the radical spin trap, α-phenyl-N-t-butylnitrone (PBN), both the incidence and severity of limb defects were significantly reduced at term with an L-NAME dose of 25 mg/kg but not at 50 mg/kg (TABLE 5). Examination of fetuses 4 hours after treatment showed severe hemorrhages in the limbs, and that hemorrhage could be dramatically reduced by coadministration of PBN. This finding was supportive of the role of ROS in the limb toxicity of L-NAME and possibly that of other vasoactive exposures.

Subsequent preliminary study found that two other drugs significantly reduced the limb effects of L-NAME (TABLE 6). These were aminoguanidine, a relatively specific inhibitor of the inducible isoform of nitric oxide synthase, and allopurinol, a xanthine oxidase inhibitor. We then performed a preliminary electron paramagnetic resonance study of the limbs of fetuses exposed to L-NAME. Using the spin trap, MGD, we found evidence of increased formation of nitric oxide in limbs. We also found significantly increased nitrotyrosine formation in L-NAME–exposed limbs and that this increase could be significantly ameliorated by cotreatment of gravidas with either aminoguanidine or allopurinol.[28] Our most recent studies have considered teratogenicity and changes in xanthine oxidase activity in the limbs of fetuses exposed to L-NAME and cotreated with allopurinol. Cotreatment with allopurinol results in dose-responsive increases in digital length at term and significant reductions in hemorrhage severity. While L-NAME significantly increased xanthine oxidase activity compared to saline-treated controls, allopurinol co-treatment restored activity to control levels.[29]

CONCLUSIONS

The rat embryo undergoes profound metabolic changes presumably related to the availability and utilization of oxygen between gestational days 10 and 14, with normal development taking place within a changing but narrow range. The initiation of these changes is most likely associated with the increase in oxygen made available to the embryo by the rapid development of the chorioallantoic placenta, which establishes a uteroplacental blood flow. Correspondingly, this is the period of major organogenesis and greatest sensitivity to environmental teratogens.

Mitochondrial morphology changes during embryonic development and these changes appear to be responsive to oxygenation. Prior to gestational day 10, oxidative metabolism is low and may be relatively unimportant to embryonic growth and development, but after that the electron-transport systems and associated phosphorylation processes increase rapidly. If the developing embryo is exposed to hyperoxic conditions, premature mitochondrial maturation may result in defects in neurulation.

Exposures that cause transient episodes of local and/or uteroplacental hypoperfusion in fetal life have been repeatedly associated with limb and central nervous system malformations. Limb reduction defects occur in approximately 0.22 out of 1000 live births, with 33% attributed to vascular causes. These malformations appear to be preceded by prompt hemorrhage and edema. We developed an *in vitro* model to study the late embryonic toxicity of cocaine and ischemia/reperfusion that is observed *in vivo*. When gd-14 embryos were exposed to episodes of hypoxia, a significant incidence of limb abnormalities was observed that resembled those resulting from multiple exposure to cocaine *in vivo*. From these results, we proposed that developing limbs were insulted by reactive oxygen species generated by reoxygenation *in vitro* that modeled reperfusion *in vivo*.

To explain the disparity in sensitivity to hypoxia/reperfusion we examined several components of the electron transport system in sensitive and insensitive fetal tissues and adult tissues. No systematic differences were observed except for the inverse relationship between superoxide generation by ETP from teratogenically sensitive and insensitive tissues and the SOD activity of homogenates of these tissues. This relationship appears to remain consistent across developmental stages and regions and therefore represents an important finding that can explain both teratogenic sensitivity and superoxide generation.

Finally, exposure of rat gravidas to the NOS inhibitor L-NAME resulted in prompt vascular engorgement and hemorrhage with dose-responsive limb reduction defects observed at term. In addition, protein nitration and xanthine oxidase activities were augmented in fetuses from gravidas exposed to L-NAME. Because limb responses to exposure via the fetal intraamniotic or maternal intraperitoneal route were comparable, we conclude that L-NAME most likely acts directly on the fetus, and that maternal hemodynamic changes are of limited pathogenic importance.

Limb reduction defects associated with fetal exposure to NOS inhibitors *in utero* can be significantly moderated by cotreatment with the antioxidant, PBN, the iNOS inhibitor, aminoguanidine, or the xanthine oxidase inhibitor, allopurinol.

Together these results suggest that L-NAME acts directly on the fetal vasculature by depleting NO, causing vascular engorgement and leakage. After this initial depletion, NO concentrations increase, most likely as a consequence of induction of iNOS during ischemia/reperfusion. The reaction products from the excesses of NO and superoxide can nitrate and oxidize macromolecules in the limb, resulting in the observed reduction defects.

ACKNOWLEDGMENTS

We wish to thank Dr. Tom Shepard, Dr. Bruce Mackler, Negin Nekahi, Louis Stamps, Ruslan Tumbic, Charles Barber, Dat Nguyen, and Tung Tran for their efforts in producing much of the work described in this review. This work was sponsored by NIH Grant ES 06361.

REFERENCES

1. MORRISS, G.M. & D.A.T. NEW 1979. Effect of oxygen concentration on morphogenesis of cranial neural folds and neural crest in cultured rat embryos. J. Embryol. Exp. Morphol. **54:** 17–35.
2. NEW, D.A.T. 1967. Development of explanted rat embryos in circulating medium. J. Embryol. Exp. Morphol. **17:** 513–525.
3. SHEPARD, T.H., L.A. MUFFLEY & L.T. SMITH. 1998. Ultrastructural study of mitochondria and their cristae in embryonic rats and primate (*N. nemestrina*). Anat. Rec. **252:** 383–392.
4. SHEPARD, T.H, L.A. MUFFLEY & L.T. SMITH. 2000. Mitochondrial ultrastructure in embryos after implantation. Hum. Reprod. **15** (Suppl. 2): 218–228.
5. TANIMURA, T. & T.H. SHEPARD. 1970. Glucose metabolism by rat embryos in vitro. Proc. Soc. Exp. Biol. Med. **135:** 51–54.
6. MACKLER, B., R. GRACE, B. HAYNES, G.J. BARGMAN & T.H. SHEPARD. 1973. Studies of mitochondrial energy systems during embryogenesis in the rat. Arch. Biochem. Biophys. **158:** 662–668.
7. LEIST, K.H. & J. GRAUWILER. 1974. Fetal pathology following uterine-vessel clamping on day 14 of gestation. Teratology **10:**55–68.
8. BARR, M, A.K. POZANSKI & R.D. SCHMICKEL. 1974. Digital hypoplasia and anticonvulsants during gestation, a teratogenic syndrome. J. Pediatr. **4:** 254–256.
9. HILL, R.M., *et al.* 1974. Infants exposed in utero to antiepileptic drugs. Am. J. Dis. Child. **127:** 645–653.
10. BURTON, B.K., C.J. SCHULZ & L.I. BURD. 1992. Limb anomalies associated with chorionic villus sampling. Obstet. Gynecol. **79:** 726–730.
11. FIRTH, H.V., *et al.* 1991. Severe limb abnormalities after chorionic villus sampling at 56–66 days' gestation. Lancet **337:** 762–763.
12. MASTRIACOVO, P. & L.D. BOTTO. 1994. Chorionic villus sampling and transverse limb deficiencies: maternal age is not a confounder. Am J. Med. Genet. **53:** 182–186.
13. OLNEY, R.S., *et al.* 1995. Increased risk for transverse digital deficiency after chorionic villus sampling: results of the United States Multistate-Control Study, 1998–1992. Teratology **51:** 20–29.

14. HOYME, H.E., et al. 1990. Prenatal cocaine exposure and fetal vascular disruption. Pediatrics **85:** 743–747.
15. WEBSTER, W.S. & P.D.C. BROWN-WOODMAN. 1990. Cocaine as a cause of congenital malformations of vascular origin: experimental evidence in the rat. Teratology **41:** 689–697.
16. FANTEL, A.G., C.V. BARBER & B. MACKLER. 1992. Ischemia/reperfusion: a new hypothesis for the developmental toxicity of cocaine. Teratology **46:** 285–292.
17. FANTEL, A.G., et al. 1992. Studies of the role of ischemia/reperfusion and superoxide anion radical production in the teratogenicity of cocaine. Teratology **46:** 293–300.
18. Fantel, A.G., et al. 1995. Studies of mitochondria in oxidative embryotoxicity. Teratology **52:** 190–195.
19. MACKLER, B., R.E. PERSON, T.-D. NGUYEN & A.G. FANTEL. 1998. Studies of the cellular localization of superoxide dismutases in adult and fetal rat tissues. Free Radic. Res. **28:** 125–129.
20. FRANK, L., J.R. BUCHER & R.J. ROBERTS. 1978. Oxygen toxicity in neonatal and adult animals of various species. J. Appl. Physiol. **45:** 699–704.
21. FRANK, L. & E.E. GROSCLOSE. 1984. Preparation for birth into an O_2-rich environment: the antioxidant enzymes in the developing rabbit lung. Pediatr. Res. **18:** 240–244.
22. FRANK, L. 1991. Developmental aspects of experimental pulmonary oxygen toxicity. Free Radic. Biol. Med. **11:** 463–494.
23. RICKETT, G.W. & F.J. KELLY. 1990. Developmental expression of antioxidant enzymes in guinea pig lung and liver. Development **108:** 331–336.
24. DICKET, A.L., et al. 1994. Nitric oxide inhibition causes intrauterine growth retardation and hind-limb disruptions in rats. Am. J. Obstet. Gynecol. **171:** 243–1250.
25. PIERCE, R.L., et al. 1995. Limb reduction defects after prenatal inhibition of nitric oxide synthase in rats. Pediatr. Res. **38:** 905–911.
26. FANTEL, A.G., et al. 1997. The teratogenicity of N^G-nitro-L-Arginine Methyl Ester (L-NAME), a nitric oxide synthase inhibitor in rats. Reprod. Toxicol. **11:** 709–717.
27. GREENBERG, S.S., et al.. 1997. Effects of NO synthase inhibitors, arginine-deficient diet, and amiloride in pregnant rats. Am. J. Physiol. **273:** 1031–1045.
28. FANTEL, A.G., et al. 1999. Role of free radicals in the limb teratogenicity of L-NAME: A new mechanistic model of vascular disruption. Teratology **60:** 151–160.
29. FANTEL, A.G. & R.E. PERSON. 2002. Further evidence for the role of free radicals in the limb teratogenicity of L-NAME. Teratology. In press.

Frequent Intracellular Clonal Expansions of Somatic mtDNA Mutations

Significance and Mechanisms

HILARY A. COLLER,[a] NATALYA D. BODYAK,[b] AND KONSTANTIN KHRAPKO[b]

[a]*Fred Hutchinson Cancer Research Center, Seattle, Washington 98119, USA*
[b]*Beth Israel Deaconess Medical Center, and Harvard Medical School, Boston, Massachusetts 02115, USA*

ABSTRACT: It has been proposed that age-dependent accumulation of somatic mutations in mtDNA is responsible for some aspects of the aging process. However, most cells contain hundreds to thousands of mtDNA molecules. Any nascent somatic mutant therefore appears as a single copy among a majority of wild-type species. A single mutant molecule is unlikely to influence the physiology of the cell and thus cannot play a role in the aging process. To affect cellular physiology, the nascent somatic mutants must somehow accumulate clonally in the cell to significant levels. The evidence supporting the view that, indeed, clonal expansion of mtDNA mutations is a widespread process in various human tissues, and the mechanisms by which clonal expansions may affect the aging process, are reviewed. Originally, clonal expansion was demonstrated for mtDNA with large deletions in muscle. Cell-by-cell analysis of human cardiomyocytes and buccal epithelial cells revealed that clonal expansion affects point mtDNA mutations as well as deletions. Expansions are not limited to muscle, but likely are present in most tissues, and almost every cell of an aged tissue is likely to be affected by an expansion. While the very existence of clonal expansion is beyond doubt, the mechanisms driving this process are largely controversial. The hypotheses explaining expansion includes random or various selective mechanisms, or both. We show that the spectra of expanded point mutations are drastically different in cardiomyocytes and epithelial cells. This suggests that the mechanisms of expansion in these tissues are different. In particular, we propose random segregation and positive selection models for epithelial and muscle cells, respectively.

KEYWORDS: somatic mutations; clonal expansion; point mutations; mtDNA

INTRODUCTION

As early as 1972, it was proposed by Harman[1] that the aging process may depend in part on the accumulation of alterations in mtDNA functions. Almost two decades later this idea was revived in a more explicit form: mutations in mtDNA were direct-

Address for correspondence: K. Khrapko, Harvard Institutes of Medicine, Suite 921, 330 Brookline Ave., Boston, MA 02215. Voice: 617-667-0973; fax: 617-667-0980.
khrapko@hms.harvard.edu

ly blamed for causing human aging and death.[2–4] It has been recognized,[2] however, that involvement of somatic mtDNA mutations in cellular physiology in general, and in the aging process in particular, would require that these mutants clonally accumulate in cells to significant levels. The rationale for such a requirement is intuitively obvious: every somatic mutation initially arises as a random event on a single DNA copy. Since every human cell contains hundreds or thousands of mtDNA copies, this initial mutant copy will have to compete with a huge excess of fully functional wild-type copies and therefore is unlikely to affect the physiology of the cell. This expectation has been confirmed in subsequent studies which demonstrated that, indeed, the extent of physiological deficiency of a cell caused by a mutation in its mtDNA is at most proportional to the fraction of such a mutation.[5] In most cases, the situation is even less favorable for the mutation: it appears that the effect of a mutation is subject to a threshold effect, that is, a mutation has almost no effect until its fraction in the cell reaches a certain threshold level, 60% or higher, depending on the type of mutation[5–8] as well as other factors.[9] Furthermore, sequential accumulation of different random mutants is not sufficient, because different mutants will likely compensate for each other's deficiencies[10–13] (see, however, Ref. 14), and therefore mutants would need to accumulate via clonal expansion of a single initial mutant.

It should be noted, however, that one cannot exclude certain "dominant negative" schemes of phenotypic expression of mtDNA mutations. For example, even a single defective mitochondrion in an otherwise normal cell might be quite damaging. For example, a mutation in mtDNA may facilitate a permeability transition of the mitochondrion.[15,16] Even a single mitochondrion containing such a mutation may theoretically put the whole cell at risk for premature apoptosis despite a huge excess of normal mitochondria. Indeed, the rupture of this single defective mitochondrion and the resulting release of cytochrome c and/or other apoptotic factors is potentially sufficient to kill the whole cell. Even in this extreme example, however, some clonal expansion is still necessary: the mutant mtDNA must have taken over a mitochondrion, which is believed to contain 2–10 mtDNA molecules.[17,18,19] Interestingly, it has been shown recently that an increased mutational rate (in the mitochondrial genome only) in the heart of a transgenic mouse resulted in a severe cardiomyopathy.[20] The early onset of cardiomyopathy (2 months), however, suggests that nascent mutations most probably did not have enough chance to reach homoplasmy in the cells of the heart. It is possible therefore, that cardiomyopathy in this case was induced via some sort of "dominant negative" effect.

Intracellular accumulation of mutant mtDNA was soon discovered in muscle fibers of individuals with mitochondrial myopathies either with mtDNA deletions,[21,22] or point mutations.[7,23] In normal aging, however, detection of mutations is complicated by the fact that mutations are rare and heterogeneous. Nevertheless, it was possible to demonstrate clonal expansions of somatic deletions of mtDNA of normal aged muscle.[24] This latter discovery has been confirmed by a large number of investigators,[25–27] using several different approaches. Interestingly, even very short deleted mtDNA species with almost all of the genome missing (including the light strand origin of replication) appear to be capable of expanding clonally, possibly via a partially duplicated form.[28]

It has been convincingly demonstrated that clonal expansions of somatic mtDNA mutations cause mitochondrial dysfunction in aged tissues that is limited to individual cells or fibers.[24,26] Moreover, it looks like at least in some cases, most if not all such mitochondrial function defects in tissue are caused by expanded mtDNA deletions.[29] However, the fraction of cells (or muscle fiber segments) containing a significant proportion of clonally expanded deletions is quite low, on the order of 1%, though reported values vary a lot. The obvious question is whether such a low fraction of defects could be relevant to the aging process. At least two plausible noncompeting mechanisms have been suggested that explain how infrequent clonal expansions of mtDNA deletions may play a role in the aging process, despite their low abundance. In one, clonal expansions in small segments of a muscle fiber are postulated to be associated with thinning and breakage of the fiber, which ultimately leads to its elimination. In this way, a relatively small number of defective segments can be responsible for sarcopenia, a significant age-associated loss of muscle fibers. Data in support of this mechanism were obtained in rats[29] and monkeys.[30] According to the other mechanism,[31,32] cells with a defect in oxidative phosphorylation caused by an expansion of a mtDNA mutation resort to glycolysis, which creates an intracellular excess of NADH. The oxidative recycling of NADH at the cellular membrane by plasma membrane oxireductase is proposed to result in extracellular superoxide production and oxidation of circulating material like low density lipoprotein (LDL). This would ultimately increase systemic oxidative stress in the organism, which is a prominent hallmark of the aging process.

Although clonal expansions of deleted mtDNA were studied in some detail in muscle and heart, it is not known whether expansions are present in other tissues, nor whether somatic point mutations are also subject to expansion. It has been shown, though, that, *in vivo*, the presence of two genotypes in various somatic cells (intracellular heteroplasmy), including intestinal epithelium[33] and hair follicles,[34] has a tendency to resolve to intracellular homoplasmy over an organism's life span. *In vitro*, various heteroplasmic cell lines also resolve to homoplasmy[35] or at least change the proportions of the two genotypes abruptly.[36] Resolution to homoplasmy is in fact an expansion of one of the genotypes constituting heteroplasmy at the expense of the other, even though the expansion may not be clonal since it does not necessarily start with a single copy. Interestingly, *in vivo*, the expanded mitochondrial DNA genotype appears to be shared by most or all cells in a turnover unit (such as an intestinal crypt[33] or a hair follicle).[34] This implies that the expansions took place in the stem cells responsible for maintenance of the corresponding turnover units. Clonal expansions of mtDNA in the germ line were demonstrated using artificial[37] or natural heteroplasmy of a point mutation[38] or a mtDNA rearrangement.[39]

In conclusion, clonal expansions of somatic deletions in mtDNA have been extensively studied, and much theory and some hard evidence[29] suggests that they may play some role in the aging process. There is no information, however, about clonal expansions of somatic point mutations, and no studies have been performed in nonmuscle somatic tissue. A number of studies of heteroplasmy *in vivo* and *in vitro* suggest that such expansions are likely to exist.

In this communication, we will present our data demonstrating that clonal expansion of somatic point mutations in mtDNA is expected to be a general process occurring in many tissues. These data are discussed with respect to the role of mtDNA in the aging process and to the mechanisms of clonal expansion.

RESULTS AND DISCUSSION

Detection of Clonal Expansions by Single Cell Sequencing

We sought to determine whether point mutations in mtDNA are capable of clonal expansion *in vivo*, as observed for mitochondrial deletions. The total load of mtDNA somatic point mutations in aged human tissues is very high, roughly on the order of one mutation per mitochondrial genome.[40,41] It was not known, however, whether these mutations were distributed randomly, or were clustered in individual cells. In the former case every cell would contain a complex mixture of mutants. In the latter, every cell would contain one kind of mutant in each of its multiple copies of mtDNA, while another cell would contain mutants of another kind, and so on. The latter situation is expected to arise if (and only if!) mutants are capable of clonal expansion. Since there is about one mutation per copy, there would be about one mutation per cell on average, with the actual number of mutations per cell distributed according to the Poisson distribution. We reasoned that if (and only if) a significant proportion of mutations were clustered, then we would be able to detect mutations by straightforward sequencing of DNA from individual cells. If, however, mutants were distributed randomly, then no mutants would be detected by sequencing, because each of the many mutants would be present at a low fraction, well below the sensitivity of sequencing. In conclusion, sequencing of DNA from individual cells is a practical test for the *in vivo* presence of clonal expansions of point mutations.

Clonal Expansions of Point Mutations are Common and Tissue Specific

We used single cell sequencing to look for clonal expansions in two very different human tissues: highly proliferative buccal epithelium and postmitotic myocardium. Cells were isolated using published protocols,[27] and their DNA was amplified using two pairs of primers covering the entire control region of the mitochondrial genome. We concentrated on the control region, because the incidence of somatic mutations per nucleotide in this region is about 10-fold higher than anywhere else in the genome. In our experiments each of the two tissues was represented by 36 cells collected from three unrelated individuals over 50 years of age (12 cells per individual). The results of single cell sequencing (performed from at least two independent PCR amplifications of cellular DNA to exclude PCR artifacts) are presented in TABLE 1.

Amazingly, about 30% of cells in both tissues contained a somatic mutation somewhere in the control region at a fraction of 50% or above. It is reasonable to assume that we have missed some expanded mutations in the unsequenced part of mtDNA, so the actual fraction of cells with expanded mutations may be even higher. We anticipate therefore that most cells contain clonal expansions. Preliminary data indicate that clonal expansions are also present at comparable frequency in neurons and skeletal muscle fibers. Another striking feature of expanded mutations is tissue specificity. While the vast majority of mutations in epithelium are length changes in the stretch of consecutive cytosines starting at bp 303, almost all heart mutations cluster within a narrow area, 16028–16054. This difference is highly significant with overall P-value less than 10^{-5}. We believe that these findings have important implications for the biology of somatic mtDNA mutations.

TABLE 1. Clonally expanded mutations in individual cells

	Buccal epithelium		Cardiomyocytes	
	Position	Change	Position	Change
1	*198*	C→T	*189*	A→G
2	*214*	A→G	*189*	A→G
3	251	G→C	555	A→G
4	*252*	T→C	16028	T→C
5	*303*	ins 2,3,4C	16029	T→C
6	*303*	del C	16033	T→C
7	*303*	del C	16035	G→A
8	*303*	ins C	16035	G→A
9	*303*	del C	16036	G→A
10	*303*	del C ins C	16036	G→A
11	*303*	ins 1,2C	16036	G→A
12	*303*	ins 1,2C	16049	G→A
13			16052	del C
14			16054	A→G

NOTE: For each tissue, 36 cells from 3 individuals (12 cells each) were analyzed. Changes in *italics* are identical to neutral human polymorphisms.

Implications for the Dynamics of Intracellular mtDNA Populations

Obviously, the finding of abundant somatic mutations in individual cells implies that at least some point mutations in mitochondrial DNA are capable of clonal expansion. The importance of these findings, however, goes beyond that. What emerges is a general picture of highly dynamic intracellular populations of mitochondrial genomes. These populations appear to be frequently (and or continuously) swept by clonal expansions, which leave the cell mainly populated with progeny of a single ancestral mitochondrial genome. At this time it is not clear whether clonal expansions were actually caused by the mutations we observed, or, in general, whether the process of expansion is mechanistically related to any mutations at all (see discussion below). We would like to propose, however, that, whatever the mechanisms, the finding that clonal expansions are so common, implies that essentially *any* somatic mutation has a chance to be propelled to significant intracellular levels (unless it negatively affects its own propagation).

Indeed, all the mutants present in a cell at the time of the onset of an expansion (roughly one per mtDNA molecule) have an equal chance to be on the "lucky" mtDNA molecule that is expanded. The progeny of that mutant will take over the whole population of mitochondrial genomes in that cell after the expansion is complete (of course, at the expense of the other mutants present in the cell at the onset of expansion, which will perish). In other cells subject to expansion, other mutants will be expanded. Overall, the frequency distribution of homoplasmic mutations in a tissue is expected, to a first approximation, to reproduce to the pre-expansion distribution of mutants, with the exception of those mutants that are selected either for or against during the expansion process.

Implications for the Mitochondrial Theory of Aging

We believe that our findings support the view that clonal expansions may not be limited to particular types of mutations (such as large deletions or relatively mild disease-associated point mutations) and particular types of tissues (in particular postmitotic), but rather represent a very general phenomenon. This, in turn, tempts us to speculate about possible alternative mechanisms by which mtDNA mutations may influence the aging process.

Relatively little attention has been paid to the role of mitochondrial mutations in aging of proliferating tissues, because it has been recognized for a while that deletions, the most studied type of mtDNA mutations, do not seem to accumulate in these tissues. We note, however, that at least in some proliferating tissues the overall rate of point mutations is no lower than in postmitotic ones and is very high in absolute terms.[40,41] We further note that the widespread impression that point mutations in mtDNA are relatively benign may come from the fact that most known pathogenic mutations are compatible with life and development, since most of them were discovered in people either with inherited mtDNA mutations or mutations that happened very early in development. Such mutations are present at high frequency in one or more tissues, and thus are easy to detect. Somatic mutations are not subject to this restriction and thus some of them may be rather devastating. It has been argued, for example, that certain mutations in complex I subunits may be deadly for neurons.[42] Such disruptive mutations could be expected to arise with certain frequency in mtDNA and would then be expected to undergo clonal expansion in accordance with their mutant fraction. When expanded, these mutants may cause, for example, age-dependent death of stem cells in epithelial tissues or cardiomyocytes in the heart.

IMPLICATIONS FOR MECHANISMS OF CLONAL EXPANSION

Multiple Hypotheses of the Expansion Mechanisms

The mechanisms driving clonal expansions of mtDNA mutations have been studied since the late 1980s, when it became clear that deleted mtDNA molecules possess an advantage over the wild type during propagation in muscle fibers.[43] Since that time many hypotheses have been suggested to explain this phenomenon (recently critically reviewed[44]), and some of them were generalized to include point mutations. It is important for our purposes to divide these hypotheses into three broad classes (the first two following the classification in Ref. 44). We assert that our data regarding expansions of point mutation in various tissues, especially the striking contrast between mutational spectra in buccal epithelium and in cardiomyocytes, can be helpful in discriminating between these hypotheses.

"Structural" hypotheses postulate that mutant mtDNA molecules have certain advantages in propagation, due to changes in DNA sequence, without any reference to the function of the proteins that could have been affected by such changes. Examples are the hypothesis that shorter length and the resulting shorter time of replication could result in an advantage for deleted mtDNA.[43] Alternatively, mutations (including point mutations) have been proposed to alter specific control sequences (e.g., destroy *cis*-inhibitory sequences), which also could result in a replication advantage for mutant mtDNA.[22]

"Phenotype-based" hypotheses consider how changes in activities of mitochondrial enzymes caused by mutations in mtDNA could result in a propagation advantage for the mutant. One hypothesis assumed that proliferation of mitochondria is controlled by the local concentration of ATP (a plausible compensatory mechanism). Low intramitochondrial ATP levels resulting from a defect in oxidative phosphorylation caused by a mutation will then stimulate the proliferation of the defective mitochondrion.[22] An elegant recent hypothesis maintains that dysfunctional mutant mitochondria accumulate less damage and thus are less likely to be turned over in the lysosomes than the wild type, which results in an advantage, though from the negative side.[45]

"Random segregation" hypotheses appeal to random distribution of mutant copies between daughter cells during mitosis in proliferative tissues or between the "pool to be degraded" and the "pool to be propagated" in mitochondrial turnover in postmitotic cells. Mitotic segregation of mutant mtDNA copies was suggested as a means by which aging tissue becomes a mosaic of cells with different capacities for oxidative phosphorylation, to justify the mitochondrial theory of aging.[2] Recently, this approach has been developed in much greater detail with respect to a post-mitotic tissue (myocardium),[46] cultured cells,[36] and for a proliferative tissue, colonic epithelium,[41] and pancreas.[47]

Expansions in Epithelium: Random Segregation

The spectra of control region mutations in buccal epithelial cells appears to be rather simple: it consists almost exclusively of one to two nucleotide deletions and insertions in the tract of seven to nine consecutive cytosines starting at base pair 303 of the mitochondrial genome (the C-tract). Importantly, these mutations are most likely to be neutral, since these mutations are identical to frequent polymorphisms, which apparently have no physiological consequences. At least three of four non-C-tract mutations—C198T, A214G, and T252C—are also identical to neutral polymorphisms, according to our Genbank search. This suggests random segregation as an expansion mechanism. We cannot decisively rule out the possibility that each of the neutral mutations was expanded because it happened to co-segregate with a mutation that is subject to positive selection and situated outside control region so that it was not detected by sequencing. However, this hypothesis appears to be unnecessary: the expansion of C-tract mutations can be readily explained by random segregation.

We have developed a computer model describing the behavior of the mitochondrial genomes during cell proliferation in epithelial tissues.[41] This model assumes that a tissue is composed of turnover units, each containing a single stem cell, which is the progenitor of all cells in the unit. The genotype of the stem cell defines the genotype of all cells in the turnover unit, so we concentrated on the processes taking place in the stem cell only. Segregation of mtDNA mutations takes place when half of the genomes are distributed to a transition cell, which is ultimately destined to

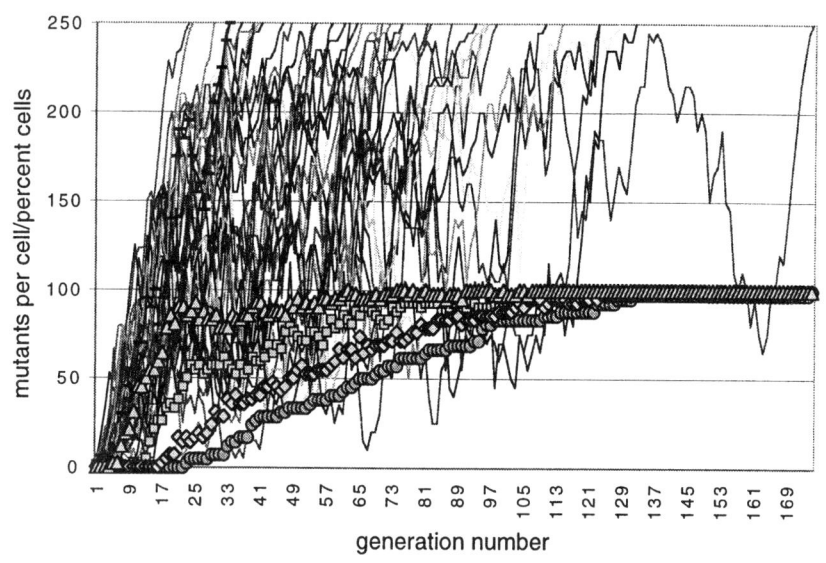

FIGURE 1. Dynamics of clonal expansion via random segregation: 10,000 mutants were randomly distributed among 10,000 cells at generation 1, and simulated segregation was run for the number of generations sufficient for the segregation process to conclude in all cells. Each cell contained 250 copies of mtDNA (50 mitochondria, 5 copies each). Forty-two cells ultimately became completely mutant, while all the rest turned completely wild type. *Thin curves*: the fraction of mutants in each of the 42 cells destined to homoplasmy. *Symbolized curves*: the percentage of the 42 cells that accumulated particular fraction of mutants (*circles*, 100%; *diamonds*, 75%; *squares*, 50%; and *triangles*, 25%). See text for details.

differentiation and death. The other half of the genomes remains in the stem cell lineage. We assume that if any mutants are present in the stem cell, then, during each division, their number will change as a result of randomly uneven distribution of mutants between daughter cells. The number of mutants per cell performs a random walk, which can stop only if the cell reaches one of the two possible "stable" states: all-mutant or all-wild type. In this model, one of the stable states will be ultimately reached given sufficient number of generations; the question is: how fast is this process?

The dynamics of mitochondrial genomes, as modeled by the computer, is presented in FIGURE 1, where the intracellular fractions of 42 mutants (all ultimately destined to reach homoplasmy in a given numeric experiment) are plotted as lines of different weights. This picture gives the flavor of randomness of the process. Note that most of mutants (249 of 250 on average for a cell containing 250 mitochondrial copies prior to mtDNA duplication) are lost from the lineage, and the corresponding tracks are not shown in the figure. The data presented in FIGURE 1 demonstrate that the anticipated dynamics of attaining intracellular homoplasmy via random segregation in epithelial cells is expected to be very rapid. For example, it takes only about 30 generations for 50% of the cells destined to become homoplasmic to accumulate at least 50% of mutant copies and only about 70 generations are sufficient for 50%

of cells to reach full homoplasmy. Interestingly, as shown elsewhere, in a system with continuous generation of mutations, the number of homoplasmic mutations in a cell population tracks the number of all mutations, but lags by 70 generations.[41] Seventy generations can therefore be considered the typical time for establishing of intracellular homoplasmy.

It should be noted that segregation of mitochondrial genomes in a cell is mathematically equivalent to segregation of mitochondrial (or any asexually transmitted) genomes in a stable population of individuals, which was studied in some detail more than a decade ago.[48,49] This approach was later adapted to describe the intracellular segregation of mtDNA.[50]

The next question was whether a typical stem cell goes through enough generations (i.e., significantly more than 70) to ensure segregation of mitochondrial genomes via random segregation. Estimates of the number of stem cell generations for adult epithelial tissues based on the observed frequency of mitosis in tissue are on the order of several hundred: 200 for a colonic epithelium[41] and 300 for lung epithelium (Coller, manuscript in preparation). An independent approach based on measuring microsatellite length variances gave an estimate of 52–280 divisions, even for tissues of a four-year-old child, with little variation between different tissues.[51] We therefore believe that it is safe to conclude that the number of lineal cell divisions in normal epithelial tissues is more than sufficient to drive somatic point mutations to homoplasmy.

Number of Segregation Units and the Rate of Segregation

The rate of random segregation strongly depends on the number of segregation units in the cell. The number of generations necessary to reach a particular level of segregation is, other factors equal, approximately proportional to the number of segregation units, whatever definition of the level of segregation is used. Summarized in FIGURE 2 are the results of modeling by several groups.[48–50] and ourselves.[41] Despite the fact that the quantities measured in each model were different, the general tendency and proportionality applies to all of them. As a rule of thumb, the number of generations necessary for half of the cells in a population to become homoplasmic is approximately equal to the number of segregation units.

In our simulations, we assumed that a cell containing 250 mitochondrial genomes is the haploid state. We assumed that a single mitochondrion contains five copies of mtDNA, which we believe is a reasonable simulation of *in vivo* estimates.[17,18] We also assumed that a segregation unit is represented by a single mitochondrion, that is, all mtDNA genomes contained within a mitochondrion are transmitted exclusively to its daughters and there is no DNA exchange between mitochondria in the cell. This resulted in 50 segregation units per cell. Furthermore, we assumed that mtDNA genomes are distributed randomly between the daughter mitochondria during proliferation of mitochondria. This latter assumption results in a very rapid segregation of genotypes between mitochondria within the cell, so that each mitochondrion for practical purposes can be considered homoplasmic at all times.

The assumption that the mitochondrion is a homoplasmic segregation unit is supported by recent data demonstrating, by means of single mitochondrion PCR, intramitochondrial homoplasmy of a heteroplasmic cell line.[19] Furthermore, a number of studies reported the lack of functional complementation between com-

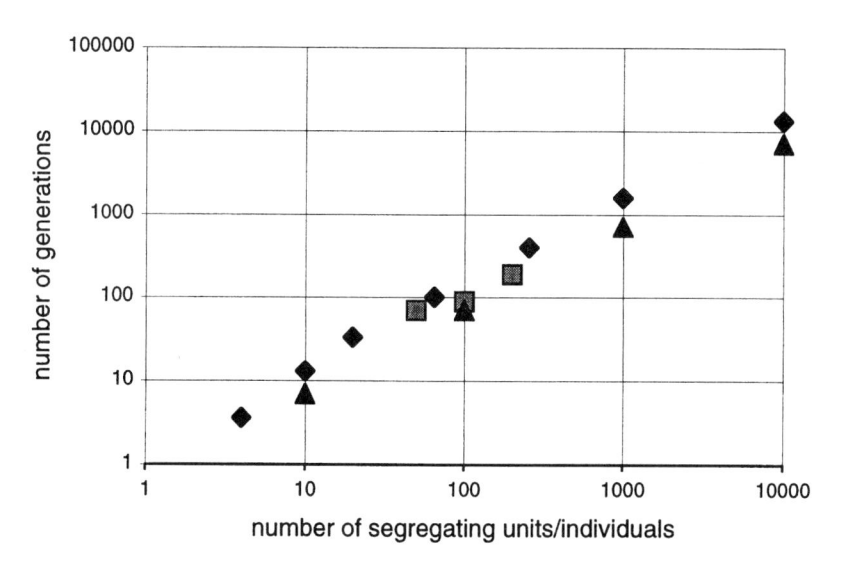

FIGURE 2. The number of generations necessary to reach a certain level of segregation is proportional to the number of segregation units per cell. The levels of segregation are defined as *diamonds*, 50% probability of survival of two or more mitochondrial lineages in a population of *N* individuals;[48] *triangles*, midpoint of distribution variance of the fraction of one of the two forms of mtDNA that originally coexisted in a cell;[49,50] *squares*, in a system with continuously generated mutations, the lag between the lines representing all mutants in a tissue and clonally expanded mutations only.[41]

plementary mtDNA mutations introduced into the cell within separate mitochondria,[11,14] which likely excludes the possibility of intermitochondrial exchange of genetic information.

There are, however, arguments against considering a mitochondrion to be the segregating unit during propagation of mtDNA. Rapid intermixing of genomes was observed upon transfection of mitochondria.[12] Furthermore, in contrast with studies cited above, efficient complementation between mitochondrial genomes mixed within a cell has been observed in other studies.[11,13,52] These findings do not exclude the possibility that the mitochondrion represents the segregating unit, but they disable a very powerful argument in its favor: if genomes within the cell do not interact, they are most probably physically separated within nonlinked mitochondria, which are therefore well-suited to behave as segregation units. It has been suggested that the two modes of interaction can be switched depending on certain conditions,[5] or that lack of complementation could be explained by posttransfection random segregation.[50] Things were complicated even further by the idea of fatefully replicated nucleoids, which are supposed to maintain stable intramitochondrial heteroplasmy irrespectively of mitochondrial fusion.[36]

The source of discrepancy between the different studies is not clear yet. We would like to point out, however, that all the above referenced studies were performed *in vitro* and little is known about the *in vivo* situation. Given the reported sensitivity of mitochondrial architecture to various stresses,[53,54] *in vitro* conditions may lead to artifacts. We believe that frequent intracellular clonal expansions in human tissues reported herein, especially those of neutral mutations in buccal epithelium, supports the possibility that the mitochondrion rather than a single mitochondrial genome is the segregating unit. Indeed, if a single genome were the segregating unit, approximately 10-fold more generations of the stem cell would be required to establish the observed extent of segregation. Although not impossible (the lack of knowledge allows a lot of flexibility), this looks like a much less probable scenario.

Expansions in the Heart: A "Structural" Mechanism?

Myocardium is a classical postmitotic tissue, in which deletions of mtDNA seem to be the dominant type of mutations and phenotype-based mechanisms were considered the best explanation for the observed clonal expansions.[45] Recently, this paradigm was challenged by an assertion that random segregation is sufficient to account for clonal expansion in the heart.[46] Ironically, the spectra of clonally expanded mtDNA point mutations in the heart do not seem to support (but do not reject) either of these hypotheses and in turn suggest that at least some clonal expansions in the heart are driven by the "structural" mechanism. It is possible that several mechanisms are responsible for the different classes of clonal expansions in the heart.

As shown in TABLE 1, almost all clonally expanded mutations detected in the heart fall within a narrow region less than 30 nucleotides long (16,028–16,054). Unlike the C-tract mutations of buccal epithelium, neither of these mutations is identical to a neutral polymorphism; in fact, all positions are conserved through great apes, which suggests that the nucleotides involved may be of some functional significance. The dimensions of the target suggests that these mutations may be affecting a binding site of a protein or a sequence responsible for the formation of a particular DNA structure. Interestingly, this region is immediately adjacent to a strong hotspot for mtDNA deletion breakpoints (around bp 16070), which are observed both in disease[55] and in normal aging.[28,56] An increased level of these deletions has been recently associated with a defect in a mitochondrial protein with structural similarity to a primase/helicase.[57]

The fact that almost all mutations are located in this area implies that these mutations are probably directly responsible for the expansion. An alternative explanation would be that the region in question is merely a mutational hotspot (caused, for instance, by a peculiar local DNA structure). The expansion of mutations in this scenario would be explained either by random segregation or by co-expansion with another mutation present on the same DNA molecule that is directly responsible for the expansion. We believe that the diversity of mutation types (G→A, A→G, C→T, del C) makes the idea of a common local hotspot, which would imply a common mechanism, unlikely.

CONCLUSION

The data on clonal expansions of mtDNA point mutations in individual cardiomyocytes and buccal epithelial cells supports the view that expansion of mtDNA mutations is a general and common process. The mechanisms responsible for clonal expansions are most probably diverse.

ACKNOWLEDGMENTS

This work was supported, in part, by Grants AG18536 and ES11343 from the National Institutes of Health (to K.K.). H.A.C. is a Jane Coffin Child Memorial Fund Fellow.

REFERENCES

1. HARMAN, D. 1972. The biologic clock: the mitochondria? J. Am. Geriatr. Soc. **20:** 145–147.
2. LINNANE, A.W., S. MARZUKI, T. OZAWA & M. TANAKA. 1989. Mitochondrial DNA mutations as an important contributor to ageing and degenerative diseases. Lancet **1:** 642–645.
3. KADENBACH, B. & J. MULLER-HOCKER. 1990. Mutations of mitochondrial DNA and human death. Naturwissenschaften **77:** 221–225.
4. WALLACE, D.C. 1992. Mitochondrial genetics: a paradigm for aging and degenerative diseases? Science **256:** 628–632.
5. ATTARDI, G., M. YONEDA & A. CHOMYN. 1995. Complementation and segregation behavior of disease-causing mitochondrial DNA mutations in cellular model systems. Biochim. Biophys. Acta **1271:** 241–248.
6. HAYASHI, J., et al. 1991. Introduction of disease-related mitochondrial DNA deletions into HeLa cells lacking mitochondrial DNA results in mitochondrial dysfunction. Proc. Natl. Acad. Sci. USA **88:** 10614–10618.
7. MORAES, C.T., et al. 1993. A mitochondrial tRNA anticodon swap associated with a muscle disease. Nat. Genet. **4:** 284–288.
8. DUNBAR, D.R., P.A. MOONIE, M. ZEVIANI & I.J. HOLT. 1996. Complex I deficiency is associated with 3243G: C mitochondrial DNA in osteosarcoma cell cybrids. Hum. Mol. Genet. **5:** 123–129.
9. KOGA, Y., et al. 2000. Single-fiber analysis of mitochondrial A3243G mutation in four different phenotypes. Acta Neuropathol. (Berl.) **99:** 186–190.
10. HAMMANS, S.R. et al. 1992. Evidence for intramitochondrial complementation between deleted and normal mitochondrial DNA in some patients with mitochondrial myopathy. J. Neurol.Sci .**107:** 87–92.
11. YONEDA, M., T. MIYATAKE & G. ATTARDI. 1994. Complementation of mutant and wild-type human mitochondrial DNAs coexisting since the mutation event and lack of complementation of DNAs introduced separately into a cell within distinct organelles. Mol. Cell. Biol. **14:** 2699–2712.
12. HAYASHI, J., M. TAKEMITSU, Y. GOTO & I. NONAKA. 1994. Human mitochondria and mitochondrial genome function as a single dynamic cellular unit. J. Cell Biol. **125:** 43–50.
13. TAKAI, D., K. ISOBE & J. HAYASHI. 1999. Transcomplementation between different types of respiration-deficient mitochondria with different pathogenic mutant mitochondrial DNAs. J. Biol. Chem. **274:** 11199–11202.
14. ENRIQUEZ, J.A., J. CABEZAS-HERRERA, M.P. BAYONA-BAFALUY & G. ATTARDI. 2000. Very rare complementation between mitochondria carrying different mitochondrial DNA mutations points to intrinsic genetic autonomy of the organelles in cultured human cells. J. Biol. Chem. **275:** 11207–11215.
15. CORTOPASSI, G.A. & A. WONG. 1999. Mitochondria in organismal aging and degeneration. Biochim. Biophys. Acta **1410:** 183–193.
16. WANG-LARSSON, J., et al. 2001. Increased in vivo apoptosis in cells lacking mitochondrial DNA gene expression. Proc. Natl. Acad. Sci USA **98:** 4038–4043.
17. BOGENHAGEN, D. & D.A. CLAYTON. 1974. The number of mitochondrial deoxyribonucleic acid genomes in mouse L and human HeLa cells: quantitative isolation of mitochondrial deoxyribonucleic acid. J. Biol. Chem. **249:** 7991–7995.
18. SATOH, M. & T. KUROIWA. 1991. Organization of multiple nucleoids and DNA molecules in mitochondria of a human cell. Exp. Cell Res. **196:** 137–140.

19. CAVELIER, L., A. JOHANNISSON & U. GYLLENSTEN. 2000. Analysis of mtDNA copy number and composition of single mitochondrial particles using flow cytometry and PCR. Exp. Cell Res. **259:** 79–85.
20. ZHANG-ZASSENHAUS, D., et al. 2000. Construction of transgenic mice with tissue-specific acceleration of mitochondrial DNA mutagenesis. Genomics **69:** 151–161.
21. MITA, S., et al. 1989. Detection of mitochondrial genomes in cytochrome-c oxidase-deficient muscle fibers of a patient with Kearns-Sayre syndrome. Proc. Natl. Acad. Sci. USA **86:** 9509–9513.
22. SHOUBRIDGE, E.A., G. KARPATI & K.E. HASTINGS. 1990. Deletion mutants are functionally dominant over wild-type mitochondrial genomes in skeletal muscle fiber segments in mitochondrial disease. Cell **62:** 43–49.
23. MORAES, C.T., et al. 1993. Two novel pathogenic mitochondrial DNA mutations affecting organelle number and protein synthesis: is the tRNA(Leu(UUR)) gene an etiologic hot spot? J. Clin. Invest. **92:** 2906–2915.
24. MULLER-HOCKER, J., P. SEIBEL, K. SCHNEIDERBANGER & B. KADENBACH. 1993. Different in situ hybridization patterns of mitochondrial DNA in cytochrome c oxidase-deficient extraocular muscle fibres in the elderly. Virchows Arch. A Pathol. Anat. Histopathol. **422:** 7–15.
25. LEE, C.M., M.E. LOPEZ, R. WEINDRUCH & J.M. AIKEN. 1998. Association of age-related mitochondrial abnormalities with skeletal muscle fiber atrophy. Free Radic. Biol. Med. **25:** 964–972.
26. BRIERLEY, E.J., et al. 1998. Role of mitochondrial DNA mutations in human aging: implications for the central nervous system and muscle. Ann. Neurol. **43:** 217–223.
27. KHRAPKO, K., et al. 1999. Cell-by-cell scanning of whole mitochondrial genomes in aged human heart reveals a significant fraction of myocytes with clonally expanded deletions. Nucleic Acids Res. **27:** 2434–2441.
28. BODYAK, N.D., E. NEKHAEVA, J.Y. WEI & K. KHRAPKO. 2001. Quantification and sequencing of somatic deleted mtDNA in single cells: evidence for partially duplicated mtDNA in aged human tissues. Hum. Mol. Genet. **10:** 17–24.
29. WANAGAT, J., Z. CAO, P. PATHARE & J.M. AIKEN. 2001. Mitochondrial DNA deletion mutations colocalize with segmental electron transport system abnormalities, muscle fiber atrophy, fiber splitting, and oxidative damage in sarcopenia. FASEB J. **15:** 322–332.
30. LOPEZ, M.E., et al. 2000. Cellular phenotypes of age-associated skeletal muscle mitochondrial abnormalities in rhesus monkeys. Mutat. Res. **452:** 123–138.
31. DE GREY, A. 1998. A mechanism proposed to explain the rise in oxidative stress during aging. J. Anti-Aging Med. **1:** 53–66.
32. DE GREY, A.D. 2000. The reductive hotspot hypothesis: an update. Arch. Biochem. Biophys. **373:** 295–301.
33. JENUTH, J.P., A.C. PETERSON. & E.A. SHOUBRIDGE. 1997. MtDNA segregation in colonic crypts: tissue-specific selection for different mtDNA genotypes in heteroplasmic mice. Nat. Genet. **16:** 93–95.
34. WILSON, M.R., et al. 1997. A family exhibiting heteroplasmy in the human mitochondrial DNA control region reveals both somatic mosaicism and pronounced segregation of mitotypes. Hum. Genet. **100:** 167–171.
35. YONEDA, M., et al. 1992. Marked replicative advantage of human mtDNA carrying a point mutation that causes the MELAS encephalomyopathy. Proc. Natl. Acad. Sci. USA **89:** 11164–11168.
36. LEHTINEN, S.K., et al. 2000. Genotypic stability, segregation and selection in heteroplasmic human cell lines containing np 3243 mutant mtDNA. Genetics **154:** 363–380.
37. JENUTH, J.P., A.C. PETERSON, K. FU & E.A. SHOUBRIDGE. 1996. Random genetic drift in the female germline explains the rapid segregation of mammalian mitochondrial DNA [see comments]. Nat. Genet. **14:** 146–151.
38. MARCHINGTON, D.R., G.M. HARTSHORNE, D. BARLOW & J. POULTON. 1997. Homopolymeric tract heteroplasmy in mtDNA from tissues and single oocytes: support for a genetic bottleneck. Am. J. Hum. Genet. **60:** 408–416.
39. MARCHINGTON, D.R., et al. 1998. Evidence from human oocytes for a genetic bottleneck in an mtDNA disease. Am. J. Hum. Genet. **63:** 769–775.

40. KHRAPKO, K., *et al.* 1997. Mitochondrial mutational spectra in human cells and tissues. Proc. Natl. Acad. Sci. USA **94:** 13798–13803.
41. COLLER, H., *et al.* 2001. High frequency of homoplasmic mitochondrial DNA mutations in human tumors can be explained without selection. Nat. Genet. **28:** 147–150.
42. CORTOPASSI, G. & E. WANG. 1995. Modelling the effects of age-related mtDNA mutation accumulation: complex I deficiency, superoxide and cell death. Biochim. Biophys. Acta **1271:** 171–176.
43. WALLACE, D.C. 1989. Mitochondrial DNA mutations and neuromuscular disease. Trends Genet. **5:** 9–13.
44. DE GREY, A. 2002. Mechanisms underlying the age-related accumulation of mutant mitochondrial DNA: a critical review. *In* Genetics of Mitochondrial Disease. I.J. Holt, Ed. Oxford University Press. In press.
45. DE GREY, A. 1997. A proposed refinement of the mitochondrial free radical theory of aging. BioEssays **19:** 161–166.
46. ELSON, J., D. SAMUELS, D. TURNBULL & P. CHINNERY. 2001. Random intracellular drift explains the clonal expansion of mitochondrial dna mutations with age. Am. J. Hum. Genet. **68:** 802–806.
47. JONES, J.B., *et al.* 2001. Detection of mitochondrial DNA mutations in pancreatic cancer offers a "mass"ive advantage over detection of nuclear DNA mutations. Cancer Res. **61:** 1299–1304.
48. AVISE, J.C., J.E. NEIGEL & J. ARNOLD. 1984. Demographic influences on mitochondrial DNA lineage survivorship in animal populations. J. Mol. Evol. **20:** 99–105.
49. SOLIGNAC, M., J. GENERMONT, M. MONNEROT & J.-C. MOUNOLOU. 1984. Genetics of mitochondria in *Drosophila*: mtDNA inheritance in heteroplasmic strains of *Drosophila mauritiana*. Mol. Gen. Genet. **197:** 183–188.
50. PREISS, T., S.A. LOWERSON, K. WEBER & R.N. LIGHTOWLERS. 1995. Human mitochondria: distinct organelles or dynamic network? Trends Genet. **11:** 211–212.
51. VILKKI, S., *et al.* 2001. Extensive somatic microsatellite mutations in normal human tissue. Cancer Res. **61:** 4541–4544.
52. TAKAI, D., *et al.* 1997. The interorganellar interaction between distinct human mitochondria with deletion mutant mtDNA from a patient with mitochondrial disease and with HeLa mtDNA. J. Biol. Chem. **272:** 6028–6033.
53. WAKABAYASHI, T., *et al.* 1997. Suppression of the formation of megamitochondria by scavengers for free radicals. Mol. Aspects Med. **18:** S51–61.
54. SOLTYS, B.J. & R.S. GUPTA. 1994. Changes in mitochondrial shape and distribution induced by ethacrynic acid and the transient formation of a mitochondrial reticulum. J. Cell Physiol. **159:** 281–294.
55. ZEVIANI, M., *et al.* 1989. An autosomal dominant disorder with multiple deletions of mitochondrial DNA starting at the D-loop region. Nature **339:** 309–311.
56. KAJANDER, O.A., *et al.* 2000. Human mtDNA sublimons resemble rearranged mitochondrial genoms found in pathological states. Hum. Mol. Genet. **9:** 2821–2835.
57. SPELBRINK, J.N., *et al.* 2001. Human mitochondrial DNA deletions associated with mutations in the gene encoding Twinkle, a phage T7 gene 4-like protein localized in mitochondria. Nat. Genet. **28:** 223–231.

Mitochondrial Damage in Aging and Apoptosis

JUAN SASTRE, CONSUELO BORRÁS, DAVID GARCÍA-SALA, ANA LLORET, FEDERICO V. PALLARDÓ, AND JOSÉ VIÑA

Departamento de Fisiología, Facultad de Medicina, Universidad de Valencia, Avda. Blasco Ibañez 17, 46010 Valencia, Spain

> ABSTRACT: Mitochondria are essential to cellular aging, and free radical production by mitochondria is increased with aging. The rate of oxidant production by mitochondria correlates inversely with maximal life span of species. In many species, females live longer than males. We report that mitochondrial oxidant production by females is significantly lower than that of males. However, mitochondria from ovariectomized females have a similar oxidant production as those of males. Thus, gender difference in life span can be explained, at least in part, by different oxidant generation by mitochondria. Administration of antioxidants, such as vitamins C and E, or a *Ginkgo biloba* extract, protects against age-associated oxidative damage to mitochondrial DNA, oxidation of glutathione, and other signs of oxidative damage to mitochondria.
>
> KEYWORDS: mitochondria; aging; free radicals; antioxidants; vitamins

MITOCHONDRIAL OXIDATIVE STRESS AND AGING

According to the free radical theory of aging, proposed by Harman[1] in the 1950s,[1] oxygen-derived free radicals are responsible for age-associated impairment at the cellular and tissue levels. This theory was developed in the early 1980s by Miquel and Fleming,[2] who suggested that oxygen free radicals produced by mitochondria play a key role in cellular aging. The continuous generation of reactive oxygen species (ROS) by mitochondria throughout cell life produces an age-related "chronic" oxidative stress, especially in mitochondria.[3,4] Moreover, the rate of mitochondrial ROS correlates inversely with the maximal life span of species.[5–7] Mitochondria are at the same time the source and the target of ROS.[8] Thus, oxidative damage to mitochondrial DNA (mtDNA), proteins, and lipids accumulates upon aging.[3,4,9] Furthermore, oxidative damage to mtDNA, but not to nuclear DNA, correlates inversely with maximum life span in eight species.[10]

Mitochondrial reduced glutathione (GSH) plays a key role in the protection against damage to mtDNA. In fact, we have shown that the age-associated oxidative damage to mtDNA correlates with an oxidation of mitochondrial glutathione.[3] Glutathione oxidation increases with age in mitochondria from liver, kidney, and brain of rats.[3] It is striking that this increase was much higher in mitochondria than in

---

Address for correspondence: Dr. José Viña, Departamento de Fisiología, Facultad de Medicina, Universitat de Valencia, Avda. Blasco Ibañez 17, 46010 Valencia, Spain. Voice: +34–96-386-46-46; fax: +34-96-386-46-42.

jose.vina@uv.es

Ann. N.Y. Acad. Sci. 959: 448–451 (2002). © 2002 New York Academy of Sciences.

whole cells. These results outline the role of mitochondria as primary targets of oxidative damage associated with aging.[2]

A common feature among many species is a gender difference in longevity. Thus, life expectancy of women is higher than that of men, a common finding in several animal species, such as rats or mice. In view of the fact that mitochondrial oxidant production has been related to longevity,[6,7] we have measured the rate of peroxide production in liver mitochondria as well as in synaptic and nonsynaptic brain mitochondria from male, female, and ovariectomized female young Wistar rats.

In the present paper, we report that synaptic, nonsynaptic, and liver mitochondria from male rats exhibit a higher rate of peroxide production than do those from females. Mitochondria from ovariectomized females have a similar rate of peroxide production as males. GSH levels in mitochondria from male rats were lower than those in females. Ovariectomy decreases GSH levels in liver mitochondria. Therefore, the gender difference in mean life span could be explained, at least in part, by the different rate of oxidant agents generated in mitochondria and by differences in mitochondrial antioxidant capacity.

We have previously shown that mitochondrial size increases and mitochondrial membrane potential decreases with age in brain and liver.[4,11,12] This may reduce the energy supply in old cells since the mitochondrial membrane potential is the driving force for ATP synthesis. Oxidative stress is involved in the age-associated deficits in mitochondrial function as well as in changes in mitochondrial morphology.[4,9] When oxidative stress was prevented by antioxidant treatment, both the age-related decrease in mitochondrial membrane potential and increase in mitochondrial size were also prevented.[4]

We also studied biochemical pathways that depend on mitochondrial function in isolated hepatocytes and found that gluconeogenesis from lactate plus pyruvate, but not from glycerol or fructose, decreases upon aging.[11] Gluconeogenesis from lactate involves mitochondria, whereas from glycerol or fructose it does not. The lower rate of gluconeogenesis from lactate plus pyruvate is due to an impaired transport of malate across mitochondrial membrane using the dicarboxylate carrier.[11] Posttranscriptional modifications appear to be involved in the age-related impairment of such a carrier, since its gene expression does not change with age.[11]

The free radical theory of aging proposed by Harman[1] is specially atractive because it provides a rationale for intervention (i.e., antioxidant administration may slow the aging process). We have shown that administration of some antioxidants, such as sulfur-containing antioxidants, vitamins C and E, or *Ginkgo biloba* extract EGb 761, protects against age-associated oxidative damage to mitochondrial DNA and oxidation of mitochondrial glutathione.[3,4] The EGb 761 extract also prevents changes in mitochondrial morphology and membrane potential associated with aging of the brain and liver. Thus, mitochondrial aging may be prevented by some antioxidants. Furthermore, we found an inverse relationship between motor coordination and oxidative damage to brain mitochondrial DNA in mice.[13] Thus, late-onset administration of antioxidants is also able to prevent the impairment in physiological performance, particularly motor coordination, that occurs upon aging. Our results suggest that antioxidants exhibit beneficial effects on mitochondrial aging by preventing the chronic oxidative stress associated with this process. To pursue studies in humans, the practical importance of an effective antioxidant treatment that started late in life should be emphasized.

The facts reported here underline the role of oxidative stress, and particularly oxidative damage to mtDNA, in aging at tissue and whole-organism levels. Hence, experimental evidence gives support to Miquel's hypothesis of the key role of mitochondrial oxidative damage in the aging process[2] as well as to Sohal's hypothesis of the rate of pro-oxidant generation as a key factor in the rate of aging.[5]

ROLE OF MITOCHONDRIA IN APOPTOSIS: RELEVANCE IN AGING

Mitochondria are key mediators of apoptosis because mitochondrial permeability transition (PT) is a critical step in apoptosis.[14] Indeed, opening of the mitochondrial PT pore causes release of apoptogenic factors, such as cytochrome c and the apoptosis-inducing factor (AIF), towards the cytosol.[14] We have recently found that mitochondrial oxidative stress is an early event in apoptosis.[15] In fact, mitochondrial glutathione oxidation occurs prior to DNA fragmentation. Hence, mitochondrial oxidative stress may cause mitochondrial PT. We have also found a decrease in mitochondrial membrane potential from apoptotic fibroblasts and an increase in the peroxide content of apoptotic fibrobasts.[15]

There are few reports on the effect of aging on apoptosis, but it has been proposed that the efficiency of apoptosis may inversely correlate with the rate of aging. Experimental studies on rats have suggested that apoptotic cell death provides protective mechanisms by removing senescent or damaged cells that might undergo neoplastic transformation.[16]

On the other hand, some common features of apoptotic cells and of cells from old animals include an increased mitochondrial peroxide production, oxidation of glutathione, and oxidation of mitochondrial DNA.[15] However, a relationship between aging and apoptosis has not been established yet.

REFERENCES

1. HARMAN, D. 1956. Aging: a theory based on free radical and radiation chemistry. J. Gerontol. **11:** 298–300.
2. MIQUEL, J., A.C. ECONOMOS, J. FLEMING, et al. 1980. Mitochondrial role in cell aging. Exp. Gerontol. **15:** 579–591.
3. GARCÍA DE LA ASUNCIÓN, J., A. MILLÁN, R. PLÁ, et al. 1996. Mitochondrial glutathione oxidation correlates with age-associated oxidative damage to mitochondrial DNA. FASEB J. **10:** 333–338.
4. SASTRE, J., A. MILLÁN, J. GARCÍA DE LA ASUNCIÓN, et al. 1998. A *Ginkgo biloba* extract (EGb 761) prevents mitochondrial aging by protecting against oxidative stress. Free Radic. Biol. Med. **24:** 298–304.
5. SOHAL, R.S. 1991. Hydrogen peroxide production by mitochondria may be a biomarker of aging. Mech. Age. Dev. **60:** 189–198.
6. KU, H., U.T. BRUNK & R.S. SOHAL. 1993. Relationship between mitochondrial superoxide and hydroperoxide production and longevity of mammalian species. Free Radic. Biol. Med. **15:** 621–627.
7. BARJA. G. 2000. The flux of free radical attack through mitochondrial DNA is related to aging rate. Aging Clin. Exp. Res. **12:** 342–355.
8. RICHTER, C., M. SCHWEIZER, A. COSSARIZZA, et al. 1996. Control of apoptosis by the cellular ATP level. FEBS Lett. **378:** 107–110.
9. SHIGENAGA, M.K., T.M. HAGEN & B.N. AMES. 1994. Oxidative damage and mitochondrial decay in aging. Proc. Natl. Acad. Sci. USA **91:** 10771–10778.

10. BARJA, G. & A. HERRERO. 2000. Oxidative damage to mitochondrial DNA is inversely related to maximum life span in the heart and brain of mammals. FASEB J. **14:** 312–318.
11. SASTRE, J., F.V. PALLARDÓ, R. PLÁ, *et al.* 1996. Aging of the liver: age-associated mitochondrial damage in intact hepatocytes. Hepatology **24:** 1199–1205.
12. HAGEN, T.M., D.L. YOWE, J.C. BARTHOLOMEW, *et al.* 1997. Mitochondrial decay in hepatocytes from old rats: membrane potential declines, heterogeneity and oxidants increase. Proc. Natl. Acad. Sci USA **94:** 3064–3069.
13. PALLARDÓ, F.V., M. ASENSI, J. GARCÍA DE LA ASUNCIÓN, *et al.* 1998. Late onset administration of oral antioxidants prevents age-related loss of motor co-ordination and brain mitochondrial DNA damage. Free Radic. Res. **29:** 617–623.
14. KROEMER, G., B. DALLAPORTA & M. RESCHE-RIGON. 1998. The mitochondrial death/life regulator in apoptosis and necrosis. Annu. Rev. Physiol. **60:** 619–642.
15. ESTEVE, J., J. MOMPÓ, J. GARCÍA DE LA ASUNCIÓN, *et al.* 1999. Oxidative damage to mitochondrial DNA and glutathione oxidation in apoptosis: studies *in vivo* and *in vitro*. FASEB J. **13:** 1055–1064.
16. MONTI, D., L. TROIANO, F. TROPEA, *et al.* 1992. Apoptosis–programmed cell death: a role in the aging process? Am. J. Clin. Nutr. **55:** 1208S–1214S.

Time to Talk SENS: Critiquing the Immutability of Human Aging

AUBREY D. N. J. DE GREY,[a] BRUCE N. AMES,[b] JULIE K. ANDERSEN,[c] ANDRZEJ BARTKE,[d] JUDITH CAMPISI,[e] CHRISTOPHER B. HEWARD,[f] ROGER J. M. McCARTER,[g] AND GREGORY STOCK[h]

[a]*Department of Genetics, University of Cambridge, Cambridge, UK*

[b]*Department of Biochemistry and Molecular Biology, University of California, Berkeley, Berkeley, California, USA*

[c]*Buck Institute for Aging Research, Novato, California, USA*

[d]*Department of Physiology, Southern Illinois University School of Medicine, Carbondale, Illinois, USA*

[e]*Life Sciences Division, Lawrence Berkeley National Laboratory, Berkeley, California, USA*

[f]*The Kronos Group, Phoenix, Arizona, USA*

[g]*Department of Physiology, University of Texas Health Sciences Center at San Antonio, San Antonio, Texas, USA*

[h]*Department of Neuropsychiatry and Biobehavior, University of California, Los Angeles, Los Angeles, California, USA*

ABSTRACT: Aging is a three-stage process: metabolism, damage, and pathology. The biochemical processes that sustain life generate toxins as an intrinsic side effect. These toxins cause damage, of which a small proportion cannot be removed by any endogenous repair process and thus accumulates. This accumulating damage ultimately drives age-related degeneration. Interventions can be designed at all three stages. However, intervention in metabolism can only modestly postpone pathology, because production of toxins is so intrinsic a property of metabolic processes that greatly reducing that production would entail fundamental redesign of those processes. Similarly, intervention in pathology is a "losing battle" if the damage that drives it is accumulating unabated. By contrast, intervention to remove the accumulating damage would sever the link between metabolism and pathology, and so has the potential to postpone aging indefinitely. We survey the major categories of such damage and the ways in which, with current or foreseeable biotechnology, they could be reversed. Such ways exist in all cases, implying that indefinite postponement of aging—which we term "engineered negligible senescence"—may be within sight. Given the major demographic consequences if it came about, this possibility merits urgent debate.

Address for correspondence: Aubrey D.N.J. de Grey, Department of Genetics, University of Cambridge, Downing Street, Cambridge CB2 3EH, UK. Voice: +44-1223-333963; fax: +44-1223-333992.

ag24@gen.cam.ac.uk

KEYWORDS: negligible senescence; exercise; hormone restoration; cell therapy; gene therapy; AGE breakers; telomerase manipulation; mitochondrial mutations; lysosomal aggregates

The term "negligible senescence" was coined[1] to denote the absence of a statistically detectable increase with organismal age in a species' mortality rate. It is accepted as the best operational definition of the absence of aging, since aging is itself best defined as an increase with time in the organism's susceptibility to life-threatening challenges. It has been compellingly shown to exist only in one metazoan, *Hydra*;[2] certain cold-blooded vertebrates may exhibit negligible senescence, but limitations of sample size leave the question open;[1] and it has not been suggested that any warm-blooded animal (homeotherm) does so. Indeed, humans are among the slowest-aging homeotherms.

Since Gilgamesh, civilization has sought to emulate *Hydra*—to achieve a perpetually youthful physiological state—by intervention to combat the aging process. Such efforts may appropriately be termed "strategies for engineered negligible senescence" (SENS). This phrase makes explicit the inevitable exposure to extrinsic, age-independent causes of death (which is blurred by more populist terms such as "immortality" or "eternal youth"), while also stressing the goal-driven, clinical nature of the task (in contrast to the basic-science tenor of, for example, "interventive biogerontology"). Here we discuss the feasibility, within about a decade, of substantive progress toward that goal.

PLAUSIBILITY OF ENGINEERED NEGLIGIBLE SENESCENCE

It is worth stressing, at the outset, civilization's considerable untapped ability to increase mean life span. One of us (B.N.A.) has devoted much energy to spreading awareness of the extremely cheap and straightforward measures already available for reducing one's age-specific susceptibility to the major life-threatening diseases, particularly cancer, by micronutrient supplementation.[3] In poorer societies, micronutrient deficiency is endemic due to poor diet; efforts to induce better dietary habits (particularly the greater consumption of fruit and vegetables) have been notably unsuccessful. However, such dietary shortfalls can also be avoided with a daily multivitamin costing just 3 cents. A large increase in such societies' mean healthy life span should result, just as has been achieved by public health measures in the past century.

Given our failure to exploit existing opportunities to maximize *average* life span, it is perhaps unsurprising that progress in extending *maximum* life span has been extremely limited (albeit non-zero[4]), at least if measured by the most established statistic, the age at death of the longest-lived subset (typically 10%) of the population. By contrast, our progress in understanding aging has continued to accelerate. This dichotomy underlies the virtual absence of serious antiaging biotechnology: while success in understanding aging has bred enthusiasm, failure in intervention has engendered disillusionment, which extends to the general public. In our view, this disillusionment has brought about an unwarranted neglect of interventive biogerontology, manifest as a deep-seated but unjustified reluctance to aim high.

The claim that this reluctance is unjustified is bold and controversial, and the main purpose of this article is to examine it in detail. One side of the argument is entirely uncontested within the biogerontology community (though perhaps less well appreciated by other biomedical experts, and certainly by the public): that *if* efforts to engineer negligible senescence have any real chance of success, then investment in such efforts is incomparably the most cost-effective long-term approach to diminishing the incidence of age-related diseases. This is a direct corollary of the exponential rise with age in the susceptibility of individuals to all such ailments. What is controversial is the premise that there is any real chance of such progress, however great the investment. The prevalence of pessimism in this regard leaves a vacuum that allows—indeed, arguably promotes—the diversion of much public and private money into putatively antiaging therapies whose availability is immediate but whose efficacy is evidently negligible.

A popular source of pessimism regarding antiaging research is that, as noted above, all homeotherms age. Does this mean that the quest to engineer negligible senescence in humans is illusory, as noted gerontologists have suggested?[5,6] No. Natural selection optimizes each species' rate of aging for its evolutionary niche, and that optimum is thought never to be infinitesimal[7]—in other words, negligible senescence is always suboptimal. (*Hydra* escape the logic underlying this generalization because their lack of long-lived cells means that the "maintenance cost" of living indefinitely is no more than that of living a few months.) Thus, the nonexistence of negligibly-senescing homeotherms in nature does not prove that attempts to engineer one are forever bound to fail.

Another central reason why biogerontologists have doubted that negligible senescence can be engineered is because it necessarily involves *reversing* any age-related decline that has already occurred, not merely retarding or postponing further decline. Reversing a process is, intuitively, enormously harder than retarding it; hence, the goal of reversing aging—when we are presently so powerless to postpone it—is deemed unreasonable. We note several critical flaws in this logic.

One derives from the fact that the public is simply not inspired by the idea of retarding aging, especially when it is presented as the *ultimate* goal of biogerontology research. This is understandable, since the public remains poorly aware that antiaging research is not simply antideath research, but that it seeks to diminish, not extend, age-related debilitation. By contrast, reversing aging—restoring the vitality and function whose progressive loss attends (and, to a greater or lesser degree, haunts) everyone over 50—is a goal which everyone understands and nearly everyone actively desires. In our view, this greater public appeal (and consequent fundability) of such work far outweighs any greater ambition and difficulty that it may possess.

A further criticism of the view that reversing aging is not yet appropriate for serious consideration is the most direct: we suggest that **reversing mammalian aging is not necessarily any harder than dramatically postponing it**. The most influential molecular changes in age-related decline, such as accumulation of mutations and undegradable material in long-lived cells, are irreversible by natural cellular processes. Moreover, the pathways by which they arise begin as intrinsic side effects of fundamental metabolic processes such as respiration and DNA replication. Cells already possess prodigiously intricate defenses against these side effects; it may be unrealistic to suppose that those defenses can be appreciably improved and aging thereby retarded (though studies with novel dietary antioxidants continue to attract interest[8,9]). On the other hand, reversing changes that cells cannot reverse is not tantamount to being cleverer than evolution, given our possession of technology that cells lack—particularly, our increasingly sophisticated ability to alter an organism's DNA sequence (and hence the gene expression of some or all of its cells) to an extent that evolution, in the time it has had, could not. In mice, retarding aging by a large amount—much more than human aging has been retarded by 20th-century medicine[4] —appears much easier than reversing it,[10,11] but this may be a peculiarity of short-lived laboratory strains.[12,13]

Finally, we warn against overestimating the difficulty of implementing interventions that rely on somatic gene therapy. Several measures whose pursuit we advocate below are in this category; moreover, they require the particularly challenging transfection of most of our postmitotic cells. Transgenic interventions are always developed in short-lived mammals (particularly mice) before any attempt is made to translate them to humans, and germline transformation of mice is already routine. Conversely, gene therapy has enormous potential in areas of medicine that do not face the same obstacle of public and professional pessimism that confronts antiaging research, with the result that (despite well-publicized setbacks) efforts to improve its versatility continue apace in numerous laboratories worldwide. Furthermore, we contend that the impact on public opinion and (inevitably) public policy of unambiguous aging-reversal in mice would be so great that whatever work remained necessary at that time to achieve adequate somatic gene therapy would be hugely accelerated. For these reasons, while acknowledging the formidable hurdles remaining in the way of truly comprehensive gene therapy, we choose to focus on mice, rather than humans, as the target organism for developing antiaging interventions that require genetic manipulation. We accept that the distinctive life span–limiting pathologies of different mammals may sometimes recommend other model organisms; however, the interventions discussed below target highly ubiquitous aspects of mammalian aging, lessening the need to study unfamiliar species.

COMPONENTS OF A STRATEGY FOR ENGINEERED NEGLIGIBLE SENESCENCE

We next survey several specific interventions that we feel are especially promising medium-term approaches to reversing age-related decline (TABLE 1). In each case we anticipate that adequately funded efforts to develop such technology have a good chance of success in mice within ten years, and in some cases much sooner; moreover, we argue below that translation of it to humans may occur rapidly thereafter.

A low-technology, but nonetheless important, aging-reversal strategy with considerable promise is appropriate exercise. Though conventional sporting activity will not extend maximum life span, other regimes (particularly pliometric contraction, where the muscle is extended while in tension) have the potential to restore both muscle mass and bone density, and are indeed used by bodybuilders. This appears to operate by releasing a splice variant of liver IGF-1 that is secreted by skeletal muscle and operates in an autocrine and paracrine fashion.[14]

TABLE 1. Major molecular and cellular changes associated with aging and feasible methods for their reversal

Damage rising with age	Effects reversible by:
Nuclear mutations	Telomerase gene deletion in quiescent cell types; angiostasis; autologous vaccines
Cell senescence	Ablation of senescent cells
Mitochondrial mutations	Allotopic expression of normally mtDNA-encoded proteins
Diverse lysosomal aggregates	Addition of bacterial hydrolase genes
Extracellular aggregates	Phagocytosis via immune stimulation
Extracellular cross-links	AGE-breaking small molecules; stimulated phagocytosis of aggregates
Cell loss	Exercise combined with gene therapy; stem cell therapy; growth factor–induced cell replacement
Immune system decline	IL-7-stimulated thymopoiesis
Hormone secretion decline	Genetically engineered muscle

NOTE: Some are already feasible in humans; the remainder can presently be developed only in mice, but will become applicable to humans as and when comprehensive somatic gene therapy is available. For details, see text.

Muscle and bone are also rejuvenated by hormone supplementation, since hormonal changes underlie (for example) the change in relative activity of osteoblasts and osteoclasts that causes loss of bone density and eventually osteoporosis.[15] Similarly, growth factor–induced reversal of thymic involution has been reported recently[16] and may comprehensively restore youthful immune function.[17] Such supplementation has side effects which many find unacceptable.[18] Logically, however, these must arise from the coexistence of a youthful level of the relevant hormones with an aged state of other aspects of physiology. Coordinated restoration of all hormones and growth factors to youthful levels may thus be anticipated to induce more widespread reversal of age-related gene expression changes, particularly if supplementation is administered by a slow-release delivery system that closely mirrors natural patterns of hormone release. In some cases that pattern is inducible or rhythmic, especially circadian;[19] this should also be feasible to emulate (if that is found to be necessary) by placing transgenes under the regulatory regions of genes whose natural expression has a similar profile. Such delivery systems must initially be developed in mice; genetic engineering of muscle to express hormones shows great promise in this regard.[20]

On the other hand, there is strong evidence that youthful levels of some hormones and growth factors promote cancer; thus, such intervention in isolation might well be life shortening. The extended life span of mice deficient for growth hormone or its receptor[21] indicates, because most laboratory mice die of cancer, that cancer appears and/or grows more slowly in a growth hormone–deficient environment. Growth hormone also promotes other pathologic conditions, including insulin resistance.[22] We therefore advocate further judicious testing of low-dose, late-onset supplementation of growth factors in combination with other interventions, and the countering of side effects by other means (discussed below). An important hormone whose levels typically rise, not fall, with age is insulin.[23] In this case the process that declines is the response to the hormone, so the hormone level itself is not the appropriate target for rejuvenating intervention.

Importantly, the ability of muscle mass to respond to growth factors or to exercise depends on the availability of muscle precursor cells (myoblasts, or satellite cells). Endogenous myoblasts are confined within the basal lamina of muscle fibers, so new myocytes can be laid down only if other cell types are induced to differentiate into myoblasts.[24] Such cells could be engineered and cultured *ex vivo* and introduced into the body before differentiation. This technique has been applied, with physiological benefits, even in the heart (which lacks natural precursor cells[25]). Similar therapy is already known to be effective for pancreatic islets[26] in modulating diabetes, of which the non-insulin-dependent variety is another major disease of (which is to say, component of) aging.

Loss of muscle mass and function with age is not limited to muscle fibers, however: the greatest proportional change is in the number of motor neurons controlling those fibers.[27] Loss of neurons also underlies various neurodegenerative diseases. Neural stem cells, cultured *ex vivo*, have been induced to differentiate and replace lost neurons after injection into the brain.[28] We feel that such technology presently shows more promise for reversing age-related neurodegeneration than the better-known discovery of neural progenitor cells within the adult brain, since the latter's capacity to replace lost neurons appears inadequate.

Perhaps even more promising, especially in the short term, as a technique to reverse age-related neural decline, is to induce regrowth of lost synapses in neurons that, though still alive, have lost many of their connections to other neurons (or to muscle), resulting in functional impairment. Neurons of most brain areas are now known not to be greatly depleted with age except in neurodegenerative diseases (though white matter volume does decrease[29]), so the window of opportunity for such treatment is substantial; successful regrowth in response to growth factors, with associated cognitive benefits, has already been reported in rats.[30] This concept extends previous successes in rodents of technically simpler interventions to restore bioenergetic capacity and resistance to atrophy.[31,32]

Cell senescence, the finite replicative potential and associated gene-expression changes seen in cell culture, has been suggested to underlie many aspects of aging and to be treatable by telomerase activation.[33] However, senescent cells are very rare *in vivo* and may often arise by telomere-independent pathways.[34] We therefore feel that any proaging role of cell senescence arises from intercellular toxicity and would be best combated by selective ablation of senescent cells. Proapoptotic signals can realistically be designed to target cells expressing surface markers diagnostic of the senescent state.

Attention to cellular aging has sometimes distracted attention from the important role of extracellular age-related changes. These include deposition of undegradable aggregates such as amyloid in the brain and elsewhere,[35,36] discussed below, and protein–protein cross-linking impairing elasticity-dependent functions such as vascular tone.[37] Small molecules that selectively cleave sugar-induced cross-links show remarkable efficacy *in vivo* in restoring youthful elasticity.[38,39]

While many aspects of aging revolve around loss of cells, others are caused by the opposite—unconstrained proliferation of cells that should be quiescent, the most extreme manifestation of which is cancer. Though many ingenious and promising anticancer therapies (including angiogenesis inhibitors[40] and autologous vaccines[41]) are being pursued, we fear that they, like the body's natural defenses, will ultimately be outsmarted by the intra-organismal natural selection that generates a cancerous cell. But the absolute requirement of telomere maintenance (generally by telomerase reactivation) for indefinite cell division gives us cause for optimism. Only our germ line and stem cell pools actually need telomere maintenance for lifelong function; if the gene encoding a telomerase subunit could be deleted from all other cells, cancer progression would be powerfully impeded. This would be therapeutically equivalent to repairing all somatic mutations in tumor-suppression genes, but whereas such repair is wholly impractical, gene deletion can be performed by comprehensive gene therapy (simulated in mice by germline transformation). Gene therapy is normally considered as a means of introducing replacement genes into cells that harbor mutations in them, but this unconventional application of it is equally feasible. It could also be used for any secondary telomere maintenance mechanisms that we may discover; one, termed ALT, is already known.[42]

Gene deletion is not the only unorthodox use of gene therapy that has antiaging potential. Another is allotopic expression of normally mitochondrial DNA (mtDNA)-encoded proteins from suitably modified nuclear transgenes. Most of the several hundred mitochondrial proteins are nuclear-coded and imported from the cytosol; only 13 (totaling fewer than 4000 amino acids) are encoded in the mtDNA, so it is both conceptually simple and realistic to engineer them to be synthesized by the majority pathway. Such transgenes would complement the spontaneous mutations that accumulate in our mtDNA, a phenomenon whose role as the nexus of respiration-driven (i.e., oxidative damage–mediated) aging has been suggested for nearly 30 years.[43,44] Success in this approach was first reported in 1986,[45] but subsequent progress has been slow; that this is largely due to lack of funding rather than intrinsic technical difficulties is shown by the recent successful allotopic expression (conferring rescue of the inactive mtDNA-encoded copy) of a medium-sized such protein in a mammalian system.[46]

Finally we consider augmentation of the mammalian genome with genes conferring functions that we entirely lack. The antiaging potential of such manipulation resides mainly in the incomplete (though impressive) ability of our lysosomes to degrade all the damaged and cross-linked substances which arise within cells as a side effect of normal metabolism. While small-molecule drugs can (as noted above) cleave the most prevalent extracellular cross-links that accumulate with age, which are molecularly well characterized, the immensely heterogeneous lipid and protein aggregates that accumulate in lysosomes are not realistically amenable to such an approach. It remains controversial[47,48] whether the best studied such aggregate, lipofuscin, is truly deleterious to the function of cells in which it accumulates to high levels (such as motor neurons and cardiomyocytes), but there is no such doubt regarding the corresponding substances found in the pigmented epithelium of the retina[49] and in arterial macrophages,[50] leading respectively to macular degeneration[49] and atherosclerosis.[51] Such aggregates are, like mtDNA mutations, plausible mediators of respiration-driven aging.[52] It is also likely that the lysosomal inclusions associated with various neurodegenerative diseases contribute substantially to the course of those pathologies;[53] finally, endocytosis of extracellular aggregates can be promoted by immune stimulation.[54] Soil bacteria such as *Rhodococcus* demonstrate a stunning variety of hydrolytic capabilities, including the commercially relevant breakdown of fuels, solvents, plastics, and even explosives such as TNT.[55] It is by no means fanciful to identify strains that break down pathologically significant aggregates, isolate the relevant enzymes, and introduce them transgenically into mammalian lysosomes. Lysosomal integrity should not be compromised, since the lysosomal membrane's robustness against mammalian hydrolases derives from a specialized molecular structure very unlike these target materials.[56] Bacteria that appear able to digest lipofuscin have indeed proven easy to isolate;[57] different aggregates will doubtless require different hydrolases, but such aggregates are few in number.

We fully appreciate that it is easy, in the case of most of the interventions discussed above, to identify potential obstacles to success. That is true of any highly innovative technological venture. We claim, however, that in no case is there a foreseeable obstacle of a magnitude that justifies delaying the attempt to develop these interventions. We argue that now is the time to heed the old adage "nothing ventured, nothing gained."

ANTICIPATED IMPACT ON PUBLIC OPINION AND ASPIRATIONS: POLICY IMPLICATIONS

The transgenic measures above are mostly achievable far more quickly in mice than in humans. Mouse transgenics, however, since it involves germline transformation, usually demonstrates only retardation of aging, not its reversal, and so may fail to ignite great public interest. We therefore urge that these techniques be tested not only in the simplest manner, by arranging for the manipulation to be active throughout the organism's lifetime, but also in an inducible context (such as the increasingly widespread hormone- or drug-induced Cre-*loxP* system[58]) so that the intervention more directly emulates the possible effects of somatic gene therapy in a middle-aged or elderly adult. Increasing mouse life span by only a year, but with a panel of interventions that was activated only when the treated mice had an expected 6 months to live, would be a far more spectacular result than a two-year increase in life span resulting from a lifelong intervention. We feel that this justifies the greater complexity of such studies. This would also have an impact on the highly active social and policy debate surrounding human germline transformation.[59]

Direct evidence that mammalian aging can be reversed is, plainly, still lacking. On the other hand, obtaining such evidence is tantamount to achieving that reversal, and the ever-accelerating pace of progress in biology and medicine frequently reminds us that judgements of what will be feasible in a few years tend to be very overconservative. Nonetheless, our optimism that the above measures jointly have the potential to bring aging reversal about needs careful justification. It does not arise simply because those measures are numerous: it is because they are comprehensive. We believe that few major features of mammalian aging are omitted from the above survey and would thus be in danger of continuing unabated even if the interventions we have discussed were all implemented successfully. Nuclear mutations other than those leading to cancer, for example, have been compellingly excluded from relevance to mammalian aging within anything approaching a normal life span.[60] Accordingly, while we accept that implementation of only a subset of the measures we have discussed may not truly restore youthful physiology, coordinated implementation of them all should indeed do so—albeit, initially, only in mice. Since none requires enormous advances in either our understanding of aging or our biotechnological arsenal, engineered negligible senescence may finally be within reach. We therefore urge abandonment of the despondency that currently prevails with regard to engineering negligible senescence. We acutely recognize the social upheavals that such progress may well bring about,[61] and join with others[62] in stressing the need to prepare for them as best we can. However, apprehension of that transition must not divert us from pursuing a goal that, after millennia of frustration, may now be within sight.

REFERENCES

1. FINCH, C. E. 1990. Longevity, Senescence and the Genome. University of Chicago Press. Chicago, IL.
2. MARTINEZ, D. 1998. Mortality patterns suggest lack of senescence in hydra. Exp. Gerontol. **33:** 217–225.
3. AMES, B.N. 1998. Micronutrients prevent cancer and delay aging. Toxicol. Lett. **102-103:** 5–18.
4. CHRISTENSEN, K. & J.W. VAUPEL. 1996. Determinants of longevity: genetic, environmental and medical factors. J. Intern. Med. **240:** 333–341.
5. HOLLIDAY, R. 1995. Understanding Ageing. Cambridge University Press. Cambridge, UK.
6. MASORO, E.J. 1996. The biological mechanism of aging: Is it still an enigma? AGE **19:** 141–145.
7. KIRKWOOD, T.B.L. & M.R. ROSE. 1991. Evolution of senescence: late survival sacrificed for reproduction. Phil. Trans. Roy. Soc. Lond. B. **332:** 15–24.
8. HAGEN, T.M., R.T. INGERSOLL, J. LYKKESFELDT, et al. 1999. (R)-alpha-lipoic acid-supplemented old rats have improved mitochondrial function, decreased oxidative damage, and increased metabolic rate. FASEB J. **13:** 411–418.
9. MELOV, S., J. RAVENSCROFT, S. MALIK, et al. 2000. Extension of life-span with superoxide dismutase/catalase mimetics. Science **289:** 1567–1569.
10. BROWN-BORG, H.M., K.E. BORG, C.J. MELISKA, et al. 1996. Dwarf mice and the ageing process. Nature **384:** 33.
11. MIGLIACCIO, E., M. GIORGIO, S. MELE, et al. 1999. The p66[shc] adaptor protein controls oxidative stress response and life span in mammals. Nature **402:** 309–313.
12. ANDERSEN, J.K. & G.J. LITHGOW. 2000. The real Dorian Gray mouse. BioEssays **22:** 410–413.
13. AUSTAD, S.N. 2000. Nontraditional but highly useful vertebrate models for the study of aging. Gerontologist **40** (special issue): abstract 357.
14. MCKOY, G., W. ASHLEY, J. MANDER, et al. 1999. Expression of insulin growth factor-1 splice variants and structural genes in rabbit skeletal muscle induced by stretch and stimulation. J. Physiol. **516:** 583–592.
15. HUGHES, D.E., A. DAI., J.C. TIFFEE, et al. 1996. Estrogen promotes apoptosis of murine osteoclasts mediated by TGF-beta. Nature Med. **2:** 1132–1136.
16. ASPINALL, R. & D. ANDREW. 2000. Thymic atrophy in the mouse is a soluble problem of the thymic environment. Vaccine **18:** 1629–1637.
17. ASPINALL, R. & D. ANDREW. 2000. Thymic involution in aging. J. Clin. Immunol. **20:** 250–256.
18. BUTLER, R. N., M. FOSSEL, C.X. PAN, et al. 2000. Anti-aging medicine. 2. Efficacy and safety of hormones and antioxidants. Geriatrics **55:** 48–58.
19. CZEISLER, C.A. & E.B. KLERMAN. 1999. Circadian and sleep-dependent regulation of hormone release in humans. Recent Progr. Horm. Res. **54:** 97–132.
20. MACCOLL, G.S., G. GOLDSPINK & P. M. BOULOUX. 1999. Using skeletal muscle as an artificial endocrine tissue. J. Endocrinol. **162:** 1–9.

21. COSCHIGANO, K.T., D. CLEMMONS, L.L. BELLUSH, et al. 2000. Assessment of growth parameters and life span of GHR/BP gene-disrupted mice. Endocrinology **141**: 2608–2613.
22. THORNER, M. O., I.M. CHAPMAN, B.D. GAYLINN, et al. 1997. Growth hormone-releasing hormone and growth hormone-releasing peptide as therapeutic agents to enhance growth hormone secretion in disease and aging. Recent Progr. Horm. Res. **52**: 215–244.
23. FACCHINI, F.S., N.W. HUA, G.M. REAVEN, et al. 2000. Hyperinsulinemia: the missing link among oxidative stress and age-related diseases? Free Rad. Biol. Med. **29**: 1302–1306.
24. DRAKONTIDES, A.B., M.J. DANON & S. LEVINE. 1999. Heterotopic neogenesis of skeletal muscle induced in the adult rat diaphragmatic peritoneum: ultrastructural and transplantation studies. Histol. Histopathol. **14**: 1135–1143.
25. TAYLOR, D.A., B.Z. ATKINS, P. HUNGSPREUGS, et al. 1998. Regenerating functional myocardium: improved performance after skeletal myoblast transplantation. Nature Med. **4**: 929–933.
26. SHAPIRO, A.M., J.R. LAKEY, E.A. RYAN, et al. 2000. Islet transplantation in seven patients with type 1 diabetes mellitus using a glucocorticoid-free immunosuppressive regimen. N. Engl. J. Med. **343**: 230–238.
27. LUFF, A.R. 1998. Age-associated changes in the innervation of muscle fibers and changes in the mechanical properties of motor units. Ann. N.Y. Acad. Sci. **854**: 92–101.
28. ARMSTRONG, R.J.E. & C.N. SVENDSEN. 2000. Neural stem cells: from cell biology to cell replacement. Cell Transplantation **9**: 139–152.
29. KETONEN, L. M. 1998. Neuroimaging of the aging brain. Neurol. Clin. **16**: 581–598.
30. CHEN, K.S., E. MASLIAH, M. MALLORY, et al. 1995. Synaptic loss in cognitively impaired aged rats is ameliorated by chronic human nerve growth factor infusion. Neuroscience **68**: 19–27.
31. BACKMAN, C., G.M. ROSE, B.J. HOFFER, et al. 1996. Systemic administration of a nerve growth factor conjugate reverses age-related cognitive dysfunction and prevents cholinergic neuron atrophy. J. Neurosci. **16**: 5437–5442.
32. POCERNICH, C.B., M. LA FONTAINE & D.A. BUTTERFIELD. 2000. In-vivo glutathione elevation protects against hydroxyl free radical-induced protein oxidation in rat brain. Neurochem. Int. **36**: 185–191.
33. BODNAR, A.G., M. OUELLETTE, M. FROLKIS, et al. 1998. Extension of life-span by introduction of telomerase into normal human cells. Science **279**: 349–352.
34. CAMPISI, J. 2000. Cancer, aging and cellular senescence. In Vivo **14**: 183–188.
35. CZECH, C., G. TREMP & L. PRADIER. 2000. Presenilins and Alzheimer's disease: biological functions and pathogenic mechanisms. Progr. Neurobiol. **60**: 363–384.
36. JOACHIM, C.L., H. MORI & D.J. SELKOE. 1989. Amyloid beta-protein deposition in tissues other than brain in Alzheimer's disease. Nature **341**: 226–230.
37. MASSI-BENEDETTI, M. & M.O. FEDERICI. 1999. Cardiovascular risk factors in type 2 diabetes: the role of hyperglycaemia. Exp. Clin. Endocrinol. Diabetes **107 (Suppl. 4)**: S120–S123.
38. VASAN, S., X. ZHANG, X. ZHANG, et al. 1996. An agent cleaving glucose-derived protein crosslinks in vitro and in vivo. Nature **382**: 275–278.
39. ASIF, M., J. EGAN, S. VASAN, et al. 2000. An advanced glycation endproduct cross-link breaker can reverse age-related increases in myocardial stiffness. Proc. Natl. Acad. Sci. USA **97**: 2809–2813.
40. BERGERS, G., K. JAVAHERIAN, K.M. LO, et al. 1999. Effects of angiogenesis inhibitors on multistage carcinogenesis in mice. Science **284**: 808–812.
41. BERD, D., J. KAIRYS, C. DUNTON, et al. 1998. Autologous, hapten-modified vaccine as a treatment for human cancers. Semin. Oncol. **25**: 646–653.
42. BRYAN, T. M., A. ENGLEZOU, L. DALLA-POZZA, et al. 1997. Evidence for an alternative mechanism for maintaining telomere length in human tumors and tumor-derived cell lines. Nature Med. **3**: 1271–1274.
43. HARMAN, D. 1972. The biologic clock: the mitochondria? J. Am. Geriatr. Soc. **20**: 145–147.
44. DE GREY, A.D.N.J. 1999. The Mitochondrial Free Radical Theory of Aging. Landes Bioscience. Austin, TX.

45. GEARING, D.P. & P. NAGLEY. 1986. Yeast mitochondrial ATPase subunit 8, normally a mitochondrial gene product, expressed in vitro and imported back into the organelle. EMBO J. **5:** 3651–3655.
46. ZULLO, S., J.M. EISENSTADT, W.T. PARK, *et al.* 2000. Gene therapy of the mitochondrial genome: a tale of two genomes. 2nd NIH Mitochondria Minisymposium. National Institutes of Health. http://tango01.cit.nih.gov/sig/mito/webversion.pdf. pp. 12–13.
47. BRUNK, U.T., C.B. JONES & R.S. SOHAL. 1992. A novel hypothesis of lipofuscinogenesis and cellular aging based on interactions between oxidative stress and autophagocytosis. Mutat. Res. **275:** 395–403.
48. BLACKETT, A.D. & D.A. HALL. 1981. Tissue vitamin E levels and lipofuscin accumulation with age in the mouse. J. Gerontol. **36:** 529–533.
49. REINBOTH, J.J., K. GAUTSCHI, K. MUNZ, *et al.* 1997. Lipofuscin in the retina: quantitative assay for an unprecedented autofluorescent compound (pyridinium bis-retinoid, A2-E) of ocular age pigment. Exp. Eye Res. **65:** 639–643.
50. BROWN, A.J., E.L. MANDER, I.C. GELISSEN, *et al.* 2000. Cholesterol and oxysterol metabolism and subcellular distribution in macrophage foam cells: accumulation of oxidized esters in lysosomes. J. Lipid Res. **41:** 226–237.
51. LUSIS, A.J. 2000. Atherosclerosis. Nature **407:** 233–241.
52. TERMAN, A. & U.T. BRUNK. 1998. Lipofuscin: mechanisms of formation and increase with age. APMIS **106:** 265–276.
53. MAYER, R.J., C. TIPLER, J. ARNOLD, *et al.* 1996. Endosome-lysosomes, ubiquitin and neurodegeneration. Adv. Exp. Med. Biol. **389:** 261–269.
54. BRAZIL, M.I., H. CHUNG & F.R. MAXFIELD. 2000. Effects of incorporation of immunoglobulin G and complement component C1q on uptake and degradation of Alzheimer's disease amyloid fibrils by microglia. J. Biol. Chem. **275:** 16941–16947.
55. GOLOVLEVA, L.A., R.M. ALIYEVA, R.P. NAUMOVA, *et al.* 1992. Microbial bioconversion of pollutants. Rev. Environ. Contam. Toxicol. **124:** 41–78.
56. MATSUZAWA, Y. & K.Y. HOSTETLER. 1979. Degradation of bis(monoacylglycero)phosphate by an acid phosphodiesterase in rat liver lysosomes. J. Biol. Chem. **254:** 5997–6001.
57. DE GREY, A.D.N.J. & J.A.C. ARCHER. 2001. Why don't graveyards fluoresce? J. Am. Aging Assoc. **24:** 118.
58. SCHWENK, F., R. KUHN, P.O. ANGRAND, *et al.* 1998. Temporally and spatially regulated somatic mutagenesis in mice. Nucleic Acids Res. **26:** 1427–1432.
59. STOCK, G. & J. CAMPBELL, Eds. 2000. Engineering the Human Germline: An Exploration of the Science and Ethics of Altering the Genes We Pass to Our Children. Oxford University Press. Oxford, UK.
60. DOLLE, M.E., H. GIESE, C.L. HOPKINS, *et al.* 1997. Rapid accumulation of genome rearrangements in liver but not in brain of old mice. Nature Genet. **17:** 431–434.
61. HAYFLICK, L. 2000. The future of ageing. Nature **408:** 267–269.
62. HARRIS, J. 2000. Essays on science and society: Intimations of immortality. Science **288:** 59.

Nature of the Aging Process
Open Discussion

AUBREY D. N. J. DE GREY, *Moderator*

The open discussion is a perennial feature of the IABG congress, and this year's was as stimulating as ever. Contributors offered a wide range of viewpoints, ranging from the highly theoretical to the unashamedly pragmatic.

The Chinese researcher Yin Dazhong spoke first and drew attention to the role of sleep in postponing aging. He summarized the conclusions of the poster that he had presented, which suggested that melatonin might exert an antiaging action by reacting with unsaturated aldehydes, toxic "garbage" whose constant removal is necessary for slow aging. He noted that the connection between sleep and aging has not been adequately researched hitherto.

Next, Imre Zs-Nagy described an abstraction of theoretical gerontology in terms of an analogy with a computer. According to this analogy, aging occurs because we lose either the program code (the DNA), or the readout device (the synthesis of proteins), or the conditions for the readout (the cellular environment in which proteins operate). He noted that decades of research have eliminated the first two alternatives, and he concluded that it was vital to begin to study proteins in more physiological, less purified contexts than is traditionally done by biochemists. He drew particular attention to the age-related changes of viscosity of the cell membrane, in which many important proteins are embedded and so should be studied.

Franklin Rosenfeldt then showed a short series of slides summarizing work he had performed in the attempt to identify a good biochemical biomarker of aging. Being a cardiologist, he chose to correlate the candidate with a physiological measure of "biological age," namely the recovery of developed force after heart surgery. Through his association with Tony Linnane he tested the level of mitochondrial DNA mutations and found a fairly good correlation, but the very low absolute levels of the mutation led him to doubt that these mutations could be a major causal factor in aging. He then examined total mtDNA abundance (relative to nuclear DNA) and found no correlation whatever with the physiological parameter. So, he asked, is there any more reliable biochemical biomarker of biological age? de Grey responded that he didn't think so—that we are still some way from having a better test for biological age than cutting someone open and seeing how hard it is to put him back together again without getting it wrong, which is what Rosenfeldt does. Linnane stressed that the constant turnover of mitochondria may be what makes mtDNA no use as a biomarker of age.

Vitaly Koltover returned to a reference de Grey had made in his talk preceding the open discussion, to the classification of about 300 theories of aging made by Medvedev in 1990. He disputed that this was really even a classification—it was

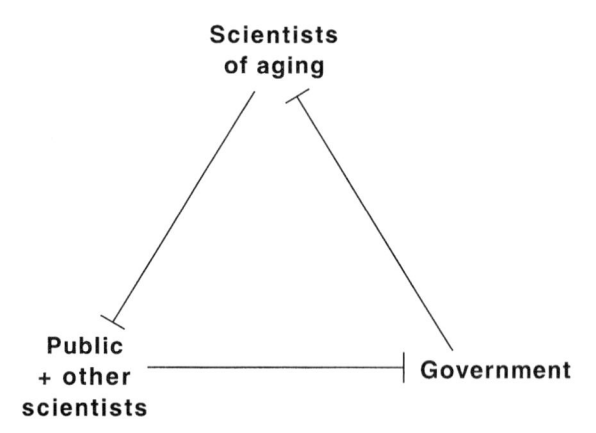

FIGURE 1. A personal opinion of how intervention in aging has become log-jammed.

more of an enumeration. He reminded us that there are two main types of mechanistic theory of aging, programmed and stochastic (and he suggested that the free radical theory is the best of the latter type). He suggested that we should reunite these theories, and that his theory of reliability of biological systems was a step towards doing this.

Jim Joseph intervened to point out that the pursuit of pet theories is less and less appropriate as a way for biogerontologists to be spending their time. He advocated a more practical, interventive approach such as had been described in de Grey's talk. Joseph noted that gerontologists owe it to the public, who ultimately funds their research, to do their best to reciprocate by developing interventions that alleviate the suffering inherent in old age.

Bob Arking pointed out that there is a causal hierarchy of degenerative events in aging, such that the "blunderbuss" policy advocated in de Grey's talk might not be the most efficient approach. He cited the success of John Phillips's group in extending *Drosophila* life span by overexpressing superoxide dismutase in only one cell type (the motor neurons). de Grey countered that this was the approach that has predominated hitherto and that it has not had conspicuous success, though he conceded that this may have been because adequate biotechnological tools have been unavailable. He suggested that there are enough researchers around that we have no reason not to try everything simultaneously.

de Grey then shifted the discussion from the expert understanding of the aging process to the public understanding of it. He made the ostensibly self-contradictory suggestion that the public are actually part of the reason why gerontologists don't work more on interventions to alleviate debilitation of old age. He outlined his reasons with the help of an overhead image (FIG. 1), in which the arrows use the gene regulation convention (that is, they are "suppressor" effects):

He explained this diagram as follows: Governments like to get reelected, so they don't finance projects that the public would regard as futile. The public, in turn, believes the consensus of public scientific opinion; in particular, if most biomedical gerontologists are publicly very pessimistic about what can be done to extend healthy life span, the public believes the pessimistic view. The circle is then closed because that *is* what biomedical gerontologists say publicly, because we like getting funded, and funding agencies don't finance projects that the public would regard as futile (nor people who advocate pursuing such projects). de Grey suggested that this logjam could most realistically be broken by gerontologists, as a community, becoming more outspoken regarding what we *really* think we might be able to do if we put our minds to it, and perhaps being a little less frightened of the consequences. He conceded that this was easy for him to say, as a theoretician with no grant to renew, but he nevertheless challenged the group to suggest an alternative.

Linnane responded that this was an unrealistic approach from the point of view of scientific social dynamics. Extraordinarily few people work on the biology of aging, ultimately because there is no coherent concept for how to attack it. This is in contrast to cardiology or diabetes, where there are enormously greater resources and greater manpower, due to the public's perception—which is not always accurate—that work in those areas can lead to real benefits in the relatively short term. He noted that he had come to think of aging as no more nor less than the sum of diseases of aging, and that this suggests that we should focus on disease therapies rather than attacking the evanescent "aging itself."

Denham Harman noted that the discussion thus far had revealed disagreement about what biomedical gerontologists should do. He stressed that extension of life expectancy at birth could no longer be achieved by better nutrition or housing, at least not in the developed world, and that the only way forward at this point was therefore to attack aging. He noted that the critical need was for testable ideas—ideas that, if correct, would suggest feasible interventions that should delay aging. In respect of the free radical theory, which he characterized as "self-administered radiation," he noted the promise of ideas such as that discussed earlier in the meeting by Mike Murphy, targeting antioxidants to mitochondria.

Arking reiterated that scientists are not an organized community—they do what they want—and that the coordinated and focused approach needed for a truly goal-directed approach to extending healthy life span is lacking.

The discussion was brought to a close by a long-standing colleague of Harman, Fred Abbo, who suggested that within 5 to 10 years it was likely that we would move beyond the treatment of a disease once it has arisen (which he termed "secondary aging"), to focus on preventing the diseases of aging from developing in the first place (treating "primary aging"). He noted that he had known Harman since they began in gerontology; at that time there was no viable biochemical theory of aging and no idea where to go. Now, by contrast, the field seemed to him to be on a firm foothold with excellent prospects.

If nothing else, this discussion clearly showed that there is still much to learn about the aging process before we can decide how to define it, to retard it, and eventually to reverse it. As the organizer of the next IABG congress, I am confident that we can look forward to a similarly lively debate at that meeting.

Oxidative Stress and Life Span Determination in the Nematode *Caenorhabditis elegans*

YOKO HONDA AND SHUJI HONDA

Tokyo Metropolitan Institute of Gerontology, Tokyo 173-0015, Japan

ABSTRACT: The free radical theory of aging proposes that oxidative stress is one of the determinants of an organism's life span. In *Caenorhabditis elegans*, genetic or environmental changes have been shown to modulate life span. Here we discuss whether changes in the generation and destruction of free radicals are implicated in these life span modulations. Changes in culture oxygen concentrations that are considered to reflect free radical generation perturb the life span. The life spans under high and low oxygen concentrations were shorter and longer, respectively, than those under normoxic conditions. Short-term exposure to high oxygen concentration lengthens the life span. This is considered to be the result of an increase in antioxidant defense induced by short-term oxidative stress. Mutations in genes such as *age-1* and *daf-2* that compose the insulin-like signaling network conferred oxidative stress resistance and an increase in Mn-SOD gene expression as well as life span extension.

KEYWORDS: oxidative stress; reactive oxygen species; life span; *Caenorhabditis elegans*; free radicals; antioxidant defense; aging

INTRODUCTION

The free radical theory of aging, first proposed by Harman,[1] is attracting considerable attention.[2,3] Reactive oxygen species (ROS), such as the superoxide radical ($O_2^{-\bullet}$), hydrogen peroxide (H_2O_2), and the hydroxyl radical ($OH^\bullet$), are generated during cellular metabolism, especially during mitochondrial energy production.[4] These ROS, in turn, cause oxidative damage to DNA[5] and to proteins.[6] This theory of aging proposes that, although the defense systems that enzymatically detoxify these ROS including superoxide dismutase (SOD), catalase, and glutathione peroxidase, have evolved,[4] not all ROS are detoxified. Oxidative damage caused by the ROS not caught by the defense systems accumulates to cause deleterious consequences in senescence.

The importance of oxidative stress in the aging processes is evidenced by the observation that the addition of SOD/catalase mimetics into the medium lengthened life span in *Caenorhabditis elegans*[7] and that overexpression of antioxidant defense enzymes extends life span in *Drosophila*.[8,9] Life span in the nematode *C. elegans*

Address for correspondence: Shuji Honda, Ph.D., Tokyo Metropolitan Institute of Gerontology, 35-2 Sakaecho, Itabashiku, Tokyo 173-0015, Japan. Voice: +813-3964-3241 ext. 3141; fax: +813-3579-4776.

hondas@center.tmig.or.jp.

Ann. N.Y. Acad. Sci. 959: 466–474 (2002). © 2002 New York Academy of Sciences.

has been shown to be modulated by genetic and environmental changes. We are interested in whether changes in ROS generation and destruction are implicated in these life span modulations.

LIFE SPAN AND ENVIRONMENTAL OXYGEN

We showed that the life span of *C. elegans* was decreased with increasing environmental oxygen concentration.[10,11] Conversely, low oxygen concentrations lengthened the life span.[11] The aging rate represented by accelerating mortality rate was also dependent on oxygen concentrations.[11] These results suggest that the environmental oxygen concentration is a life span determinant. Because ROS are thought to arise in organisms at a rate dependent on the oxygen concentration,[12] these findings suggest that ROS-mediated oxidative stress is involved in determination of life span.

On the other hand, short-term exposure to hyperoxia slightly lengthened life span.[51] This effect is thought to be a kind of hormesis. Hormesis is the phenomenon when a short-term or a low-level exposure to an agent that is harmful in the long term or at high levels causes beneficial effects such as life span extension. *C. elegans* showed hormesis in that low doses of radiation or short-term heat exposure extended life span.[13,14]

In response to oxidative stress, the level of SOD activity[15] and gene expression and oxidative stress resistance[51] increases in *C. elegans*. Hence, life span extension induced by short-term exposure to hyperoxia may be due in part to reduction in ROS-mediated oxidative stress.

LIFE EXTENSION MUTANTS

Life extension mutants of the nematode *C. elegans* have recently been isolated, and the gene network responsible for its longevity has been unraveled.[16] Mutants of each of two genes that are components of insulin-like signaling transduction, *daf-2*, a homologue of the member of the insulin or insulin-like growth factor receptor family,[17] and *age-1*, a homologue of the mammalian phosphatidylinositol-3-OH (PI3) kinase,[18] live twice as long as the wild type. That is, they display the life extension (Age) phenotype,[19,20] as well as the constitutive dauer formation (Daf-c) phenotype.[21,22] Animals proceed through four larval stages (L1–L4) to become adults. When the food supply is limited and the population density is high, however, animals at the L1 stage proceed to the dauer larva at the L2 stage. The dauer larva is a developmentally arrested dispersal stage; it is resistant to adverse environmental conditions and is adapted for long-term survival.[21] It seems that the dauer stage is nonaging, since the post-dauer life span is not affected by a prolonged dauer stage of up to two months.[23]

A number of genes that regulate dauer formation have been identified.[21] These genes have been assembled into a regulatory pathway.[21] Mutants of some genes do not undergo dauer formation under conditions in which the food supply is limited and population density is high (Daf-d phenotype), whereas mutants of other genes display the Daf-c phenotype under normal conditions. Temperature-sensitive Daf-c mutants of the *daf-2* gene, which are located in the downstream positions of the pathways, develop reproductively and display the Age phenotype at permissive temperatures that do not induce dauer formation.

By contrast, Daf-c mutations in genes located in the upstream positions of the pathways, such as *daf-1*, *daf-7*, and *daf-11*, including TGF-β signaling, do not affect the adult life span.[19,24] The simplest interpretation of these observations is that the efficient life-maintenance mechanism of long dauer survival uncouples from other dauer-formation mechanisms and is inappropriately expressed in adult *daf-2* mutants at permissive temperatures, resulting in adult life span extension.[19,24]

The Daf-d mutation in the *daf-16* gene, a homologue of an HNF3/forkhead transcription factor[25,26] and the Daf-d mutation in the *daf-18* gene, a homologue of PTEN: PIP3 phosphatase, suppress the Age phenotype of *daf-2* mutants.[19,24] Ruvkun and his collaborators suggested that PDK1 and AKT-1/AKT-2 transduce signals from AGE-1 to DAF-16 transcription factor.[27,28] These indicate that insulin-like signaling controls longevity by regulating the PIP3 level and the activity of DAF-16 transcription factor. Therefore, it seems likely that the insulin-like signaling pathway transcriptionally activates the expression of target genes, which specify the efficient life-maintenance mechanism.

The other Age mutants are those in a set of *clk* genes (*clk-1*, *clk-2*, *clk-3*, and *gro-1*), which display an altered biological timing phenotype.[29] *clk-1* is involved in the biosynthesis of ubiquinone, a substance that regulates energy production in the mitochondria.[30] The maximum period of time by which life span is extended in a *clk-1* mutant is only about 40%. However, the mean life span of the double mutant, *daf-2; clk-1*, is over five times the life span of the wild type.[29] This indicates that the *daf-2* insulin-like signaling pathway and the *clk-1* pathway interact in determining the adult life span.

ANTIOXIDANT DEFENSE ENZYMES

SOD is a major enzyme that protects against oxidative stress by catalyzing the removal of $O_2^{-\bullet}$,[4] a central ROS involved in the generation of various toxic ROS. In eukaryotes, there are three types of SODs: cytosolic CuZn-SOD, extracellular CuZn-SOD, and Mn-SOD, an enzyme located in the mitochondria, the major site of $O_2^{-\bullet}$ generation.[4] Several genes in *C. elegans* encode SOD enzymes: *sod-1* encodes cytosolic CuZn-SOD,[31] *sod-2* and *sod-3* each encode Mn-SOD,[32-34] and *sod-4* encodes extracellular CuZn-SOD.[35] The functional differences between the two Mn-SODs in *C. elegans* are not yet known. Catalase catalyzes H_2O_2 removal. Two catalase genes are present in *C. elegans*. Taub *et al.* showed that *ctl-1* encodes a cytosolic catalase; *ctl-2* encodes a peroxisomal catalase.[36] A *ctl-1* mutation was shown to suppress the life extension phenotype of *daf-2*, *age-1*, and *clk-1* mutants.[36]

We have tried to find the genetic pathway(s) that alleviate oxidative stress in the longevity gene network of *C. elegans*. We have screened the Age mutants that are associated with the oxidative stress resistance phenotype, referred to as the Oxr phenotype. The Oxr phenotype may be determined by pathways involved in the detoxification of ROS.

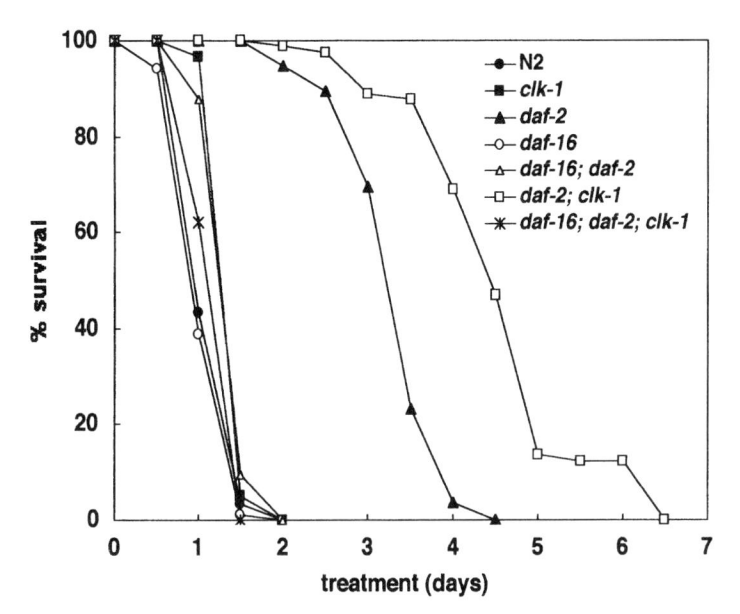

FIGURE 1. Oxidative stress resistance in various mutants of *C. elegans*. Survival period of adult *C. elegans* upon being exposed to oxidative stress. The various mutants and the wild type were exposed to 50 mM paraquat under 98% oxygen. The number of animals surviving was monitored.

OXR AND *SOD* EXPRESSION IN LIFE EXTENSION MUTANTS

For the Oxr assay, we used paraquat (PQ), an intracellular $O_2^{-\bullet}$ generator,[37] under hyperoxia. The *daf-2* mutants that display the Age phenotype survived for a longer period of time than the wild type in the presence of PQ under hyperoxia (FIG. 1).[38] The *daf-2* mutant showed a greater resistance to 20 mM menadione, another intracellular $O_2^{-\bullet}$ generator, under hyperoxia than the wild type.[38] These results indicate that the *daf-2* mutants have the Oxr phenotype. A mutation in *daf-16* and *daf-18*, each completely suppressed the Oxr phenotype of the *daf-2* mutant (FIG. 1),[38] indicating that *daf-16* and *daf-18* act downstream of *daf-2* to confer Oxr as well as Age.[19,24]

Daf-c and Non-Age mutants, such as *daf-1*, *daf-7*, and *daf-11*, did not display the Oxr phenotype.[38] This indicates that there is a correlation between the Age[19,24] and Oxr phenotypes[31,52] among Daf-c mutants.

The level of *sod-3* mRNA in the *daf-2* mutants was significantly higher than that in the wild type.[38] The levels of mRNA transcripts of *sod-1*, *sod-2*, and catalase in *daf-2* were similar to those in the wild type.[38] The elevated level of *sod-3* mRNA in the *daf-2* mutant was suppressed by the *daf-16* mutation and the *daf-18* mutation.[38] Correlation between Age and Oxr phenotype and *sod-3* expression is also shown in the *age-1* mutant.[51] These indicate that the insulin-like signaling pathway regulates the expression of the *sod-3* gene (FIG. 2).

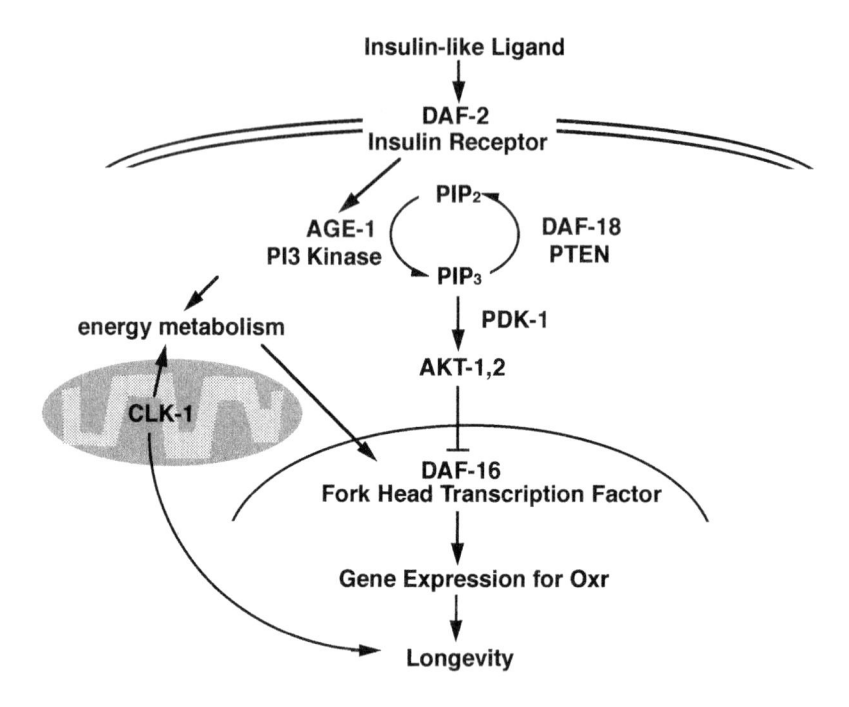

FIGURE 2. A model of pathways for life span determination.

INSULIN SIGNALING AND ROS

The biological significance of the relationship between insulin signaling and Mn-SOD gene expression is not clearly understood at the present time. In vertebrates, insulin is involved in the cellular regulation of glucose uptake and energy metabolism.[39] If the insulin-like signaling system in *C. elegans* is similar to that in vertebrates, defects in insulin-like signaling due to a *daf-2* mutation may be responsible for these metabolic changes. In fact, Kimura, et al.[17] pointed out that the protein sequence of the insulin receptor in an insulin-resistant patient had the same amino acid substitution[40] as that in the *daf-2(e1391)* mutant of *C. elegans*. In mammals, the glucose level affects the redox state of the mitochondria,[41] which, in turn, is associated with the level of ROS generation.[42] In cultured mouse astrocytes[43] and human breast carcinoma cells,[44] glucose deprivation induces oxidative stress; this suggests that glucose metabolism affects ROS generation.

It has been shown in a variety of eukaryotes that ROS induce the gene expression of Mn-SOD.[45] Interestingly, there is an intriguing link between an insulin-signaling defect and the gene expression of Mn-SOD in vertebrates: TNF-α, which interferes with insulin-receptor signaling,[46] induces the gene expression of Mn-SOD.[47] ROS, especially H_2O_2, have been found to be involved in insulin or insulin-like growth factor signaling.[48] The link between insulin signaling and ROS could have been conserved among diverse species.

DAUER AND LONGEVITY

The mechanism responsible for *daf-2* mutants having an extended adult life span may be a dauer subprogram for efficient life maintenance that uncouples from other aspects of dauer formation at permissive temperatures, induced in the adult stage.[19,24] The mechanism responsible for the Oxr phenotype is a candidate for this subprogram. Dauer larvae are resistant to H_2O_2, and have elevated levels of SOD and catalase activity.[49] We found that *daf-7*, a Daf-c and Non-Age ts mutant, has an elevated level of *sod-3* mRNA at the dauer stage, but that it does not have an elevated level of *sod-3* mRNA nor the Oxr phenotype at the adult stage.[38] This result supports the idea that the efficient life-maintenance subprogram including *sod-3* is incorporated into the dauer-formation program in Daf-c, Non-Age, and Non-Oxr mutants, such as the *daf-7* mutant; these mutants in the adult stage would display neither the Age nor Oxr phenotypes.

It is interesting that *C. elegans* has two Mn-SOD genes, *sod-2* and *sod-3*, since other eukaryotes are known to have one.[4] *sod-2* is expressed at almost the same level in both the adult and dauer stages, whereas *sod-3* is expressed specifically in the dauer stage of Non-Age worms.[38] Taken together with the above results, we can suppose that *sod-3* comprises part of the efficient life-maintenance subprogram and switches on at the dauer stage. It may be possible that *sod-2* has an antioxidant function under normal conditions defining the wild-type adult life span and that *sod-3* could represent another life span–determining program usually executed at the dauer stage.

CLK-1 AND MN-SOD

The other Age mutant, *clk-1*, did not display the Oxr phenotype (FIG. 1) and did not have an elevated level of *sod-3* mRNA.[38] Interestingly, the *clk-1* mutation greatly enhanced Oxr (FIG. 1) and the level of *sod-3* mRNA in the *daf-2* mutant.[38] It was found that the *clk-1* and *daf-2* mutations synergistically extend adult life span.[29] These results suggest that the *clk-1* mutation potentiates the Age phenotype in the *daf-2* mutant, through the same mechanism that regulates the Oxr phenotype and *sod-3* mRNA level.

The *clk-1* gene function is involved in the synthesis of ubiquinone in the mitochondria, and therefore may regulate cellular energy metabolism.[30] In our model (FIG. 2), the defect in insulin-like signaling caused by the *daf-2* mutation activates the regulatory system of Mn-SOD gene expression. This system may be regulated by the level of cellular energy metabolism, for example, glucose concentration or mitochondrial redox level, using the analogy that in mammals glucose levels affect the regulation of the expression of various genes by insulin.[50] We can speculate that the synergistic action of the *clk-1* and *daf-2* mutations on life extension may be executed through the pathway in which changes in mitochondrial energy metabolism, induced by the *clk-1* mutation, affect the regulatory system of Mn-SOD gene expression. Further studies are needed to confirm this model.

CONCLUSION

There is accumulating evidence that suggests the involvement of ROS in the aging process of *C. elegans*. We showed that changes in environmental oxygen concentrations perturbed life span, suggesting that ROS-mediated oxidative stress was involved in determination of life span. We also found a close correlation between the Age and Oxr phenotypes and the increased level of *sod-3* mRNA in the gene network for longevity in *C. elegans*. This suggests that life extension in the life-extension mutant may result in part from a slowing in the rate of accumulation of oxidative damage caused by normal metabolism, especially mitochondrial energy production.

ACKNOWLEDGMENTS

Some *C. elegans* strains were obtained from Caenorhabditis Genetic Center, which is supported by the National Institutes of Health National Center for Research Resources. This work was supported in part by grants-in-aid from the Ministry of Education, Culture, Sports, Science and Technology and the Ministry of Health, Labour and Welfare of Japan.

REFERENCES

1. HARMAN, D. 1956. Aging: a theory based on free radical and radiation chemistry. J. Gerontol. **11:** 298–300.
2. HARMAN, D. 2001. Aging: Overview. Ann. N.Y. Acad. Sci. **928:** 1–21.
3. BECKMAN, K.B. & B.N. AMES. 1998. The free radical theory of aging matures. Physiol. Rev. **78:** 547–581.
4. FRIDOVICH, I. 1995. Superoxide radical and superoxide dismutases. Annu. Rev. Biochem. **64:** 97–112.
5. BECKMAN, K.B. & B.N. AMES. 1997. Oxidative decay of DNA. J. Biol. Chem. **272:** 19633–19636.
6. STADTMAN, E.R. 1992. Protein oxidation and aging. Science **257:** 1220–1224.
7. MELOV, S., J. RAVENSCROFT, S. MALIK, *et al.* 2000. Extension of life-span with superoxide dismutase/catalase mimetics. Science **289:** 1567–1569.
8. ORR, W.C. & R.S. SOHAL. 1994. Extension of life-span by overexpression of superoxide dismutase and catalase in *Drosophila melanogaster*. Science **263:** 1128–1130.
9. PARKES, T.L., A.J. ELIA, D. DICKINSON, *et al.* 1998. Extension of *Drosophila* lifespan by overexpression of human SOD1 in motorneurons. Nat. Genet. **19:** 171–174.
10. HONDA, S. & M. MATSUO. 1992. Lifespan shortening of the nematode *Caenorhabditis elegans* under higher concentrations of oxygen. Mech. Age. Dev. **63:** 235–246.
11. HONDA, S., N. ISHII, K. SUZUKI & M. MATSUO. 1993. Oxygen-dependent perturbation of life span and aging rate in the nematode. J. Gerontol. **48:** B57–B61.
12. FREEMAN, B.A. & J.D. CRAPO. 1981. Hyperoxia increases oxygen radical production in rat lungs and lung mitochondria. J. Biol. Chem. **256:** 10986–10992.
13. JOHNSON, T.E. & P.S. HARTMAN. 1988. Radiation effects on life span in *Caenorhabditis elegans*. J. Gerontol. **43:** B137–141.
14. LITHGOW, G.J., T.M. WHITE, S. MELOV & T.E. JOHNSON. 1995. Thermotolerance and extended life-span conferred by single-gene mutations and induced by thermal stress. Proc. Natl. Acad. Sci. USA **92:** 7540–7544.
15. DARR, D. & I. FRIDOVICH. 1995. Adaptation to oxidative stress in young, but not in mature or old, *Caenorhabditis elegans*. Free Radic. Biol. Med. **18:** 195–201.
16. GUARENTE, L. & C. KENYON. 2000. Genetic pathways that regulate ageing in model organisms. Nature (Lond.) **408:** 255–262.

17. KIMURA, K.D., H.A. TISSENBAUM, Y. LIU & G. RUVKUN. 1997. daf-2, an insulin receptor-like gene that regulates longevity and diapause in Caenorhabditis elegans. Science 277: 942–946.
18. MORRIS, J.Z., H.A. TISSENBAUM & G. RUVKUN. 1996. A phosphatidylinositol-3-OH kinase family member regulating longevity and diapause in Caenorhabditis elegans. Nature (Lond.) 382: 536–539.
19. KENYON, C., J. CHANG, E. GENSCH, et al. 1993. A C. elegans mutant that lives twice as long as wild type. Nature (Lond.) 366: 461–464.
20. FRIEDMAN, D.B. & T.E. JOHNSON. 1988. A mutation in the age-1 gene in Caenorhabditis elegans lengthens life and reduces hermaphrodite fertility. Genetics 118: 75–86.
21. RIDDLE, D.L. & P.S. ALBERT. 1997. Genetic and environmental regulation of dauer larva development. In C. elegans II. D.L. Riddle, T. Blumenthal, B.J. Meyer & J.R. Priess, Eds.: 739–768. Cold Spring Harbor Press. Plainview, NY.
22. DORMAN, J.B., B. ALBINDER, T. SHROYER & C. KENYON. 1995. The age-1 and daf-2 genes function in a common pathway to control the lifespan of Caenorhabditis elegans. Genetics 141: 1399–1406.
23. KLASS, M. & D. HIRSH. 1976. Non-ageing developmental variant of Caenorhabditis elegans. Nature (Lond.) 260: 523–525.
24. LARSEN, P.L., P.S. ALBERT & D.L. RIDDLE. 1995. Genes that regulate both development and longevity in Caenorhabditis elegans. Genetics 139: 1567–1583.
25. OGG, S., S. PARADIS, S. GOTTLIEB, et al. 1997. The Fork head transcription factor DAF-16 transduces insulin-like metabolic and longevity signals in C. elegans. Nature (Lond.) 389: 994–999.
26. LIN, K., J.B. DORMAN, A. RODAN & C. KENYON. 1997. daf-16: an HNF-3/forkhead family member that can function to double the life-span of Caenorhabditis elegans. Science 278: 1319–1322.
27. PARADIS, S. & G. RUVKUN. 1998. Caenorhabditis elegans Akt/PKB transduces insulin receptor-like signals from AGE-1 PI3 kinase to the DAF-16 transcription factor. Genes Dev. 12: 2488–2498.
28. PARADIS, S., M. AILION, A. TOKER, et al. 1999. A PDK1 homolog is necessary and sufficient to transduce AGE-1 PI3 kinase signals that regulate diapause in Caenorhabditis elegans. Genes Dev. 13: 1438–1452.
29. LAKOWSKI, B. & S. HEKIMI. 1996. Determination of life-span in Caenorhabditis elegans by four clock genes. Science 272: 1010–1013.
30. JONASSEN, T., M. PROFT, F. RANDEZ-GIL, et al. 1998. Yeast clk-1 homologue (Coq7/Cat5) is a mitochondrial protein in coenzyme Q synthesis. J. Biol. Chem. 273: 3351–3357.
31. LARSEN, P.L. 1993. Aging and resistance to oxidative damage in Caenorhabditis elegans. Proc. Natl. Acad. Sci. USA 90: 8905–8909.
32. SUZUKI, N., K. INOKUMA, K. YASUDA & N. ISHII. 1996. Cloning, sequencing and mapping of a manganese superoxide dismutase gene of the nematode Caenorhabditis elegans. DNA Res. 3: 171–174.
33. GIGLIO, M.P., T. HUNTER, J.V. BANNISTER, et al. 1994. The manganese superoxide dismutase gene of Caenorhabditis elegans. Biochem. Mol. Biol. Int. 33: 37–40.
34. HUNTER, T., W.H. BANNISTER & G.J. HUNTER. 1997. Cloning, expression, and characterization of two manganese superoxide dismutases from Caenorhabditis elegans. J. Biol. Chem. 272: 28652–28659.
35. FUJII, M., N. ISHII, A. JOGUCHI, et al. 1998. A novel superoxide dismutase gene encoding membrane-bound and extracellular isoforms by alternative splicing in Caenorhabditis elegans. DNA Res. 5: 25–30.
36. TAUB, J., J.F. LAU, C. MA, et al. 1999. A cytosolic catalase is needed to extend adult lifespan in C. elegans daf-C and clk-1 mutants. Nature (Lond.) 399: 162–166.
37. HASSAN, H.M. & I. FRIDOVICH. 1978. Superoxide radical and the oxygen enhancement of the toxicity of paraquat in Escherichia coli. J. Biol. Chem. 253: 8143–8148.
38. HONDA, Y. & S. HONDA. 1999. The daf-2 gene network for longevity regulates oxidative stress resistance and Mn-superoxide dismutase gene expression in Caenorhabditis elegans. FASEB J. 13: 1385–1393.
39. WHITE, M.F. & C.R. KAHN. 1994. Molecular aspects of insulin action. In Joslin's Diabetes Mellitus. 13th edit. C.R. Kahn & G.C. Weir, Eds.: 139–162. Lea & Febiger. Philadelphia.

40. KIM, H., H. KADOWAKI, M. SAKURA, *et al.* 1992. Detection of mutations in the insulin receptor gene in patients with insulin resistance by analysis of single-stranded conformational polymorphisms. Diabetologia **35:** 261–266.
41. RAMIREZ, R., A. SENER & W.J. MALAISSE. 1995. Hexose metabolism in pancreatic islets: effect of D-glucose on the mitochondrial redox state. Mol. Cell. Biochem. **142:** 43–48.
42. TAKESHIGE, K. & S. MINAKAMI. 1979. NADH- and NADPH-dependent formation of superoxide anions by bovine heart submitochondrial particles and NADH-ubiquinone reductase preparation. Biochem. J. **180:** 129–135.
43. PAPADOPOULOS, M.C., I.L. KOUMENIS, L.L. DUGAN & R.G. GIFFARD. 1997. Vulnerability to glucose deprivation injury correlates with glutathione levels in astrocytes. Brain Res. **748:** 151–156.
44. LEE, Y. J., S.S. GALOFOLO, C.M. BERNS, *et al.* 1998. Glucose deprivation-induced cytotoxicity and alterations in mitogen-activated protein kinase activation are mediated by oxidative stress in multidrug-resistant human breast carcinoma cells. J. Biol. Chem. **273:** 5294–5299.
45. HO, Y.-S., M.S. DEY & J.D. CRAPO. 1996. Antioxidant enzyme expression in rat lungs during hyperoxia. Am. J. Physiol. **270:** L810–818.
46. UYSAL, K.T., S.M. WIESBROCK, M.W. MARINO & G.S. HOTAMISLIGIL. 1997. Protection from obesity-induced insulin resistance in mice lacking TNF-α function. Nature (Lond.) **389:** 610–614.
47. WONG, G.H.W. & D.V. GOEDDEL. 1988. Induction of manganous superoxide dismutase by tumor necrosis factor: possible protective mechanism. Science **242:** 941–944.
48. KRIEGER-BRAUER, H.I., P. MEDDA & H. KATHER. 1997. Insulin-induced activation of NADPH-dependent H_2O_2 generation in human adipocyte plasma membranes is mediated by Gi2 J. Biol. Chem. **272:** 10135–10143.
49. ANDERSON, G.L. 1981. Superoxide dismutase activity in dauer larvae of *Caenorhabditis elegans* (Nematoda: Rhabditidae). Can. J. Zool. **60:** 288–291.
50. VAULONT, S. & A. KAHN. 1994. Transcriptional control of metabolic regulation genes by carbohydrates. FASEB J. **8:** 28–35.
51. HONDA, S. & Y. HONDA. Life span extentions associated with upregulation of gene expression of antioxidant enzymes in *Caenorhabditis elegans*; Studies of mutation in the *age-1*, PI3 kinase homologue and short-term exposure to hypoxia. J. Am. Aging Assoc. In press.
52. VANFLETEREN, J.R. 1993. Oxidative stress and ageing in *Caenorhabditis elegans*. Biochem. J. **292:** 605–608.

Membrane Fatty Acid Unsaturation, Protection against Oxidative Stress, and Maximum Life Span

A Homeoviscous-longevity Adaptation?

REINALD PAMPLONA,[a] GUSTAVO BARJA,[b] AND MANUEL PORTERO-OTÍN[a]

[a]*Metabolic Physiopathology Research Group, Department of Basic Medical Sciences, Faculty of Medicine, University of Lleida, Lleida 25198, Spain*

[b]*Department of Animal Biology-II (Animal Physiology), Faculty of Biology, Complutense University, Madrid 28040, Spain*

ABSTRACT: Aging is a progressive and universal process originating endogenously that manifests during postmaturational life. Available comparative evidence supporting the mitochondrial free radical theory of aging consistently indicates that two basic molecular traits are associated with the rate of aging and thus with the maximum life span: the presence of low rates of mitochondrial oxygen radical production and low degrees of fatty acid unsaturation of cellular membranes in postmitotic tissues of long-lived homeothermic vertebrates in relation to those of short-lived ones. Recent research shows that steady-state levels of free radical–derived damage to mitochondrial DNA (mtDNA) and, in some cases, to proteins are lower in long- than in short-lived animals. Thus, nonenzymatic oxidative modification of tissue macromolecules is related to the rate of aging. The low degree of fatty acid unsaturation in biomembranes of long-lived animals may confer advantage by decreasing their sensitivity to lipid peroxidation. Furthermore, this may prevent lipoxidation-derived damage to other macromolecules. Taking into account the fatty acid distribution pattern, the origin of the low degree of membrane unsaturation in long-lived species seems to be the presence of species-specific desaturation pathways that determine membrane composition while an appropriate environment for membrane function is maintained. Mechanisms that prevent or decrease the generation of endogenous damage during the evolution of long-lived animals seem to be more important than trying to intercept those damaging agents or repairing the damage already inflicted. Here, the physiological meaning of these findings and the effects of experimental manipulations such as dietary stress, caloric restriction, and endocrine control in relation to aging and longevity are discussed.

KEYWORDS: advanced maillard products; aging; antioxidants; arachidonic acid; diets; double-bond index; DNA oxidation; docosahexaonic acid; free radicals; 8-hydroxy-deoxyguanosine; linoleic acid; longevity; malondialdehyde; mitochondria; protein oxidation

Address for correspondence: Dr. Reinald Pamplona, Departament de Ciències Mèdiques Bàsiques, Facultat de Medicina, Universitat de Lleida, Av. Rovira Roure, 44, 25198 Lleida, Spain. Voice: +34-973-702408; fax: +34-973-702426.
   manuel.portero@cmb.udl.es.

Ann. N.Y. Acad. Sci. 959: 475–490 (2002). © 2002 New York Academy of Sciences.

INTRODUCTION

The aging process causes a multitude of detrimental changes in the organism at all levels of biological organization, especially limiting maximum functional capacities, decreasing homeostasis, and increasing the probability of death. All those changes are thought to originate from a smaller number of causes continuously operating throughout life. The early proposal that free radicals,[1] especially of mitochondrial origin,[2,3] are among the main causes of aging is increasingly receiving support from scientific studies;[4] but any theory of aging should fit with at least two main characteristics of this process: aging is progressive and endogenous.[5] True aging changes occur throughout life at an approximately similar rate. Thus, the causes of aging cannot be present exclusively in old individuals, they must be present already in young adult individuals, otherwise the young would not become old. They must be present during the whole life span, both in youth and at old age, at roughly the same levels. On the other hand, aging is an endogenous process. This means that exogenous factors like dietary-dependent antioxidants, radiation, or external sources of stress cannot be the causes of aging. It also means that the aging rate of each animal species, and thus maximum longevity (MLSP), is mainly determined by the genes, not by the environment.[6,7] The endogenous character of aging explains why different animal species age at widely different rates under similar environments (varying more than 40-fold among mammalian species) and why the intrinsic aging rate of a given species (unlike its age at death due to external stress) is similar in widely different environments. Survival rate in stressful environments should not be confused with aging. The external environmental conditions strongly modify survival and thus mean life span, whereas genetically determined progressive and endogenous processes mainly control the rate of aging and the longevity of species. Available comparative evidence consistently indicates that there are two basic molecular traits linking aging and oxidative stress: the rate of generation of oxygen radicals (ROS) in mitochondria and the degree of unsaturation of membrane fatty acids. Both are, or lead to, endogenously determined processes that occur continuously throughout life at a characteristic rate in each animal species depending on its longevity.

ANTIOXIDANTS, MITOCHONDRIAL ROS PRODUCTION, AND MAXIMUM LIFE SPAN

Synoptically, the main findings relating antioxidants and free radical production with maximum longevity are the following (FIG. 1):

(1) Endogenous antioxidant enzymes and low-molecular-weight antioxidants are negatively correlated with maximum longevity; that is, long-lived animals, either mammals, birds, or vertebrates in general share a common trait: they have very low levels of endogenous tissue antioxidants. Furthermore, experimental supplementation with antioxidants does not slow the intrinsic aging process. Hence, antioxidants cannot determine longevity (reviewed in Pérez-Campo et al.[8]).

(2) All the comparative studies performed thus far show that the rate of mitochondrial oxygen radical generation is lower in long-lived than in short-lived animals. This occurs in all kinds of species, comparing animals following the "rate of living theory" [9–11] (the inverse relationship between maximum longevity and meta-

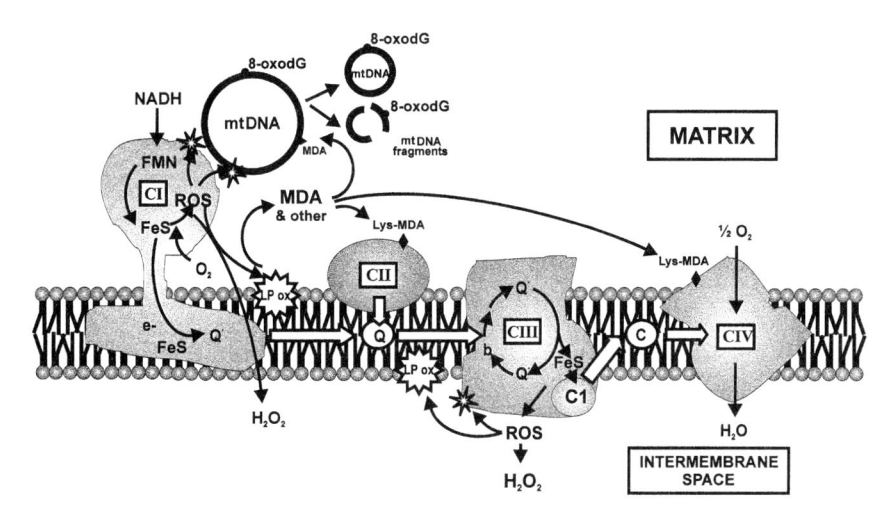

FIGURE 1. Although heart mitochondria can produce ROS at both complexes I and III, the longevity-related difference has been located at complex I in rat versus pigeon.[13] Recent results discard the flavin and suggest that iron–sulphur clusters (FeS) are the ROS generators of complex I.[17] Caloric restriction also decreases mitochondrial ROS generation of rat heart mitochondria specifically at complex I.[18] ROS production causes oxidative damage to mtDNA and to polyunsaturated fatty acids, leading to the formation of carbonyl compounds that, in turn, damage other macromolecules.

bolic rate), as well as in comparisons between animals showing differences in longevity that cannot be explained on the basis of their metabolic rates (e.g., mammals vs. birds).[12–15] Therefore, the rate of mitochondrial ROS generation is a better correlate of maximum longevity and aging rate than the basal rate of oxygen consumption. This is logical since, after all, the potentially damaging agents are the ROS, not ground-state oxygen. Furthermore, it is interesting to note that ROS production does not increase in proportion to the increase in oxygen consumption during state 4 to state 3 energy transition, which can explain the paradox that exercise does not shorten rodent or human longevity.[16] This is so because the degree of reduction of the electron carriers in the respiratory chain, including those containing the ROS generators, increases when electron flow decreases; and the larger the degree of reduction of the generator, the higher will be its rate of ROS production.[16] So, mitochondrial ROS production does not necessarily increase in proportion to mitochondrial oxygen consumption, either across species or in a single species under different physiological conditions, because the free radical leak (the percent of total electron flow leading to univalent O_2 reduction) in the respiratory chain is not a constant. It remains to be tested whether a decrease in the rate of mitochondrial ROS generation in a given species, performed experimentally without deleterious effects, can slow down the aging rate.

(3) Localization studies in heart mitochondria show that complexes I and III can produce H_2O_2 in state 4, but the lower mitochondrial ROS production of pigeons (MLSP, 35 years) in relation to rats (MLSP, 4 years) is localized exclusively at complex I.[13] Recent results discard the flavin and suggest that the iron–sulphur

clusters are the ROS generators of complex I.[17] Interestingly, it has been recently found that the only manipulation that consistently slows down aging, caloric restriction (CR), also decreases mitochondrial ROS generation of rat heart mitochondria specifically at complex I.[18]

(4) It has been recently found that the steady-state levels of oxidative damage in mtDNA (not in nDNA), measured as 8-oxodG in the heart and brain of homeothermic animals (mammals or birds), are also negatively correlated with maximum longevity.[19,20] Mitochondrial ROS damage mtDNA more intensely than nDNA in the heart and brain of homeothermic vertebrates because of the proximity between the source of damage and the target. Thus, the attack rate of mitochondrial ROS against mtDNA can be a major determinant of aging rate.[21–23] This can occur through the repeatedly described accumulation of mtDNA mutations during rodent and human aging.[24,25] The rate of accumulation of those somatic age-related mutations is much quicker in short- than in long-lived animals.[26,27] The hypothesis emerges that the rate of mitochondrial ROS production of each animal determines the rate of ROS attack and flux of oxidative damage through mtDNA[23] and thus the rate of accumulation of mtDNA mutations and the aging rate. Furthermore, it has been found that CR also decreases 8-oxodG in heart mtDNA (not in nDNA) in agreement with a CR-induced decrease in mitochondrial ROS production.[18] Thus, a common mechanism seems to be responsible, at least in part, for decreases in aging rate in a given species (after CR) and between different animal species: a decrease in ROS generation at complex I.

(5) Proteins are also directly modified by ROS, leading to the formation of oxidatively modified amino acids. Furthermore, proteins are indirectly modified by reactive carbonyl compounds resulting from oxidation of carbohydrates and polyunsaturated fatty acids, with the final formation of advanced maillard products (AMPs).[28] Several fundamental findings relate this protein damage and aging rate: (a) the accumulation of protein damage during aging in extracellular matrix and tissues;[28,29] (b) the concentration[30,31] and the rate of accumulation[32] of protein damage is higher in short- than in long-lived animal species; and (c) the concentration[33] and rate of accumulation[32] of protein damage is lower in food-restricted than in *ad libitum*–fed animals.

MEMBRANE FATTY ACID UNSATURATION AND MAXIMUM LIFE SPAN

The available comparative studies indicate that maximum longevity is inversely related to mitochondrial free radical production and mtDNA and tissue protein oxidative damage. Although these very important characteristics are consistent with the free radical theory of aging, additional factors related to other macromolecules can also lead to a low level of oxidative damage in long- versus short-lived animal species.

Among cellular macromolecules, polyunsaturated fatty acids (PUFA) exhibit the highest sensitivity to ROS-induced damage, their sensitivity to oxidation exponentially increasing as a function of the number of double bonds per fatty acid molecule.[34] A low degree of fatty acid unsaturation in cellular membranes, and particularly in the inner mitochondrial membrane, may be advantageous by decreasing their sensitivity to lipid peroxidation. This would also protect other molecules

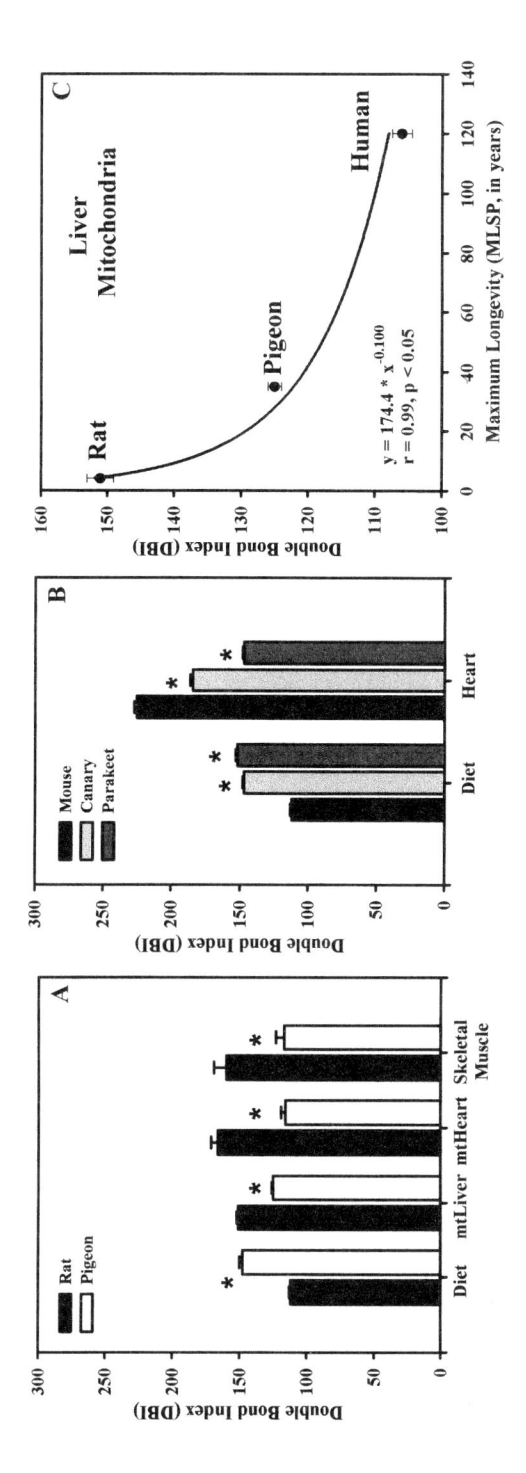

FIGURE 2. (A) Double-bond index (DBI) of fatty acid present in the diet and tissue lipids (liver[35] and heart[30] mitochondria and skeletal muscle) of rats (MLSP, 4 years) and pigeons (MLSP, 35 years). (B) DBI of fatty acids present in the diet and heart lipids of mice (MLSP, 3.5 years), canaries (MLSP, 24 years), and parakeets (MLSP, 21 years).[37] (C) Relationship between liver mitochondria DBI and maximum longevity (MLSP, in years) in vertebrate species (DBI was calculated from data in Ref. 35). DBI = [(Smol% monoenoic × 1) + (Smol% dienoic × 2) + (Smol% trienoic × 3) + (Smol% tetraenoic × 4) + (Smol% pentaenoic × 5) + (Smol% hexaenoic × 6)].

against lipoxidation-derived damage. In agreement with this, it has been found that long-lived animals have a lower degree of total tissue and mitochondrial fatty acid unsaturation (low double-bond index [DBI]) than short-lived ones. Thus, an early study found that the DBI of liver mitochondrial phospholipids was lower in pigeons (MLSP, 35 years) than in rats (MLSP, 4 years) and was also lower in humans (MLSP, 122 years) than in pigeons (FIG. 2C).[35] These results were later confirmed by another independent laboratory.[36] Further, also comparing rat versus pigeon, the same result was obtained in heart mitochondria[33] and skeletal muscle (unpublished results) (FIG. 2A). Nevertheless, the possibility remained that the low DBI found in pigeon (order *Columbiformes*) has a physiological significance unrelated to MLSP. To discern whether a low DBI is a general characteristic of these highly long-lived animals, additional bird species were studied. It was then observed that the DBI in heart of both canary (MLSP, 24 years; order *Passeriformes*) and parakeet (MLSP, 21 years; order *Psittaciformes*) was lower than that of mice (MLSP, 3.5 years) (FIG. 2B).[37] A negative correlation between DBI and MLSP was also obtained in mitochondrial phospholipids[38,39] and heart[40] (FIG. 3) and liver[32] total phospholipids of mammals with different longevities.

Concerning the physiological meaning of the decrease in the degree of unsaturation in long-lived animals, various possibilities have been presented. Some authors[41] have proposed that mammals of large body size have a low DBI in order to decrease their metabolic rates, because the lower the DBI of a membrane, the lower is its permeability to ions (and ion pumping is one of the main determinants of metabolic rate). The permeability to Na^+ and K^+ in liver hepatocytes[42] and to H^+ in the inner mitochondrial membranes[43] also correlates negatively with body size. Whereas this possibility could be true for mammals of different sizes, it cannot explain the low DBI of birds because they have a metabolic rate similar or even higher than that of mammals of similar size. But the studied birds and the mammals of large body size share a common trait: their maximum longevity is very high (they age slowly). Thus, it can be hypothesized that the low DBI of long-lived homeotherms (either mammals or birds) could have been selected during evolution to decrease membrane lipid peroxidation and its lipoxidative consequences to other cellular macromolecules including proteins[44] and DNA.[45] Thus, the low fatty acid unsaturation of long-lived mammals of large body size would protect their tissues against oxidative damage, and, simultaneously, it could contribute to lowering their metabolic rate. But the more general relationship in all homeotherms (either mammals or birds) is the negative association between DBI and MLSP, not between DBI and metabolic rate. The low DBI of birds does not fit with their very high metabolic rates, whereas it does fit

FIGURE 3. Relationship between maximum longevity (MLSP) and double-bond index (DBI, *upper left*), *in vivo* lipid peroxidation (*upper right*), *in vitro* lipid peroxidation (*lower left*), and the lipoxidation-derived protein damage marker malondialdehyde-lysine (*lower right*) in heart phospholipids of eight mammalian species. The MLSP of the selected species are the following: mouse (*Mus musculus*), 3.5 years; rat (*Rattus norvegicus*), 4 years; guinea pig (*Cavia porcellus*), 8 years; rabbit (*Oryctolagus caniculus*), 13 years; sheep (*Ovis aries*), 20 years; pig (*Sus scrofa*), 27 years; cow (*Bos taurus*), 30 years; and horse (*Equus caballus*), 46 years. Values are means ± SEM. Data for DBI, and *in vivo* and *in vitro* lipid peroxidation have been obtained from Ref. 40.

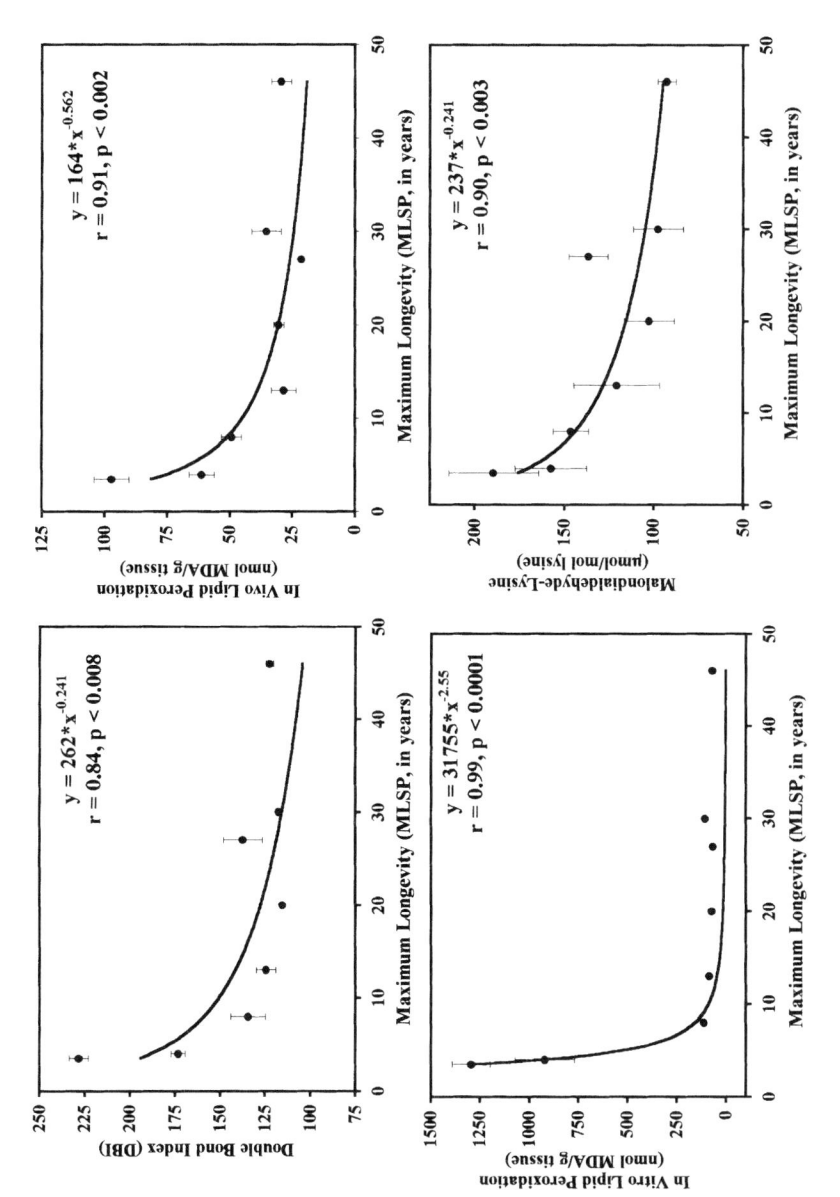

FIGURE 3. *See preceding page for legend.*

with their high longevity. Undoubtedly, factors other than DBI must be responsible for the high metabolic activity of birds.

Oxidation of PUFA leads to the formation of hydroperoxides and endoperoxides, which undergo fragmentation to yield a broad range of reactive intermediates, including alkanals, alkenals, hydroxyalkenals, glyoxal, and malondialdehyde (MDA).[46] These carbonyl compounds, and possibly their peroxide precursors, react with nucleophilic groups in proteins, resulting in chemical modification of the protein. The modification of amino acids in proteins by products of lipid peroxidation results in the chemical, nonenzymatic formation of a variety of adducts, including malondialdehyde-lysine (MDA-lys) and N^e-carboxymethyllysine (CML) among others,[28] which may be useful as indicators of protein oxidative stress *in vivo*. In this context, it has been demonstrated that in long-lived animal species a low degree of total tissue and mitochondrial fatty acid unsaturation (low DBI) is accompanied by a low sensitivity to *in vivo* and *in vitro* lipid peroxidation[32,33,35,37,40] and a low concentration of the lipoxidation-derived adducts MDA-lys and CML in several tissues and mitochondrial proteins[32,33] (see FIG. 3 for heart phospholipids). Independent experiments have also demonstrated a negative correlation between sensitivity to lipid autoxidation and MLSP in brain and kidney homogenates from different mammalian species.[47]

Because correlation does not imply causation, in order to ascertain whether the low DBI protects mitochondria of long-lived animals by decreasing lipid oxidation and protein lipoxidation, an experimental dietary study of *in vivo* modification of the DBI of rat heart mitochondria was performed. The diets used were specially designed to partially circumvent the homeostatic system of compensation of dietary-induced changes in DBI that operates at tissue level. For this purpose, Wistar rats were fed for 7 weeks with semipurified AIN-93G diets containing 10% menhaden oil (rich in n-3; UFA group), or 9.5% hydrogenated coconut plus 0.5% corn oil (SAT group) as the sole source of fat. The addition of 0.5% corn oil in the SAT group was included to avoid homeostatic (DBI) reactive increases in mead acid (20:3n-9) in the SAT group. The analysis of heart mitochondria showed that the dietary manipulation was successful, since the DBI was lower in the SAT than in UFA group (FIG. 4, left panel). The decrease in the DBI significantly lowered *in vivo* levels of lipid peroxidation, protein carbonyls, MDA-lysine, and CML in heart mitochondria[48] (FIG. 4). These observations demonstrate that lowering the DBI of tissue cellular membranes protects against lipid and lipoxidation-derived protein peroxidation. This strengthens the notion that the relatively low DBI of the membranes of long-lived animals could have evolved to protect them from oxidative damage.

The fatty acid profiles of the mammals and birds studied indicate that their biological membranes maintain a similar fatty acid average chain length (around 18 carbon atoms), and a similar ratio of saturated versus unsaturated fatty acids irrespective of animal longevity. The low DBI observed in long-lived species is obtained by modulating the type of unsaturated fatty acid that participates in membrane composition. So, there is a systematic redistribution between the types of PUFAs present from the highly unsaturated arachidonic (20:4n-6, AA) and docosahexaenoic (22:6n-3, DHA) acids in short-lived animals to the less unsaturated linoleic acid (18:2n-6, LA), and, in some cases, to linolenic acid (18:3n-3, LNA) in the long-lived ones at the mitochondrial and tissue levels[32,33,35,37-40] (see FIG. 5 for LA and DHA).

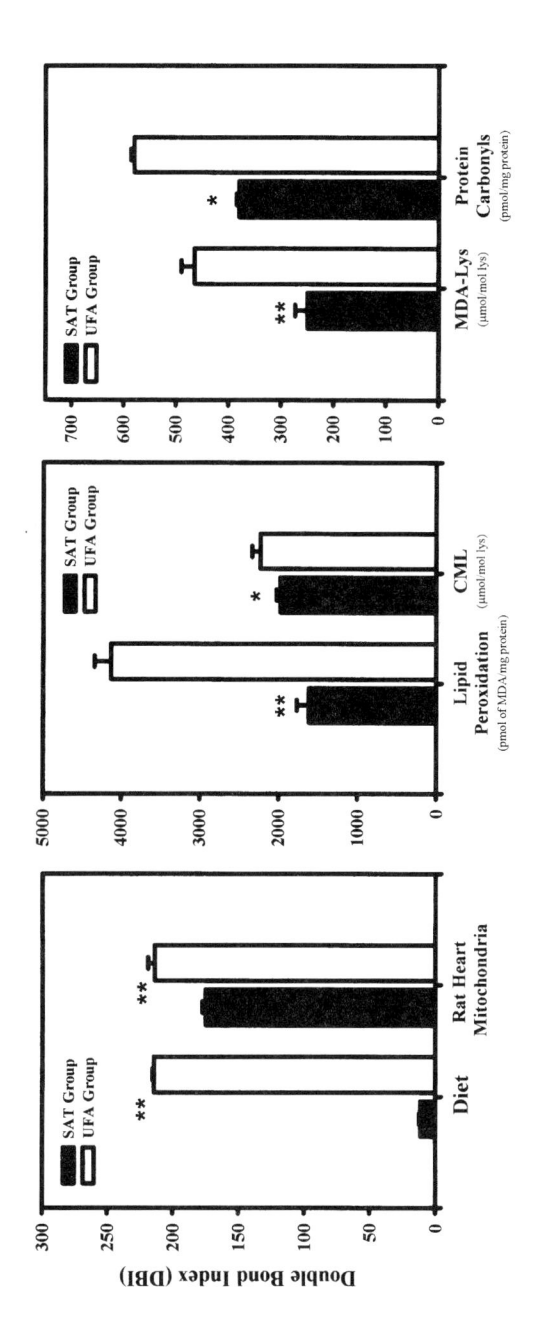

FIGURE 4. *Left*: double-bond index (DBI) of the dietary fats and total phospholipids in heart mitochondria of rats fed saturated or unsaturated diets.[48] *Right*: lipid and protein peroxidation markers in heart mitochondria of rats fed saturated or unsaturated diets.[48] Values are means ± SEM.

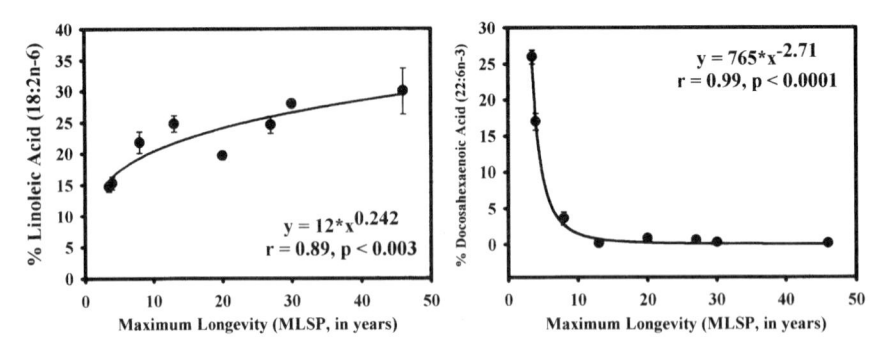

FIGURE 5. Relationship between maximum longevity (MLSP) and linoleic acid (18:2n-6) and docosahexaenoic acid (22:6n-3) contents in heart phospholipids of eight mammalian species.[40] The MLSP of the selected species are indicated in the figure legend of FIGURE 3. Values are means ± SEM.

Furthermore, we have shown that the interspecies differences were not due in any case to dietary PUFAs, since diet DBI did not correlate with MLSP.

Although those findings had never been described as a function of MLSP, two previous comparative reports existed in mammals relating fatty acid unsaturation to body size. In the first one, it was observed that DHA acutely decreased as body size increased in the order mouse–rat–rabbit–man–whale,[49] which is also an order of increasing MLSP, although this was not commented on by the authors. In the second report,[41] it was found that the DBI was negatively correlated with body size in the heart, skeletal muscle, and kidney cortex of five species (mouse–rat–rabbit–sheep–cattle); whereas in the liver the negative trend did not reach statistical significance, and in the brain no correlation was observed. The fatty acids mainly responsible for these differences were again DHA and AA, which decreased as body size increased, and LA, which showed progressively larger levels in animals of larger size.

These results suggest that cellular and/or subcellular mechanisms exist to bring about the observed distinctive distribution of acyl groups in the cellular and mitochondrial membrane phospholipids among different vertebrates. Two mechanisms may be implied in determining the fatty acid profile observed in tissue and mitochondrial total lipids or phospholipid classes: the fatty acid desaturation pathway and the deacylation–reacylation cycle. The estimation of delta-5 and delta-6 desaturase activities indicated that they were various magnitudes lower in long-lived species compared with short-lived ones.[32,33,40] This can explain why DHA and AA decrease and LA and/or LNA increase from short- to long-lived animals. The same was also postulated in the studies referred to above, since desaturases are the limiting enzymes in the pathways of n-3 and n-6 synthesis of the highly unsaturated PUFAs AA (20:4n-6) and DHA (22:6n-3) from their dietary precursors, LA (18:2n-6) and LNA (18:3n-3), respectively. The authors concluded that the main factor responsible for the different DBIs was the possession of low delta-5/-6 desaturase activities in animals of large body size.[41] Thus, desaturation pathways would make available *in situ* the n-6 and n-3 fatty acids to phospholipid acyltransferases in order to remodel the phospholipid acyl groups, postulating the presence of constitutively low species-specific desaturase activities in long-lived animals.[32,33,40] The finding that the acyltransferase to n-6 desaturase activity ratio is about 10:1 in tissues[50] also suggests that the desaturases are the main limiting factor responsible for the observed DBI–longevity relationship.[32,33,40]

The presence of constitutively low desaturase activities in long-lived animals can explain why feeding corn oil (rich in LA) to primates increases mainly LA (to 30% of total fatty acids) instead of AA (only to 10% of total) in their tissues,[51] whereas in short-lived rodents dietary LA leads to strong increases in AA. Similarly to those primates, human monastic communities that chronically consume only corn oil as the main dietary fat source (67% rich in LA) have lipid profiles with around 30% LA but only 9% AA in their lipoproteins.[52] Also, standard diets of mammals (i.e., rats, mice, cows, and horses) and even of birds contain the precursors in the n-6 and n-3 PUFA families LA and LNA at similar levels (35–41% and 1–2%, respectively, in the four species) and do not contain DHA (this extremely unsaturated fatty acid is not added to commercial diets because it oxidizes too easily to be stable at room temperature). However, tissue DHA reached 10% in mice and 3.6% in rats, whereas it was below 0.6–0.3% in cows and horses, which also showed low AA/LA ratios.

The low DBI of long-lived animals is based in a redistribution between types of PUFAS without any alteration in the total (%) PUFA content or in the average chain length. This is an elegant evolutionary strategy, since it allows the reduction of sensitivity to lipid peroxidation and lipoxidation-derived damage to cellular macromolecules without altering fluidity/microviscosity, a fundamental property of cellular membranes for the proper function of receptors, ion pumps, and transport of metabolites, among other functions. This occurs because membrane fluidity is known to increase strongly with the formation of the first and (less) with the second double bonds by means of their introduction of "kinks" in the fatty acid molecule, whereas additional (the third and subsequent) double bonds cause few further variations in fluidity.[53] This is so because the kink has a larger impact on fluidity when the double bond is situated near the center of the fatty acid chain (first double bond) than when it is situated progressively nearer to its extremes (next double bond additions). In the case of sensitivity to lipid peroxidation, however, double bonds increase it irrespective of being situated at the center or laterally on the fatty acids. Thus, by substituting fatty acids with four or six double bonds with those having only two (or sometimes three) double bonds, the sensitivity to lipid peroxidation is strongly decreased in long-lived animals; whereas the fluidity of the membrane is essentially maintained. We call this phenomenon, reminiscent of membrane acclimation to temperature at PUFA level in poikilotherms, the *homeoviscous longevity adaptation in homeotherms*.

The adjustment of the DBI of each organ and species independently of the diet indicates that it is an endogenous trait under genome control. This occurs through PUFA-induced repression of the expression of genes controlling PUFA synthesis, whereas PUFA-deficient diets increase the expression of those genes.[54] These genome-based mechanisms are responsible for the decreases in PUFAn-6 induced by diets rich in PUFAn-3 as well as for the reverse, which occur mainly trough variations in delta-5/-6 activities.[55] If both n-3 and n-6 PUFA are absent from the diet, the unusual fatty acid mead acid (20:3n-9) can still be synthesized from oleic acid (18:1n-9, OA), a process also controlled by delta-5/6 desaturases.[56] In that situation 20:3n-9 can reach a level as high as 15% of total fatty acids to maintain the tissue DBI. These compensations are overlooked in dietary-based studies in which only the fatty acid composition of the diets, but not that of the tissues, is measured. Their unnoticed occurrence can be a reason why some studies on the effects of dietary oils differing in their PUFA content have resulted in the lack of or small changes in tissue oxidative damage[57] or survival,[58] and they stress the need for genetic manipulations to actually alter the DBI of the tissues to a large extent.

Many previous studies have shown that increased levels of very unsaturated fatty acids like AA and DHA can have detrimental effects in various tissues. Examples of this include decreases in respiratory control and increases in proton leak in mitochondria, increased mitochondrial breakage and dysfunction, peroxisome proliferation, fatal ventricular fibrillation in rats, neurological damage, increased lipid peroxidation in association with various diseases, increased incidence of death from apoplexy, or sudden cardiac death in humans. Increases of more than one order of magnitude in AA (to 500 mM) occur in the brain during ischemia and even concentrations of AA and eicosapentaenoic acid (20:5n-3, EPA) in the much lower 20–40 mM range uncouple mitochondria and cause tissue edema.[59] Hypermetabolic uncoupling effects of thyroid hormones on rat liver mitochondria are due, to a great extent, to increased AA/LA ratios caused by increases in desaturase activities induced by the hormone, whereas LA is considered a "proton plug" or coupler (see Ref. 60 for review). Furthermore, the largest amounts of unsaturated fats in the healthy human diet must be present as OA or LA, fatty acids with low degrees of unsaturation; whereas beneficial levels of dietary n-3 PUFAs (the n-3 "paradox") occur only at low 1% optimum dietary levels. These beneficial effects, which seem mainly related to avoidance of blood coagulation and perhaps to promotion of apoptosis of heavily damaged cells,[61] are observed in humans, whose low delta-5/-6 desaturase activities limit the conversion of dietary LNA to the highly unsaturated fatty acids like DHA.

Finally, there are other observations that suggest a role for fatty acid desaturation in the determination of aging rate: (1) Decreases in the less unsaturated LA and LNA and increases in the highly unsaturated AA, 22:4n-3, 22:5n-3, and DHA membrane fatty acids have been described during aging in rat liver[62,63] and heart[49]; whereas fasting decreases delta-5/-6 desaturases, and caloric restriction avoided the age-related increases in DBI by increasing OA and LA and decreasing 22:4n-3, 22:5n-3, DHA, and the peroxidizability index in rat liver microsomal and mitochondrial phospholipids.[62] (2) The senescent accelerated prone mouse (SAM-P) has higher levels of the very unsaturated AA and DHA and peroxidizability index and lower levels of LA than SAM-resistant controls.[64] (3) Most interestingly, Eskimos are human populations showing unusually low incidence of coronary heart disease, psoriasis, rheumatoid arthritis, and asthma and have very low levels of AA in plasma phospholipids due to a genetic lack of delta-5 desaturase activity that persists even after changing them to an LA-rich diet.[65] All these facts raise the possibility that variations in desaturase activities can explain part of the changes in aging rate occurring in those models.

In summary, up to now, only two oxidative stress–related traits correlate with the maximum longevity of animals in the appropriate sense: the rate of mitochondrial oxygen radical generation and the degree of unsaturation of membrane fatty acids (FIG. 6). These two molecular traits are significantly lower in all the long-lived homeothermic vertebrates so far studied when compared to short-lived ones, and their values can be main causes of the low aging rate of long-lived animals. The two

LONG-LIVED ANIMALS

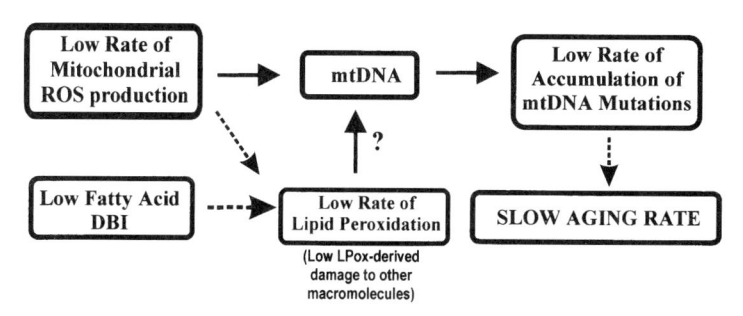

FIGURE 6. Long-lived animals show low rates of mitochondrial ROS production,[15] low steady-state levels of oxidative attack to mtDNA,[19] and low rates of accumulation of mtDNA mutations.[26,27] The low double-bond content (DBI) of cellular membranes in long-lived animals[35–40] can also contribute to a decrease in aging rate by lowering lipoxidation-derived damage to proteins and mtDNA.

MLSP-related traits are species specific, and they are thus genetically determined characteristics that would continuously cause a slow rate of accumulation of irreversible damage in long-lived animals. Thus, they fit with the concept that causes of aging must be endogenous and must operate progressively. Both work through a common mechanism: they decrease the rate generation of endogenous damage. This makes sense evolutionarily, since those kinds of mechanisms are less energetically expensive and much more efficient than increasing antioxidants or repair in order to keep a high MLSP.[23] Furthermore, both determine rate processes (rates of ROS production and of lipid- or lipoxidation-derived peroxidation), which is consistent with their hypothesized role of also controlling a rate process: aging.

ACKNOWLEDGMENTS

The investigations described in this article were supported by grants from the National Health Research Foundation (Nos. 98/0752 and 00/0753 to R. Pamplona and Nos. 93/0145, 96/1253, and 99/1049 to G. Barja).

REFERENCES

1. HARMAN, D. 1956. Aging: a theory based on free radical and radiation chemistry. J. Gerontol. **11:** 298–300.
2. HARMAN, D. 1972. The biological clock: the mitochondria? J. Am. Geriatr. Soc. **20:** 145–147.
3. MIQUEL, J. & A.C. ECONOMOS. 1980. Mitochondrial role in cell aging. Exp. Gerontol. **15:** 575–591.
4. CADENAS, E. & L. PACKER, Eds. 1999. Understanding the Process of Aging. Marcel Dekker, Inc. New York.
5. STREHLER, B.L. 1962. Time, cells and aging. Academic Press. New York.

6. FINCH, C.E. & R.E. TANZI. 1997. Genetics of aging. Science **27:** 407–411.
7. MARTIN, G.M., S.N. AUSTAD & T.E. JOHNSON. 1996. Genetic analysis of ageing: role of oxidative damage and environmental stresses. Nat. Genet. **13:** 25–34.
8. PÉREZ-CAMPO, R., M. LÓPEZ-TORRES, S. CADENAS, *et al.* 1998. The rate of free radical production as a determinant of the rate of aging: evidence from the comparative approach. J. Comp. Physiol. B. **168:** 149–158.
9. RUBNER, M. 1908. *In* Das Problem der Lebensdauer und seine Beziehungen zu Wachstum und Ernährung. R. Oldenburg, Ed. München.
10. PEARL, R. 1928. The Rate of Living. University of London Press. London.
11. SOHAL, R.S., I. SVENSSON & U.T. BRUNK. 1990. Hydrogen peroxide production by liver mitochondria in different species. Mech. Ageing Dev. **53:** 209–215.
12. BARJA, G., S. CADENAS, C. ROJAS, *et al.* 1994. Low mitochondrial free radical production per unit O_2 consumption can explain the simultaneous presence of high longevity and high aerobic metabolic rate in birds. Free Radic. Res. **21:** 317–328.
13. HERRERO, A. & G. BARJA. 1997. Sites and mechanisms responsible for the low rate of free radical production of heart mitochondria in the long-lived pigeon. Mech. Ageing Dev. **98:** 95–111.
14. HERRERO, A. & G. BARJA. 1998. H_2O_2 production of heart mitochondria and aging rate are slower in canaries and parakeets than in mice: sites of free radical generation and mechanisms involved. Mech. Ageing Dev. **103:** 133–146.
15. BARJA, G. 1999. Mitochondrial free radical generation: sites of production in states 4 and 3, organ specificity and relationship with aging rate. J. Bioenerg. Biomembr. **31:** 347–366.
16. HERRERO, A. & G. BARJA. 1997. ADP-regulation of mitochondrial free radical production is different with complex I- or complex II-linked substrates: implications for the exercise paradox and brain hypermetabolism. J. Bioenerg. Biomembr. **29:** 241–249.
17. HERRERO, A. & G. BARJA. 2000. Localization of the site of oxygen radical generation inside the complex I of heart and nonsynaptic brain mammalian mitochondria. J. Bioenerg. Biomembr. **32:** 609–615.
18. GREDILLA, R., A. SANZ, M. LOPEZ-TORRES & G. BARJA. 2001. Caloric restriction decreases mitochondrial free radical generation at complex I and lowers oxidative damage to mitochondrial DNA in the rat heart. FASEB J. **15:** 1589–1591.
19. BARJA, G. & A. HERRERO. 2000. Oxidative damage to mitochondrial DNA is inversely related to maximum life span in the heart and brain of mammals. FASEB J. **14:** 312–318.
20. HERRERO, A. & G. BARJA. 1999. 8-Oxodeoxyguanosine levels in heart and brain mitochondrial and nuclear DNA of two mammals and three birds in relation to their different rates of aging. Aging Clin. Exp. Res. **11:** 294–300.
21. BARJA, G., S. CADENAS, C. ROJAS, *et al.* 1994. A decrease of free radical production near critical sites as the main cause of maximum longevity in animals. Comp. Biochem. Physiol. **108B:** 501–512.
22. BARJA, G. 1998. Mitochondrial free radical production and aging in mammals and birds. Ann. N.Y. Acad. Sci. **854:** 224–238.
23. BARJA, G. 2000. The flux of free radical attack through mitochondrial DNA is related to aging rate. Aging Clin. Exp. Res. **12:** 342–355.
24. NAPIWOTZKI, J., A. REITH, A. BECKER, *et al.* 1999. Quantitative analysis of mutations of mitochondrial DNA during human aging. *In* Understanding the Process of Aging. E. Cadenas & L. Packer, Eds.: 251–264. Marcel Dekker. New York.
25. NAGLEY, P. & C. ZHANG. 1998. Mitochondrial DNA mutations in aging. *In* Mitochondrial DNA Mutations in Aging, Disease and Cancer. K.K. Singh, Ed.: 205–238. Springer. Berlin.
26. WANG, E., A. WONG & G. CORTOPASSI. 1997. The rate of mitochondrial mutagenesis is faster in mice than in humans. Mutat. Res. **377:** 157–166.
27. MELOV, S., P.E. COSKUN & D.C. WALLACE. 1999. Mouse models of mitochondrial disease, oxidative stress, and senescence. Mutat. Res. **434:** 233–247.
28. DEGENHARDT, T.P., E. BRINKMANN-FRYE, S.R. THORPE & J.W. BAYNES. 1998. Role of carbonyl stress in aging and age-related diseases. *In* The Maillard Reaction in Foods

and Medicine. J. O'Brien, H.E. Nursten, M.J.C. Crabbe & J.M. Ames, Eds.: 3–10. The Royal Society of Chemistry. Cambridge, UK.
29. STADTMAN, E.R. & R.L. LEVINE. 2000. Protein oxidation. Ann. N.Y. Acad. Sci. **899:** 191–208.
30. PAMPLONA, R., M. PORTERO-OTÍN, J.R. REQUENA, et al. 1999. A low degree of fatty acid unsaturation leads to lower lipid peroxidation and lipoxidation-derived protein modification in heart mitochondria of the longevous pigeon than in the short-lived rat. Mech. Ageing Dev. **106:** 283–296.
31. PAMPLONA, R., M. PORTERO-OTÍN, D. RIBA, et al. 2000. Low fatty acid unsaturation: a mechanism for lowered lipoperoxidative modification of tissue proteins in mammalian species with long life span. J. Gerontol. **55A:** B286–B291.
32. SELL, D.R., M.A. LANE, W.A. JOHNSON, et al. 1996. Longevity and the genetic determination of collagen glycoxidation kinetics in mammalian senescence. Proc. Natl. Acad. Sci. USA **93:** 485–490.
33. PAMPLONA, R., M. PORTERO-OTÍN, M.J. BELLMUNT, et al. 2001. Aging increases N^ε-(carboxymethyl)-lysine and caloric restriction decreases N^ε-(carboxyethyl)-lysine and N^ε-(malondialdehyde)-lysine in rat heart mitochondrial proteins. Free Radic. Res. **36:** 47–54.
34. BIELSKI, B.H.J., R.I. ARUDI & M.W. SUTHERLAND. 1983. A study of the reactivity of $HO_2/O_2^{\bullet-}$ with unsaturated fatty acids. J. Biol. Chem. **258:** 4759š4761.
35. PAMPLONA, R., J. PRAT, S. CADENAS, et al. 1996. Low fatty acid unsaturation protects against lipid peroxidation in liver mitochondria from longevous species: the pigeon and human case. Mech. Ageing Dev. **86:** 53–66.
36. GUTIERREZ, A.M., G.R. REBOREDO, C.J. ARCEMIS & A. CATALÁ. 1997. Non-enzymatic lipid peroxidation of microsomes and mitochondria isolated from liver and heart of pigeon and rat. Int. J. Biochem. Cell Biol. **32:** 73–79.
37. PAMPLONA, R., M. PORTERO-OTÍN, D. RIBA, et al. 1999. Heart fatty acid unsaturation and lipid peroxidation, and aging rate, are lower in the canary and the parakeet than in the mouse. Aging Clin. Exp. Res. **11:** 44–49.
38. PAMPLONA, R., M. PORTERO-OTÍN, C. RUIZ, et al. 1998. Mitochondrial membrane peroxidizability index is inversely related to maximum life span in mammals. J. Lipid Res. **39:** 1989–1994.
39. PORTERO-OTÍN, M., M.J. BELLMUNT, M.C. RUIZ, et al. 2001. Correlation of fatty acid unsaturation of the major liver mitochondrial phospholipid classes in mammals to their potential life span. Lipids **36:** 491–498.
40. PAMPLONA, R., M. PORTERO-OTÍN, C. RUIZ, et al. 1999. Double bond content of phospholipids and lipid peroxidation negatively correlate with maximum longevity in the heart of mammals. Mech. Ageing Dev. **112:** 169–183.
41. COUTURE, P. & A.J. HULBERT. 1995. Membrane fatty acid composition of tissues is related to body mass of mammals. J. Membr. Biol. **148:** 27–39.
42. PORTER, R.K. & M.D. BRAND. 1995. Causes of differences in respiration rate of hepatocytes from mammals of different body mass. Am. J. Physiol. **269:** R1213–R1224.
43. PORTER, R.K. & M.D. BRAND. 1993. Body mass dependence of H^+ leak in mitochondria and its relevance to metabolic rate. Nature **362:** 628–629.
44. REFSGAARD, H.H.F., L. TSAI & E.R. STADTMAN. 2000. Modifications of proteins by polyunsaturated fatty acid peroxidation products. Proc. Natl. Acad. Sci. USA **97:** 611–616.
45. DRAPER, H.H. 1995. Effects of peroxidative stress and age on the concentration of a deoxyguanosine-malondialdehyde adduct in rat DNA. Lipids **30:** 959–961.
46. ESTERBAUER, H., R.J. SCHAUR & H. ZOLLNER. 1991. Chemistry and biochemistry of 4-hydroxynonenal, malondialdehyde and related aldehydes. Free Radic. Biol. Med. **11:** 81–128.
47. CUTLER, R.G. 1985. Peroxide-producing potential of tissues: inverse correlation with longevity of mammalian species. Proc. Natl. Acad. Sci. USA **82:** 4798–4802.
48. HERRERO, A., M. PORTERO-OTÍN, M.J. BELLMUNT, et al. 2001. Effect of the degree of fatty acid unsaturation of rat heart mitochondria on their rates of H_2O_2 production and lipid and protein oxidative damage. Mech. Ageing Dev. **122:** 427–443.

49. GUDBJARNASON, S. 1989. Dynamics of n-3 and n-6 fatty acids in phospholipids of heart muscle. J. Intern. Med. **225:** 117–128.
50. IVANETICH, K.M., J.J. BRADSHAW & M.R. ZIMAN. 1996. delta-6 desaturase: improved methodology and analysis of the kinetics in a multi-enzyme system. Biochim. Biophys. Acta **1292:** 120–132.
51. CHARNOCK, J.S., M.Y. ABEYWARDENA, V.M. POLETTI & P.L. MCLENNAN. 1992. Differences in fatty acid composition of various tissues of the marmosset monkey (*Callithrix jacchus*) after different lipid-supplemented diets. Comp. Biochem. Physiol. **101A:** 387–393.
52. SOLÀ, R., A.E. LA VILLE, J.L. RICHARD, *et al.* 1997. Oleic acid rich diet protects against the oxidative modification of high density lipoprotein. Free Radic. Biol. Med. **22:** 1037–1045.
53. BRENNER, R.R. 1984. Effect of unsaturated fatty acids on membrane structure and enzyme kinetics. Progr. Lipid Res. **23:** 69–96.
54. SESSLER, A. & J.B. NTAMBI. 1998. Polyunsaturated fatty acid regulation of gene expression. J. Nutr. **128:** 923–926.
55. NAKAMURA, M.T., H.P. CHO & S.D. CLARKE. 2000. Regulation of hepatic delta-6 desaturase expression and its role in the polyunsaturated fatty acid inhibition of fatty acid synthase gene expression in mice. J. Nutr. **130:** 1561–1565.
56. COOK, H.W. 1996. Fatty acid desaturation and chain elongation in eukaryotes. *In* Biochemistry of Lipids, Lipoproteins and Biomembranes. D.E. Vance & J.E. Vance, Eds.: 129–152. Elsevier. Amsterdam.
57. LOFT, S., E.B. THORLING & H.E. POULSEN. 1998. High fat diet induced damage estimated by 8-oxo-7,8-dihydro-2′-deoxyguanosine excretion in rats. Free Radic. Res. **29:** 595–600.
58. HARMAN, D. 1971. Free radical theory of aging: effect of the amount and degree of unsaturation of dietary fat on mortality rate. J. Gerontol. **26:** 451–457.
59. TAKEUCHI, Y., H. MORII, M. TAMURA, *et al.* 1991. A possible mechanism of mitochondrial dysfunction during cerebral ischemia: inhibition of mitochondrial respiratory activity by arachidonic acid. Arch. Biochem. Biophys. **289:** 33–38.
60. HOCH, F.L. 1992. Cardiolipins and membrane function. Biochim. Biophys. Acta. **1113:** 71–133.
61. TROYER, D. & G. FERNANDES. 1996. Nutrition and apoptosis. Nutr. Res. **16:** 1959–1987.
62. LAGANIERE, S. & B.P. YU. 1993. Modulation of membrane phospholipid fatty acid composition by food age and food restriction. Gerontology **39:** 7–18.
63. YU, B.P., J.J. CHEN, C.M. KANG, *et al.* 1996. Mitochondrial aging and lipoperoxidative products. Ann. N.Y. Acad. Sci. **786:** 44–56.
64. CHOI, J.H., J. KIM, Y.S. MOON, *et al.* 1996. Analysis of lipid composition and hydroxyl radicals in brain membranes of senescent-accelerated mice. Age **19:** 1–5.
65. HORROBIN, D.F. & M.S. MANKU. 1987. Genetically low arachidonic acid and high dihomogammalinolenic acid levels in Eskimos may contribute to low incidence of coronary heart disease, psoriasis, arthritis and asthma. *In* Polyunsaturated Fatty Acids and Eicosanoids. W.E.M. Lands, Ed.: 413–415. American Oil Chemists Society. Champaign, IL.

Mitochondrial Decay in the Aging Rat Heart

Evidence for Improvement by Dietary Supplementation with Acetyl-L-Carnitine and/or Lipoic Acid

TORY M. HAGEN, RÉGIS MOREAU, JUNG H. SUH, AND FRANCESCO VISIOLI

Department of Biochemistry and Biophysics, Linus Pauling Institute, Oregon State University, Corvallis, Oregon 97331, USA

ABSTRACT: Mitochondrial decay has been postulated to be a significant underlying part of the aging process. Decline in mitochondrial function may lead to cellular energy deficits, especially in times of greater energy demand, and compromise vital ATP-dependent cellular operations, including detoxification, repair systems, DNA replication, and osmotic balance. Mitochondrial decay may also lead to enhanced oxidant production and thus render the cell more prone to oxidative insult. In particular, the heart may be especially susceptible to mitochondrial dysfunction due to myocardial dependency on β-oxidation of fatty acids for energy and the postmitotic nature of cardiac myocytes, which would allow for greater accumulation of mitochondrial mutations and deletions. Thus, maintenance of mitochondrial function may be important to maintain overall myocardial function. Herein, we review the major age-related changes that occur to mitochondria in the aging heart and the evidence that two such supplements, acetyl-L-carnitine (ALCAR) and (R)-α-lipoic acid, may improve myocardial bioenergetics and lower the increased oxidative stress associated with aging. We and others have shown that feeding old rats ALCAR reverses the age-related decline in carnitine levels and improves mitochondrial β-oxidation in a number of tissues studied. However, ALCAR supplementation does not appear to reverse the age-related decline in cardiac antioxidant status and thus may not substantially alter indices of oxidative stress. Lipoic acid, a potent thiol antioxidant and mitochondrial metabolite, appears to increase low molecular weight antioxidant status and thereby decreases age-associated oxidative insult. Thus, ALCAR along with lipoic acid may be effective supplemental regimens to maintain myocardial function.

KEYWORDS: aging; mitochondria; heart; oxidative stress

AGE-ASSOCIATED CHANGES IN THE HEART

Aging is associated with an increased incidence of cardiac arrythmias and diastolic and systolic dysfunction, which may ultimately lead to heart failure. Heart fail-

---

Address for correspondence: Tory M. Hagen, Linus Pauling Institute, Department of Biochemistry and Biophysics, 571 Weniger Hall, Oregon State University, Corvallis, OR 97331. Voice: 541-737-5083; fax: 541-737-5077.
tory.hagen@orst.edu

ure alone is the leading cause of hospitalization, permanent disability, and death over the age of 65 in the United States.[1] Because of the enormous suffering and healthcare burden that cardiac dysfunction causes, much effort has gone into understanding the mechanisms leading to age-related myocardial decline. Nevertheless, it has thus far been difficult to separate the effects of aging *per se* from those of age-associated diseases (atherosclerosis, diabetes, hypertension) on cardiac performance. Thus, the relative contribution of aging to myocardial dysfunction is not well defined. Despite this problem, two major detrimental age-associated changes to the heart have been identified that would markedly affect myocardial performance. First, the heart becomes "stiff" with age due to increased collagen content,[2–6] fragmentation of elastin fibers,[7] and fibrotic scarring on the endo- and epi-cardial surfaces.[8] This decreases cardiac distensibility and increases diastolic pressure, prolonging the time needed to fill the ventricle with blood. Second, there is extensive age-related myocardial tissue remodeling. The number of cardiac myocytes declines significantly with age in both rats and humans.[4] For example, this myocardial atrophy has been attributed to oxidative damage that eventually causes cellular necrosis or apoptosis (see Refs. 9–11 for reviews). Atrophy is followed by compensatory hypertrophy of the remaining cardiac myocytes. Remodeling affects the heart in contraction (systolic function), but more acutely during relaxation (diastolic function) because of an abnormal diastolic pressure/volume relationship that reduces the ability of the ventricle to fill with blood without increased atrial and ventricular filling pressure.[12]

These general age-related changes to the heart have all been implicated as underlying events that account for increased cardiac arrhythmias, diastolic dysfunction, and heart failure.[2,4,12,13] Although the mechanism(s) leading to these alterations in the heart are not well understood, there are several reasons to suggest that mitochondrial decay may significantly contribute to myocardial dysfunction with age.

CONTRIBUTION OF MITOCHONDRIAL DECAY TO AGE-RELATED CARDIAC DYSFUNCTION

Mitochondrial Contribution to Cardiac Stiffness

The heart is dependent on high-energy phosphates supplied by the mitochondria to carry out both contraction and relaxation.[2,14,15] To maintain myocardial function, a constant supply of ATP is required, but few reserves are maintained. Thus, when energy supply is interrupted (ischemia) or impaired (aging), ATP levels decline rapidly. Like systolic contraction, diastolic relaxation also requires high levels of ATP because ATP acts as an allosteric effector to disassociate actin from myosin[16] (FIG. 1, path I). Thus, any decrement in mitochondrial ATP synthesis affects cardiac stiffness appreciably. Decline in ATP synthesis also compromises Ca^{2+} reuptake into the sarcoplasmic reticulum from the cytosol, again affecting myocardial relaxation[17,18] (FIG. 1, path II). The Na^+/Ca^{2+} transporter is also energy-dependent, and a decline in myocardial ATP levels would thus slow cardiac relaxation by decreasing the rate of Ca^{2+} removal from the cytosol.[18,19] It is notable that a general attribute of myocardial aging is a prolonged cytosolic calcium transient pulse and slower myocardial relaxation rate.[19,20]

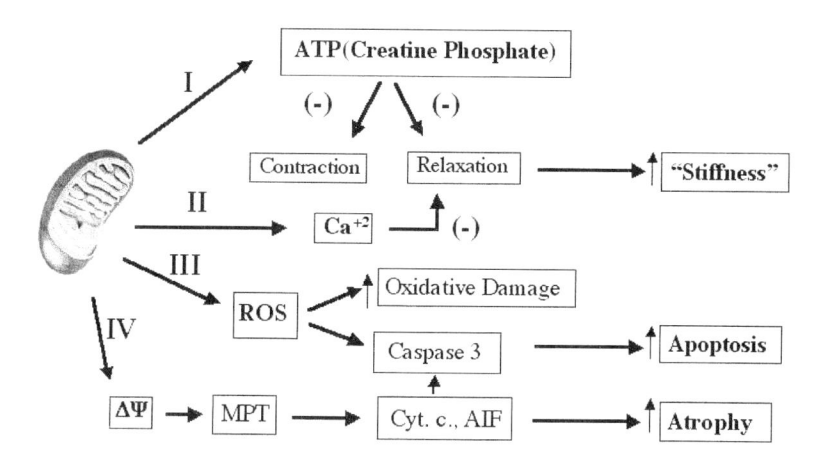

FIGURE 1. Theoretical ways that mitochondrial decay may affect cardiac function. (I) Loss of ATP production would affect both contraction and relaxation characteristics, leading to overall loss of cardiac distensibility. (II) Mitochondrial decay could affect calcium homeostasis and buffering capacity, which would also affect cardiac contraction and relaxation. (III) Altered coupling of electron transport to ATP production would lead to increased oxidant production, increasing the likelihood of enhanced oxidative stress and activation of the apoptotic cascade. (IV) Loss of $\Delta\Psi$ may lead to the opening of the mitochondrial megachannel and the release of apoptogenic factors, again increasing the propensity of cell loss and cardiac atrophy.

Mitochondrial Contribution to Myocardial Oxidative Stress

Mitochondria constantly produce significant amounts of reactive oxygen species (ROS) as by-products of electron transport; these not only damage mitochondria but also other cellular biomolecules due to oxidant leakage into the cytoplasm[21–23] (FIG. 1, path III). Mitochondrial DNA (mtDNA) is particularly susceptible to oxidant-induced damage due to its proximity to the source of ROS production and the lack of protecting histones.[21] mtDNA damage, if not repaired, may be converted into mutations. These mutations would affect electron transport, thereby further reducing the capacity to synthesize ATP and increasing ROS production. Direct oxidative modification of proteins has also been observed and may also contribute to heightened mitochondrial dysfunction and possibly increased oxidant production. Thus, aging results in a vicious cycle of higher oxidative damage followed by lower coupling of electron transport to ATP synthesis, which eventually leads to elevated cellular damage from ever-increasing levels of oxidants leaking from compromised mitochondria. Increased oxidant stress would thereby contribute to cardiac atrophy via necrosis or apoptosis, both of which can be triggered by oxidants.[9–11]

Mitochondrial Contribution to Apoptosis and Myocardial Atrophy

Mitochondrial decay may, in part, cause the profound age-related atrophy of the heart through enhanced apoptosis or programmed cell death. Although apoptosis can be initiated by a variety of endogenous and exogenous signals (including increased mitochondrial-derived oxidants), it now appears that these diverse pathways converge into a few "gate-keeping" mechanisms that, if entered, lead to a "point-of-no-return," and cell death ensues.[24] Currently, mitochondria are considered one of the principal gatekeepers that govern whether a cell irreversibly undergoes apoptosis (FIG. 1, path IV). Principally, disruption and collapse of the inner mitochondrial transmembrane potential ($\Delta\Psi$) causes cells to undergo apoptosis. Measurement of the mitochondrial $\Delta\Psi$ (the driving force for ATP synthesis) by fluorescent dyes such as rhodamine 123 (R123) reveals that cells destined for programmed cell death have a significantly lower $\Delta\Psi$ than normal cells.[25] In relation to aging, we have reported that hepatocytes[26,27] and cardiac myocytes[28] from old rats exhibited a lower average $\Delta\Psi$ than that observed in cells from young rats. This significant ($P = 0.03$) decline in R123 fluorescence is not due to changes in cell size or shape because measurement of forward light scatter, which reflects cellular morphology, did not change with age. Loss of $\Delta\Psi$ would be expected to increase apoptosis vis-à-vis opening of a mitochondrial pore, which markedly affects permeability.[29,30] This so-called "mitochondrial permeability transition" (MPT) appears to be a hallmark of cells entering into irreversible apoptosis,[24] including those of the heart. MPT indirectly activates caspase-3 through release of cytochrome c and other apoptogenic factors. Caspase-3 is an aspartyl protease that has been called the "death protease" because its activation is believed to be one of the first committed steps leading to cell death.[30] Thus, age-dependent loss of $\Delta\Psi$ sets up conditions where proapoptogenic signals, which would otherwise lower but not collapse $\Delta\Psi$ in cells in young animals, may cause MPT leading to "unscheduled" apoptosis and loss of cardiac myocytes in the aging heart.

In summary, mitochondrial decay contributes to the major alterations occurring in the aging heart: myocardial stiffness, atrophy, and tissue remodeling. Experimental evidence for a decline in mitochondrial function in both humans and experimental animals, however, has been surprisingly difficult to discern and quantify.

EXPERIMENTAL EVIDENCE FOR MITOCHONDRIAL DECAY IN THE HEART

Structural Changes

A number of age-related structural and morphological changes occur in heart mitochondria. There is a small age-associated decline (10 to 18%) in the number of cardiac mitochondria in both rats and humans;[31] however, the volume that mitochondria occupy in myocardial tissue, which approaches 30% of total cellular volume,[32] does not change.[33] This indicates that there is an increase in mitochondrial size with age.[34] Mitochondria lose cristae, and the inner mitochondrial membrane becomes less invaginated, suggesting an overall age-associated decline in oxidative capacity and reduced myocardial energy supply.[35] Electron micrographs also show mitochondria becoming more "electron dense" with age; this change may be caused by accumulation of oxidized lipids, proteins, carbohydrates, and redox-active metal ions.[35]

There are also significant age-related changes to the inner mitochondrial membrane. The fatty acids in phospholipids comprising the inner mitochondrial membrane become shorter and more unsaturated, making them prone to lipid peroxidation.[36] These structural changes also reportedly affect membrane fluidity and alter conformation of key substrate transport proteins.[37] Levels of cardiolipin, an important phospholipid cofactor for a number of mitochondrial transport enzymes,[38] also decline significantly with age. Loss of cardiolipin during aging markedly decreases substrate transport in isolated mitochondrial preparations and lowers cytochrome c oxidase activity.[39] Thus, significant age-related biophysical changes occur in cardiac mitochondria that would be expected to markedly affect overall mitochondrial and, in turn, cellular function.

Functional Changes

Levels of myocardial carnitine, an amino acid necessary for shuttling fatty acyl moieties from the cytosol into the mitochondria for β-oxidation, decline significantly in the rat heart with age.[40] This leads to a significant loss in β-oxidation of fatty acids and suggests that mitochondria become deprived of their major source for ATP synthesis.[41] ATP levels, which are normally sufficient to supply the needs of the heart for only a few minutes,[42] would be expected to decrease, creating energy deficits and cardiac dysfunction. Direct measurement of mitochondrial ATP synthesis indicates that there may be a decline in the capacity to generate ATP, but the extent and significance of these changes are difficult to assess because of the inconsistent results reported.[43–45] There is a similar lack of consensus about the extent of age-related changes in adenine nucleotide exchange, with loss in exchange rates reported to be anywhere from relatively minor to major.[43–46] As for age-related changes to the mitochondrial electron transport chain: there may or may not be changes in the levels of mitochondrial cytochrome content with age, depending on the study.[47–49] Complex I of the oxidation/phosphorylation chain is generally reported to be impaired with age in cardiac mitochondria, but the extent of this impairment is not yet established.[47–51] Activities of complexes III and IV have been variously shown to decline or remain unchanged with age.[47,48,52] Activity of complex II, the succinate dehydrogenase, may decline,[53] remain unchanged,[49,54] or increase[55,56] in old rats, although the predominant view supports a lack of age-related loss in activity for complex II. There is equally conflicting evidence either arguing for or against changes in F_0F_1 ATPase activity with age.[51,52,57,58] In summary, aging appears to result in a loss of fatty acid- and glutamate-supported (complex I) oxidative capacity, but due to inconsistent results, it is difficult to gauge the extent or nature of other functional changes to mitochondria.

Coupling of electron transport to ATP synthesis, measured as the respiratory control (RCR) and ADP/O ratios, has variously been reported to decline or remain similar to that found for isolated cardiac mitochondria from young rats.[54–57,59,60] Myocardial ATP concentrations do not appear to be altered with age, indicating that glycolysis plays a greater role in supplying ATP to the myocardium. However, this hypothesis is not, as yet, supported by experimental evidence because glycolytic[57,58] and citric acid cycle[50,52,55,60–65] enzymes, including pyruvate dehydrogenase,[66] are variously reported to decline or remain unchanged during aging.

In support of the view that there is a metabolic decline in the aging heart muscle, we recently showed that cellular O_2 consumption in isolated cardiac myocytes declines from 718 ± 12 μmol O_2/min per 10^6 cells in young rats ($n = 3$) to 299 ± 43 μmol O_2/min per 10^6 cells ($n = 2$) in old rats (FIG. 2). These results suggest a similar

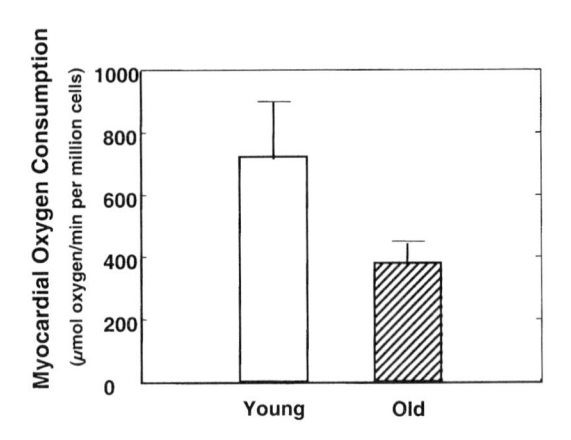

FIGURE 2. Oxygen consumption in isolated cardiac myocytes declines with age. O_2 consumption in isolated cardiac myocytes from young and old rats was monitored using an oxygen electrode. Results show that O_2 consumption, an indicator of cellular metabolic rate, declines sharply with age. Results are expressed as mean ± SEM for cells from young rats ($n = 3$) and the mean ± range ($n = 2$) for cells from old rats.

age-related loss of metabolic rate in isolated cardiac myocytes, as we previously observed in isolated hepatocytes from old rats.[67]

Changes in Oxidant Production and Oxidative Damage

It is generally agreed that isolated mitochondrial preparations from old versus young heart produce more ROS, reflecting an age-related decline in electron transport efficiency. Nohl and Hegner[68] showed that the rate of ROS production by heart mitochondria from old rats increased twofold over the rate observed in heart mitochondria from young rats. Other studies also reported increased superoxide and hydrogen peroxide production.[69,70] Recent data from Hansford and coworkers,[71] however, indicate that increased age-related oxidant production might be an artifact stemming from the assay conditions used in earlier studies. Under their conditions, they showed no age-related increase in ROS production in isolated mitochondrial preparations from rat hearts. Thus, it is no longer clear whether ROS production increases in the heart with age. If these results are confirmed, the increased accumulation of oxidative damage evident in the heart with age may be caused by a decline in cellular repair capacity or antioxidant status rather than increased oxidant production *per se*.

To further address this question, we recently examined mitochondrial oxidant production in isolated cardiac myocytes. For these studies, cells were incubated with dichlorofluorescein diacetate (DCF), a compound that becomes fluorescent upon oxidation, which allows observation of ROS/RNS production in intact cells. We observed that the rate of DCF oxidation increased by 31% in cells from old compared to young rats (FIG. 3). This increase in oxidant production was even more pronounced when normalized to oxygen consumption (FIG. 3B). On this basis, the rate of DCF fluorescence per µmol O_2 consumed in cardiac myocytes from old rats was

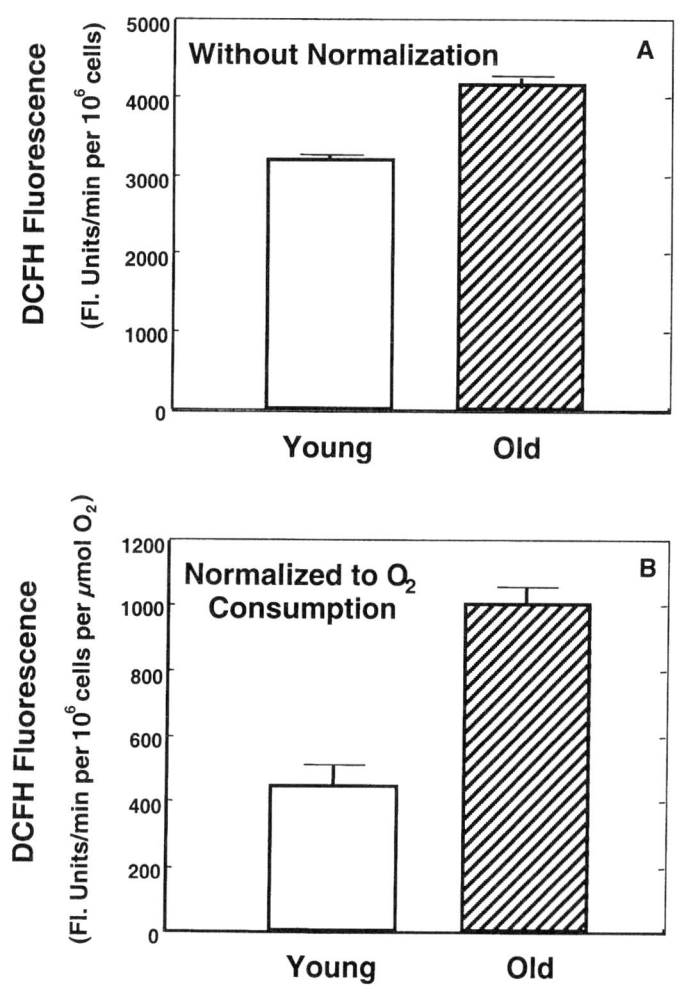

FIGURE 3. Cardiac myocytes produce significantly more oxidants with age. Isolated cells (1.0×10^4) were incubated with DCFH (0.01 mg/mL), and oxidant appearance was measured using a fluorescent plate reader (Cytofluor). **(A)** Cells from old rats (24 month) produce ~30% more oxidants, as measured by DCF fluorescence, than cells from young (3 month) rats. **(B)** The rate of oxidant production is even more marked when oxidant production is normalized to the cellular rate of O_2 consumption. Results are expressed as the mean ± SEM of four experiments.

2.7-fold higher than for cells from young rats. Because oxidation of DCF cannot distinguish the source or type of oxidizing species, it is not possible to define whether the increase in oxidant appearance was from mitochondria or other sources. However, these findings suggest that the aging heart muscle is experiencing a more oxidizing environment than that seen in cells from young animals.

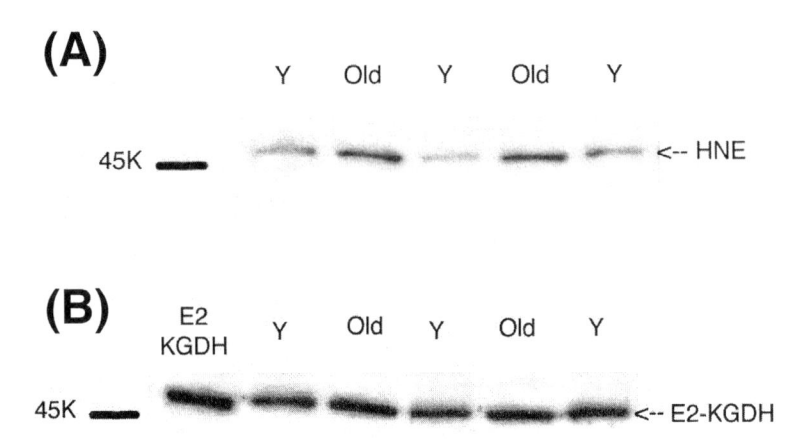

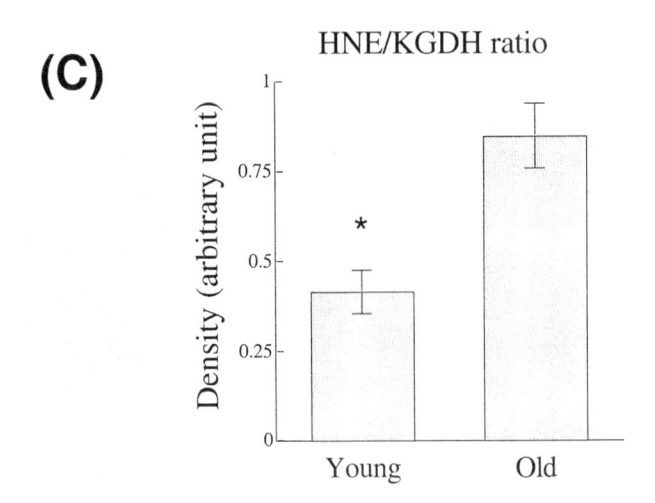

FIGURE 4. Age-related increase in protein modification to mitochondrial E2 component of α-ketoglutarate dehydrogenase (KGDH) by 4-hydroxynonenal (HNE). Immunoblot analysis of subsarcolemmal mitochondrial proteins isolated from young (3–4 month) and old (24–28 month) rat myocardium. Proteins (73 µg) were loaded onto SDS-PAGE gels and transblotted onto nitrocellulose membranes. Membranes were incubated with anti-HNE IgG (**A**) then stripped and incubated with bovine KGDH antiserum. (**B**) Antibody binding was visualized using ECL™ Western Blotting System. (**C**) A ratio of integrated density (HNE/E2 of KGDH) was plotted for each age group. Data are mean ± SD for 5–7 animals (* $P \leq 0.01$).

During the aging process biomolecules appear increasingly damaged by oxidative modifications that affect their function. The degree of oxidative modification is proportional to the proximity to sites of oxidant production and inversely correlated with its rate of turnover. Thus, a long-lived protein such as collagen will accumulate oxidative damage over time. As a major site of oxidant generation, it is anticipated that mitochondria will also accumulate oxidative damage. In fact, studies have reported higher levels of oxidative damage to mtDNA,[72,73] myocardial accumulation of lipofuscin,[74] mitochondrial lipid peroxidation,[75] and protein glycation[76–78] with age. In particular, there is evidence of an age-related increase in protein–carbonyl adducts. Reactive carbonyl compounds, which may arise from carbohydrates, lipids, and amino acids, form covalent bonds with polypeptide amino and thiol groups and eventually produce advanced glycation end products (AGE) and/or advanced lipoxidation end products (ALE).[79,80] In the myocardium of aging rats, we have identified posttranslational modification to a key enzyme of the mitochondrial NADH generating machinery, α-ketoglutarate dehydrogenase (KGDH). KGDH was found to be increasingly adducted by 4-hydroxynonenal (4-HNE), a peroxidation product of arachidonic acid in old rats (FIG. 4). The finding of 4-HNE-KGDH adduct *in vivo* indicates that KGDH is prone to oxidative damage, as suggested earlier.[81] Further *in vitro* studies showed that 4-HNE adduction is followed by a decline in KGDH activity.[82,83] Thus, oxidative damage to KGDH and, potentially, other key enzymes involved in bioenergetics may be a significant underlying event in age-related mitochondrial decay, which could adversely impact how mitochondria may meet cellular energy demands and combat increased oxidant appearance.

Taken together, the experimental evidence (reviewed above) indicates that there are a number of age-related mitochondrial changes in the heart. Structural changes are severe, suggesting acute attenuation of mitochondrial function. However, there is no consensus about the extent or precise nature of the *functional* alterations in mitochondria with age. It is interesting to note that strong evidence for mitochondrial decay in the heart mainly comes from studies using histology to assess age-related changes, whereas variable and inconsistent results are obtained when isolated mitochondria are used.

IMPROVEMENT OF MITOCHONDRIAL FUNCTION THROUGH DIETARY SUPPLEMENTATION OF ACETYL-L-CARNITINE AND LIPOIC ACID

Effects of Acetyl-L-Carnitine on Mitochondrial Bioenergetics

As discussed above, the extent and nature of mitochondrial functional decay in the aging heart are unclear, but there are a number of structural changes that would be expected to affect overall mitochondrial function. Myocardial carnitine levels exhibit an age-related decline, thereby affecting fatty acid uptake for mitochondrial fatty acid β-oxidation.[38,41,60,75] It has been shown that administration of carnitine, particularly acetyl-L-carnitine (ALCAR), can slow or reverse a number of parameters of mitochondrial decay in many tissues.[26,84–88] Dietary ALCAR is readily taken up from the gastrointestinal tract into the blood and is well tolerated, even in high doses.[89]

Dietary supplementation of ALCAR to rats reverses the decline in liver[26] and heart[85–87] cardiolipin levels. As noted above, cardiolipin serves as a key cofactor for a number of mitochondrial substrate transport proteins, for example, cytochrome c oxidase, F_0F_1 ATPase, and the phosphate carrier (reviewed in Ref. 38); and increased levels of cardiolipin would allow mitochondria to more readily generate ATP for cardiac work. ALCAR administration to rats reverses the age-related decline in cytochrome c oxidase[86] and phosphate carrier activity[90] in heart mitochondria and lowers accumulation of lipofuscin in Purkinje fibers.[91] ALCAR also increases mtD-A transcription back to levels seen in tissue from young animals.[88] These results suggest that ALCAR administration has multiple effects on mitochondria, all serving to increase the capacity to generate ATP. These multiplicative effects of ALCAR may be attributable to its ability to deliver acetyl-CoA equivalents to the citric acid cycle and to facilitate mitochondrial β-oxidation of fatty acids, as noted above.

Carnitine and its derivatives (ALCAR and proprionyl-carnitine [ProCAR]) have been subjected to a number of clinical studies relevant to pathologic conditions of the heart. In a double-blind, placebo-controlled trial, L-carnitine improved indices of myocardial metabolism and cardiac recovery in patients after heart bypass surgery.[91] In another randomized, double-blind, placebo-controlled trial, the effect of carnitine (2 g/day for 28 days) supplementation on the management of cardiac recovery following suspected acute myocardial infarction was examined. Results showed that patients given carnitine had decreased infarct size and lower levels of serum transaminases and lipid peroxides when compared to the placebo group.[92] In a similar trial where patients were given carnitine for one year following myocardial infarction, the carnitine-supplemented group had attenuated left ventricular dilation and decreased incidence of deaths and congestive heart failure. While epidemiological studies or clinical trials have yet to be performed to directly examine the effects of carnitine on indices of the aging heart in humans, evidence to date suggests that therapeutic treatment of carnitine effectively improves cardiac performance following a number of pathophysiological insults.

Despite the benefits of ALCAR treatment, there are also potential adverse effects. While ALCAR supplementation reversed many of the altered characteristics evident in mitochondrial metabolism with age, the rate of oxidant production, as measured by DCF fluorescence, was higher in the liver of supplemented old rats when compared to cells from untreated old rats.[26] We also showed that antioxidant status declines, oxidant production increases, and oxidative damage is elevated in isolated hepatocytes from old but not young rats when given 1.5% (wt/vol) ALCAR in the drinking water.[26] Lower doses of ALCAR, that is, below 1.0% (wt/vol) in the drinking water did not increase hepatocellular oxidative stress (B.N. Ames, personal communication). Thus, while ALCAR supplementation may enhance overall mitochondrial electron transport activity in livers of old rats, it also raises hepatocellular oxidative stress at high supplemental concentrations.

To determine whether providing 1.5% ALCAR to rats caused a similar increased oxidative stress in the myocardium, rats were given ALCAR for one month before sacrifice. Results showed that there were no alterations in oxidant production in isolated cardiac myocytes under the same feeding regimen (data not shown), suggesting that ALCAR supplementation may increase oxidative insult in livers but not hearts

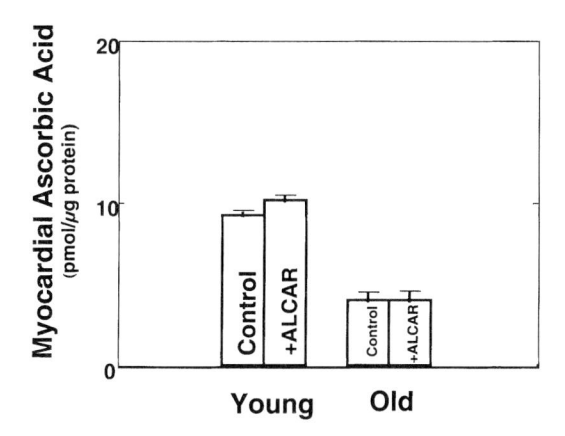

FIGURE 5. ALCAR supplementation does not affect the age-related myocardial decline in tissue ascorbic acid levels. ALCAR (1.5% [wt/vol] in the drinking water) was fed to rats for 1 month before sacrifice. Myocardial ascorbic acid levels were determined by HPLC with electrochemical detection. Results show that, unlike in hepatocytes, ALCAR supplementation does not induce a further decline in ascorbic acid concentrations in either young or old rats. Results are expressed as the mean ± SEM; $n = 6$ for old rats; $n = 3$ for young rats.

of old rats. Furthermore, myocardial levels of ascorbic acid, which decline significantly ($P < 0.02$) with age (FIG. 5) did not exhibit a further ALCAR-induced decline (FIG. 5). Ascorbic acid concentrations declined from 9.25 ± 0.31 ($n = 3$) to 3.98 ± 0.67 pmol/µg protein in young compared to old rats, respectively, reflecting a 2.3-fold loss of this important antioxidant. In contrast to the studies on liver, we did not see a further ALCAR-induced decline in tissue ascorbate concentrations (FIG. 5). The reasons for this apparent difference in the two tissues are not clear, but may be due to differential uptake and/or clearance from the different organs.

Effects of Lipoic Acid Supplementation

We further found that the age-related and ALCAR-induced increase in oxidant production and oxidative damage can be reversed by co-supplementation with (R)-α-lipoic acid (LA), a disulfide compound found naturally in plants and animals that has been identified as a potent antioxidant. The disulfide form of lipoic acid is reduced in mitochondria by specific dehydrogenases, and its supplementation would thus "target" an antioxidant to the mitochondria, the major site of ROS production.[93] Supplementation with LA may also boost mitochondrial function because it is a cofactor for pyruvate and α-ketoglutarate dehydrogenase[94,95] and, as such, may be a useful dietary supplement in its own right to increase overall mitochondrial metabolism. LA has been given as a therapy for many diseases associated with impaired energy utilization and/or increased oxidative stress, such as type II diabetes,[95,96] diabetic polyneuropathies,[97,98] and ischemia/reperfusion injury in the heart.[99] To a degree, the same type(s) of metabolic impairment and increased oxidative stress seen

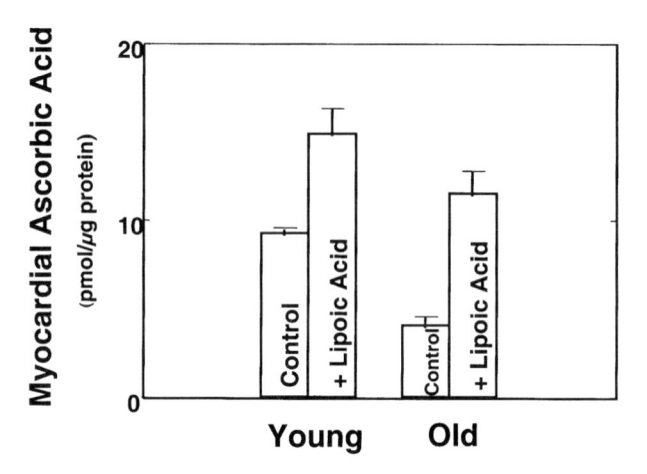

FIGURE 6. Lipoic acid supplementation reverses the age-related decline in myocardial ascorbic acid levels. Myocardial ascorbic acid levels declined significantly with age ($P = 0.001$). A 2-week feeding regimen of LA (0.5% [wt/vol]) reversed this age-related decline and also resulted in increased myocardial ascorbic acid concentration in young animals ($P = 0.041$).

in these conditions may also occur in the aging heart. Lipoic acid supplementation may thus be useful to either slow or prevent the age-related decline in cardiac metabolism and increase antioxidant defenses against putative increased mitochondrial oxidant production.

The effect of LA supplementation on myocardial ascorbate levels has been recently examined. Our preliminary evidence reveals that feeding rats lipoic acid effectively reverses the age-related decline in ascorbic acid levels (FIG. 6). Myocardial ascorbic acid concentrations in LA-treated young rats were 14.9 ± 1.43 pmol/μg protein ($n = 5$), which was 61% higher than that for unsupplemented young rats (FIG. 6). Ascorbic acid values in LA-treated old rats were 11.5 ± 1.29 pmol/μg protein ($n = 5$), reflecting a significant ($P = 0.001$) 2.9-fold increase over those of untreated old rats. These levels were not significantly different from and, in fact, were higher than the ascorbic acid levels found in untreated young animals ($P = 0.67$) (FIG. 6).

Currently, experiments are under way whereby ALCAR and LA are cosupplemented to young and old rats to determine whether the combination of these compounds can effectively increase myocardial metabolism without a concomitant increase in oxidative stress.

SUMMARY

Our studies using isolated cardiac myocytes indicate that mitochondrial function is adversely affected to a significant degree in the aging rat heart, but ALCAR and LA supplementation reverses a number of indices of mitochondrial decay. These results on cardiac myocytes add to the substantial evidence gathered on hepatocellular mitochondrial decay and strongly support our hypotheses that (1) there is a significant age-related mitochondrial decay in cardiac myocytes and (2) ALCAR and/or LA supplementation can ameliorate this decay. A summation of the results indicates significant age-related mitochondrial decay in rat hepatocytes. In support of our central hypotheses, preliminary studies suggest similar extensive mitochondrial decay in isolated cardiac myocytes from old rats. Moreover, feeding rats ALCAR and/or LA markedly either improves mitochondrial function or increases cellular antioxidant status. The only exception to this is that ALCAR feeding increases oxidative stress in the liver but not the heart of old rats; however, preliminary evidence shows that this potential problem can be rectified using LA as a cosupplement. We are now preparing to conduct detailed studies on cardiac myocytes analogous to those already performed.

ACKNOWLEDGMENTS

The authors would like to thank Brian Dixon for careful reading of the manuscript. This work was supported by National Institute on Aging Grant RIAG17141A.

REFERENCES

1. COHN, J.N., M.R. BRISTOW, *et al.* 1997. Report of the National Heart, Lung, and Blood Institute Special Emphasis Panel on Heart Failure Research. Circulation **95:** 766–770.
2. KATZ, A.M. 1988. Cellular mechanisms of heart failure. Am. J. Cardiol. **62:** 3A–8A.
3. LEUKJEWICZ, J.E., M.J. DAVIES, *et al.* 1972. Collagen in human myocardium as a function of age. Cardiovasc. Res. **11:** 463–470.
4. COLUCCI, W.S. 1997. Molecular and cellular mechanisms of myocardial failure. Am. J. Cardiol. **80:** 15L–25L.
5. CORNWELL, G.G., B.P. THOMAS, *et al.* 1991. Myocardial fibrosis in aging germ-free and conventional Lobund-Wistar rats: the protective effect of diet restriction. J. Gerontol. **46:** B167–B170.
6. YANG, C.M., V. KONDASWAMY, *et al.* 1997. Changes in collagen phenotypes during progression and regression of cardiac hypertrophy. Cardiovasc. Res. **36:** 236–245.
7. SHAROV, V.G., H.N. SABBAH, *et al.* 1997. Abnormalities of cardiomyocytes in regions bordering fibrous scars of dogs with heart failure. Int. J. Cardiol. **60:** 273–279.
8. SVANBORG, A. 1997. Age-related changes in cardiac physiology. Can they be postponed or treated with drugs? Drugs Aging **10:** 463–472.
9. HAUNSTETTER, A. & S. IZUMO. 1998. Apoptosis: basic mechanisms and implications for cardiovascular disease. Circ. Res. **82:** 1111–1129.
10. HETTS, S.W. 1998. To die or not to die. An overview of apoptosis and its role in disease. J. Am. Med. Assoc. **279:** 300–307.
11. JAMES, T.N. 1998. Normal and abnormal consequences of apoptosis in the human heart. Annu. Rev. Physiol. **60:** 309–325.
12. TRESCH, D.D. & M.F. MCGOUGH. 1995. Heart failure with normal systolic function: a common disorder in older people. J. Am. Gerontol. Soc. **43:** 1035–1042.
13. CARRÉ, F., F. RANNOU, *et al.* 1993. Arrythmogenicity of the hypertrophied and senescent heart and relationship to membrane proteins involved in the altered calcium handling. Cardiovasc. Res. **27:** 1784–1789.
14. GRYNBERG, A. & L. DEMAISON. 1996. Fatty acid oxidation in the heart. J. Cardiovasc. Pharmacol. **28**(Suppl.): S11–S17.
15. NEELEY, J.R. & H.E. MORGAN. 1974. Relationship between carbohydrate and lipid metabolism and energy balance of heart muscle. Annu. Rev. Physiol. **36:** 413–459.

16. KATZ, A.M. 1991. Energetics and the failing heart. Hosp. Pract. **26:** 78–80.
17. MORGAN, J.P., R.E. ERNY, et al. 1990. Abnormal intracellular calcium handling, a major cause of systolic and diastolic dysfunction in ventricular myocardium from patients with heart failure. Circulation **81**(Suppl. III): 21–23.
18. NEGRETTI, N., S.C. O'NEILL, et al. 1993. The relative contributions of different intracellular and sarcolemmal systems to relaxation in rat ventricular myocytes. Cardiovasc. Res. **27:** 1826–1830.
19. FROLKIS, V.V., R.A. FROLKIS, et al. 1988. Contractile function in Ca^{2+} transport system of myocardium in ageing. Gerontology **34:** 64–74.
20. SIRI, F.M., J. KRUEGER, et al. 1991. Depressed intracellular calcium transients and contraction in myocytes from hypertrophied and failing guinea pig hearts. Am. J. Physiol. **261**(Heart Circ. Physiol.) **30:** H514–H530.
21. SHIGENAGA, M.K., T.M. HAGEN, et al. 1994. Oxidative damage and mitochondrial decay in aging. Proc. Natl. Acad. Sci. USA **91:** 10,771–10,778.
22. SOHAL, R.S. 1993. Aging, cytochrome oxidase activity, and hydrogen peroxide release by mitochondria. Free Radic. Biol. Med. **14:** 583–588.
23. MUSCARI, C., F. MIRELLA, et al. 1990. Mitochondrial function and superoxide generation from submitochondrial particles of aged rat hearts. Biochim. Biophys. Acta **1015:** 200–204.
24. PETIT, P.X., N. ZAMZAMI, et al. 1997. Implication of mitochondria in apoptosis. Mol. Cell. Biochem. **174:** 185–188.
25. ZAMZAMI, N., P. MARCHETTI, et al. 1995. Reduction in mitochondrial potential constitutes an early irreversible step of programmed lymphocyte death in vivo. J. Exp. Med. **181:** 1661–1672.
26. HAGEN, T.M., R.T. INGERSOLL, et al. 1998. Acetyl-L-carnitine fed to old rats partially restores mitochondrial function and ambulatory activity. Proc. Natl. Acad. Sci. USA **95:** 9562–9566.
27. HAGEN, T.M., D.L. YOWE, et al. 1997. Mitochondrial decay in hepatocytes: membrane potential decline, heterogeneity and oxidants increase. Proc. Natl. Acad. Sci. USA **94:** 3064–3069.
28. HAGEN, T.M. 2001. Increased mitochondrial decay and oxidative stress in the aging rat heart: improvement by dietary supplementation with (R)-α-lipoic acid. *In* Free Radicals in Chemistry, Biology and Medicine. T. Yoshikawa, S. Toyokuni, et al., Eds.: 262–271. OICA International. London.
29. ZORATTI, M. & I. SZABO. 1995. The mitochondrial permeability transition. Biochim. Biophys. Acta **1241:** 139–176.
30. CAI, J. & D.P. JONES. 1998. Superoxide in apoptosis. Mitochondrial generation triggered by cytochrome *c* loss. J. Biol. Chem. **273:** 11401–11404.
31. SACHS, H.G., J.A. GOLGAN, et al. 1977. Ultrastructure of the aging myocardium: a morphometric approach. Am. J. Anat. **150:** 63–72.
32. FERRARI, R. 1996. The role of mitochondria in ischemic heart disease. J. Cardiovasc. Pharmacol. **28**(Suppl. 1): S1–S10.
33. FLEISCHER, M., M. WARMUTH, et al. 1978. Ultrastructural morphometric analysis of normally loaded human myocardial left ventricals from young and old patients. Virchows Arch. [Pathol. Anat.] **380:** 123–133.
34. DAVID, H., A. BOZNER, et al. 1981. Pre- and postnatal development and ageing of the heart. Ultrastructural results and quantitative data. Exp. Pathol. Suppl. **7:** 1–176.
35. TATE, E.L. & G.H. HERBENER. 1976. A morphometric study of the density of mitochondrial cristae in heart and liver of aging mice. J. Gerontol. **31:** 129–134.
36. LAGANIERE, S. & B.P. YU. 1993. Modulation of membrane phospholipid fatty acid composition by age and food restriction. Gerontology **39:** 7–18.
37. HEGNER, D. 1980. Age-dependence of molecular and functional changes in biological membrane properties. Mech. Ageing Dev. **14:** 101–118.
38. HOCH, F.L. 1992. Cardiolipins and biomembrane function. Biochim. Biophys. Acta **1113:** 71–133.
39. PARADIES, G., F.M. RUGGIERO, et al. 1993. Age-dependent decrease in the cytochrome *c* oxidase activity and changes in phospholipids in rat heart mitochondria. Arch. Gerontol. Geriatr. **16:** 263–272.

40. HANSFORD, R. & F. CASTROL. 1982. Age-linked changes in the activity of enzymes of the tricarboxylic acid cycle and lipid oxidation, and of carnitine content, in muscles of the rat. Mech. Ageing Dev. **19:** 191–200.
41. MCMILLIN, J.B., G.E. TAFFET, et al. 1993. Mitochondrial metabolism and substrate competition in the aging Fischer rat heart. Cardiovasc. Res. **27:** 2222–2228.
42. HANSFORD, R.G. 1980. Metabolism and energy production. Aging **12:** 25–76.
43. NOHL, H. & R. KRAMER. 1980. Molecular basis of age-dependent changes in the activity of adenine nucleotide translocase. Mech. Ageing Dev. **14:** 137–144.
44. GUERRIERI, F., G. VENDENIALE, et al. 1996. Alteration in F_oF_1 ATPase during aging. Possible involvement of oxygen free radicals. Ann. N.Y. Acad. Sci. **786:** 62–71.
45. CLANDININ, M.T. & S.M. INNIS. 1983. Does mitochondrial ATP synthesis decline as a function of change in the membrane environment with ageing. Mech. Ageing Dev. **22:** 205–208.
46. KIM, J., E. SHRAGO, et al. 1988. Age-related changes in respiration coupled to phosphorylation. II. Cardiac mitochondria. Mech. Ageing Dev. **46:** 279–290.
47. CASTELLUCIO, C., A. BARACCA, et al. 1994. Mitochondrial activities of rat heart during aging. Mech. Ageing Dev. **76:** 73–88.
48. ABU-ERREISH, G.M. & D.R. SANADI. 1978. Age-related changes in cytochrome concentration of myocardial mitochondria. Mech. Ageing Dev. **7:** 425–432.
49. SUGIYAMA, S., M. TAKASAWA, et al. 1993. Changes in skeletal muscle, heart and liver mitochondrial electron transport activities in rats and dogs of various ages. Biochem. Mol. Biol. Int. **30:** 937–944.
50. GENOVA, M.L., C. CASTELLUCIO, et al. 1995. Major changes in complex I activity in mitochondria from aged rats may not be detected by direct assay of NADH:coenzyme Q reductase. Biochem. J. **311:** 105–109.
51. LENAZ, G., C. BOVINA, et al. 1997. Mitochondrial complex I defects in aging. Mol. Cell. Biochem. **174:** 329–333.
52. MULLER-HOCKER, J., S. SCHAFER, et al. 1996. Defects of the respiratory chain in various tissues of old monkeys: a cytochemical-immunocytochemical study. **86:** 197–213.
53. TELESARA, C.L. & R. ARORA. 1994. Age related changes in gastrocnemius, diaphragm and heart muscles with special reference to SDH and m-ATPase. Indian J. Exp. Biol. **32:** 772–780.
54. GOLD, P.H., M.V. GEE, et al. 1968. Effect of age on oxidative phosphorylation in the rat. J. Gerontol. **23:** 509–513.
55. CHEN, J.C., J.B. WARSHAW, et al. 1972. Regulation of mitochondrial respiration in senescence. J. Cell Physiol. **80:** 141–145.
56. VITORICA, J. & A. MACHADO. 1981. Comparison between developmental and senescent changes in enzyme activities linked to energy metabolism in rat heart. Mech. Ageing Dev. **16:** 105–116.
57. GUERRI, F., G. CAPOZZA, et al. 1993. Functional and molecular changes in F_0F_1 ATP-synthase of cardiac muscle during aging. Cardioscience **4:** 93–98.
58. BAROGI, S., A. BARACCA, et al. 1995. Lack of major changes in ATPase activity in mitochondria from liver, heart, and skeletal muscle of rats upon ageing. Mech. Ageing Dev. **84:** 139–150.
59. NOHL, H., V. BREUNINGER, et al. 1978. Influence of mitochondrial radical formation on energy-linked respiration. Eur. J. Biochem. **90:** 385–390.
60. PARADIES, G., F.M. RUGGIERO, et al. 1992. Decreased activity of the phosphate carrier and modification of lipids in cardiac mitochondria from senescent rats. Int. J. Biochem. **24:** 783–787.
61. FROLKIS, V.V. & L.N. BOGATSKAYA. 1968. The energy metabolism of myocardium and its regulation in animals of various age. Exp. Gerontol. **3:** 199–210.
62. BRANDSTRUP, N., J.E. KIRK, et al. 1957. The hexokinase and phosphoglucoisomerase activities of aortic and pulmonary artery tissue in individuals of various ages. J. Gerontol. **12:** 166–171.
63. JI, L.L., D. DILLON, et al. 1991. Myocardial aging: antioxidant enzyme systems and related biochemical properties. Am. J. Physiol. **261:** R386–R392.
64. ERMINI, M. 1976. Ageing changes in mammalian skeletal muscle: biochemical studies. Gerontology **22:** 301–316.

65. RUMSEY, W.L., Z.V. KENDRICK, et al. 1987. Bioenergetics in the aging Fischer 344 rat: effects of exercise and food restriction. Exp. Gerontol. **22:** 272–287.
66. NAKAI, N., Y. SATO, et al. 1997. Effects of aging on the activities of pyruvate dehydrogenase complex and its kinase in rat heart. Life Sci. **60:** 2309–2314.
67. SUH, J.H., E.T. SHIGENO, et al. 2001. Oxidative stress in the aging rat heart is reversed by supplementation with (R)-α-lipoic acid. FASEB J. **15:** 700–706.
68. NOHL, H. & D. HEGNER. 1978. Do mitochondria produce oxygen radicals in vivo? Eur. J. Biochem. **82:** 563–567.
69. SAWADA, M. & J.C. CARLSON. 1987. Changes in superoxide radical and lipid peroxide formation in the brain, heart, and liver during the lifetime of the rat. Mech. Aging Dev. **41:** 125–137.
70. SOHAL, R.S., H.H. KU, et al. 1994. Oxidative damage, mitochondrial oxidant generation and antioxidant defenses during aging and in response to food restriction in the mouse. Mech. Ageing Dev. **74:** 121–133.
71. HANSFORD, R.G., B.A. HOGUE, et al. 1997. Dependence of H_2O_2 formation by rat heart mitochondria on substrate availability and donor age. J. Bioenerg. Biomemb. **29:** 89–95.
72. YOWE, D.L. & B.N. AMES. 1998. Quantitation of age-related mitochondrial DNA deletions in rat tissues shows that their pattern of accumulation differs from that of humans. Gene **209:** 23–30.
73. MUSCARI, C., A. GIACCARI, et al. 1996. Presence of a DNA-4236 bp deletion and 8-hydroxy-deoxyguanosine in mouse cardiac mitochondrial DNA during aging. Aging (Milano) **8:** 429–433.
74. NAKANO, M., F. OENZIL, et al. 1995. Age-related changes in the lipofuscin accumulation of brain and heart. Gerontology **41**(Suppl. 2): 69–79.
75. PARADIES, G., F.M. RUGGIERO, et al. 1998. Peroxidative damage to cardiac mitochondria: cytochrome oxidase and cardiolipin alterations. FEBS Lett. **424:** 155–158.
76. MUNCH, G., J. THOME, et al. 1997. Advanced glycation endproducts in ageing and Alzheimer's disease. Brain Res. Rev. **23:** 134–143.
77. SCHLEIDER, E.D., E. WAGNER, et al. 1997. Increased accumulation of the glycoxidation product N(epsilon)-(carboxymethyl)lysine in human tissues in diabetes and aging. J. Clin. Invest. **99:** 457–468.
78. SAXENA, A.K., P. SAXENA, et al. 1999. Protein aging by carboxymethylation of lysines generates sites for divalent metal and redox active copper binding: relevance to diseases of glycoxidative stress. Biochem. Biophys. Res. Commun. **260:** 332–338.
79. MIYATA, T., K. KUROKAWA, et al. 2000. Advanced glycation and lipoxidation end products: role of reactive carbonyl compounds generated during carbohydrate and lipid metabolism. J. Am. Soc. Nephrol. **11:** 1744–1752.
80. SINGH, R., A. BARDEN, et al. 2001. Advanced glycation end-products: a review. Diabetologia **44:** 129–146.
81. UCHIDA, K., L.I. SZWEDA, et al. 1993. Immunochemical detection of 4-hydroxynonenal protein adducts in oxidized hepatocytes. Proc. Natl. Acad. Sci. USA **90:** 8742–8746.
82. HUMPHRIES, K.M. & L.I. SZWEDA. 1998. Selective inactivation of α-ketoglutarate and pyruvate dehydrogenase: reaction of lipoic acid with 4-hydroxy-2-nonenal. Biochemistry **37:** 15835–15841.
83. HUMPHRIES, K.M., Y. YOO, et al. 1998. Inhibition of NADH-linked mitochondrial respiration by 4-hydroxy-2-nonenal. Biochemistry **37:** 552–557.
84. TAGLIALATELA, G., A. CAPRIOLI, et al. 1996. Spatial memory and NGF levels in aged rats: natural variability and effects of acetyl-L-carnitine. Exp. Gerontol. **31:** 577–587.
85. PARADIES, G., F.M. RUGGIERO, et al. 1995. Carnitine-acylcarnitine translocase activity in cardiac mitochondria from aged rats: the effect of acetyl-L-carnitine. Mech. Ageing Dev. **84:** 103–112.
86. PARADIES, G., F.M. RUGGIERO, et al. 1994. Effect of aging and acetyl-L-carnitine on the activity of cytochrome oxidase and adenine nucleotide translocase in rat heart mitochondria. FEBS Lett. **350:** 213–215.
87. PARADIES, G., F.M. RUGGIERO, et al. 1994. The effect of aging and acetyl-L-carnitine on the function and on the lipid composition of rat heart mitochondria. Ann. N.Y. Acad. Sci. **717:** 233–243.

88. GADALETA, M.N., V. PETRUZZELLA, et al. 1994. Mitochondrial DNA transcription and translation in aged rat. Effect of acetyl-L-carnitine. Ann. N.Y. Acad. Sci. **717:** 150–160.
89. GROSS, C.J. & D.A. SAVAIANO. 1993. Effect of development and nutritional state on the uptake, metabolism and release of free and acetyl-L-carnitine by the rodent small intestine. Biochim. Biophys. Acta **1170:** 265–274.
90. PARADIES, G., F.M. RUGGIERO, et al. 1992. The effect of aging and acetyl-L-carnitine on the phosphate carrier and on the phospholipid composition in rat heart mitochondria. Biochim. Biophys. Acta **1103:** 324–326.
91. PASTORIS, O., M. DOSSENA, et al. 1998. Effect of L-carnitine on myocardial metabolism: results of a balanced, placebo-controlled, double-blind study in patients undergoing open heart surgery. Pharmacol. Res. **37:** 115–122.
92. SINGH, R.B., M.A. NIAZ, et al. 1996. A randomised, double-blind, placebo-controlled trial of L-carnitine in suspected acute myocardial infarction. Postgrad. Med. J. **72:** 45–50.
93. HARAMAKI, N., D. HAN, et al. 1997. Cytosolic and mitochondrial systems for NADH- and NADPH-dependent reduction of alpha-lipoic acid. Free Radic. Res. Med. **22:** 535–542.
94. ROY, S. & L. PACKER. 1998. Redox regulation of cell functions by alpha-lipoate: biochemical and molecular aspects. Biofactors **7:** 263–267.
95. BUSTAMENTE, J., J.K. LODGE, et al. 1998. α-Lipoic acid in liver metabolism and disease. Free Radic. Biol. Med. **24:** 1023–1039.
96. JACOB, S., E.J. HENRIKSEN, et al. 1996. Improvement of insulin-stimulated glucose disposal in type 2 diabetes after repeated parenteral administration of thioctic acid. Exp. Clin. Endocrinol. Diabet. **104:** 284–288.
97. SACHSE, G. & B. WILLMS. 1980. Efficacy of thioctic acid in the therapy of peripheral diabetic neuropathy. Horm. Metab. Res. Suppl. **9:** 105–107.
98. ZIEGLER, D., M. HANEFELD, et al. 1995. Treatment of symptomatic diabetic peripheral neuropathy with the antioxidant α-lipoic acid. A 3-week multicentre randomized controlled trial (ALADIN study). Diabetologia **38:** 1425–1433.
99. ZIMMER, G., T.K. BEIKLER, et al. 1995. Dose/response curves of lipoic acid R- and S-forms in the working rat heart during reoxygenation: superiority of the R-enantiomer in enhancement of aortic flow. J. Mol. Cell. Cardiol. **27:** 1895–1903.

Can Antioxidant Diet Supplementation Protect against Age-related Mitochondrial Damage?

JAIME MIQUEL

Department of Biotechnology, University of Alicante, E-03080 Alicante, Spain

ABSTRACT: Harman's free radical theory of aging and our electron-microscopic finding of an age-related mitochondrial degeneration in the somatic tissues of the insect *Drosophila melanogaster* as well as in the fixed postmitotic Leydig and Sertoli cells of the mouse testis led us to propose a mitochondrial theory of aging, according to which metazoan senescence may be linked to oxygen stress-injury to the genome and membranes of the mitochondria of somatic differentiated cells. These concepts attract a great deal of attention, since, according to recent work, the mitochondrial damage caused by reactive oxygen species (ROS) and concomitant decline in ATP synthesis seem to play a key role not only in aging, but also in the fundamental cellular process of apoptosis. Although diet supplementation with antioxidants has not been able to increase consistently the species-characteristic maximum life span, it results in significant extension of the mean life span of laboratory animals. Moreover, diets containing high levels of antioxidants such as vitamins C and E seem able to reduce the risk of suffering age-related immune dysfunctions and arteriosclerosis. Presently, the focus of age-related antioxidant research is on compounds, such as deprenyl, coenzyme Q_{10}, alpha-lipoic acid, and the glutathione-precursors thioproline and *N*-acetylcysteine, which may be able to neutralize the ROS at their sites of production in the mitochondria. Diet supplementation with these antioxidants may protect the mitochondria against respiration-linked oxygen stress, with preservation of the genomic and structural integrity of these energy-producing organelles and concomitant increase in functional life span.

KEYWORDS: free radicals; free radical theory of aging; oxygen stress; mitochondria; mitochondrial mutation theory of aging; aging of differentiated cells; antioxidants; deprenyl; ubiquinol-10 (CoQ_{10}); alpha-lipoic acid; glutathione; thiazolidine carboxylic acid; *N*-acetylcysteine; life extension; longevity

INTRODUCTION

The free radical theory of aging farsightedly proposed by Harman in 1956[1] assumes that senescence is caused by "the deleterious, irreversible changes produced by free radical reactions." Therefore, according to this concept, the damage by reactive oxygen species (ROS) plays a key role in the determination of life span, and experiments in which endogenous free radical reactions are lowered by antioxidants lend support to the above theory and may result in significant longevity gains.

Address for correspondence: Dr. Jaime Miquel, C. Marqués de Campo, 66 (Farmacia), 03700 Denia (Alicante), Spain. Voice: +34-96-5788495; fax: +34-96-5780641.

In support of this theory, early research on diet supplementation with antioxidants reviewed elsewhere[2] was able to increase the mean life span of diverse experimental animals, including rotifers, mice, and rats. Among the antioxidants used, those containing thiol groups were quite effective. Thus, according to work from our laboratory,[3] diet supplementation with the antioxidants sodium and magnesium L-thiazolidine-4-carboxylate increased both the mean and maximum life span of mice and *Drosophila* and had a protective action against the senescent decline of their physiological competence. Since that pioneering work, many attempts have been made to increase life span with limited success, because usually mean life span, but not maximum life span, is increased.

Some pitfalls of antioxidant research have been pointed out by Yu,[4] regarding the influence on experiment interpretation of cellular antioxidant homeostasis (with resulting compensatory actions among the various antioxidants) and of the possible conversion of the antioxidants ascorbate and carotenoids to prooxidants under certain physiological conditions. Nevertheless, there is a growing consensus that diets enriched with antioxidant vitamins or vitamin E–sparing coantioxidants may protect against serious age-related processes, especially immune dysfunction[5,6] and arteriosclerosis,[7,8] the pathogenesis of which, according to Harman,[9] is linked to the injurious effects of oxygen free radicals and progressive blood lipid peroxidation.[10] Thus, the data from present research agree with Harman's view:[11] "The probability of developing these 'free radical diseases' should be decreased by lowering the free radical reaction level by any means, i.e., food restriction, antioxidants, increase in glutathione peroxidase or superoxide dismutase."

In contrast to this, the above compounds seem unable to provide a consistent increase in maximum life span, which would require a favorable modulation of the fundamental mechanisms of cell aging. Thus Rottkamp *et al.*[12] state that antioxidant therapies show scant effects on modification of the aging process, but they point out that "our current inability to incorporate these apparent shortcomings do not necessarily have to discount the importance of oxidative stress, but may have more to do with our incomplete understanding of how oxidative homeostasis is maintained. In other words, the antioxidant therapies that have been developed and tested to date may be *incorrectly targeted*" [italics added].

In agreement with the above, we feel that the growing acceptance of the central role of mitochondrial damage in cell aging justifies a more selective antioxidant diet supplementation aimed at protecting these organelles against chronic oxidative stress. This may preserve high levels of ATP synthesis and physiological functions, thus yielding more significant increases in functional life span than those achieved by means of what Yu[4] calls "the 'shotgun' approach" at antiaging intervention.

THE ROS STRESS–MITOCHONDRIAL MUTATION THEORY OF AGING

The main justification for present attempts to increase longevity through improved mitochondria-based antioxidant protection can be found in Harman's[13] concept of free radical attack on mitochondria as the biological clock of aging, as well as in our finding of mitochondrial degeneration, which increases with age, in the somatic tissues of the insect *Drosophila melanogaster*[14,15] and in the fixed postmitotic (irreversibly differentiated) Sertoli and Leydig cells of the mouse testis.[16] These observations provide experimental support for the oxygen stress-mitochondrial mutation theory of aging (or mitochondrial theory of aging of differentiated cells; FIG. 1). According to this concept, first proposed in 1980 by Miquel et al.[17] and expanded in further publications from our laboratory,[18–21] ROS-linked mutagenic injury to the mitochondrial genome (mtDNA) of differentiated cells (which lack the mitochondria-regenerating power of frequent mitosis) with concomitant bioenergetic decline is the fundamental cause of aging. More specifically, we hypothesize that, because of its oxidative and mutagenic environment, the mitochondrial genome (mtDNA) of fixed postmitotic cells (and to a lesser degree that of other differentiated cells) suffers accumulative mutations and deletions and/or unspecific oxidative damage, with resulting membrane disorder. These genetic and structural injuries impair the maintenance, renewal, and function of the mitochondria, with resulting cell-bioenergetic decline and progressive loss of physiological functions.

Support for this theory can be found in the above-cited publications as well as in similar concepts and data from other laboratories, the review of which is beyond the scope of the present article. Nevertheless, it is worth noting that the main prediction of the mitochondrial theory of aging, that is, the presence of age-related mtDNA damage, has been fulfilled by the finding of an accumulation of deletions and point mutations of the mtDNA in various tissues of aged subjects.[22,23] Moreover, work presented by Wei at the 8th Congress of the International Association of Biomedical Gerontology and reported by Suh et al.[24] shows an age-related increase in human mitochondrial genomes with a 4977-bp deletion. The involvement of oxidative stress in these mtDNA changes is suggested by the observation that, by constructing a series of cytoplast hybrids (cybrids) containing mitochondria with this deletion, the fraction of mutated mtDNA correlates with raised oxidative damage and decreased respiratory function.

TREATMENTS THAT MAY INCREASE FUNCTIONAL LIFE SPAN BY MEANS OF MITOCHONDRIAL ANTIOXIDANT PROTECTION

Until now the only intervention capable of achieving striking increases in both mean and maximum life span, probably through mitochondria-protecting mechanisms, is caloric restriction. Nevertheless, a fast-increasing amount of data suggests that a number of antioxidants, including these briefly discussed below, might be able to retard mitochondrial senescence. Probably, these mitochondria-targeted antioxidant treatments will delay the functional losses associated with normal aging, thus preventing some of the age-associated diseases and increasing maximum life span.

Deprenyl

As pointed out by Maruyama et al.,[25] deprenyl attenuates the progressive degeneration of dopaminergic neurons in the nigrostriatum during aging and in Parkinson's disease by mechanisms including a specific protection of mitochondria against respiratory chain–dependent oxygen stress. This is probably due to the fact that, in addition to its direct antioxidant action,[26] deprenyl enhances the activity of mitochondria-protecting SOD and catalase,[27] increases the expression of glutathione peroxidase, and preserves the mitochondrial membrane potential.[28] Because mito-

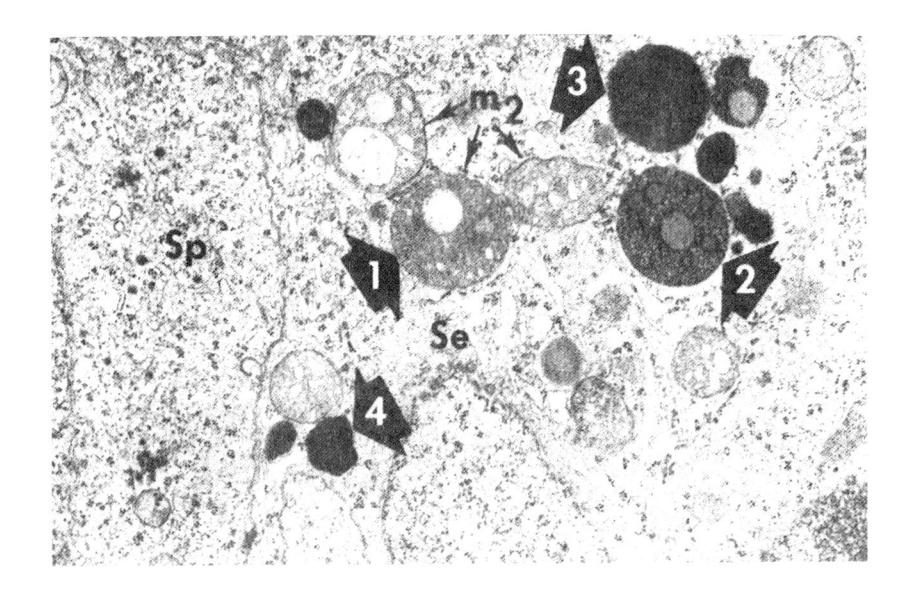

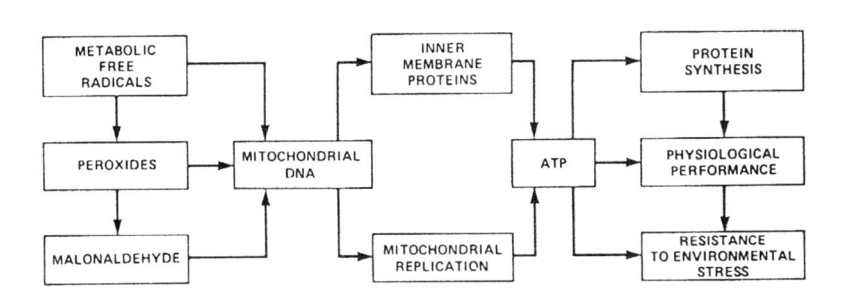

FIGURE 1. *Top panel*: Electron micrograph of the testis of a 4-month-old mouse that shows the apparent vulnerability of the mitochondria of somatic differentiated cells to ROS stress. The irreversibly differentiated (fixed postmitotic) Sertoli cell (Se; *right side*) contains structurally normal mitochondria (1; m_2), an altered osmiophilic (fat-containing) mitochondrion (2), and smaller dense bodies (most of which result from peroxidative and lysosomal attack on mitochondrial membranes). This suggests that, even at this young age, the Sertoli cells may suffer a process of mitochondrial degeneration. By contrast, the spermatogonion (Sp; *on the left*) does not show any structural signs of ROS-related damage because of its very effective protective mechanisms that include frequent mitosis-linked "rejuvenation" of the organelles and the very small volume of the mitochondrial compartment in comparison to cellular size. This ensures that the nuclear and mitochondrial genomes of spermatogonia (which play a key role in reproduction-dependent species survival) suffer a minimum of exposure to the mutagenic ROS released in the respiratory chain. (×18,200). (Reproduced from Miquel *et al.*[16]) *Lower panel*: Main proposed mechanisms of our ROS stress–mitochondrial theory of aging, from the molecular to the functional levels. (Reproduced by permission from Miquel and Fleming.[19])

chondrial dysfunction is centrally involved in triggering apoptosis, an effective prevention of mitochondrial oxidative damage by deprenyl may provide a reasonable explanation for its antiapoptotic effect in models of neuronal apoptosis.[25,28]

Coenzyme Q_{10}

It is well known that coenzyme Q_{10} (ubiquinol-10) acts as an electron carrier of the mitochondrial respiratory chain. Moreover, the mitochondria-protecting action of ubiquinol-10 was confirmed by the finding that ubiquinone reduced to ubiquinol in the electron transport chain strongly inhibits lipid peroxidation in isolated organelles. As summarized by Frei et al.,[29] "The data of this study and all the evidence for antioxidant function of ubiquinol published over the last three decades strongly suggest that ubiquinol-10 contributes significantly to antioxidant defenses in biology, complementing the antioxidant activities of α-tocopherol by scavenging free lipid radicals and, possibly, by recycling α-tocopherol."

More recently, Bliznakov[30] comments that since the mitochondrial theory of aging has gained considerable acceptance, attention should be paid by gerontologists to the importance of coenzyme Q_{10} in both its roles, that is, support of ATP biosynthesis in the mitochondrial inner membrane (thus preserving cellular integrity and function) and very effective scavenging of ROS.

Alpha-Lipoic Acid

This is a very interesting compound, because it is a normal component of mitochondria, where it forms the prostethic group of coenzyme-A (CoA). Alpha-lipoic acid (ALA) is a relatively small molecule (MW 206), very hydrophobic, and with an -S-S- group, the antioxidant action of which was shown by the finding that ALA prevents the pathological results of vitamin C deficiency in guinea pigs and of vitamin E in rats.[31] As recently reviewed by Packer et al.,[32] several studies in various model systems have shown that ALA is a powerful neutralizer of ROS such as the OH• free radical, hypochlorous acid, and singlet oxygen. Moreover, ALA has preventive effects on diabetic microangiopathy[33] and protects against skin senescence and age-related cognitive deficits.[34] In view of the above, we feel that the probable protective effects of ALA on intramitochondrial thiol-redox homeostasis (and related mitochondrial biogenesis and bioenergetic function) deserve further in-depth investigation.

Glutathione, Thiazolidine Carboxylic Acid, and N-Acetylcysteine

The use of these three antioxidants in aging research derives from the finding reviewed elsewhere[35,36] and confirmed by recent studies[37–39] that aging is accompanied by a progressive oxidation of glutathione and other thiolic compounds in the tissues of both vertebrates and invertebrates. This results in changes of the redox (GSSG/GSH) ratio that are much more striking in the mitochondria than in the extramitochondrial compartment and lead to oxidative damage of the mtDNA.[37,38] In our opinion, the above justifies the attempts to modulate the mitochondrial rate of aging, thus increasing maximum life span, by dietary administration of glutathione and related thiol-containing compounds that have been shown to prevent excessive oxidation of the sulfur pool. Among these, thiazolidine carboxylic acid (thioprolin, TP) and *N*-acetylcysteine (NAC) stand out because, upon dietary administration, they raise the tissue levels of the main physiological thiols (glutathione and cysteine) and are effective in the treatment of ROS-related hepatic syndromes.[40]

TP is a cyclic sulfur amino acid similar in structure to proline that acts as an antioxidant and free radical scavenger[40] and, according to our above-mentioned work, has favorable effects on both longevity and physiological functions in *Drosophila* and mice.[3] This early thiol-antioxidant work has been expanded by the finding that dietary administration of sulfur-containing antioxidants, such as GSH or a TP derivative (ATCM) to mice prevents the age-related loss of performance in a tightrope test,[41,42] as well as two effects of aging on brain mitochondria, that is, increase in the GSSG/GSH ratio and oxidative damage to mtDNA. Another mitochondria-protecting effect of the thiolic antioxidants is a significant preservation of the activity of the liver respiratory enzymes of aging mice fed a NAC-supplemented diet.[43]

Further research on thiol-antioxidants involves the immune system, which is very sensitive to both the age-related injurious action of oxygen stress[44] and the anti-aging (redox homeostasis-preserving) effects of thiol supplementation.[5] The functions of this system require a delicate balance between prooxidant and the antioxidant mechanisms in which GSH plays a central role. Therefore, a thiol-rich diet may contribute to preserving that balance in the aged, with concomitant prevention of the injury caused by oxygen stress[45] and protection against the apoptosis of immune cells.[46] In agreement with the above, the administration of thiol compounds has a favorable effect on the immune cells of senescing mice.[6,48,49] As shown by De la Fuente *et al.*,[48] even a short-term (5 weeks) dietary intake of one of these antioxidants, that is, TP, to aged mice stimulates the main functions of lymphocytes.

It is interesting in light of possible clinical application of the thiolic antioxidants that recent work from De la Fuente's laboratory[50] has shown that in a model of premature mouse aging linked to high anxiety levels (which interfere with performance in a behavioral test[51]), the favorable immuno-modulating action of diet supplementation with thioproline was more evident in the prematurely aged mice than in those showing normal aging. This is in agreement with the view that antioxidants do not indiscriminately stimulate the immune functions, but instead they exert a protective inmunomodulation, maintaining those functions at adequate levels despite the age-related oxidative stress.[6] As previously discussed,[52] the immunoprotective action of TP may be related to a favorable effect of this thiolic antioxidant on mitochondrial homeostasis, with concomitant protection against the senescent impairment in the bioenergetic competence of the mitochondria of aged immune cells. Accordingly, De la Fuente (personal communication) has observed good preservation of mitochondrial structure in lymphocyte cultures from aged mice in medium supplemented with TC.

Because immune decline contributes significantly to morbidity and mortality in the elderly,[53] the finding that administration of TP to mice for only five weeks improves several immune functions recommends this compound for clinical study of its potential contribution to the attainment of a longer and healthier human life span.

ACKNOWLEDGMENTS

This work was supported in part by FISss Grant No. 99/1264.

REFERENCES

1. HARMAN, D. 1956. Aging: a theory based on free radical and radiation chemistry. J. Gerontol. **11:** 298–300.
2. WEBER, H. & J. MIQUEL. 1986. Antioxidant supplementation and longevity. *In* Nutritional Aspects of Aging. Vol. 1. L.H. Chen, Ed.: 2–49. CRC Press. Boca Raton, FL.
3. MIQUEL, J. & A.C. ECONOMOS. 1979. Favorable effects of the antioxidants sodium and magnesium thiazolidine carboxylate on the vitality and life span of *Drosophila* and mice. Exp. Gerontol. **14:** 279–285.
4. YU, B.P. 1999. Approaches to anti-aging interventions: the promises and the uncertainties. Mech. Ageing Dev. **111:** 73–87.
5. DE LA FUENTE, M. & V.M. VÍCTOR. 2000. Anti-oxidants as modulators of immune function. Immunol. Cell Biol. **78:** 49–54.
6. MEYDANI, S.N., M. MEYDANI, J.B. BLUMBERG, *et al.* 1997. Vitamin E supplementation and in vivo immune response in healthy elderly subjects. J. Am. Med. Assoc. **277:** 1380–1386.
7. RAMÍREZ-BOSCÁ, A., M.A. CARRIÓN-GUTIÉRREZ, A. SOLER, *et al.* 1997. Effects of the antioxidant turmeric on lipoprotein peroxides: implications for the prevention of atherosclerosis. Age **29:** 165–168.
8. WITTING, P.K., K. PETTERSON, A-M. ÖSTLUND-LINDQVIST, *et al.* 1999. Inhibition by a coantioxidant of aortic lipoprotein lipid peroxidation and atherosclerosis in apolipotein E and low density lipoprotein receptor gene double knockout mice. FASEB J. **13:** 667–675.
9. HARMAN, D. 1960. Atherosclerosis: oxidation of serum lipoproteins and its relationship to pathogenesis. Clin. Res. **8:** 108.
10. MIQUEL, J., A. RAMÍREZ-BOSCÁ & A. SOLER. 1998. Increase with age of serum lipid peroxides: implications for the prevention of atherosclerosis. Mech. Ageing Dev. **100:** 17–24.
11. HARMAN, D. 1986. Free radical theory of aging: role of free radicals in the origination and evolution of life, aging, and disease processes. *In* Free Radicals, Aging and Degenerative Diseases. J.E. Johnson, Jr., R. Walford, D. Harman & J. Miquel, Eds.: 3–49. Alan R. Liss. New York.
12. ROTTKAMP, C.A., A. NUNOMURA, K. HIRAI, *et al.* 2000. Will antioxidants fulfill their expectations for the treatment of Alzheimer disease? Mech. Ageing Dev. **116:** 169–179.
13. HARMAN, D. 1972. The biological clock: The mitochondria? J. Am. Geriatr. Soc. **20:** 145–147.
14. MIQUEL, J. 1971. Aging of male *Drosophila melanogaster:* histological, histochemical and ultrastructural observations. *In* Advances in Gerontological Research. Vol. 3. B.L. Strehler, Ed.: 39–71. Academic Press. New York.
15. MIQUEL, J., A.L. TAPPEL & C.J. DILLARD. 1974. Fluorescent products and lysosomal components in aging *Drosophila melanogaster.* J. Gerontol. **29:** 622–637.
16. MIQUEL, J., P.R. LUNDGREN & J.E. JOHNSON. 1978. Spectrophotometric and electron microscopic study of lipofuscin accumulation in the testis of aging mice. J. Gerontol. **33:** 5–19.
17. MIQUEL, J.E., A.C. ECONOMOS, J. FLEMING, *et al.* 1980. Mitochondrial role in cell aging. Exp. Gerontol. **15:** 579–591.
18. FLEMING, J.E., J. MIQUEL & L.S. COTTRELL. 1982. Is cell aging caused by respiration-dependent injury to the mitochondrial genome? Gerontology **28:** 44–53.
19. MIQUEL, J. & J. FLEMING. 1986. Theoretical and experimental support for an "oxygen radical–mitochondrial injury" hypothesis of cell aging. *In* Free Radicals, Aging, and Degenerative Diseases. J.E. Johnson, Jr., D. Harman, R. Walford & J. Miquel, Eds.: 51–74. Alan R. Liss. New York.
20. MIQUEL, J. 1991. An integrated theory of aging as the result of mitochondrial DNA mutation in differentiated cells. Arch. Gerontol. Geriatr. **12:** 99–117.
21. MIQUEL, J. 1998. An update on the oxygen stress–mitochondrial mutation theory of aging: genetic and evolutionary implications. Exp. Gerontol. **33:** 113–126.

22. HATTORI, K., M. TANAKA, S. SUJIYAMA, et al. 1991. Age-dependent increase in deleted mitochondrial DNA in the human heart: possible contributory factor to presbycardia. Am. Heart J. **121:** 1735–1742.
23. KOVALENKO, S.A., G. KOPSIDAS, M.M. ISLAM, et al. 1998. The age associated decrease in the amount of amplifiable full lenght mitochondrial DNA in human skeletal muscle. Biochem. Mol. Biol. Int. **46:** 1233–1241.
24. SUH, Y., W.Y. PARK & S.C. PARK. 2000. The 8th Congress of the International Association of Biomedical Gerontology. Mech. Ageing Dev. **116:** 47–57.
25. MARUYAMA, W., T. TAKAHASHI & M. NAOI. 1998. (–)-Deprenyl protects human dopaminergic neuroblastoma SH-SY5Y cells. J. Neurochem. **70:** 2510–2515.
26. WU, R.M., C.C. CHIUEH, A. PERT, et al. 1993. Apparent antioxidant effect of (–)-deprenyl on hydroxyl radical formation and nigral injury elicited by MPP in vivo. Eur. J. Pharmacol. **243:** 231–247.
27. CARRILLO, M.C., S. KANAI, M. NOKUBO, et al. 1992. Deprenyl increases the activities of superoxide dismutase and catalase in striatum but not in hippocampus: the sex and age-related differences in the optimal dose in the rat. Exp. Neurol. **116:** 286–294.
28. WADIA, J.S., R.M.E. CHALMERS-REDMAN, W.J.H. WU, et al. 1998. Mitochondrial membrane potential and nuclear changes in apoptosis caused by serum and nerve growth factor withdrawal: time course and modification by (–)-deprenyl. J. Neurosci. **18:** 932–947.
29. FREI, B., M.C. KIM & B.N. AMES. 1990. Ubiquinol-10 is an effective lipid-soluble antioxidant at physiological concentrations. Proc. Natl. Sci. USA **87:** 4879–4883.
30. BLIZNAKOV, E.G. 1999. Aging, mitochondria, and coenzyme Q_{10}: the neglected relationship. Biochimie **81:** 1131–1132.
31. ROSENBERG, H.R. & R. CULIK. 1959. Effect of α-lipoic acid on vitamin C and vitamin E deficiencies. Arch. Biochem. Biophys. **80:** 86–93.
32. PACKER, L., E.H. WITT & H.J. TRITACHLER. 1995. Alpha-lipoic acid as a biological antioxidant. Free Radic. Biol. Med. **19:** 227–250.
33. GUILLASSEAU, P.J. 1994. Preventive treatment of diabetic microangiopathy: blocking the pathogenic mechanisms. Diabete Metabol. **20:** 219–228.
34. STOLL, S., H. HARTMANN, S.A. COHEN, et al. 1993. The potent free radical scavenger α-lipoic acid improves memory in aged mice: putative relationships to NMDA receptor deficits. Pharmacol. Biochem. Behav. **46:** 799–805
35. MIQUEL, J. & H. WEBER. 1990. Aging and increased oxidation of the sulfur pool. In Glutathione: Metabolism and Physiological Functions. J. Viña, Ed.: 187–192. CRC Press. Boca Raton, FL.
36. VIÑA, J.R., G.T. SÁEZ & J. VIÑA. 1989. The physiological functions of glutathione. In Handbook of Free Radicals and Antioxidants in Biomedicine. Vol. 2. J. Miquel, A.T. Quintanilha & H. Weber, Eds.: 121–132. CRC Press. Boca Raton, FL.
37. GARCÍA DE LA ASUNCIÓN, J., A. MILLÁN, R. PLA, et al. 1996. Mitochondrial glutathione oxidation correlates with age-associated oxidative damage to mitochondrial DNA. FASEB J. **20:** 333–338.
38. SASTRE, J., F.V. PALLARDÓ, J. GARCÍA DE LA ASUNCIÓN, et al. 2000. Mitochondria, oxidative stress and aging. Free Radic. Res. **32:** 189–198.
39. CHEN, T.S., J.P. RICHIE JR., H.T. NAGASAWA, et al. 2000. Glutathione monoethyl ester against glutathione deficiencies due to aging and acetaminophen in mice. Mech. Ageing Dev. **120:** 127–139.
40. DANSETTE, P.M., A. SASSI, C. DESCHAMPS, et al. 1990. Sulfur containing compounds as antioxidants. In Antioxidants in Therapy and Preventive Medicine. I. Emerit, L. Packer & C. Auclair, Eds.: 209–215. Plenum Press. New York and London.
41. PALLARDÓ, E.V., M. ASENSI, J. GARCÍA DE LA ASUNCIÓN, et al. 1998. Late onset administration of oral antioxidants prevents age-related loss of motor coordination and brain mitochondrial DNA damage. Free Radic. Res. **29:** 617–623.
42. MIQUEL, J. & M. BLASCO. 1978. A simple technique for evaluation of vitality loss in aging mice, by testing their muscular coordination and vigor. Exp. Gerontol. **13:** 389–396.
43. MIQUEL, J., M.L. FERRANDIS, E. DE JUAN, et al. 1995. N-Acetylcysteine protects against age-related decline of oxidative phosphorylation in liver mitochondria. Eur. J. Pharmacol. (Environ. Toxicol. Pharmacol. Sect.) **292:** 333–335.

44. STOHS, S.J., F.H. EL-RASHIDY, T. LAWSON, et al. 1984. Changes in glutathione and glutathione metabolizing enzymes in human erythrocytes and lymphocytes as a function of age of donor. Age **7:** 3–7.
45. SÁEZ, G.T., W.H. BANNISTER & J.V. BANNISTER. 1990. Free radicals and thiol compounds—the role of glutathione against free radical toxicity. *In* Glutathione: Metabolism and Physiological Functions. J. Viña, Ed.: 237–254. CRC Press. Boca Raton, FL.
46. ESTEVE, J., J. MOMPÓ, J. GARCÍA DE LA ASUNCIÓN, et al. 1999. Oxidative damage to mitochondrial DNA and glutathione in apoptosis: studies *in vivo* and *in vitro*. FASEB J. **13:** 1055–1064.
47. PIERI, C.F., F. MORONI & R. RECCHIONI. 1992. Glutathione influences the proliferation as well as the extent of mitochondrial activation in rat splenocytes. Cell. Immunol. **145:** 210–217.
48. DE LA FUENTE, M., M.D. FERRÁNDEZ, M. DEL RIO, et al. 1998. Enhancement of leukocyte functions in aged mice supplemented with the antioxidant thioproline. Mech. Ageing Dev. **104:** 213–225.
49. FERRÁNDEZ, M.D., R. CORREA, M. DEL RÍO, et al. 1999. Effects in vitro of several antioxidants on the natural killer function of aging mice. Exp. Gerontol. **34:** 675–685.
50. CORREA, R., B. BLANCO, M. DEL RÍO, et al. 1999. Effect of a diet supplemented with thioproline on murine macrophage function in a model of premature ageing. Biofactors **10:** 195–200.
51. DE LA FUENTE, M., M. MIÑANO, V.M. VICTOR, et al. 1998. Relation between exploratory activity and immune function in aged mice: a preliminary study. Mech. Ageing Dev. **102:** 263–272.
52. VERITY, M.A., C.F. TAM, C. CHEUNG, et al. 1983. Delayed phytohemagglutinin-stimulated production of adenine trisphosphate by aged human lymphocytes: possible relation to mitochondrial dysfunction. Mech. Ageing Dev. **23:** 53–65.
53. PAWELEC, G. 1995. Molecular and cell biological studies of ageing and their application to considerations of Y lymphocyte immunosenescence. Mech. Ageing Dev. **79:** 1232–1237.

The First Six Years at the National Institute for Longevity Sciences, Japan

KENICHI KITANI

Distinguished Guest Scientist, Ex–Director General,
National Institute for Longevity Sciences, Aichi 474-8522, Japan

ABSTRACT: The National Institute for Longevity Sciences (NILS) of Japan opened on July 7, 1995, 15 years after the Science Council of Japan recommended the establishment of the National Center for Aging and Geriatric Illnesses (the provisional name for NILS) in 1980. During the first four years of operation, 8 separate research departments, containing 21 laboratories, were established. NILS has both research departments for biomedical sciences, such as dementia research, molecular genetics, and geriatric research, and also departments of gerontechnology and the care of the elderly, which engage in research directed toward the comprehensive improvement of the health and well-being of the elderly. On July 9, 1995, the day of the opening ceremonies, NILS employed only three staff members, including the director general. At the end of fiscal year 2000 (March 31, 2001), the institute comprised a staff of more than 200 people, including 30 senior science staff and about 50 junior scientists. The Japanese government has recently decided to expand NILS to double its present size by the end of fiscal year 2004 (March 2005).

KEYWORDS: aging; geriatric diseases; research center; longitudinal study; dementia

HISTORY

Although the National Institute for Longevity Sciences (NILS) is only 6 years old, it had been in the planning stages for 15 years (TABLE 1). In 1980, the Science Council of Japan officially recommended the establishment of a national research center for aging and geriatric illnesses. At that point the Ministry of Health and Welfare of Japan started to plan the construction of the Research Center for the Science of Aging and Health (the provisional name) by organizing committees at various levels and discussing the plan. TABLE 1 is a brief summary of events that occurred during the 15 years and illustrates how quickly the Japanese government acted.

Address for correspondence: Kenichi Kitani, M.D., Ph.D., Distinguished Guest Scientist, Ex–Director General, National Institute for Longevity Sciences, 36-3, Gengo Moriokacho, Obu-shi, Aichi 474-8522, Japan. Fax: +81-562-45-0184.
  kitani@nils.go.jp

TABLE 1. History of NILS

November 1980	The Science Council of Japan recommended the establishment of the National Aging and Geriatric Illnesses Center (provisional name).
May 1989	The Ministry of Health and Welfare established the study group for the Research Center for the Science of Aging and Health (Chairman: Teruhiko Saburi, member of the Examination Committee of Social Insurance).
November 1989	The study group of the Ministry of Health and Welfare for the Research Center for the Science of Aging and Health presented its report, "Toward the Establishment of the Research Center for the Science of Aging and Health," to the Minister of Health and Welfare: the decision was made to locate the Center in Aichi Prefecture.
December 1989	The government compiled a ten-year strategy to promote health care and welfare for the aged (original called the Gold Plan).
March 1993	Construction began on the National Longevity Sciences Center (provisional name).
March 1995	Construction was completed on the National Longevity Sciences Center (provisional name).
July 1995	The National Institute for Longevity Sciences opened in Chubu National Hospital.
October 1997	Aichi Health Village was opened.
1998	Original organizations were completed: eight research departments and twenty-one laboratories.
October 2000	Postgraduate Medical School, Nagoya University Basic Science of Aging, opened in NILS.
2005	To be upgraded to the Research Institute for the National Center for Longevity Sciences (twelve research departments and forty-seven laboratories being planned).

THE INAUGURATION

On July 1, 1995, NILS was inaugurated as a branch organization of the National Chubu Hospital in Obu city, Aichi Prefecture, Japan. It has a six-floor main building with about 8000 m^2 of floor space and a two-floor building with 1400 m^2 for studying and housing experimental animals (FIG. 1).

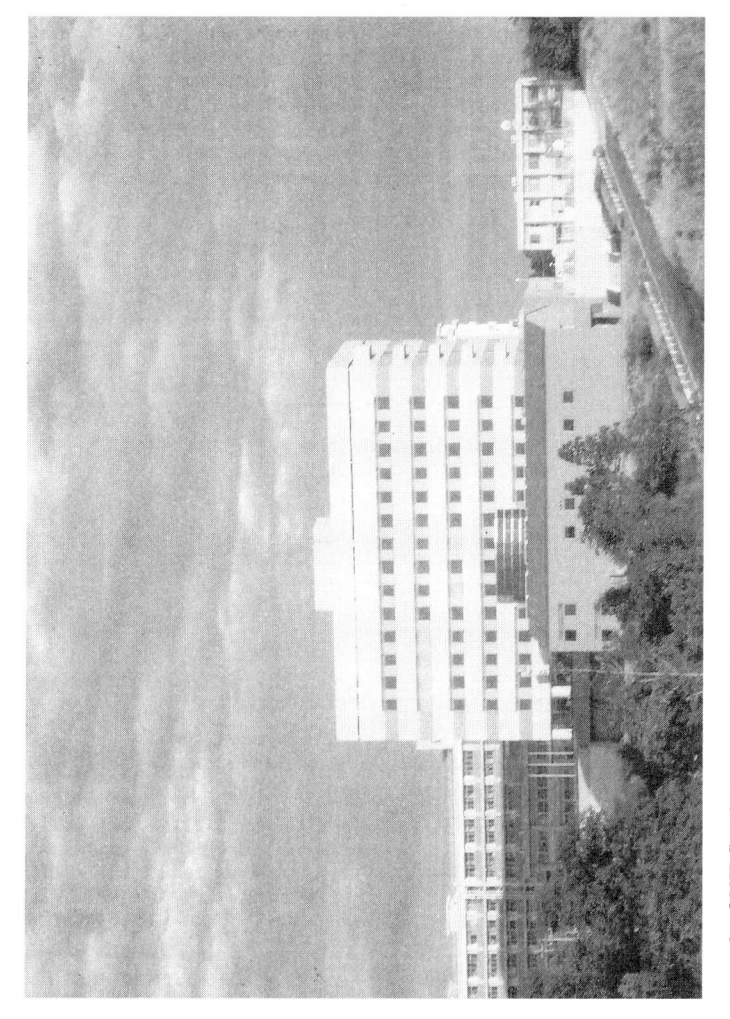

FIGURE 1. Photograph of NILS (*white square building in the middle*). The front building with the dark roof is an annex building for experimental animals.

ORGANIZATION

FIGURE 2 illustrates the organization of NILS, which consists of 8 research departments and 21 laboratories. These departments, which were originally planned before the inauguration of NILS, were successively opened in the first four years. In 1995, four departments (Basic Gerontology, Dementia Research, Geriatric Research, and Imaging Sciences) were opened. In 1996, two more departments (Molecular Genetic and Epidemiology) were opened. In the third year, 1997, the Department for the Care of the Aged opened, and finally in 1998, the Department of Gerontechnology was opened. At the time of the opening ceremony for NILS, only three senior staff members, including myself, the director general, were presented to the participants of the ceremony. At the end of fiscal year 2000, when I retired, more than 200 people were working at NILS, including 30 senior scientists and about 50 junior scientists (postdoctoral fellows).

BUDGET

Initial investments totaled about US$100 million for building construction ($800 million) and equipment ($20 million), which was received between 1993 and 1995. Another $20 million for equipment was received between 1995 and 1997. The annual budget, which comes from the Ministry of Health and Welfare (MHW), is about $15 million, which primarily covers salaries and maintenance. Only about $1 million comes from this source as research money (annual basic research funds). The rest of the research money is obtained from grants for research projects of various kinds, mainly from the MHW or the Science and Technology Agency, and since 1999, the Ministry of Education and Culture (MEC).

Naturally, during the first fiscal year, 1995, NILS had very little money, inasmuch as the basic research funds from the MHW were quite limited (about half a million dollars in this fiscal year), and there was no chance for scientists at NILS to apply for other research funds for this fiscal year, since in Japan scientists apply for research grants by the end of the previous fiscal year. Worse yet, a grant that was approved by the MEC in that fiscal year had to be abandoned when scientists from universities that belonged to the MEC came to NILS, which itself belongs to the MHW: in Japan this is known as the "bureaucratic organizational gap."

Fortunately, the government began to reorganize the research budget system, primarily by increasing the amount of research money for the following fiscal year, and NILS was marginally in time to benefit from this change in the grant system. For the next fiscal year, 1996, scientists at NILS began to apply for, and obtain, research funds (more or less similar to the system used at the NIH in the United States). In 1996, NILS received research funding for just under $2 million, and every year the amount continued to rise, with the amount close to $10 million in 2000. The rapid rise of research grant money in the past five years also signifies that research activities at NILS is rapidly being recognized among Japanese scientific communities.

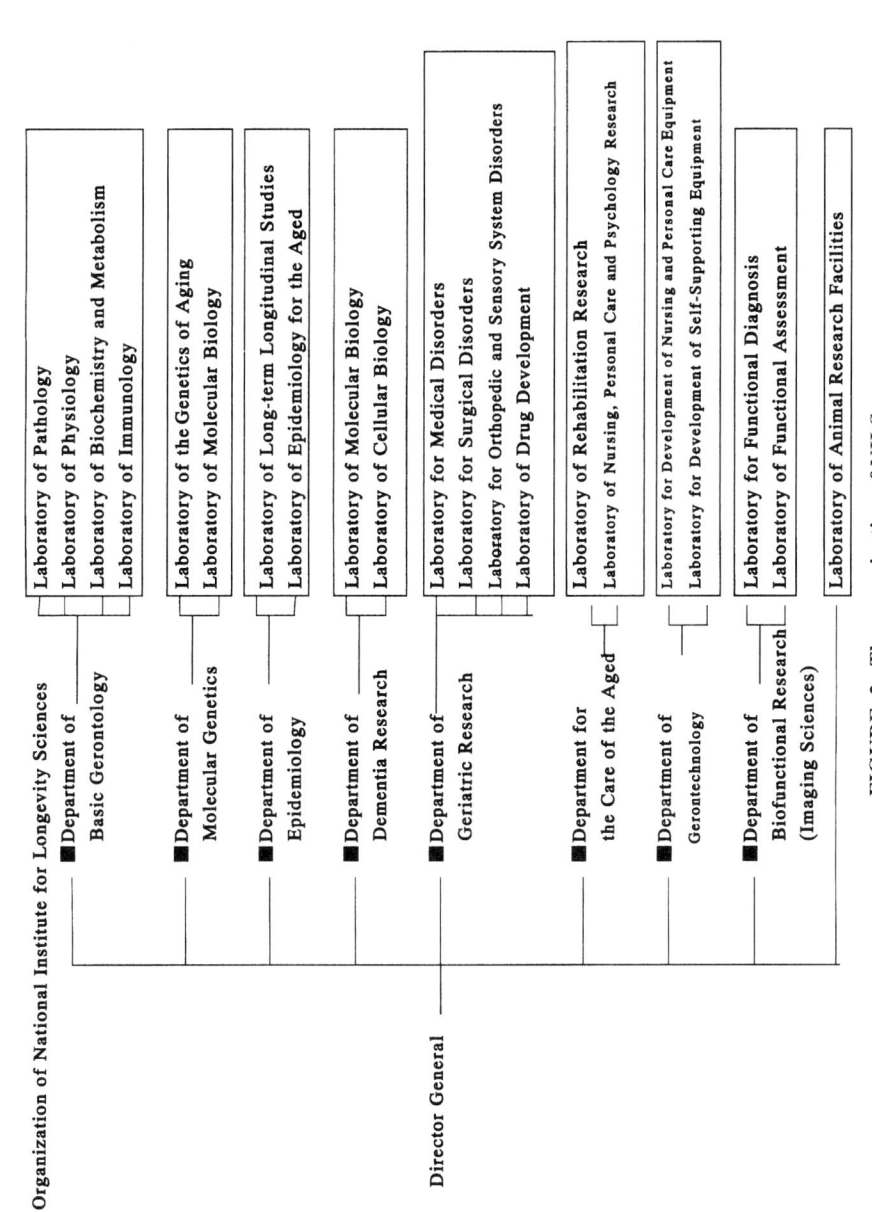

Organization of National Institute for Longevity Sciences

Director General
- Department of Basic Gerontology
  - Laboratory of Pathology
  - Laboratory of Physiology
  - Laboratory of Biochemistry and Metabolism
  - Laboratory of Immunology
- Department of Molecular Genetics
  - Laboratory of the Genetics of Aging
  - Laboratory of Molecular Biology
- Department of Epidemiology
  - Laboratory of Long-term Longitudinal Studies
  - Laboratory of Epidemiology for the Aged
- Department of Dementia Research
  - Laboratory of Molecular Biology
  - Laboratory of Cellular Biology
- Department of Geriatric Research
  - Laboratory for Medical Disorders
  - Laboratory for Surgical Disorders
  - Laboratory for Orthopedic and Sensory System Disorders
  - Laboratory of Drug Development
- Department for the Care of the Aged
  - Laboratory of Rehabilitation Research
  - Laboratory of Nursing, Personal Care and Psychology Research
- Department of Gerontechnology
  - Laboratory for Development of Nursing and Personal Care Equipment
  - Laboratory for Development of Self-Supporting Equipment
- Department of Biofunctional Research (Imaging Sciences)
  - Laboratory for Functional Diagnosis
  - Laboratory of Functional Assessment
- Laboratory of Animal Research Facilities

FIGURE 2. The organization of NILS.

RESEARCH ACTIVITIES

Space does not allow me to describe in detail all of the research activities at NILS. Here I will describe, however, the activities of several departments.

The Department of Epidemiology is carrying out a unique longitudinal study of aging that began in late 1997. Every two years the study examines 2400 randomly chosen individuals (from resident registration lists) over the age of 40 who reside in Obu city and Higashiura-cho, which are close to NILS. Four days every week, 6 or 7 individuals visit NILS and are examined. The examinations include a routine physical examination; blood chemistry laboratory tests; an ECG and other physiology examinations; exercise tests; ear, nose, and (especially) eye tests; nutritional examinations; and psychological evaluations. The number of procedures, including questionnaires, numbers more than 1000. The first wave, including the test run, started in November 1997 and ended in March 2000. The second wave, which started in April 2000, is to be completed in March 2002. This is the Japanese counterpart to the famous Baltimore Longitudinal Study of Aging, and we hope to obtain many similar, but also some groundbreaking results. It is expected that results of longitudinal studies of NILS will answer many questions, for example, regarding differences among different ethnic groups. We have an advantage over the Baltimore study, in that we are now accumulating a lot of molecular genetic data as well as data that can be acquired only by means of the most advanced technologies. For example, we are taking MRI brain images of all participants in this project, which will be longitudinally studied every two years. The results of the first wave are comprehensively summarized and available in a monograph on the internet (http://www.nils.go.jp/organ/ep/monograph.htm).

It is quite difficult to understand from its name what the Department of Biofunctional Research actually does, inasmuch as this title is a direct translation of the official Japanese name for this department. Actually, the department's function can be better understood if we call it the Department of Imaging Sciences. It occupies the entire first floor of the institute and is engaged in brain research and diagnosis for elderly individuals and patients. The department is capable of performing several procedures, including the positron emission tomography (PET), MRI, CT, as well as magnetic encephalography (MEG). By combining information obtained from these different modalities, the department is collecting data on anatomical and functional alterations in the brains of elderly Japanese, including data devoted to the longitudinal study by the Department of Epidemiology.

The Department of Geriatric Research is primarily working on the molecular genetics, pathogenesis, pathophysiology, treatment, and prevention of osteoporosis and has many advanced research achievements in this field.

The Department of Dementia Research, which began operations in the opening year is one of the departments that has made the most rapid and significant progress in its research. This department has been primarily involved in the pathogenesis of Alzheimer's disease and has been examining three major areas: (1) the role of presenilin in the generation of $A\beta$; (2) GM_1 ganglioside-bound $A\beta$ formation, and (3) $apoE_4$ and cholesterol homeostasis, all leading to neuronal death in Alzheimer's disease. This department is making significant progress in understanding the pathogenesis of Alzheimer's disease.

As was emphasized earlier, NILS is not only a biomedical institute but is also an organization active in new research areas for the health and welfare of the elderly. Our newest department is the Department of Gerontechnology. Scientists here are working primarily on two major projects: the first is developing equipment (the wires of which do not touch the subjects) for monitoring movements and physiological functions of elderly individuals. The other project uses robotics technology to develop assistive devices that can substitute as caregivers in the daily life of elderly persons. The activities of this department are being performed in collaboration with hospital staff as well as with many research and development groups of local and nationwide industries. As of the end of fiscal year 2001, I can now proudly say that research activities at NILS are in full bloom.

All updated research output from NILS can be viewed on the internet home page (www.nils.go.jp). In 2000, about 150 original research papers in English were published from NILS in peer-reviewed journals of different disciplines. Because of the diversity of research activities at NILS, its entire research contributions cannot be easily appreciated in scientific journals of any given specialized research field. However, I believe that the diverse research activities performed on at NILS fulfil the mission of this institute, one that will ultimately lead to the promotion of the health and welfare of the elderly not only in Japan but worldwide.

INTERNATIONAL ACTIVITIES

Without a long history of recognition, it is not an easy task for a new research institute to develop international activities. Despite these difficulties, we have made a major effort to interact internationally by (1) organizing international scientific meetings with invited scientists from abroad and by (2) visiting renowned institutions throughout the world, expecially in the United States.

In the first category we organized Tokyo Gerontology Week in August 1995, which occurred right after the inauguration of NILS. This took place in Makuhari, Chiba, Japan and consisted of two successive meetings: the Sixth Congress of the International Association of Biomedical Gerontology[1] and the Fifth International Symposium on Ceroid and Lipofuscin Pigments.[2] Right after these two meetings, a special lecture was given by Professor Denham Harman to celebrate the opening of NILS (FIG. 3). Since 1996, five successive International Workshops on Longevity Sciences have been held in Obu with the support of the Japan Foundation of Aging and Health. The titles of these workshops, held, respectively, from 1996 to 2000, were as follows: The Role of Molecular Genetics in Longevity Sciences,[3] The Role of Proteins in Longevity Sciences,[4] Interventions in Aging and Associated Disorders,[5] Interventions, Part II,[6] and Interventions, Part III.[7] In addition, we also organized another workshop in 1997: the First Japan–Germany Workshop on Longevity Sciences in Nagoya, with the sponsorship of the Science and Technology Agency of Japan. Further, in collaboration with the National Institute on Aging in the United States, in June 2000, we sponsored a joint Japan–USA Workshop at NILS entitled Non-Human Primate Models in Aging. All of these meetings helped to promote the advancement of research in longevity sciences as well as inform the international scientific community about NILS.

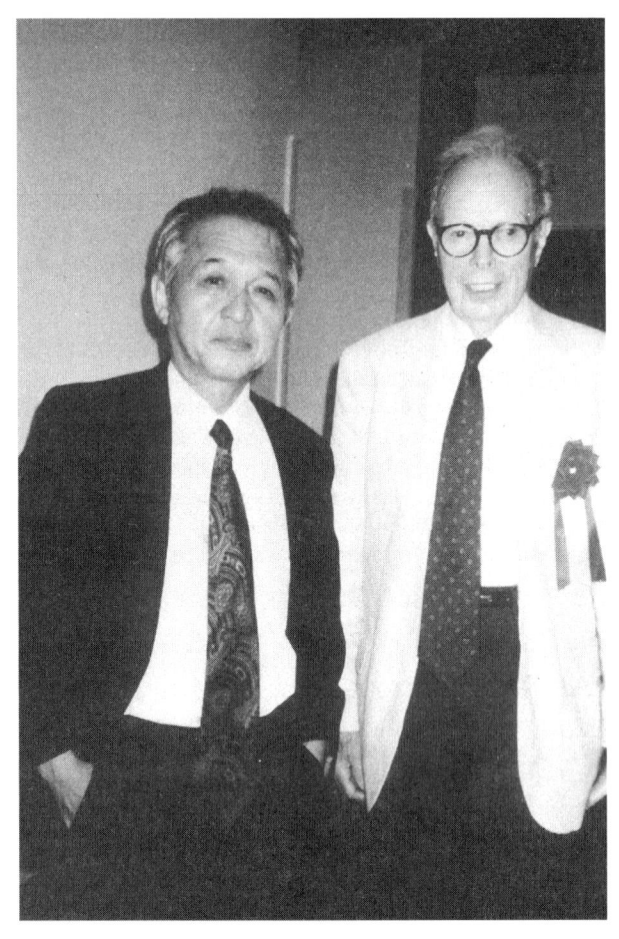

FIGURE 3. Professor Denham Harman (*right*) and the author (*left*) at the time of a special invited lecture by Dr. Harman celebrating the inauguration of NILS (August 1995).

Supported by the Japan Foundation of Aging and Health, we have sent scientists specializing in the fields of geriatrics and gerontology to the United States as well as to European countries for the purpose of mutually exchanging knowledge and information and promoting the activities of NILS. Institutions visited included the National Institute on Aging (NIA), Baltimore; the Mount Sinai Hospital, New York; the Department of Gerontology, Harvard Medical School, Boston; the USDA Human Nutrition Research Center on Aging at Tufts University, Boston; the University of Texas, San Antonio; and the Arizona Center on Aging at Arizona State University. Institutions we visited in Europe included the Institute for the Health of the Elderly in Newcastle upon Tyne, England; the University of London; the University of Heidelberg; the Max Plank Institute for Psychiatry in Munich; the University of Mainz and the University of Würzburg in Germany; the Institute of Aging, Leiden, the Netherlands; and many other institutes, hospitals, and facilities for the elderly. I would like to thank all of the institutions that we visited; they received us so kindly, even when our visit came at an inconvenient time. Our visits have helped to further inform Japanese scientists in their ongoing research in gerontology and geriatrics.

CONCLUSION AND FUTURE PERSPECTIVES

In summary, the first six years of NILS have passed very quickly, especially given its many problems during the first months. Despite these difficulties, NILS still continues to grow rapidly in 2002, which gives me much joy to see. Recently, the government made a decision to expand NILS and to change its name to Research Institute for the National Center for Longevity Sciences. By the end of fiscal year, 2004 (March 2005), it will double in size and a new geriatric hospital will be constructed. It is my personal view, however, that without exception, at least in Japan, increasing the size of an organization decreases its efficiency, whether it be a company, a government, or a research institute. It is my sincere hope, however, that all will go well and that NILS will grow to be even more efficient and productive in the field of longevity science in the twenty-first century.

ACKNOWLEDGMENTS

The author deeply appreciates the careful reading of the manuscript by Dr. G. O. Ivy. The excellent secretarial work of Ms. T. Ohara is gratefully acknowledged.

REFERENCES

1. KITANI, K., A. AOBA & S. GOTO, EDS. 1996. Pharmacological Intervention in Aging and Age-associated Disorders. Annals of the New York Academy of Sciences. Vol. 786. New York.
2. KITANI, K., G.O. IVY & H. SHIMASAKI, EDS. 1995. Gerontology 41.s2.95, Lipofuscin and Ceroid Pigments. State of the Art. S. Karger AG. Basel.
3. KITANI, K. & J. VIJG, EDS. 1997. Roles of Molecular Genetics in Longevity Sciences. Mech. Ageing Dev. Vol. 98(3) Elsevier. Amsterdam.
4. KITANI, K. & S. GOTO, EDS. 1999. Roles of Proteins in Ageing and Age-associated Disorders. Mech. Ageing Dev. Vol. 107(3) Elsevier. Amsterdam.
5. KITANI, K. & W. MARUYAMA, EDS. 1999. Intervention in Aging and Age-associated Disorders. Mech. Ageing Dev. Vol. 111(2,3) Elsevier. Amsterdam.
6. KITANI, K., Y. YAMADA & K. IKEDA, EDS. 2000. Interventions. Part II: Mech. Ageing Dev. Vol. 116(2,3) Elsevier. Amsterdam.
7. KITANI, K., ED. 2002. Interventions. Part III: Mech. Ageing Dev. Elsevier. Amsterdam. In press.

Index of Contributors

Abe, K., 275–284
Ahn, J.S., 45–49
Aiken, J., 412–423
Ames, B.N., 133–166, 452–462
Andersen, J.K., 452–462
Araki, S., 50–56
Arking, R., 251–262
Atamna, H., 133–166

Barja, G., 475–490
Bartke, A., 452–462
Baynes, J.W., 360–367
Bertani, M.F., 285–294
Block, G., 180–187
Bodyak, N.D., 434–447
Borrás, C., 448–451
Bovina, C., 199–213
Brownlee, M., 368–383
Brownson, C., 285–294
Bua, E., 412–423
Buck, S., 251–262

Campisi, J., 452–462
Cao, Z.J., 412–423
Carrillo, M.-C., 295–307
Castelli, G.P., 199–213
Cavalieri, E.L., 341–354
Cho, K-A, 45–49
Coller, H.A., 434–447

D'Aurelio, M., 199–213
de Grey, A.D.N.J., 452–462, 463–465
Dirks, A., 93–107
Drew, B., 66–81
Durham, W.J., 108–116

Eastwood, H., 396–411
El-Sawi, M.R., 238–250
Esmore, D., 355–359

Fantel, A.G., 424–433
Fato, R., 199–213
Ferro, A., 285–294

Floyd, R.A., 321–329
Formiggini, G., 199–213
Forster, M.J., 321–329
Fossel, M., 14–23
Fukui, K., 275–284

Galli, R.L., 128–132
Gane, A.M., 263–274
García-Sala, D., 448–451
Genova, M.L., 199–213
Giuliano, G., 199–213
Goto, S., 50–56
Graves, S., 396–411

Hagen, T.M., 491–507
Harman, D., xi–xii, 384–395
Hayasaka, T., 275–284
Hensley, K., 321–329
Heward, C.B., 452–462
Hipkiss, A.R., 285–294
Honda, S., 466–474
Honda, Y., 466–474
Hughes, G., 263–274
Hwangbo, D.-S., 251–262

Ivy, G.O., 295–307

Jang, I.S., 45–49
Ji, L.L., 82–92
Joseph, J.A., 128–132

Kagan, V.E., 188–198
Kanai, S., 295–307
Kawai, K., 188–198
Kelleher-Anderson, J.A., 321–329
Kelso, G.F., 263–274
Keylock, K.T., 117–127
Khrapko, K., 434–447
Kisin, E.R., 188–198
Kitani, K., 295–307, 517–525
Kopsidas, G., 396–411
Korol, D.L., 167–179
Kovalenko, S., 396–411

Kuratsune, H., 133–166

Lane, M., 251–262
Ledgerwood, E.C., 263–274
Leeuwenburgh, C., 66–81, 93–107
Lenaz, G., 199–213
Linnane, A.W., 355–359, 396–411
Liu, J., 133–166
Lloret, A., 448–451
Lopez, M., 412–423
Lowder, T.W., 117–127
Lyon, W., 355–359

Manchester, L.C., 238–250
Marasco, S., 355–359
McCarter, R.J.M., 452–462
McKenzie, D., 412–423
McKiernan, S., 412–423
Melov, S., 330–340
Minami, C., 295–307
Miquel, J., 508–516
Moreau, R., 491–507
Murphy, M.P., 263–274

Nagley, P., 355–359
Nakamoto, H., 50–56

Omoi, N.-O., 275–284
Osipov, A.N., 188–198
Ou, R., 355–359

Pallardó, F.V., 448–451
Pamplona, R., 475–490
Paolucci, U., 199–213
Papakostopoulos, P., 396–411
Park, J.-S., 45–49
Park, S.C., 45–49
Park, W.-Y., 45–49
Pepe, S., 355–359
Perls, T., 1–13
Person, R.E., 424–433
Phaneuf, S., 93–107
Pich, M.M., 199–213
Pollack, M., 93–107
Porta, E.A., 57–65
Porteous, C.M., 263–274
Portero-Otín, M., 475–490

Reid, M.B., 108–116
Reiter, R.J., 238–250
Richardson, M., 396–411
Rogan, E.G., 341–354
Rosenfeldt, F.L., 355–359
Rowland, M., 355–359
Ruiz, E., 285–294
Russell, J.W., 368–383

Saretzki, G., 24–29
Sastre, J., 448–451
Serbinova, E.A., 188–198
Serinkan, B.F., 188–198
Shinnkai, T., 275–284
Shukitt-Hale, B., 128–132
Shvedova, A.A., 188–198
Skulachev, V.P., 214–237
Smith, R.A.J., 263–274
Spiteller, G., 30–44
Stock, G., 452–462
Suh, J.H., 491–507
Suzuki, S., 275–284

Takahashi, R., 50–56
Tan, D.X., 238–250

Urano, S., 275–284

Ventura, B., 199–213
Viña, J., 448–451
Vincent, A.M., 368–383
Visioli, F., 491–507
von Zglinicki, T., 24–29

Wanagat, J., 412–423
Wolinsky, I., 188–198
Wood, P.L., 321–329
Woods, J.A., 117–127

Yamamoto, T., 295–307
Yarovaya, N., 396–411
Youdim, K.A., 128–132

Zhang, C., 396–411
Zs.-Nagy, I., 308–320